Marine Natural Product Chemistry: A Themed Issue Dedicated to Prof. Dr. Peter Proksch on His Research Career

Marine Natural Product Chemistry: A Themed Issue Dedicated to Prof. Dr. Peter Proksch on His Research Career

Editors

Bin-Gui Wang
RuAngelie Edrada-Ebel
Chang-Yun Wang

MDPI • Basel • Beijing • Wuhan • Barcelona • Belgrade • Manchester • Tokyo • Cluj • Tianjin

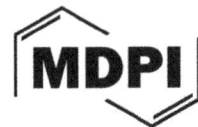

Editors

Bin-Gui Wang
Chinese Academy of Sciences
China

RuAngelie Edrada-Ebel
University of Strathclyde
UK

Chang-Yun Wang
Ocean University of China
China

Editorial Office
MDPI
St. Alban-Anlage 66
4052 Basel, Switzerland

This is a reprint of articles from the Special Issue published online in the open access journal *Marine Drugs* (ISSN 1660-3397) (available at: https://www.mdpi.com/journal/marinedrugs/special_issues/Professor_Peter_Proksch_Marine_Drugs).

For citation purposes, cite each article independently as indicated on the article page online and as indicated below:

LastName, A.A.; LastName, B.B.; LastName, C.C. Article Title. *Journal Name* **Year**, *Volume Number*, Page Range.

ISBN 978-3-0365-6161-5 (Hbk)
ISBN 978-3-0365-6162-2 (PDF)

© 2023 by the authors. Articles in this book are Open Access and distributed under the Creative Commons Attribution (CC BY) license, which allows users to download, copy and build upon published articles, as long as the author and publisher are properly credited, which ensures maximum dissemination and a wider impact of our publications.

The book as a whole is distributed by MDPI under the terms and conditions of the Creative Commons license CC BY-NC-ND.

Contents

About the Editors . . . . **vii**

Preface to "Marine Natural Product Chemistry: A Themed Issue Dedicated to Prof. Dr. Peter Proksch on His Research Career" . . . . **ix**

Peter Proksch
Looking Back at My Years in Marine Natural Products Chemistry
Reprinted from: *Mar. Drugs* **2022**, *20*, 161, doi:10.3390/md20030161 . . . . **1**

Flore Caudal, Nathalie Tapissier-Bontemps and Ru Angelie Edrada-Ebel
Impact of Co-Culture on the Metabolism of Marine Microorganisms
Reprinted from: *Mar. Drugs* **2022**, *20*, 153, doi:10.3390/md20020153 . . . . **3**

Noora Barzkar, Saeid Tamadoni Jahromi and Fabio Vianello
Marine Microbial Fibrinolytic Enzymes: An Overview of Source, Production, Biochemical Properties and Thrombolytic Activity
Reprinted from: *Mar. Drugs* **2022**, *20*, 46, doi:10.3390/md20010046 . . . . **27**

Muh. Ade Artasasta, Yanwirasti Yanwirasti, Muhammad Taher, Akmal Djamaan, Ni Putu Ariantari, Ru Angelie Edrada-Ebel and Dian Handayani
Apoptotic Activity of New Oxisterigmatocystin Derivatives from the Marine-Derived Fungus *Aspergillus nomius* NC06
Reprinted from: *Mar. Drugs* **2021**, *19*, 631, doi:10.3390/md19110631 . . . . **41**

Zhi-Hui He, Jia Wu, Lin Xu, Man-Yi Hu, Ming-Ming Xie, You-Jia Hao, Shu-Jin Li, et al.
Chemical Constituents of the Deep-Sea-Derived *Penicillium solitum*
Reprinted from: *Mar. Drugs* **2021**, *19*, 580, doi:10.3390/md19100580 . . . . **51**

Wencong Yang, Qi Tan, Yihao Yin, Yan Chen, Yi Zhang, Jianying Wu, Leyao Gao, et al.
Secondary Metabolites with α-Glucosidase Inhibitory Activity from Mangrove Endophytic Fungus *Talaromyces* sp. CY-3
Reprinted from: *Mar. Drugs* **2021**, *19*, 492, doi:10.3390/md19090492 . . . . **59**

Lichuan Wu, Ke Ye, Sheng Jiang and Guangbiao Zhou
Marine Power on Cancer: Drugs, Lead Compounds, and Mechanisms
Reprinted from: *Mar. Drugs* **2021**, *19*, 488, doi:10.3390/md19090488 . . . . **73**

Joana D. M. de Sá, José A. Pereira, Tida Dethoup, Honorina Cidade, Maria Emília Sousa, Inês C. Rodrigues, Paulo M. Costa, et al.
Anthraquinones, Diphenyl Ethers, and Their Derivatives from the Culture of the Marine Sponge-Associated Fungus *Neosartorya spinosa* KUFA 1047 [†]
Reprinted from: *Mar. Drugs* **2021**, *19*, 457, doi:10.3390/md19080457 . . . . **93**

Zhiqiang Song, Yage Hou, Qingrong Yang, Xinpeng Li and Shaohua Wu
Structures and Biological Activities of Diketopiperazines from Marine Organisms: A Review
Reprinted from: *Mar. Drugs* **2021**, *19*, 403, doi:10.3390/md19080403 . . . . **115**

Chengwen Wei, Chunxiao Sun, Zhao Feng, Xuexia Zhang and Jing Xu
Four New Chromones from the Endophytic Fungus *Phomopsis asparagi* DHS-48 Isolated from the Chinese Mangrove Plant *Rhizophora mangle*
Reprinted from: *Mar. Drugs* **2021**, *19*, 348, doi:10.3390/md19060348 . . . . **151**

Ying Sun, Xiaoli Ma and Hao Hu
Marine Polysaccharides as a Versatile Biomass for the Construction of Nano Drug Delivery Systems
Reprinted from: *Mar. Drugs* **2021**, *19*, 345, doi:10.3390/md19060345 . . . . **161**

Raha Orfali, Shagufta Perveen, Muhammad Farooq Khan, Atallah F. Ahmed, Mohammad A. Wadaan, Areej Mohammad Al-Taweel, Ali S. Alqahtani, et al.
Antiproliferative Illudalane Sesquiterpenes from the Marine Sediment Ascomycete *Aspergillus oryzae*
Reprinted from: *Mar. Drugs* **2021**, *19*, 333, doi:10.3390/md19060333 . . . . **177**

Pengrui Wang, Jiapeng Chen, Lujing Chen, Li Shi and Hongbing Liu
Characteristic Volatile Composition of Seven Seaweeds from the Yellow Sea of China
Reprinted from: *Mar. Drugs* **2021**, *19*, 192, doi:10.3390/md19040192 . . . . **187**

Yan Chen, Ge Zou, Wencong Yang, Yingying Zhao, Qi Tan, Lin Chen, Jinmei Wang, et al.
Metabolites with Anti-Inflammatory Activity from the Mangrove Endophytic Fungus *Diaporthe* sp. QYM12
Reprinted from: *Mar. Drugs* **2021**, *19*, 56, doi:10.3390/md19020056 . . . . **201**

Tao Chen, Yun Huang, Junxian Hong, Xikang Wei, Fang Zeng, Jialin Li, Geting Ye, et al.
Preparation, COX-2 Inhibition and Anticancer Activity of Sclerotiorin Derivatives
Reprinted from: *Mar. Drugs* **2021**, *19*, 12, doi:10.3390/md19010012 . . . . **211**

Ya-Ping Liu, Sheng-Tao Fang, Zhen-Zhen Shi, Bin-Gui Wang, Xiao-Nian Li and Nai-Yun Ji
Phenylhydrazone and Quinazoline Derivatives from the Cold-Seep-Derived Fungus *Penicillium oxalicum*
Reprinted from: *Mar. Drugs* **2021**, *19*, 9, doi:10.3390/md19010009 . . . . **229**

Lu-Jia Yang, Xiao-Yue Peng, Ya-Hui Zhang, Zhi-Qing Liu, Xin Li, Yu-Cheng Gu, Chang-Lun Shao, et al.
Antimicrobial and Antioxidant Polyketides from a Deep-Sea-Derived Fungus *Aspergillus versicolor* SH0105
Reprinted from: *Mar. Drugs* **2020**, *18*, 636, doi:10.3390/md18120636 . . . . **239**

Ya-Nan Wang, Ling-Hong Meng and Bin-Gui Wang
Progress in Research on Bioactive Secondary Metabolites from Deep-Sea Derived Microorganisms
Reprinted from: *Mar. Drugs* **2020**, *18*, 614, doi:10.3390/md18120614 . . . . **251**

Yan-He Li, Xiao-Ming Li, Xin Li, Sui-Qun Yang, Xiao-Shan Shi, Hong-Lei Li and Bin-Gui Wang
Antibacterial Alkaloids and Polyketide Derivatives from the Deep Sea-Derived Fungus *Penicillium cyclopium* SD-413
Reprinted from: *Mar. Drugs* **2020**, *18*, 553, doi:10.3390/md18110553 . . . . **277**

Yu Dai, Kunlong Li, Jianglian She, Yanbo Zeng, Hao Wang, Shengrong Liao, Xiuping Lin, et al.
Lipopeptide Epimers and a Phthalide Glycerol Ether with AChE Inhibitory Activities from the Marine-Derived Fungus *Cochliobolus Lunatus* SCSIO41401
Reprinted from: *Mar. Drugs* **2020**, *18*, 547, doi:10.3390/md18110547 . . . . **285**

About the Editors

Bin-Gui Wang

Bin-Gui Wang is a Professor of marine natural products at the Institute of Oceanology, Chinese Academy of Sciences. He received his B.Sc. degree from the Chemistry Department of Lanzhou University in 1986 and obtained several years of experience in natural antioxidants investigation at the Xi'an Oils and Fats Institute. In 1997, he completed his Ph.D. degree in Organic Chemistry at the Chemistry Department of Lanzhou University, and was a postdoctoral fellow at the Kunming Institute of Botany of the Chinese Academy of Sciences from 1997 to 1999. He has been a DAAD fellow at the Institute of Pharmaceutical Biology and Biotechnology at Heinrich-Heine-Universität Düsseldorf in Germany from 2000 to 2002 (with Prof. Peter Proksch). His research involves studies of bioactive natural compounds from marine organisms such as marine algae, endophytic fungi, and deep-sea-sourced microbes. He has published approximately 230 research papers, reviews, and book chapters, and is a coinventor on 25 patents. He is a member of the Chinese Pharmaceutical Association and serves on the editorial boards of Biochemical Systematics and Ecology, Chemistry and Biodiversity, Marine Drugs, and Marine Life Science and Technology.

RuAngelie Edrada-Ebel

Dr. RuAngelie Edrada-Ebel currently heads the Natural Products Metabolomics Group (NPMG) at the Strathclyde Institute of Pharmacy and Biomedical Sciences and is currently author of more than 100 publications and two patents on marine natural products. She obtained her PhD (Dr. rer. nat) degree from the Julius-Maximilian-Universität Würzburg, under the supervision of Professor Peter Proksch. Her expertise comprises both natural products isolation and structure elucidation with modern spectroscopic techniques. Her current research is based on the application of metabolomics on natural products research to identify and biotechnologically optimize the production of bioactive secondary metabolites in marine-derived microorganisms.

Chang-Yun Wang

Chang-Yun Wang received his Ph.D. degree from Ocean University of China in 1999 under the supervision of Professor Huashi Guan. In 2000, he joined the research group of Prof. Peter Proksch at the Institute for Pharmaceutical Biology and Biotechnology in University of Duesseldorf, Germany, as a 'German Academic Exchange Service' (DAAD) fellow. In 2002, he returned to work at the School of Medicine and Pharmacy in Ocean University of China as a professor. His research interest focused on discovery of new bioactive ingredients from marine resources and development of marine natural products into drug-like compounds for the treatment of cancer, inflammation, infectious diseases and other human diseases.

Preface to "Marine Natural Product Chemistry: A Themed Issue Dedicated to Prof. Dr. Peter Proksch on His Research Career"

As early as 30 years ago, Professor Dr. Peter Proksch was aware that marine organisms with diverse species are a huge treasure for the discovery of marine natural products with medicinal values. Since then, he has transferred his research interest from terrestrial plants to marine animals. His attention was caught by the colorful coral reefs in the tropical seas. He focused his research work on marine invertebrates, mainly including sponges, molluscs and tunicates. With the deepening of research, he expanded his research object to symbiotic microorganisms derived from marine invertebrates. Thousands of new marine natural products have been discovered by his group from marine invertebrates and their symbiotic microorganisms, most of them having novel structures and significant biological activities. A series of lead compounds with antitumor, antiviral, and antibacterial activities have been discovered and developed.

In his academic career, Professor Dr. Peter Proksch has put forward many innovative ideas which have played a guiding role in the field of marine natural products and marine drugs. He has published more than 600 peer-reviewed original papers, review articles and book chapters. Many academic views proposed by Professor Dr. Peter Proksch have important insights and provide a reference for scholars in the domain of marine natural products and marine drugs. He explored and practiced the discovery of bioactive secondary metabolites from marine invertebrates and their symbiotic microorganisms. We are deeply impressed by his great achievements in marine natural products and marine drugs.

Professor Dr. Peter Proksch not only has a global vision, but also has a broad mind and sincere spirit of international cooperation. He has trained a large number of scholars and students from all over the world, especially from China, Indonesia, India, Vietnam, Mongolia, Egypt, Turkey, Morocco, Cameroon and Nigeria. His laboratory is therefore known as the PP international family. He spread his academic thoughts and scientific spirit and was admired and respected by scientists in the field of natural product chemistry.

On the occasion of Professor Dr. Peter Proksch finishing his academic career, we are honored to be invited to organize an album in the journal of Marine Drugs to commemorate his outstanding contribution to marine natural products and marine drugs, as well as express our admiration for him. At the same time, we also hope that the album can inspire young generation of scholars in this field to make greater contributions in the future, explore the medicinal value of marine natural products and benefit human health.

Bin-Gui Wang, RuAngelie Edrada-Ebel, and Chang-Yun Wang
Editors

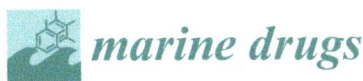

Editorial

Looking Back at My Years in Marine Natural Products Chemistry

Peter Proksch

Institute of Pharmaceutical Biology and Biotechnology, Heinrich-Heine-University Duesseldorf, 40225 Duesseldorf, Germany; proksch@uni-duesseldorf.de

When I started to work on marine natural products some thirty years ago I was attracted to this fascinating field of science by the exotic environment, the colourful shapes of (mostly) marine invertebrates and their complex ecological interactions. Having had mainly worked before on terrestrial plants the marine environment offered a totally new world for me, which has lost nothing of its thrill and fascination up to the present day. In parallel to marine macroorganisms I soon embarked on studying natural products from marine-derived microorganisms, which again opened up a new world both in terms of a huge biodiversity as well as highly unusual and complex microbial natural products, with many of them exhibiting pronounced biological activities. I consider myself very lucky for having been able to contribute to this field of science. The beauty of the marine environment and the thrill of treasure hunting for new and bioactive metabolites have never ceased to have a grip on me.

Having said this, the key point of looking back at my years in marine natural products chemistry is, however, still missing. What continues to impress me the most are the friendships with collaborators, colleagues and students from all over the world whom I was lucky to meet along the way. Many of those have contributed to this Special Issue of *Marine Drugs*, which was dedicated to me and for which I am most grateful. Friendships that span thousands of kilometers and have already lasted for decades evolved from a mutual interest in marine natural products. These friendships, which included many collaborations with the home institutions of my former associates far away, have enabled me not only to embark on new projects but become acquainted with other cultures, other ways of living and other ways of looking at life. All of this has had a marked effect on my professional career and enriched my life tremendously. If someone were to ask me today what the most important aspect of my life as a scientist has been, my answer would be: meeting highly talented people along the way, helping them to embark on their own careers as scientists and finding friends for life.

May this field of science never cease to attract young talents who help to push forward our knowledge of the sea and its hidden treasures.

Funding: This research received no external funding.

Conflicts of Interest: The authors declare no conflict of interest.

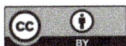

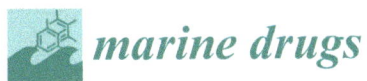

Review

Impact of Co-Culture on the Metabolism of Marine Microorganisms

Flore Caudal [1], Nathalie Tapissier-Bontemps [2,3] and Ru Angelie Edrada-Ebel [4,*]

[1] Laboratoire Biotechnologie et Chimie Marines, Université Bretagne Sud, EA3884, LBCM, IUEM, CEDEX, 56321 Lorient, France; flore.caudal@univ-ubs.fr
[2] CRIOBE, USR3278-EPHE/CNRS/UPVD/PSL, University of Perpignan via Domitia, 52 Avenue Paul Alduy, 66860 Perpignan, France; nathalie.tapissier@univ-perp.fr
[3] Laboratoire d'Excellence 'CORAIL', Moorea 98729, French Polynesia
[4] The Natural Products Metabolomics Group, Strathclyde Institute of Pharmacy and Biomedical Sciences, Faculty of Science, University of Strathclyde, The John Arbuthnott Building, 161 Cathedral Street, Glasgow G4 0RE, UK
* Correspondence: ruangelie.edrada-ebel@strath.ac.uk

Abstract: Natural products from plants have been listed for hundreds of years as a source of biologically active molecules. In recent years, the marine environment has demonstrated its ability to provide new structural entities. More than 70% of our planet's surface is covered by oceans, and with the technical advances in diving and remotely operated vehicles, it is becoming easier to collect samples. Although the risk of rediscovery is significant, the discovery of silent gene clusters and innovative analytical techniques has renewed interest in natural product research. Different strategies have been proposed to activate these silent genes, including co-culture, or mixed fermentation, a cultivation-based approach. This review highlights the potential of co-culture of marine microorganisms to induce the production of new metabolites as well as to increase the yields of respective target metabolites with pharmacological potential, and moreover to indirectly improve the biological activity of a crude extract.

Keywords: co-culture; natural products; marine bacteria; marine fungi

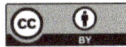

1. Introduction

Secondary metabolites are molecules found in nature that are produced by organisms from one or several primary metabolites. Secondary metabolites are not required for basic viability but are essential for the organism's survival strategies. These natural products are synthesised by many organisms, such as bacteria, fungi, plants, and sponges, and are found in all environments, both terrestrial and marine.

Natural products from terrestrial plants and microorganisms are a common source of modern drug molecules. Historically, they have been used since ancient times and in traditional medicine for the treatment of many diseases and illnesses. Natural products constitute the foundation of medicines for human health. The earliest records dating from around 2600 BC documented the use of about 1000 substances derived from plants in Mesopotamia, such as oils of *Cupressus sempevirens* (cypress) and *Glycyrrhiza glabra* (liquorice). One of the best-known documents is the "*Ebers Papyrus*", dating from 1500 BC, recording more than 700 medicines, most of them of plant origin [1–3].

Recently, Newmann and Cragg (2012) reported that between 1981 and 2010, 48.6% of the 175 small drug molecules used in cancer therapy were either natural products or derived therefrom. In other areas, such as anti-infectives, the influence of natural products as lead structures has been quite remarkable [4,5].

Regarding microorganisms, it is estimated that the number of existing microbial species would be around 10^5 to 10^6, but only several thousand have been isolated into pure cultures [6]. It is still possible to find biologically active molecules with novel structures or unprecedented carbon skeletons and unique modes of action from uncultivable and undiscovered species. Additionally, unlike macro-organisms, microorganisms have significant advantages in terms of their resilience and feasibility in terms of the cost of an industrial-scale fermentation. For the preservation of their environment of origin, the possibility to collect samples sustainably without having an impact on the biodiversity of the natural environment is of great importance. Furthermore, microorganisms are a prolific source of structurally diverse bioactive metabolites and have yielded some of the most important antibiotics in the pharmaceutical industry—one best known example is the discovery of penicillin by Fleming in 1928 [2].

Plants have also been proven to be very good sources of bioactive natural products, but in recent years, the marine environment has demonstrated its ability to provide new structural entities as well. More than 70% of our planet's surface is covered by oceans, and in certain marine ecosystems, such as coral reefs, experts estimate that the biological diversity is higher than in a tropical rainforest [7]. Exploration of the marine environment has for a very long time been limited to coasts and ocean surfaces, but with technical advances in diving and remotely operated vehicles (ROVs), it is becoming easier to take samples at deeper ocean depths. As for terrestrial microorganisms, marine bacteria and fungi quickly proved to be prolific sources of novel bioactive compounds [8].

Therapeutic molecules from the marine environment are now available in the market. In 2007, trabectedin (**1**) (Yondelis®) was the first marine-derived anti-neoplastic drug to be approved in the European Union. Trabectedin (Figure 1) was initially isolated from the Caribbean tunicate *Ecteinascida turbinata* [9]. Currently, PharmaMar commercially prepares Yondelis® by chemical synthesis [10,11]. Another example is salinosporamide A (**2**) (Marizomib®), which was isolated from a marine-derived microorganism. In 2002, Feling et al. of the Fenical and Jensen group initially isolated salinosporamide A (**2**) (Figure 1) from a sediment obligate marine actinomycete, *Salinospora tropica* [12]. Salinosporamide A (**2**) is a 20S proteasome inhibitor that was granted an orphan drug designation by the European Medicines Agency (EMA) for the treatment of multiple myeloma [13].

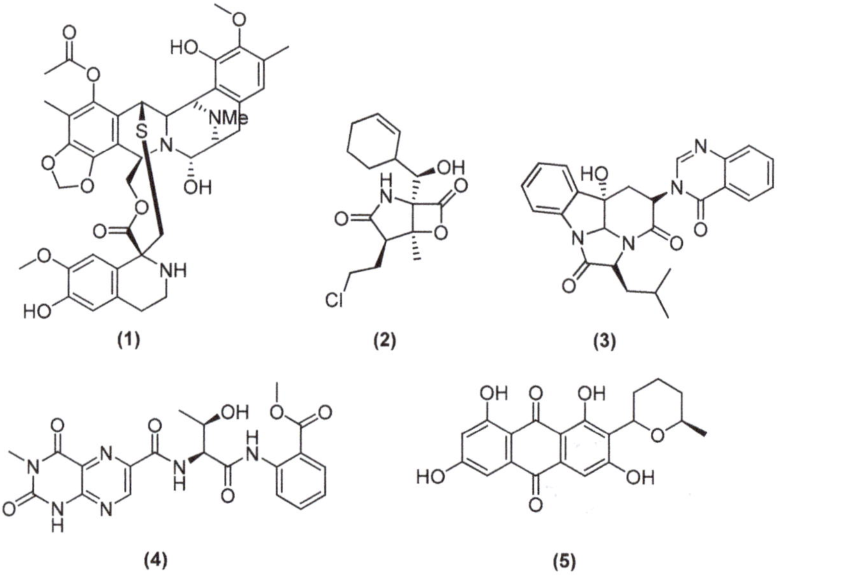

Figure 1. Chemical structures of trabectedin (**1**), salinosporamide A (**2**), isopropylchaetominine (**3**), isoterrelumamide A (**4**), and 5′-epi-averufanin (**5**).

Natural products therefore represent a non-negligible share of molecules on the market, but currently, the risk of rediscovery is always high. They have been laid aside for several years by the pharmaceutical industry in favour of synthetic molecules. However, with the discovery of silent gene clusters and the significant improvement of screening, analytical, and molecular biological techniques, a renewed interest in natural products research has been increasingly flourishing.

Whole-genome sequencing of different microorganisms has disclosed inconsistencies between the number of groups of genes identified using informatic approaches and the number of metabolites produced by the organisms [14]. The genes that are present but not expressed under laboratory conditions are called silent gene clusters. A hypothesis was then proposed for activating these silent gene clusters to potentially access new secondary metabolites that could be of pharmacological interest. Different strategies for activating these silent gene clusters are described below.

Various strategies have been put together to influence the production of secondary metabolites by microorganisms when grown in the laboratory. As described in a 2014 review paper by Bertrand et al., it is possible to explore organisms at different levels, from their genome to their metabolome via their transcriptome and proteome [15]. At the genome level, metabolic engineering was among the first techniques to be exploited, and was defined by Khosla and Keasling as "the process of rerouting metabolic pathways by genetic manipulation" [16]. In recent years, metabolic engineering has enabled the development of several techniques of genetic manipulation, the most common of which involves the biosynthesis of secondary metabolites in a heterologous host. When the natural producer of certain targeted secondary metabolites do not grow well under laboratory or industrial conditions, the biosynthetic gene cluster of interest is inserted into a different but more robust microorganism, which is selected on the basis of the involved biosynthetic pathway of targeted metabolites [17]. Mutasynthesis is another technique in which a mutant microorganism that is deficient in a key part of the biosynthetic pathway is employed and to which analogous precursors are supplemented to augment the production of new metabolites of interest [18]. These methodologies applied on the microbial genome have also been utilised along with combinatorial biosynthesis. With combinatorial biosynthesis, genes and modules of closely related synthetic pathways of secondary metabolites would be rearranged to create new congeners [17]. The success rate of combinatorial synthesis depends on the position of the introduction of the modification. Modifications at the later stages of the synthetic pathway would afford higher success rates. Indeed, there will potentially be less enzyme downstream of the point of alteration, due to having to tolerate these modifications of the substrate and complicating the process [17]. For this kind of method, it is essential that the biosynthetic gene clusters of the microorganisms are sequenced and the functions of the genes of interest are also assigned [15].

Epigenetic modification is another commonly used strategy utilised on the transcriptome and the proteome, where microorganisms were treated with epigenetic modifiers such as DNA methyl transferase or histone deacetylase inhibitors to modulate the DNA histone remodelling the chromatin for initiating the transcription of silent genes [19]. 5-Azacytidine is among the most commonly used DNA methyl transferase inhibiting molecules. Akone et al. (2016) of the Proksch group in Düsseldorf, Germany, used 5-azacytidine on fungal endophytic cultures of *Chaetomium* sp. to generate five additional polyketide congeners along with enhancing the production of targeted anticancer metabolites produced in their co-culture experiments [20]. Alternatively, the Oshima group utilised suberoyl bis-hydroxamic acid, an example of a histone deacetylase inhibitor that afforded the production of a novel series of three new prenylated tryptophan analogues known as luteorides from cultures of the entomopathogenic fungus, *Torrubiella luteorostrata* [21]. Epigenetic modification has demonstrated the accumulation of new natural products of interest.

Microbial cultures grown under laboratory conditions may afford a different metabolomic profile when found in their original environment, and therefore it is important to take into account the chemical–ecological relationships that occur in their communities [15].

Moreover, genomic data are not available for all microorganisms. Therefore, non-genome-dependent techniques have also been developed. One of the strategies often related to chemical ecology is a cultivation-based approach, namely, the "one strain many compounds" (OSMAC) technique, which underlines how a single strain can produce different molecules when grown under different inoculation and incubation conditions [14]. Different parameters can be changed, such as the salinity of the medium, its composition, the addition of different salts, elicitors, differences in temperature or agitation conditions, and many more. One of the other parameters to be taken into account is also the observed differences in metabolomic profiles between cultures grown in solid and liquid media, as illustrated in a review paper by Romano et al. (2018) of the Dobson group in Cork, Ireland [14]. An example to illustrate the OSMAC approach is a comparative study on the changes in the metabolomic profile of a sponge-associated fungus, *Aspergillus carneus* [22]. In this study, Özkaya et al. (2018) of the Proksch group isolated three new natural products (Figure 1)—isopropylchaetominine (**3**), isoterrelumamide A (**4**), and 5′-epi-averufanin (**5**)—after the fungus was inoculated on three different media. Isoterrelumamide A (**4**) was present only after fermentation on modified Czapek medium, while 5′-epi-averufanin was only afforded when incubated on solid rice medium with or without sea salt. It can thus be seen that depending on the composition of the culture medium in which the microorganism was inoculated, the detected secondary metabolites were not always the same [22].

Finally, the third option is by co-culture, also called mixed-fermentation, which is another cultivation-based approach. In this technique, two or more different microorganisms are inoculated together to mimic the natural habitat in which symbiotic or competing interactions between microorganisms are simulated and/or enhanced. Natural habitats could be characterised by limited access to resources and nutrients, as well as by an exchange of metabolites between micro- and/or macroscopic organisms. Competition between microbes is deliberately provoked by inducing stress factors, which stimulates the activation of silent gene clusters that were not expressed under classical culture conditions [8].

In this review, we focus on secondary metabolites from marine microorganisms and how co-culture techniques can induce their production. The different techniques implemented for mixed fermentations are discussed. Finally, the review is concluded through a critical enquiry on the potential for producing new metabolites by employing different novel co-culture techniques. This review, however, will not differentiate marine fungi from marine-derived fungi. Marine-derived fungi are species that do not belong to the well-documented lineages of obligate marine fungi, or when the source macro-organism cannot be conclusively identified as marine [23]. Nevertheless, these microorganisms could be isolated from oceans; ocean-dwelling animals; marine algae; and from marine–terrestrial transitional habitats, e.g., mangroves and other halophytes.

2. Co-Cultivation between Marine Microorganisms

The different results obtained from various representative examples of co-culture conditions presented in publications from 2010 to 2020 were surveyed in this review paper. The next three sections will tackle, and present publications found under the search terms: marine culture "coculture" OR "mixed fermentation" OR "co-culture" AND "fungi" OR "bacteria". Articles were then classified into the three sections according to the type of co-inoculated microorganisms: (1) bacteria–fungi, (2) between bacteria, and (3) between fungi.

2.1. Co-Cultures between Fungi and Bacteria

In this section, only the three most relevant sample articles were found to correspond to the mixed fermentation of marine fungi and bacteria. One example of the association between marine-derived fungi and a terrestrial bacterium is also presented.

Yu, Ding, and Ma (2016) co-cultured the fungus *Aspergillus flavipes* with the actinomycete *Streptomyces* sp., which were both isolated from marine coastal sediment from the Nanji Islands in China. The mixed fermentation increased the production yield of new cytochalasin analogues from the corresponding fungal monoculture [24]. This co-culture induced the production of six cytochalasans shown in Figure 2, namely, rosellichalasin (6), aspochalasin E (7), aspochalasin P (8), aspochalasin H (9), aspochalasin M (10), and 19,20-dihydro-aspochalasin D (11). These secondary metabolites were produced in monocultures of *Aspergillus flavipes* but at very low concentrations that were below the limit of quantification through HPLC-TOF-MS. Yu, Ding, and Ma (2016) detected the respective *m/z* ion peaks, demonstrating the enhancement of cytochalasan production that required physical contact between non-inactivated co-cultivated microbes. All six cytochalasans exhibited strong activity against *Streptomyces* sp. with an inhibition rate of 50–80% at concentrations between 2 and 16 µg/mL but had no effect on the fungus *A. flavipes* at the same concentration. This result indicated that the cytochalasans assisted *A. flavipes* to compete with *Streptomyces*.

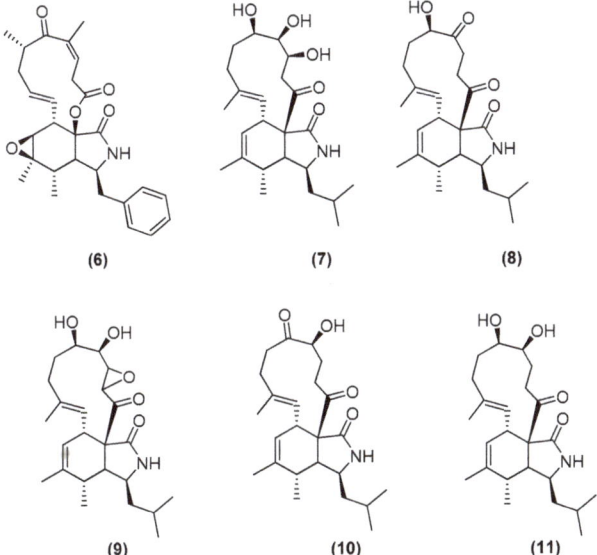

Figure 2. Chemical structures of rosellichalasin (6), aspochalasin E (7), aspochalasin P (8), aspochalasin H (9), aspochalasin M (10), and 19,20-dihydro-aspochalasin D (11).

From the same perspective, Wakefield et al. (2017) of the Jasper group in Aberdeen, United Kingdom, described co-cultures of a marine-derived fungus, *Aspergillus fumigatus* MR2012, with two hyper-arid desert bacterial isolates *Streptomyces leeuwenhoekii* strain C34 and strain C58 [25]. The co-culture with strain C34 afforded a new luteoride derivative, luteoride D (12); a new pseurotin congener, pseurotin G (13); and two known compounds, terezine D (14) and 11-O-methylpseurotin A (15), which were not found in the axenic fungal culture (Figure 3). Interestingly, some of the major fungal metabolites produced by the respective axenic cultures were suppressed. The microbial co-culture with strain C58 dramatically increased the production of chaxapeptin (16) that was already initially found in the axenic culture of the bacteria while inducing the production of a known pentalenic acid (17). It is interesting to note that the co-culture process could induce the production of new compounds and increase the yield of existing metabolites from both axenic microbial cultures and not in only one of the two microorganisms involved in the co-culture. However, co-culturing could also result in a loss of production of some major families of fungal metabolites present in its axenic culture, while none of the bacterial metabolites were proven to have antifungal effects.

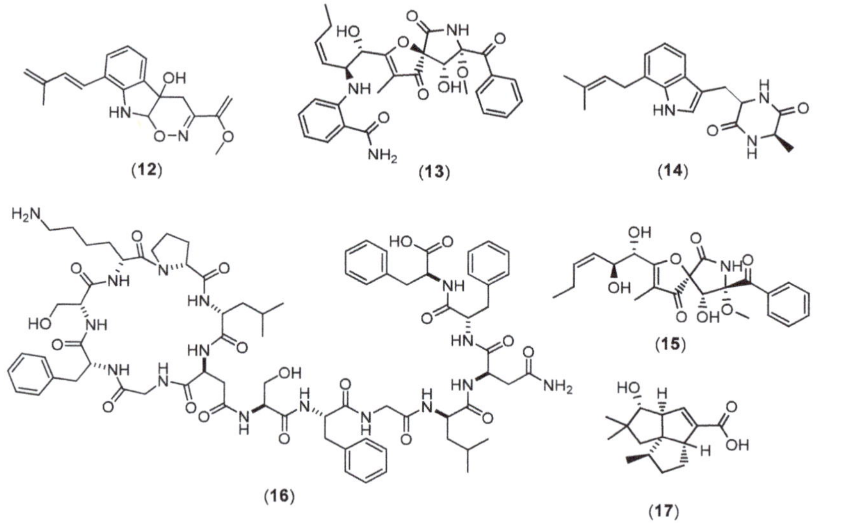

Figure 3. Chemical structures of luteoride D (**12**), pseurotin G (**13**), terezine D (**14**), 11-*O*-methylpseurotin A (**15**), chaxapeptin (**16**), and pentalenic acid (**17**).

To observe the induction of antimicrobial compounds as well as the production of biosurfactants and quorum-sensing inhibitors, Dusane et al. (2011), from Pune University in India, worked with four marine epibiotic bacteria (*Bacillus* sp. S3, *Bacillus pumilus* S8, *Bacillus licheniformis* D1, and *Serratia marcescens* V1) that exhibited bioactivity against pathogenic or biofouling fungi [26]. Dusane et al. demonstrated the induction and/or enhancement of antimicrobial activity by co-culturing marine epibiotic bacteria with *Candida albicans* and *Yarrowia lipolytica*. Except for S8, monocultures of S3, D1, and V1 displayed antifungal activity against *C. albicans*. On the other hand, none of the axenic cultures of epibiotic bacteria showed any antifungal activity against *Y. lipolytica*. However, cell-free supernatants of mixed fermentation cultures of marine *Bacillus* sp. S3 and *C. albicans* induced antifungal activity against *Y. lipolytica*, while co-cultures of D1 and *C. albicans* enhanced biosurfactant production. Dusane et al. illustrated the induction and enhancement of the production of certain metabolites of interest with specific biological activity by co-culturing microorganisms with pathogenic microbial strains.

2.2. Co-Cultures between Two Bacterial Strains

In recent years, several reports on co-cultures between bacteria have been published. Based on the search terms mentioned above, we chose the 11 most appropriate publications reported on co-cultures between marine bacteria for further evaluation, including one of the papers presented at the end of the previous section. Bacteria in the marine environment are found in numerous habitats, not only in sediments, but also in association with algae and other macro-organisms. These microbes can have a free mode of life in water or sessile in the form of a biofilm in which bacteria can communicate by quorum sensing [27].

In the last paper presented in the previous section, Dusane et al. also co-cultured four marine epibiotic bacteria with other bacteria, such as *Pseudomonas aeruginosa* PA and *Bacillus pumilus* BP [26]. The respective cell-free supernatants of co-cultures of marine *Bacillus* sp. S3 and S8 with *Ps. aeruginosa* and *B. pumilus* allowed for the induction of antifungal activity. Again, antifungal activity was evident when marine isolates were co-cultivated with either pathogenic or biofouling bacterial cultures. However, the enhancement of the antibacterial activity was less apparent when compared with the distinctive induction of antifungal activity by the cell-free supernatants of the co-cultures. Exceptionally, the antibacterial activity of *B. licheniformis* D1 against *Ps. aeruginosa* was significantly increased when co-cultured with the latter pathogen. Similarly, a significant enhancement of biosurfactant production was observed when *S. marcescens* V1 was co-cultivated with the biofouling bacteria *B. pumilus*, which was not observed when inoculated with other non-biofouling marine bacterial isolates. On the other hand, cell-free supernatants of co-cultures of *Ps. aeruginosa* and *Bacillus* sp., as well as of their respective axenic cultures, were also observed to exhibit quorum sensing inhibitory activity. Co-cultivation of marine epibiotic bacteria with pathogenic and fouling bacteria were able to either induce or enhance all the indicated bioactivity in this research paper, which signposted the production of secondary metabolites with antibiotics, anti-quorum sensing, and biosurfactant activities.

In another study, Haque et al. (2016) focused on the antifungal and anticancer activity of an ethyl acetate crude extract obtained from a co-culture of two marine *Streptomyces* sp., ANAM-5 and AIAH-10, isolated from mangrove forest soil samples of Sundarbans, Bangladesh [28]. Only crude extracts of the co-cultures were implemented for the bioassays, while no isolated purified compounds could be utilised. The crude extracts exhibited antifungal activities against both *Saccharomyces cerevisiae* and *Aspergillus niger* with an MIC value of 64 µg/mL as well as against *Candida albicans* with an MIC value of 32 µg/mL. Haque et al. evaluated the antineoplastic activity of the co-culture extracts by measuring cell growth inhibition and the enhancement of the life span of Ehrlich ascites carcinoma (EAC) cell-bearing mice. The efficiency of the activity of the crude extract was compared with the standard anticancer drug bleomycin. Co-cultured bacterial crude extracts effectively inhibited cell growth rate at 75.75% at a of dose 100 mg/kg (i.p.), which is quite comparable to that of bleomycin at 0.3 mg/kg. Crude extracts of the co-cultured bacteria also effectively increased the life span of tumour-bearing mice by 71.79% at a dose of 100 mg/kg (i.p.). In conclusion, the extract obtained from the co-culture displayed interesting antimicrobial and anti-neoplastic activity. Reported biological activity was enhanced by 70% with the crude extracts of the co-culture, but there is no record whether new compounds were generated or merely enhanced concentration of biologically active components.

Ravi et al. (2017), from VIT University in India, briefly described co-culturing marine and terrestrial actinomycetes to enhance anticancer bioactivity [29]. The co-cultured bacterial extract gave an IC$_{50}$ value of 20 µg/mL, while the extract from the monoculture afforded a weaker IC$_{50}$ of 40 µg/mL. It was interesting to perceive that the co-culture of two actinomycetes species from different ecological origin could augment the production of potential anticancer metabolites. Ravi et al. also disclosed that under co-culture conditions, albeit with the occurrence of normal and healthy actinomycete filaments, spore production was greatly suppressed.

Yu et al. (2015) of the Ma group from Zhejiang University, Hangzhou, developed a relatively simple fermentation method to increase the production of algicidal tryptamine derivatives [30]. Tryptamine derivatives, as shown in Figure 4, were initially introduced as very promising molecules for the control of harmful algal blooms, but their application and further study was halted by the low production rate of the bioactive metabolites in axenic cultures of *Bacillus mycoides*. Bacterial co-cultures were established using the OSMAC technique to optimise the production of potent algicidal tryptamine congeners. Yu et al. subjected *Streptomyces* sp. CGMCC4.7185 and *Bacillus mycoides* to mixed fermentation, and various experiments were carried out to find the best culture medium and pH to enhance the production of the desired tryptamine analogues. The mean production yields of the respective tryptamine derivatives from a 68 L fermentation culture under optimised conditions were 14.9 mg/L for *N*-acetyltryptamine (**18**), 2.8 mg/L for *N*-propanoyltryptamine (**19**), 3.0 mg/L for bacillamide A(**20**), 13.7 mg/L for bacillamide B (**21**), and 9.6 mg/L for bacillamide C (**22**). The total tryptamine yield represented more than 50% of the crude ethyl acetate extract (3.0 g in the 5.5 g total extract). Under normal axenic culture conditions, the occurrence of various tryptamine analogues was undetectable by HPLC equipped with a diode array detector at a UV range between 200 and 400 nm but perceivable by TLC when visualised with iodine vapour.

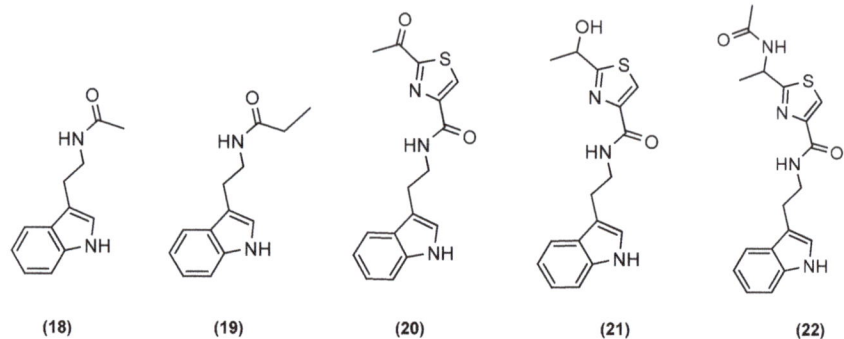

Figure 4. Chemical structures of the co-culture-induced compounds *N*-acetyltryptamine (**18**), *N*-propanoyltryptamine (**19**), bacillamide A (**20**), bacillamide B (**21**), and bacillamide C (**22**).

Low biomass yields with bacterial cultures are a frequent challenge. Under a co-culture environment, a higher production yield of the targeted secondary metabolites was facilitated. With higher yields, the various analogues can be further evaluated for their other potential activities and cytotoxicity studies. However, subsequently, for a large (industrial) scale-up, as the fermentation parameters can change and are not directly reproducible, then it may be necessary to employ other techniques or in combination with co-cultivation such as hemisynthesis or one of the metabolic engineering methods described above in Section 1.

Cho and Kim (2012), from Soon Chun Hyang University, Korea, increased the production of a target antifouling compound by co-culturing a bacterium producing the metabolite of interest with a competitor bacterium isolated from the same host macroorganism [31]. The active antifouling diterpene lobocompactol (**23**) (Figure 5) was initially isolated from the marine *Streptomyces cinnabarinus* PK209. To increase lobocompactol production, Cho and Kim selected *Alteromonas* sp. KNS-16 as the lobocompactol-resistant bacterium for a co-culture competitor. Both bacterial strains, PK209 and KNS-16, were isolated from the surface of a seaweed rhizosphere. The co-culture of these two bacterial strains resulted in a 10.4-fold increase in the production of lobocompactol compared to the PK209 monoculture (2.7 mg/L instead of 0.25 mg/L). Lobocompactol (**23**) exhibited significant antifouling activity with an EC_{50} of 0.18 µg/mL against the macroalga *Ulva pertusa* and 0.43 µg/mL against the diatom *Navicula annexa*. The extract also demonstrated its activity against the fouling bacteria. These studies from Yu et al. [30] as well as Cho and Kim [31] presented the potential of co-cultures in increasing the production of a particular target metabolite.

Co-cultures have also led to the discovery of new bioactive molecules. Shin et al. (2018) from Seoul National University elucidated a new piperazic acid-bearing cyclic peptide, dentigerumycin E (**24**) (Figure 5), afforded by the co-culture of the marine *Streptomyces* sp. JB5 and *Bacillus* sp. GN1, isolated from an intertidal mudflat in Wando, Republic of Korea [32]. *Streptomyces* sp. JB5 was co-cultivated with seven different bacterial strains including *Bacillus* sp. HR1, *Paenibacillus* sp. CC2, *Brevibacillus* sp. PTH23, *Streptomyces* sp. SD53, *Streptomyces* sp. UTZ13, *Hafnia* sp. CF1, and *Mycobacterium* sp. Myc06. However, only the co-culture with *Bacillus* sp. HR1, which is phylogenetically close to *Bacillus* sp. GN1, afforded dentigerumycin. Although the mechanism triggering the biosynthesis of dentigerumycin E (**24**) by *Bacillus* strains remains unclear, the results of these co-culture experiments imply that *Bacillus* strains, which are most closely related to *B. cereus*, may share the ability to induce production of dentigerumycin E (**24**) in *Streptomyces* sp. JB5. Full genome sequencing of *Streptomyces* sp. JB5 allowed for the identification of the BGC for dentigerumycin E (**24**), and thus it was confirmed that it was indeed produced by the *Streptomyces* strain. Different experiments have shown that dentigerumycin E had antimetastatic potential against breast cancer cells.

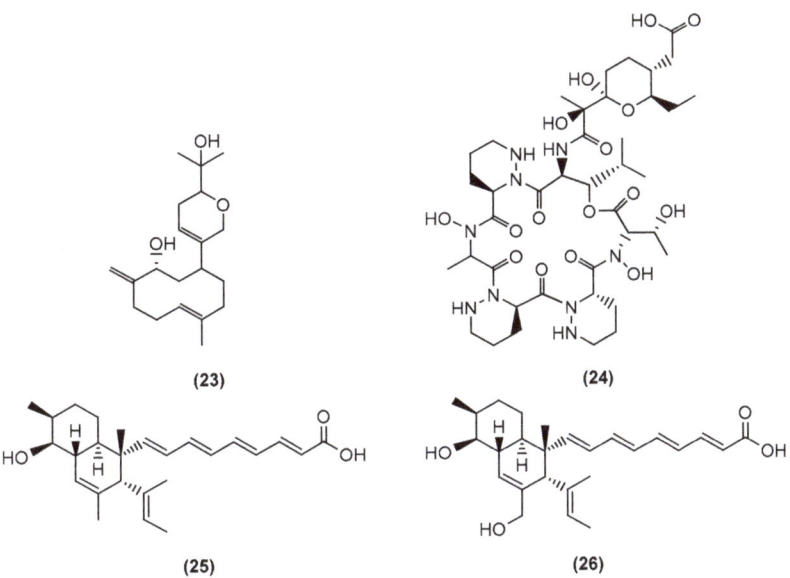

Figure 5. Chemical structures of lobocompactol (**23**), dentigerumycin E (**24**), and janthinopolyenemycins A (**25**) and B (**26**).

Anjum et al. (2018) of the Lian group from Zhejiang University, Hangzhou, isolated janthinopolyenemycins A (**25**) and B (**26**), two rare polyketides (Figure 5), from a co-culture of two *Janthinobacterium* spp. strains ZZ145 and ZZ148 obtained from a marine soil sample, and the strains were co-inoculated in different media including rice solid medium [33]. Both polyketides exhibited antifungal activity against *C. albicans* with MIC and MBC values of 15.6 and 31.25 µg/mL, respectively, although their bioactivities were less potent than the control (amphotericin B). The janthinopolyenemycin congeners were also found to be active against methicillin-resistant *Staphylococcus aureus* (MRSA) and *E. coli*. The co-culture of ZZ145 and ZZ148 induced the generation of the new janthinopolyenemycin congeners.

Many of the marine bacteria used in co-cultures were derived from soil sediment. However, the literature has also shown co-cultures of sponge-derived actinomycetes [34]. Dashti et al. (2014) of the Quinn group in Griffith University co-cultured *Nocardiopsis* sp. RV163, derived from the Mediterranean sponge *Dysidea* along with *Actinokineospora* sp. EG49 from the Red Sea sponge *Spheciospongia vagabunda* to induce the biosynthesis of three compounds (Figure 6), namely, *N*-(2-hydroxyphenyl)-acetamide (**27**), 1,6-dihydroxyphenazine (**28**), and 5a,6,11a,12-tetrahydro-5a,11a-dimethyl[1,4]benzoxazino[3,2-*b*][1,4]benzoxazine (**29**), of which compound **28** was produced at a very high yield at 12% of the crude extract weight. Dashti et al. monitored the induced production of new metabolites in the co-culture by ^{1}H NMR analysis of the respective culture extracts. The ^{1}H NMR spectral data also indicated the suppression of the production of some of the metabolites present in the axenic cultures, which was similarly observed by Wakefield et al. in 2017 [25]. All three afforded compounds (**27** to **29**) were tested for bioactivity against *Bacillus* sp. P25, *Escherichia coli* and *Fusarium* sp. P21, and human parasites *Leishmania major* and *Trypanosoma brucei*, as well as *Nocardiopsis* sp. RV163 and *Actinokineospora* sp. EG49 cultures. Only 1,6-dihydroxyphenazine (**28**) exhibited bioactivity against *Bacillus* sp.; *Trypanosoma brucei*; and, interestingly, against *Actinokineospora* sp. EG49, which may indicate that compound **28** was biosynthesised by *Nocardiopsis* sp. RV163. These last three studies demonstrated the potential of a co-culture to induce the production of new metabolites.

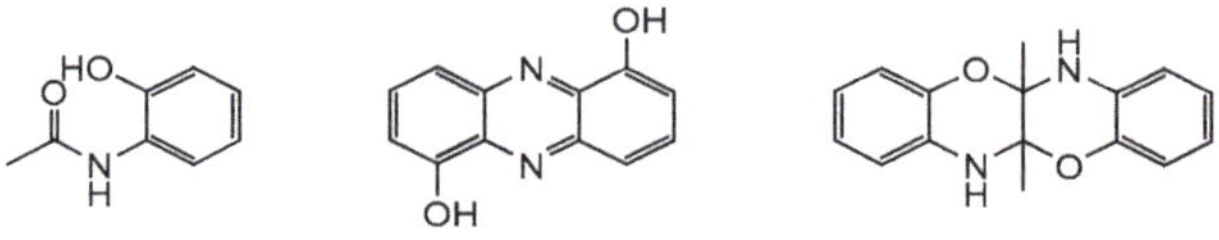

Figure 6. Chemical structures of *N*-(2-hydroxyphenyl)-acetamide (**27**), 1,6-dihydroxyphenazine (**28**), 5a,6,11a,12-tetrahydro-5a,11a-dimethyl[1,4]benzoxazino [3,2-b][1,4]benzoxazine (**29**), and keyicin (**30**).

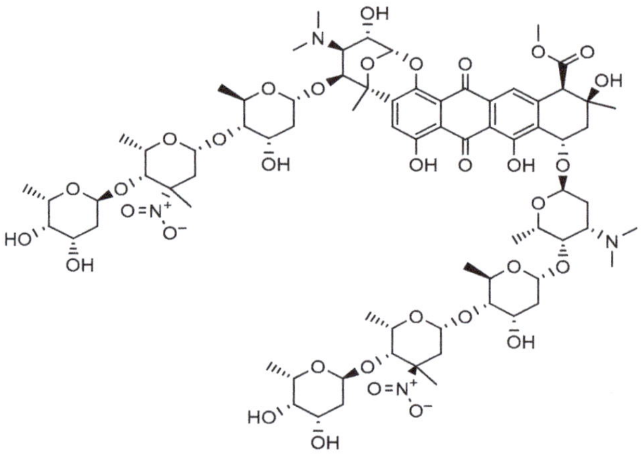

The last two studies in this section are articles by the Bugni group from the University of Wisconsin. Unlike all the previous articles, these latter studies used microscale fermentation [35]. Microscale cultivation was carried out in 96-well plates, in volumes of 500 µL. Adnani et al. (2015) selected *Mycobacterium* sp. (WMMA-183) and *Rhodococcus* sp. (WMMA-185) as co-culture strains for various species from within the multiple genera of Micromonosporaceae. From the Micromonosporaceae family, 65 species were chosen for analysis of their monoculture and co-culture metabolomic profiles. While some culture samples showed antibiotic induction, some significant limitations also occurred, as this method is likely to miss antibiotics produced in the co-culture due to the initial activity observed in axenic cultures from an unrelated antibiotic. To resolve such methodological limitations, a complementary approach by LC–MS-based metabolomics was employed to analyse the types of compounds produced during the interaction and exhibition of antibiotic activity. For the 130 co-culture combinations, a total of 12 Micromonosporaceae demonstrated discernible diversity, with six producing a unique chemistry but shared similar chemical profiles when co-cultured with *Mycobacterium* sp. or *Rhodococcus* sp., while the other six produced different metabolomic profiles that were dependent on the bacterium with which it was co-cultured. Co-cultures producing similar chemical profiles were clustered, while secondary metabolites exclusively produced in co-culture were further evaluated for novelty. As an example, co-culture of *Verrucosispora* sp. and *Rhodococcus* sp. exclusively produced a total of 29 identified compounds. Of the 29 compounds, 27 were determined to be novel, and 24 could be reproduced in the scale-up. This latter study demonstrated the ability to screen and identify the generation of new metabolites from a microscale fermentation approach.

In their article, Adnani et al. (2017) described the production of keyicin (**30**), a new *bis*-nitroglycosylated anthracycline (Figure 6), by a co-culture of a *Rhodococcus* sp. and a *Micromonospora* sp. [36]. Keyicin (**30**) was produced exclusively via mixed fermentation, but physical contact between the two bacteria was not necessary. Monocultures of the two bacterial strains were incubated in distinct chambers but were connected through a tunnel separated by a diffusible membrane allowing the exchange of metabolites without any cellular transfer between chambers. Through genome sequencing, *Micromonospora* sp. was shown to be the "true" producer of keyicin in the co-culture. Keyicin (**30**) inhibited the growth of *Mycobacterium* sp. and *Rhodococcus* sp., as well as *B. subtilis* and methicillin-sensitive *Staphylococcus aureus* (MSSA) at minimum inhibitory concentrations of 8 and 2 µg/mL, respectively. In contrast to many other anthracyclines, 20 *E. coli*-based chemical genomics studies revealed that keyicin's mechanism of action did not induce DNA damage.

In this section, it is shown that there are various types of co-culture between bacteria, and much remains to be discovered. Co-culture between bacteria has afforded interesting molecules and has made it possible to induce the production of new metabolites while increasing the production of known compounds or further enhancing their bioactivity, whether in small- to medium-sized liquid fermentation or in micro-fermentation scales. Co-culturing *Micromonospora* sp. and *Rhodococcus* sp. exclusively induced the production of the target metabolite keyicin (**30**), which was not afforded by the monocultures, although the biosynthetic gene cluster was found in *Micromonospora* sp.

2.3. Co-Cultures between Two Fungal Strains

In this last section, 14 pertinent articles were selected to describe the co-cultivation of two fungal species. Isolation of fungal samples from the marine environment has received increasing attention as a new source of interesting metabolites. As mentioned in the introduction, it is more difficult to differentiate a marine from a terrestrial fungus when compared to a bacterium. Unlike bacteria, marine fungi do not necessarily need sea salts in their culture medium to grow. Therefore, both obligate marine and marine-derived fungi will be included in this section.

Most of the literature has described fungal co-cultures between the genus *Penicillium* and/or *Aspergillus* and/or with other fungal genera. Bao et al. (2017) of the Qi group in Guangzhou, China, co-cultivated two marine gorgonian-associated fungi, *Aspergillus sclerotiorum* SCSGAF 0053 and *Penicillium citrinum* SCSGAF 0052, both isolated from *Muricella flexusa* collected from the South China Sea [37]. The development of a red pigment was only observed in the co-culture, which did not occur in either of the monocultures. Six new compounds (**31–36**) shown in Figure 7 were elucidated, including two furanone derivatives, sclerotiorumins A (**31**) and B (**32**); a novel oxadiazin derivative, sclerotiorumin C (**33**); a pyrrole derivative, 1-(4-benzyl-1*H*-pyrrol-3-yl)ethenone (**34**); and two complexes of neoaspergillic acid with aluminium (**35**) and iron (**36**) (Figure 7). Sclerotiorumin C (**33**) was the first naturally occurring 1,2,4-oxadiazin-6-one described. All compounds were tested for different activities—aluminiumneohydroxyaspergillin (**35**) showed significant selective cytotoxicity against human histiocytic lymphoma U937 cell line (IC$_{50}$ = 4.2 µM) and strong toxicity towards brine shrimp (LC$_{50}$ = 6.1 µM), and interestingly was able to increase the growth and biofilm formation of *S. aureus*.

Kossuga et al. (2013) of the Berlinck group in São Paulo co-cultivated a total of 50 fungal strains and 5 bacterial strains in 250 growth experiments. Analysis of the extracts indicated changes in the chemical profile of eight co-cultures when compared to their corresponding monocultures. However, most of the dereplicated metabolites are already known compounds. The co-cultures produced a minority of the secondary metabolites that contained novel carbon skeletons. *Penicillium* sp. Ma(M3)V co-cultured with *Trichoderma* sp. Gc(M2)1 produced a complex extract that yielded two new polyketides (Figure 8), (*Z*)-2-ethylhex-2-enedioic acid (**37**) and (*E*)-4-oxo-2-propylideneoct-7-enoic acid (**38**) [38]. Polyketides **37** and **38** are examples of unprecedented carbon skeletons.

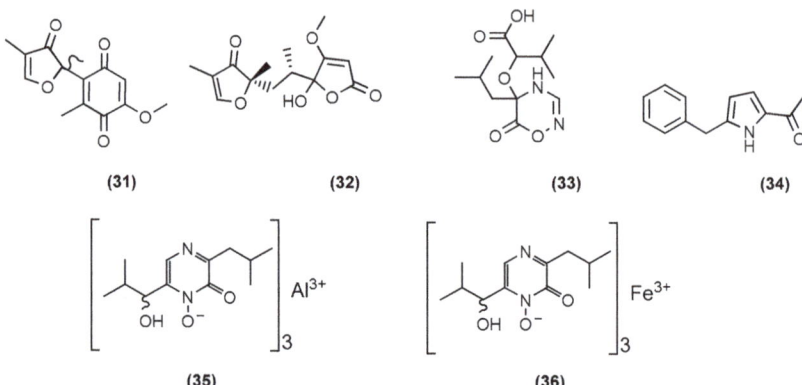

Figure 7. Chemical structures of sclerotiorumins A-B (**31** and **32**), sclerotiorumin C (**33**), 1-(4-benzyl-1*H*-pyrrol-3-yl)ethanone (**34**), aluminiumneohydroxyaspergillin (**35**), and ferrineohydroxyaspergillin (**36**).

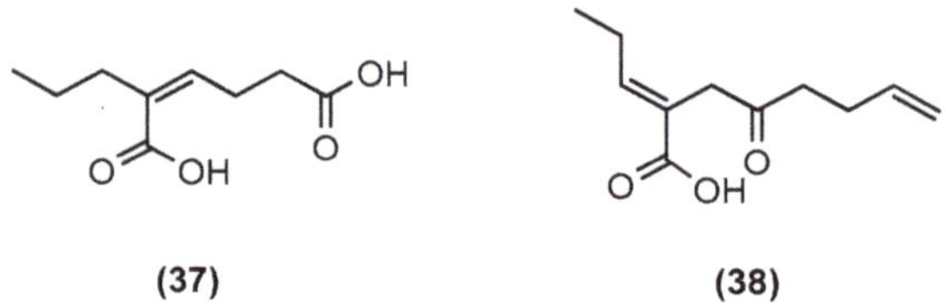

Figure 8. Chemical structures of (*Z*)-2-ethylhex-2-enedioic acid (**37**) and (*E*)-4-oxo-2-propylideneoct-7-enoic acid (**38**).

The group of Zhuravleva and Afiyatullov (2016) in Russia isolated known diorcinol congeners B to E (**39** to **42**) along with a new derivative, diorcinol J (**43**) (Figure 9), by the mixed fermentation of *Aspergillus sulphureus* KMM 4640 and *Isaria felina* KMM 4639 obtained from a muddy sand and a marine sediment, respectively [39]. Diorcinol J (**43**) was the only congener that showed cytotoxicity against Ehrlich carcinoma cells, by the membranolytic mechanism. In addition, more recently in 2018, the group of Zhuravleva and Afiyatullov isolated five new prenylated indole alkaloids (Figure 10) from the same co-culture. This included 17-hydroxynotoamide D (**44**), 17-*O*-ethylnotoamide M (**45**), 10-*O*-acetylsclerotiamide (**46**), 10-*O*-ethylsclerotiamide (**47**), and 10-*O*-ethylnotoamide R (**48**) [40]. However, 10-*O*-ethylnotoamide R (**48**) was not detected in the original extract, and thus the authors postulated that **48** might not be a natural product, but an artefact obtained during the isolation process. Zhuravleva and Afiyatullov also investigated the effect of 17-hydroxynotoamide D (**44**), 17-*O*-ethylnotoamide M (**45**), and 10-*O*-ethylnotoamide R (**48**) on the viability of human non-malignant and prostate cancer cells, as well as on the formation of colonies of human prostate cancer cells 22Rv1. 17-*O*-Ethylnotoamide M (**45**) exerted a significant effect on reducing 22Rv1 colony formation at concentrations of 10 µM by 25%. 22Rv1 cells are known to be resistant to hormone therapy, as well as to the new second-generation drugs. Therefore, drugs that are active in these cell lines may be of potential interest for further investigation in the therapy of drug-resistant human prostate cancer. Although these new molecules were produced only in the co-culture, it is worth mentioning that brevianamide F (**49**) (Figure 10), a common precursor of the afforded alkaloids, had earlier been isolated from *A. sulphureus*.

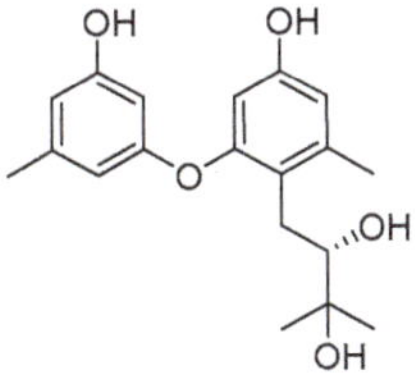

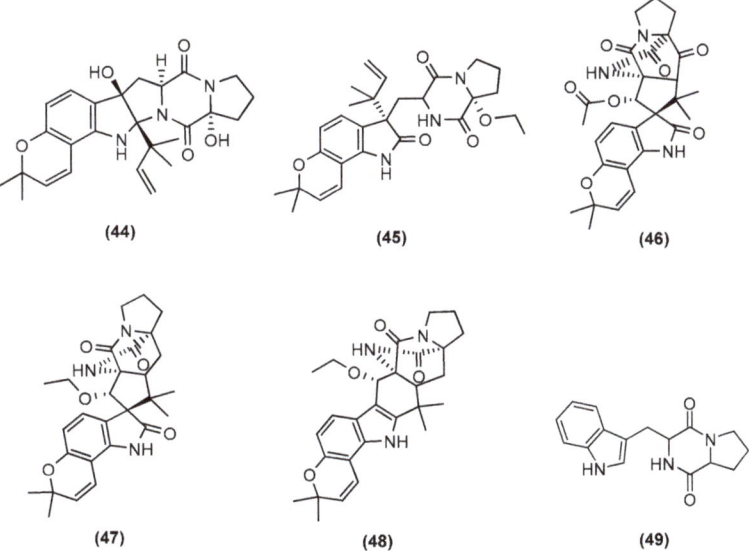

Figure 9. Chemical structures of diorcinols congeners B to E (**39** to **42**) and diorcinol J (**43**).

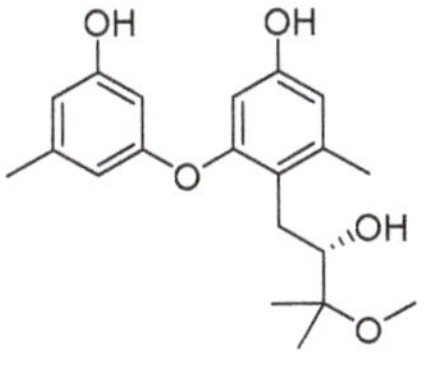

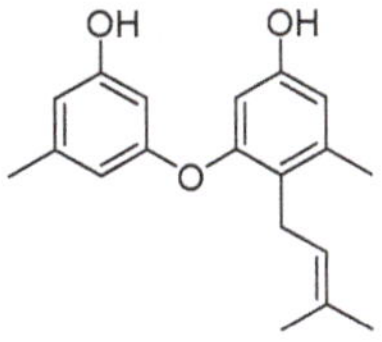

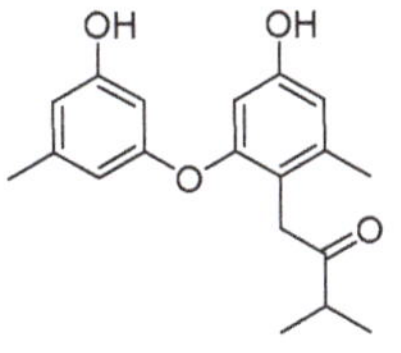

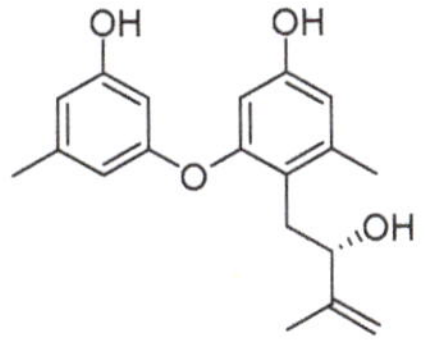

Figure 10. Chemical structures of 17-hydroxynotoamide D (**44**), 17-*O*-ethylnotoamide M (**45**), 10-*O*-acetylsclerotiamide (**46**), 10-*O*-ethylsclerotiamide (**47**), 10-*O*-ethylnotoamide R (**48**), and brevianamide F (**49**).

Ebada et al. (2014) of the Roth group in BioMar, Düsseldorf, co-cultured two marine algal-derived fungal strains of *Aspergillus* BM-05 and BM-05ML that yielded the cyclo-tripeptide psychrophilin E (**50**), along with five known compounds (protuboxepin A (**51**); oxepinamide E (**52**); and three mycotoxins, namely, sterigmatocystin (**53**), 5-methoxysterigmatocystin (**54**), and aversin (**55**)), as shown in Figure 11 [41]. Dalsgaard et al. (2004) of the Christophersen group in Copenhagen first reported the cyclotripeptide analogues, psychrophilins A to D (**56** to **59**), which were earlier isolated from a marine-derived psychrotolerant fungal species of the genus *Penicillium* [42,43]. In contrast to previously described congeners, in psychrophilin E (**50**), the α-amino group in the tryptophan residue was acetylated into an *N*-acetyl moiety, which was oxidised in psychrophilins

A to D into a nitro group. In addition, the existence of other psychrophilins in the extract could not be detected, implying that this mixed fermentation may have played a role in modifying the biosynthetic pathway by an acetylation rather than an oxidation step. All the isolated compounds from the co-culture of *Aspergillus* BM-05 and BM-05ML were assessed for their in vitro anti-proliferative activities. Psychrophilin E (**50**), sterigmatocystin (**53**), and 5-methoxysterigmatocystin (**54**) exhibited selective anti-proliferative activities towards the HCT116 (colon cancer) cell line with IC$_{50}$ values of 28.5, 10.3, and 4.4 µM, respectively, which were more active than cisplatin as a positive control (IC$_{50}$ = 33.4 µM).

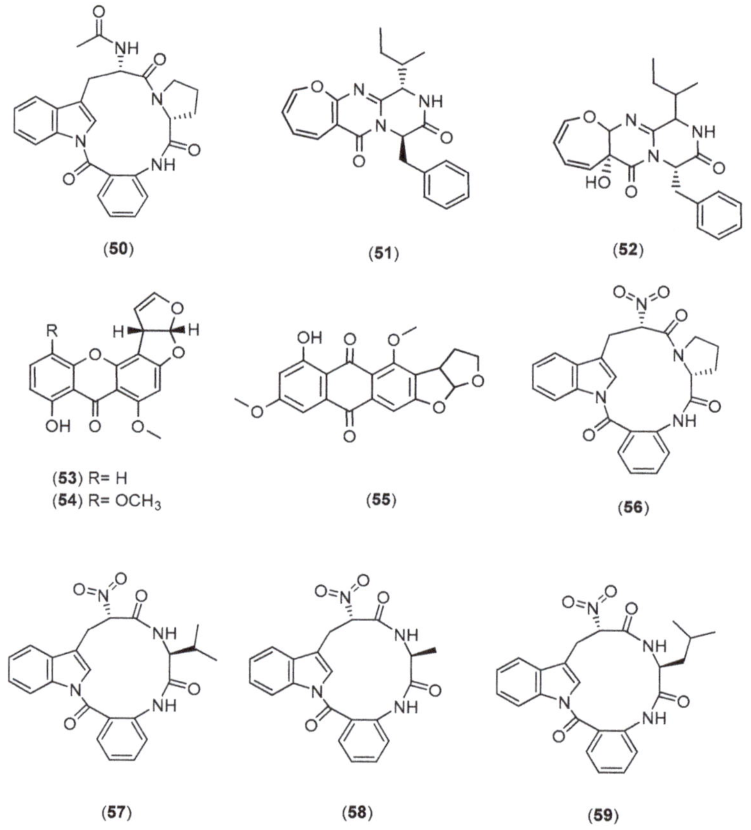

Figure 11. Chemical structures of psychrophilin E (**50**), protuboxepin A (**51**), oxepinamide E (**52**) sterigmatocystin (**53**), 5-methoxysterigmatocystin (**54**) aversin (**55**), and psychrophilin A to D (**56** to **59**).

The group of Zhu from Foshan University, China (2011), isolated aspergicin (**60**) with two know compounds (Figure 12), neoaspergillic acid (**61**) and ergosterol (**62**), from a co-culture of two mangrove *Aspergillus* epiphytes [44]. Both aspergicin (**60**) and neoaspergillic acid (**61**) showed significant inhibitory effect on three Gram-positive bacteria, *Staphylococcus aureus*, *Staphylococcus epidermidis*, and *Bacillus subtilis*, and three Gram-negative bacteria, *Bacillus dysenteriae*, *Bacillus proteus*, and *E. coli*, but with lower MICs for neoaspergillic acid (**61**).

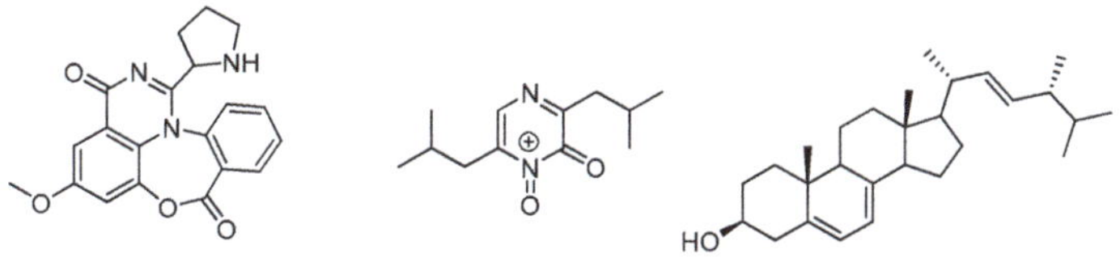

Figure 12. Chemical structures of aspergicin (**60**), neoaspergillic acid (**61**), and ergosterol (**62**).

During the last decade, several research teams in Guangzhou, China, led by She, Lin, (2010, 2011, and 2013), and Li (2014, 2015, and 2017), have been working on secondary metabolites produced by co-cultures of *Phomopsis* sp. K38 and *Alternaria* sp. E33, and were able to isolate many new compounds. All publications from the Guangzhou teams, except for Ding et al. [45], followed the same protocol. The Guangzhou research groups collected two mangrove-derived fungi, *Phomopsis* sp. K38 and *Alternaria* sp. E33, from the South China Sea coastline. The co-culture extract displayed higher cytotoxicity against Hep-2 and HepG2 cells than that of the K38 or E33 monocultures. Amongst the first molecules isolated was a new diimide derivative (Figure 13), (−)-byssochlamic acid bisdiimide (**63**) [46]. Unfortunately, the isolated purified bisdiimide exhibited weak cytotoxicity against Hep-2 and HepG2 cells, with IC_{50} values of only 45 and 51 µg/mL, respectively. The same fungal co-culture also yielded a new xanthone derivative (Figure 13), 8-hydroxy-3-methyl-9-oxo-9*H*-xanthene-1-carboxylic acid methyl ether (**64**) [47]. The new xanthone derivative (**64**) inhibited the growth of five tested microorganisms, *Gloeasporium musae*, *Blumeria graminearum*, *Fusarium oxysporum*, *Peronophthora cichoralearum*, and *Colletotrichum glocosporioides*. The co-culture also afforded a new polysubstituted benzaldehyde, ethyl 5-ethoxy-2-formyl-3-hydroxy-4-methylbenzoate (**65**) [48]. Wang et al. (2013) bioassayed the new polysubstituted benzaldehyde compound (**65**) against four plant pathogenic fungi, namely, *Fusarium graminearum*, *Gloeosporium musae*, *Rhizoctonia solani* Kuhn, and *Phytophthora sojae* Kaufmann and Gerdemann. Antifungal activities were observed at inhibitory zone diameters of 12.06, 11.57, 10.21, and 8.50 mm, respectively.

Later studies of the same co-culture strains E33 and K38 afforded two new cyclopeptides [49]. Huang et al. (2014) evaluated the in vitro antifungal activity of two cyclic tetrapeptides, cyclo (D-Pro-L-Tyr-L-Pro-L-Tyr) (**66**) and cyclo (Gly-L-Phe-L-Pro-L-Tyr) (**67**), against *C. albicans*, *G. graminis*, *R. cerealis*, *H. sativum*, and *F. graminearum*. Both peptides **66** and **67** showed moderate-to-high antifungal activities as compared with the positive control (ketoconazole), but cyclo (Gly-L-Phe-L-Pro-L-Tyr) (**67**) was more active than cyclo (D-Pro-L-Tyr-L-Pro-L-Tyr) (**66**). Li et al. (2014) found another cyclic tetrapeptide, cyclo-(L-leucyl-trans-4-hydroxy-L-prolyl-D-leucyl-trans-4-hydroxy-L-proline) (**68**), from the same fungal co-culture [50] and tested the compound against the same crop-threatening fungi except for *C. albicans*. Compound **68** showed moderate to high antifungal activities and afforded quite a comparable bioactivity to the positive control, triadimefon, against *H. sativum*. All isolated cyclopeptides **66** to **68** are shown in Figure 13.

From the same co-culture that produced the cyclic tetrapeptides, Wang et al. (2015) isolated a new 7-(γ,γ-dimethylallyloxy)-6-hydroxy-4-methylcoumarin (**69**) (Figure 13) [51], and this was also tested against the four plant pathogenic fungi. However, unlike the peptides, the compound showed no in vitro activity against these plant pathogens over a 6.00 mm inhibition zone at 250 µM.

More recently, Ding et al. (2017) elucidated a new nonadride derivative, (−)-byssochlamic acid imide (**70**) (Figure 13), from the same mangrove fungal co-cultures [45]. Chen et al. (2004) earlier reported the antifungal, phytotoxic, enzyme inhibitory, and cytotoxic activities of nonadride analogues [52]. The new nonadride derivative from the co-culture showed moderate inhibitory activity toward *Fusarium graminearum* and *F. oxysporum* with MIC values of 50 and 60 µg/mL, respectively, as compared with the positive control carbendazim (MIC 6.25 µg/mL). By adding salt to the media, changing the incubation period and temperature, Ding et al. were able to generate a new analogue that is unrelated to cyclic tetrapeptide derivatives earlier targeted by their predecessors.

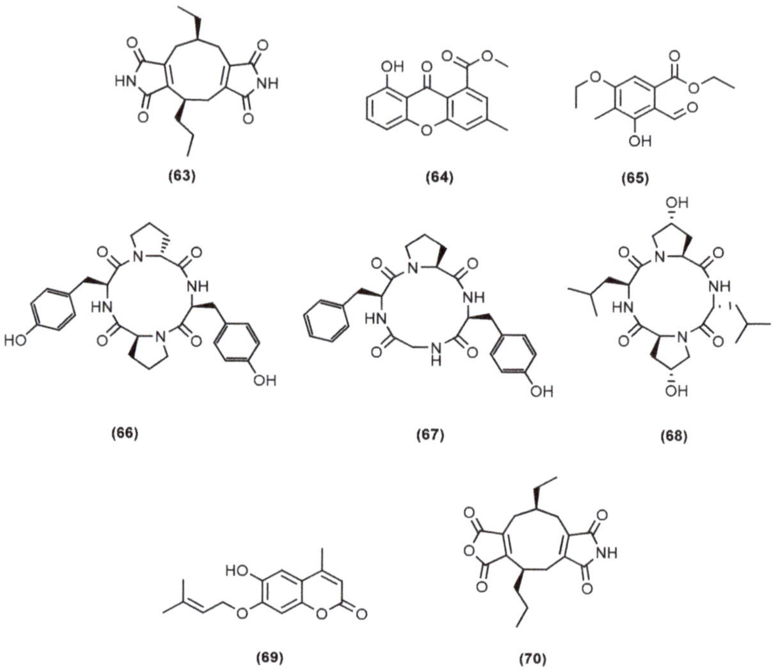

Figure 13. Chemical structures of (−)-byssochlamic acid bisdiimide (**63**), 8-hydroxy-3-methyl-9-oxo-9*H*-xanthene-1-carboxylic acid methyl ether (**64**), ethyl 5-ethoxy-2-formyl-3-hydroxy-4-methylbenzoate (**65**), cyclo (D-Pro-L-Tyr-L-Pro-L-Tyr) (**66**), cyclo (Gly-L-Phe-L-Pro-L-Tyr)s (**67**), cyclo-(L-leucyl-trans-4-hydroxy-L-prolyl-D-leucyl-trans-4-hydroxy-L-proline) (**68**), 7-(γ,γ-dimethylallyloxy)-6-hydroxy-4-methylcoumarin (**69**), and (−)-byssochlamic acid imide (**70**).

The last study presented in this section involved the co-culture of two fungal morphs of the marine algal-derived *Aspergillus alliaceus* [53]. The fungal co-culture consisted of identical strains but from different phases of development at their respective asexual and sclerotial morph stages. Both morphs produced distinct secondary metabolite patterns in monoculture, but their co-culture significantly changed the metabolic profile of the strain. Mandelare et al. (2018) of the Loesgen group in Oregon State isolated a new bianthrone dimer allianthrone A (**71**) from the co-cultures, while they observed elevated levels of nalgiolaxin (**72**) produced by the asexual morph. In parallel, Mandelare et al. found allianthrone A and its two diastereomers, allianthrones B (**73**) and C (**74**) (Figure 14), from the liquid fermentation culture at a ratio of 2:1:1. The two-week liquid cultures of the combined asexual and sclerotial morphs of *A. alliaceus* reliably produced the known compound nalgiolaxin at a higher yield. Allianthrone A showed weak cytotoxicity against the HCT-116 colon cancer and SK-Mel-5 melanoma cell lines. This study illustrated the first case of elicitation of new fungal chemistry by a co-culture approach of two different developmental stages of a homothallic *Aspergillus* species.

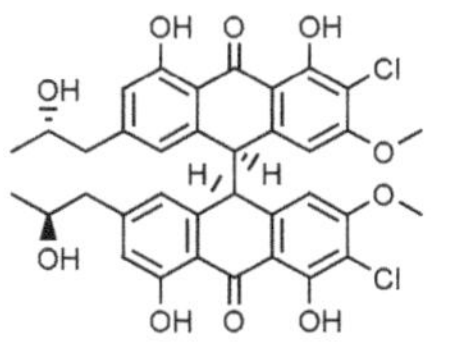

Figure 14. Chemical structures of allianthrone A (**71**), nalgiolaxin (**72**), allianthrone B (**73**), and C (**74**).

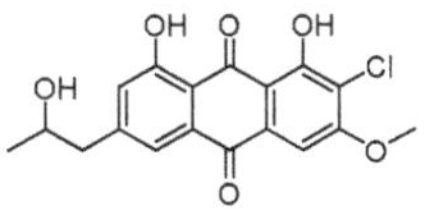

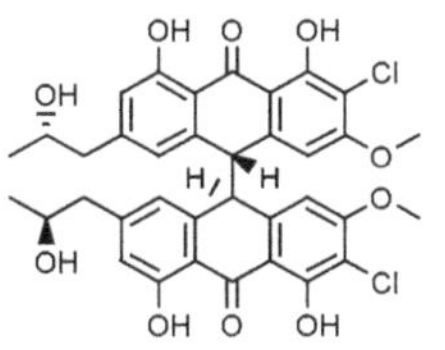

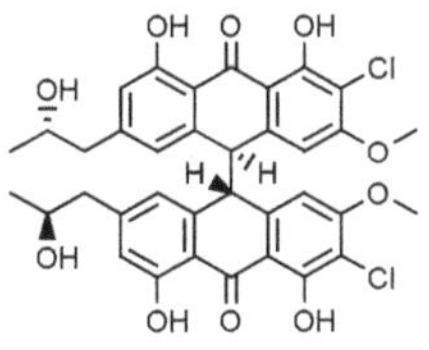

In recent publications, contrary to the previous section, it was observed that mixed fermentation between fungal species increased the discovery of new molecules, while the detection of enhanced biologically activity was less evident. Enhancing biomass yield in fungal cultures is in general easier to achieve in comparison to bacterial cultures due to their longer incubation period and life cycle. With higher biomass yield, the isolation of the metabolites is easier as well, and hence a higher rate of enhancing the production of targeted known bioactive compounds and at the same time a higher discovery rate of new compounds can be obtained but may not necessarily be active.

Nevertheless, as the utmost goal is to enhance the production yield, as well as to induce improved biological activity by stimulating the biosynthesis of new compounds, it can be discouraging that the generated new analogues may be rendered inactive. In most cases, the bioactivity seems to be at its optimum on one analogue, despite the occurrence of various new metabolites. A combination of metabolic engineering techniques needs to be considered, and this includes finding an efficient screening method to obtain the right elicitor to increase the probability of finding biologically active scaffolds. However, another limiting factor is the number of available assays in respective laboratories, and this could also be the main reason that despite the high number of new congeners being isolated, only one or two analogue(s) could be considered to exhibit potent bioactivity. The process of inducing the production of new bioactive compounds is dependent on conditions that a microorganism would need for a specific life mode to survive. There is yet much to be discovered about cryptic biosynthetic gene clusters and how they can be elicited for their expression. In this case, a full understanding of this microbial processing factory still needs to be explored.

3. Different Techniques of Co-Culture Used

In this last section, the techniques used by the different research teams presented in this literature review for various co-culture conditions are listed below in Table 1. The following are tabulated: the microorganisms used, their geographical origin, the culture medium(s) used, the conditions under which the cultures were made (static or under agitation, temperature, and incubation period), the experimental set-up, and the article from which the technique originated. The techniques are quite diverse, but generally the incubation time is longer for fungi than for bacteria and the temperature is often between 25 and 32 °C.

Table 1. Widely used co-culture techniques.

Microorganisms (Experimental Aim)	Source	Media	Conditions	Experiments	Reference
Aspergillus flavipes *Streptomyces* sp. (enhancement of cytochalasan production)	Marine sediments of the Nanji Islands, China	5 g yeast extract, 5 g glycerol, and 1 L 75% seawater (pH 7.5)	180 rpm at 28 °C, 8 days	5 mL of microbial seed broth (*A. flavipes* and *Streptomyces* sp. in a ratio of 1:4 (v/v)) was added to the 200 mL culture medium.	[24]
Aspergillus fumigatus MR2012 *Streptomyces leeuwenhoekii* (inducing the generation of new compounds and increasing the yield of existing metabolites)	Red sea sediment in Hurghada, Egypt. Hyper-arid soil of Laguna de Chaxa, Chile	ISP2 medium (4.0 g yeast extract, 10.0 g malt extract, 4.0 g dextrose in artificial sea water; pH 7.2)	180 rpm at 30 °C, 8 days	200 mL of primary seed culture of each of fungal and bacterial isolates was used to inoculate 4 L of ISP2. Inoculation of the primary fungal culture was started 2 days before bacterial inoculation.	[25]
Bacillus sp., *B. pumilus*, *B. licheniformis*, *Serratia marcescens* with *Candida albicans*, *Yarrowia lipolytica*, *Pseudomonas aeruginosa* (induction and enhancement of the production of certain bioactive metabolites)	Surfaces of the green mussel, *Perna viridis* and the coral, *Symphyllia* sp. from the nearshore regions of Kovalam and Mandapam, Tamil Nadu, India.	LB medium (10 g peptone, 10 g NaCl, 5 g yeast extract, for 1 L; pH = 7)	30 °C, 24 h	10 μL (1×10^8 cells/mL) of 12-h-old culture of inducer fungi or bacteria was added to the flasks containing 12-h-old culture of marine isolates.	[26]
Streptomyces sp. (reported biological activity was enhanced by 70% with the crude extract of the co-culture, but there is no record whether new compounds were generated or merely enhanced concentration of biologically active components)	Soil of mangrove forest Sundarbans, Bangladesh	Yeast extract glucose broth media (yeast extract 2.5 g/L, glucose 5 g/L)	220 rpm at 31 °C, 7 days	20 mL inocula (2 days of fermentation) of both fungi were mixed in a 500 mL conical flask containing 200 mL sterilised yeast-extract glucose broth media (co-culture).	[28]
Streptomyces sp. *Bacillus mycoides* (enhancement of the production of a target metabolite)	Marine sediments of the Nanji Islands, China	MM medium (5 g yeast extracts, 5 g glycerol in 1 L 75% sea water; pH 8.0)	Static incubation, 14 days	*Streptomyces* sp. was first cultivated in 500 mL Erlenmeyer flasks containing 200 mL of MM medium for 7 days, then 1% (v/v) of *B. mycoides* suspension (OD_{590} 0.5) was added.	[30]
Streptomyces cinnabarinus PK209 *Alteromonas* sp. KNS-16 (enhancement of the production of a target metabolite)	Sediments and seaweed rhizosphere, depth of 10 m along coast of Korea	TBFeC medium (3 g tryptone, 5 g casitone, 4 g of glucose, 0.04 g $Fe_2(SO_4)_3 \cdot 4H_2O$, 0.1 g KBr, and 1 L of sea water; pH 7.8)	215 rpm at 25°, 288 h	1 mL (10^5 cells) of 16-h-old KNS-16 culture in NB medium was inoculated into 1 L of 96-h-old strain PK209 in TBFeC medium in Fernbach flasks.	[31]

Table 1. Cont.

Microorganisms (Experimental Aim)	Source	Media	Conditions	Experiments	Reference
Streptomyces sp. *Bacillus* sp. (to induce production of dentigerumycin E)	Mud sample from intertidal mudflat in Wando, Republic of Korea	YEME liquid medium (4 g yeast extract, 10 g malt extract, 4 g glucose in 1 L artificial seawater)	200 rpm at 30°, 8 days	Equal volumes of 4-day cultures of both fungi were mixed (10 mL to 10 mL) and inoculated into a 500 mL baffled Erlenmeyer flask containing 200 mL of YEME liquid medium.	[32]
Janthinobacterium spp. ZZ145 and ZZ148 (to induce the generation of the new janthinopolyenemycin congeners)	Marine soil from coastal area of Sindh, Karachi, Pakistan	Rice medium (rice 40 g, sea salt 35 g, tap water 60 mL)	Under stationary state at 28°, 25 days	3.5 mL of ZZ145 in EY liquid medium and 3.5 mL of ZZ148 in B liquid medium were inoculated into rice medium in 500 mL Erlenmeyer flasks.	[33]
Actinokineospora sp. EG49 *Nocardiopsis* sp. RV163 (to induce the generation of new metabolites.)	*Spheciospongia vagabunda* (Red Sea sponge) *Dysidea avara* (Mediterranean sponge)	ISP2 medium (4.0 g yeast extract, 10.0 g malt extract, 4.0 g dextrose in artificial sea water; pH 7.2)	150 rpm at 30°, 7 days	10 mL of 5-day-old culture of *Nocardiospsis* was inoculated into 2 L Erlenmeyer flasks, each containing 1 L of ISP2m inoculated with 10 mL of 5-day old culture of *Actinokineospora*.	[34]
Mycobacterium sp. *Rhodococcus* sp. (screen and identify the generation of new metabolites)	Sponge or ascidian specimens in the Florida Keys, USA	ASW-A media (20 g soluble starch, 10 g glucose, 5 g peptone, 5 g yeast extract, 5 g $CaCO_3$ per litre of artificial seawater)	300 rpm at 30°, 14 days	In detoxified polypropylene square 96-deepwell microplates, 500 µL ASW-A was added to each well. Wells were inoculated with 15 µL of *Micromonosporaceae* and 5 µL of mycolic acid-containing bacteria.	[35]
Rhodococcus sp. *Micromonospora* sp. (to induce the generation of a new metabolite)	Marine sponge *Chondrilla nucula* and ascidian *Ecteinascidia turbinata*	ASW-D media (2 g yeast extract, 5 g malt extract, 2 g dextrose per litre of artificial seawater)	14 days	Same techniques used in [28].	[36]
Aspergillus sclerotiorum *Penicillium citrinum* (to induce the generation of new analogues)	Gorgonian *Muricella flexuosa* collected from the South China Sea, Sanya	Glucose 1.0%, $MgSO_4$ 0.1%, KH_2PO_4 0.1%, peptone 0.1%, sea salt 3.0% and pH 6.5–7.0	Static incubation at 28°, 30 days	1 mL, about 10^8 CFU/mL of *P. citrinum*, and 1 mL, about 10^4 CFU/mL of *A. sclerotiorum* were inoculated into 1 L flasks containing 300 mL of liquid medium.	[37]
Penicillium sp. *Trichoderma* sp. (to induce the generation of new analogues)	*Mycale angulosa* *Geodia corticostylifera* (marine sponges)	Malt medium (20 g malt extract, ASW 1 L; pH 8.0)	100 rpm at 25°, 12 days	8 plugs of mycelia of each fungus, grown in Petri dishes, were inoculated in 250 mL of 2% malt medium.	[38]

Table 1. Cont.

Microorganisms (Experimental Aim)	Source	Media	Conditions	Experiments	Reference
Aspergillus sulphureus Isaria eline (to induce the generation of new analogues)	Muddy sand of eastern Sakhalin shelf and sediments of South China Sea	20 g rice, 20 mg yeast extract, 10 mg KH_2PO_4, 10 mg $KNaC_4H_4O_6$ $4H_2O$ and 40 mL natural seawater	25°, 14 days	A. sulphureus was cultivated for 7 days, then inoculated with I. eline, and co-cultivated.	[39]
		20 g of rice, 20 mg yeast extract, 10 mg KH_2PO_4, and 40 mL of natural sea water	14 days	They were grown separately for 7 days and then I. eline mycelium was inoculated into 20 flasks with A. sulphureus culture.	[40]
Aspergillus sp. (to induce the generation of new analogues)	Sargassum collected off Helgoland, North Sea Germany	Peptone from soya 4 g, maize starch 10 g, $MgSO_4$ 3.6 g, NaCl 20 g, yeast extract 2 g, $CaCO_3$ 1.8 g, per 1 L demineralised water	Static incubation at 28°, 28 days	Agar plugs from plated cultures were co-cultivated in 1 L Erlenmeyer flasks (500 mL/flasks).	[41]
Aspergillus sp. (to induce the generation of new analogues)	Rotten fruit of a mangrove Avicennia marina in Zhanjiang, China	GYP medium (glucose 10 g/L, yeast extract 1 g/L, peptone 2 g/L, crude sea salt 3.5 g/L; pH 7.0)	Room temperature, 30 days	Inoculated with the mycelium of the isolate FSY-01, then inoculated with that of FSW-02 immediately.	[44]
Phomopsis sp. K38 Alternaria sp. E33 (to induce the generation of new analogues)	Mangrove in Leizhou Peninsula, Guangdong Province, China	Glucose 10 g/L, peptone 2 g/L, yeast extract 1 g/L, NaCl 30 g/L	30°, 25 days	Plugs of agar supporting mycelial growth were cut and transferred to a 250 mL Erlenmeyer flask containing 100 mL of the liquid medium. After 5–7 days, the mycelium was transferred to 500 mL Erlenmeyer flasks containing 200 mL of culture liquid.	[46–51]
		GYT medium (1% glucose, 0.1% yeast extract, 0.2% peptone, 0.2% crude sea salt)	Static incubation at 28°, 30 days	A small scrap of an agar slice with mycelium was added into a 500 mL Erlenmeyer flask containing 250 mL of GYT medium.	[45]
Aspergillus alliaceus (elicitation of new fungal chemistry)	Marine alga	Malt pH 6 buffered (malt extract 20 g/L, glucose 10 g/L, yeast extract 2 g/L, $(NH_4)_2HPO_4$ 0.5 g/L)	110 rpm at 28°, 30 days	Both developmental stages of A. alliaceus were grown on separate agar plates and used to inoculate each 50 mL of malt liquid media. After 2 weeks, the two cultures were combined into 1 L of malt-based buffered media.	[53]

EY liquid medium: yeast 1.0 g, tryptone 5.0 g, $FeCl_3·6H_2O$ 0.17 g, KH_2PO_4 0.12 g, sea salt 35 g, water 1 L. B liquid medium: soluble starch 20 g, KNO_3 1 g, K_2HPO_4 0.5 g, $MgSO_4·7H_2O$ 0.5 g, NaCl 0.5 g, $FeSO_4$ 0.01 g, water 1 L. Legend: LB medium = Luria–Bertani medium; YEME medium = yeast extract–malt extract medium; ISP2 medium = International Streptomyces Project-2 medium; ASW = artificial seawater medium.

Extremely low yielding target metabolites detected in axenic cultures may not be feasibly translated for isolation work. As illustrated by the literature reviewed in this paper [24–26,30], these metabolites could be detected but would not be quantifiable by mass spectrometry. These same metabolites would be below the limit of detection for a UV-HPLC-coupled system. In these cases, compound yields of these target metabolites in axenic culture were not measurable prior to coculturing. The authors of the reviewed papers demonstrated enhanced compound production by comparing extracted mass ion chromatograms of the target metabolites in axenic and co-culture conditions [24–26,30]. As demonstrated by references listed on Table 1, successful induction of compound production afforded a range of three- to fivefold increase in yield of the target metabolite. Except for the production of lobocompactol (**23**), Cho and Kim (2012) started with a quantifiable amount of 0.25 mg/L in axenic cultures, and they achieved a 10.4-fold increase by mixed fermentation [31]. In some publications, several techniques have been tested. The techniques that have generated the most conclusive results are shown in Table 1.

4. Conclusions

With new omics techniques and microbiological genetic data, it has been possible to identify a variety of previously unknown metabolic pathways. Microorganisms have a very high potential to produce metabolites with a high chemical diversity. As shown in this literature review, many of the microorganisms' biosynthetic genes remain silent or are not transcribed when they are grown under laboratory conditions. With co-culture or mixed fermentation for endogenous metabolite production, cryptic pathways can be stimulated through interaction and communication between microorganisms. Indeed, co-culture tries to mimic the environment where communications between microorganisms are abundant, dynamic, and complex.

From the various publications reviewed here, it was shown that co-culture can induce the production of new metabolites as well as increase the yields of respective target metabolites with pharmacological potential, and moreover can indirectly improve the biological activity of a crude extract. In parallel, mixed fermentation techniques may also suppress the production of metabolites that were found in axenic culture [34]. The diverse responses driven by the various co-culture methods could represent the potential counteracting response to the competition between the microorganisms. However, the afforded metabolites do not necessarily show activity against competing microorganisms, which indicates that the interactions could also be more complex than a simple question of competition.

The co-culture technique employed is essential, as it has been demonstrated that a single fermentation variable can have a very large impact on the production of specific metabolites [31]. When fungi and bacteria were co-cultured, it was essential to consider the incubation time needed for each to grow so that one does not take over the other. Physical contact may be necessary for the production of some metabolites, as for cytochalasin [24], but may not always be the case, as in the production of keyicin [36]. It is quite complicated to make any generalisations on the expected outcomes of certain co-culture techniques. However, techniques have been emerging, such as co-cultures in 96-well plates, which allowed for the testing of various combinations of media, buffers, and elicitors to be assessed. Innovative cultures also involved mixed fermentation of a single fungus from two different stages of development [53].

Furthermore, various other culture techniques could evolve to be associated with mixed fermentation methods, such as I-chip [54]. I-chip is a technique of in situ cultivation that utilises a device for the isolation of bacteria that are difficult to culture in the laboratory. This device contains hundreds of miniaturised diffusion chambers that are inoculated with a single bacterial cell. This device can then be placed in the natural environment of the organisms cultured in the diffusion chambers, be it in the sediment, the soil, or in the macro-organisms, as has recently been performed in a sponge [55]. I-chip allows microorganisms to grow in their natural environment, in addition to allocating microbial interactions, and affords access to the discovery of new organisms supplementing novel molecules [54].

The use of microorganisms from different geographical origins would also broaden the possibility to increase diversity, for example in the mixed fermentation of macro-algae endophytes simply from various parts of the globe. Microorganisms from the marine environment are still considered to be underexploited, and many discoveries are yet to be made. This technique can be used routinely in laboratories associated with techniques such as one strain many compounds (OSMAC). Natural marine products and the technique of co-culture can allow the discovery of new molecules of pharmacological interest and address the problem regarding the expression of silent genes clusters.

Author Contributions: Conceptualisation, R.A.E.-E.; methodology, F.C.; formal analysis, F.C.; investigation, F.C.; resources, F.C.; data curation, F.C.; writing—original draft preparation, F.C.; writing—review and editing, R.A.E.-E. and N.T.-B.; visualisation, F.C. and R.A.E.-E.; supervision, R.A.E.-E. and N.T.-B.; project administration, N.T.-B.; funding acquisition, F.C and N.T.-B. All authors have read and agreed to the published version of the manuscript.

Funding: Student placement for F.C. was funded by the Mobilité Programme Erasmus+ of the European Union 2019-1-FR01-KA103-061405.

Institutional Review Board Statement: Not applicable.

Informed Consent Statement: Not applicable.

Acknowledgments: F.C from the University of Perpignan via Domitia has carried out a mobility at the Strathclyde Institute of Pharmacy and Biomedical Sciences, Faculty of Science, University of Strathclyde, from 3 February to 23 June 2020 under the Erasmus programme—Student mobility for placements (SMP) to attain a Master 2 Certificate—Marine Science—Molécules Bioactives et Environnement Année universitaire 2019–2020.

Conflicts of Interest: The authors declare no conflict of interest.

References

1. Borchardt, J.K. The Beginnings of Drug Therapy: Ancient Mesopotamian Medicine. *Drug News Perspect.* **2002**, *15*, 187. [CrossRef] [PubMed]
2. Cragg, G.M.; Newman, D.J. Natural Products: A Continuing Source of Novel Drug Leads. *Biochim. Biophys. Acta BBA—Gen. Subj.* **2013**, *1830*, 3670–3695. [CrossRef] [PubMed]
3. Dias, D.A.; Urban, S.; Roessner, U. A Historical Overview of Natural Products in Drug Discovery. *Metabolites* **2012**, *2*, 303–336. [CrossRef] [PubMed]
4. Newman, D.J.; Cragg, G.M. Natural Products as Sources of New Drugs over the 30 Years from 1981 to 2010. *J. Nat. Prod.* **2012**, *75*, 311–335. [CrossRef]
5. Newman, D.J.; Cragg, G.M. Natural Products as Sources of New Drugs from 1981 to 2014. *J. Nat. Prod.* **2016**, *79*, 629–661. [CrossRef]
6. Kaeberlein, T. Isolating "Uncultivable" Microorganisms in Pure Culture in a Simulated Natural Environment. *Science* **2002**, *296*, 1127–1129. [CrossRef]
7. Haefner, B. Drugs from the Deep: Marine Natural Products as Drug Candidates. *Drug Discov. Today* **2003**, *8*, 536–544. [CrossRef]
8. Marmann, A.; Aly, A.; Lin, W.; Wang, B.; Proksch, P. Co-Cultivation—A Powerful Emerging Tool for Enhancing the Chemical Diversity of Microorganisms. *Mar. Drugs* **2014**, *12*, 1043–1065. [CrossRef]
9. Rinehart, K.L.; Holt, T.G.; Fregeau, N.L.; Stroh, J.G.; Keifer, P.A.; Sun, F.; Li, L.H.; Martin, D.G. Ecteinascidins 729, 743, 745, 759A, 759B, and 770: Potent Antitumor Agents from the Caribbean Tunicate Ecteinascidia Turbinata. *J. Org. Chem.* **1990**, *55*, 4512–4515. [CrossRef]
10. Carter, N.J.; Keam, S.J. Trabectedin: A Review of Its Use in Soft Tissue Sarcoma and Ovarian Cancer. *Drugs* **2010**, *70*, 335–376. [CrossRef]
11. D'Incalci, M.; Badri, N.; Galmarini, C.M.; Allavena, P. Trabectedin, a Drug Acting on Both Cancer Cells and the Tumour Microenvironment. *Br. J. Cancer* **2014**, *111*, 646–650. [CrossRef] [PubMed]
12. Feling, R.H.; Buchanan, G.O.; Mincer, T.J.; Kauffman, C.A.; Jensen, P.R.; Fenical, W. Salinosporamide A: A Highly Cytotoxic Proteasome Inhibitor from a Novel Microbial Source, a Marine Bacterium of the New Genus Salinospora. *Angew. Chem. Int. Ed.* **2003**, *42*, 355–357. [CrossRef] [PubMed]
13. Buckingham, L. EU/3/18/2119. Available online: https://www.ema.europa.eu/en/medicines/human/orphan-designations/eu3182119 (accessed on 8 May 2020).

14. Romano, S.; Jackson, S.A.; Patry, S.; Dobson, A.D.W. Extending the "One Strain Many Compounds" (OSMAC) Principle to Marine Microorganisms. *Mar. Drugs* **2018**, *16*, 244. [CrossRef] [PubMed]
15. Bertrand, S.; Bohni, N.; Schnee, S.; Schumpp, O.; Gindro, K.; Wolfender, J.-L. Metabolite Induction via Microorganism Co-Culture: A Potential Way to Enhance Chemical Diversity for Drug Discovery. *Biotechnol. Adv.* **2014**, *32*, 1180–1204. [CrossRef]
16. Khosla, C.; Keasling, J.D. Metabolic Engineering for Drug Discovery and Development. *Nat. Rev. Drug Discov.* **2003**, *2*, 1019–1025. [CrossRef]
17. Pickens, L.B.; Tang, Y.; Chooi, Y.-H. Metabolic Engineering for the Production of Natural Products. *Annu. Rev. Chem. Biomol. Eng.* **2011**, *2*, 211–236. [CrossRef]
18. Kennedy, J. Mutasynthesis, Chemobiosynthesis, and Back to Semi-Synthesis: Combining Synthetic Chemistry and Biosynthetic Engineering for Diversifying Natural Products. *Nat. Prod. Rep.* **2008**, *25*, 25–34. [CrossRef]
19. Tr, K. Co-Culture as the Novel Approach for Drug Discovery from Marine Environment. *Nov. Approaches Drug Des. Dev.* **2017**, *2*, 78–81. [CrossRef]
20. Akone, S.H.; Mándi, A.; Kurtán, T.; Hartmann, R.; Lin, W.; Daletos, G.; Proksch, P. Inducing Secondary Metabolite Production by the Endophytic Fungus Chaetomium Sp. through Fungal–Bacterial Co-Culture and Epigenetic Modification. *Tetrahedron* **2016**, *72*, 6340–6347. [CrossRef]
21. Asai, T.; Yamamoto, T.; Oshima, Y. Histone Deacetylase Inhibitor Induced the Production of Three Novel Prenylated Tryptophan Analogs in the Entomopathogenic Fungus, Torrubiella Luteorostrata. *Tetrahedron Lett.* **2011**, *52*, 7042–7045. [CrossRef]
22. Özkaya, F.C.; Ebrahim, W.; El-Neketi, M.; Tansel Tanrıkul, T.; Kalscheuer, R.; Müller, W.E.G.; Guo, Z.; Zou, K.; Liu, Z.; Proksch, P. Induction of New Metabolites from Sponge-Associated Fungus *Aspergillus carneus* by OSMAC Approach. *Fitoterapia* **2018**, *131*, 9–14. [CrossRef] [PubMed]
23. Overy, D.P.; Bayman, P.; Kerr, R.G.; Bills, G.F. An Assessment of Natural Product Discovery from Marine (Sensu Strictu) and Marine-Derived Fungi. *Mycology* **2014**, *5*, 145–167. [CrossRef]
24. Yu, L.; Ding, W.; Ma, Z. Induced Production of Cytochalasans in Co-Culture of Marine Fungus *Aspergillus Flavipes* and Actinomycete *Streptomyces* sp. *Nat. Prod. Res.* **2016**, *30*, 1718–1723. [CrossRef] [PubMed]
25. Wakefield, J.; Hassan, H.M.; Jaspars, M.; Ebel, R.; Rateb, M.E. Dual Induction of New Microbial Secondary Metabolites by Fungal Bacterial Co-Cultivation. *Front. Microbiol.* **2017**, *8*, 1284. [CrossRef]
26. Dusane, D.H.; Matkar, P.; Venugopalan, V.P.; Kumar, A.R.; Zinjarde, S.S. Cross-Species Induction of Antimicrobial Compounds, Biosurfactants and Quorum-Sensing Inhibitors in Tropical Marine Epibiotic Bacteria by Pathogens and Biofouling Microorganisms. *Curr. Microbiol.* **2011**, *62*, 974–980. [CrossRef] [PubMed]
27. Lazăr, V.; Chifiriuc, M.C. Architecture and Physiology of Microbial Biofilms. *Roum. Arch. Microbiol. Immunol.* **2010**, *69*, 95–107. [PubMed]
28. Haque, M.; Rahman, M.; Haque, M.; Sarker, A.; Islam, M. Antimicrobial and Anticancer Activities of Ethyl Acetate Extract of Co-Culture of *Streptomyces* Sp. ANAM-5 and AIAH-10 Isolated From Mangrove Forest of Sundarbans, Bangladesh. *J. Appl. Pharm. Sci.* **2016**, *6*, 51–55. [CrossRef]
29. Ravi, L.; Baskar, R.; Sarveswari, S.; Kannabiran, K. Co-Culturing of Marine and Terrestrial Actinomycetes to Obtain Novel Secondary Metabolites. *Ann. Pharmacol. Pharm.* **2017**, *2*, 1041.
30. Yu, L.; Hu, Z.; Ma, Z. Production of Bioactive Tryptamine Derivatives by Co-Culture of Marine *Streptomyces* with *Bacillus Mycoides*. *Nat. Prod. Res.* **2015**, *29*, 2087–2091. [CrossRef]
31. Cho, J.Y.; Kim, M.S. Induction of Antifouling Diterpene Production by *Streptomyces cinnabarinus* PK209 in Co-Culture with Marine-Derived *Alteromonas* Sp. KNS-16. *Biosci. Biotechnol. Biochem.* **2012**, *76*, 1849–1854. [CrossRef]
32. Shin, D.; Byun, W.S.; Moon, K.; Kwon, Y.; Bae, M.; Um, S.; Lee, S.K.; Oh, D.-C. Co-culture of Marine *Streptomyces* Sp. with *Bacillus* Sp. Produces a New Piperazic Acid-Bearing Cyclic Peptide. *Front. Chem.* **2018**, *6*, 498. [CrossRef] [PubMed]
33. Anjum, K.; Sadiq, I.; Chen, L.; Kaleem, S.; Li, X.-C.; Zhang, Z.; Lian, X.-Y. Novel Antifungal Janthinopolyenemycins A and B from a Co-Culture of Marine-Associated Janthinobacterium Spp. ZZ145 and ZZ148. *Tetrahedron Lett.* **2018**, *59*, 3490–3494. [CrossRef]
34. Dashti, Y.; Grkovic, T.; Abdelmohsen, U.; Hentschel, U.; Quinn, R. Production of Induced Secondary Metabolites by a Co-Culture of Sponge-Associated Actinomycetes, *Actinokineospora* sp. EG49 and *Nocardiopsis* sp. RV163. *Mar. Drugs* **2014**, *12*, 3046–3059. [CrossRef] [PubMed]
35. Adnani, N.; Vazquez-Rivera, E.; Adibhatla, S.; Ellis, G.; Braun, D.; Bugni, T. Investigation of Interspecies Interactions within Marine Micromonosporaceae Using an Improved Co-Culture Approach. *Mar. Drugs* **2015**, *13*, 6082–6098. [CrossRef]
36. Adnani, N.; Chevrette, M.G.; Adibhatla, S.N.; Zhang, F.; Yu, Q.; Braun, D.R.; Nelson, J.; Simpkins, S.W.; McDonald, B.R.; Myers, C.L.; et al. Co-culture of Marine Invertebrate-Associated Bacteria and Interdisciplinary Technologies Enable Biosynthesis and Discovery of a New Antibiotic, Keyicin. *ACS Chem. Biol.* **2017**, *12*, 3093–3102. [CrossRef]
37. Bao, J.; Wang, J.; Zhang, X.-Y.; Nong, X.-H.; Qi, S.-H. New Furanone Derivatives and Alkaloids from the Co-Culture of Marine-Derived Fungi *Aspergillus sclerotiorum* and *Penicillium citrinum*. *Chem. Biodivers.* **2017**, *14*, e1600387. [CrossRef]
38. Kossuga, M.H.; Ferreira, A.G.; Sette, L.D.; Berlinck, R.G.S. Two Polyketides from a Co-Culture of Two Marine-Derived Fungal Strains. *Nat. Prod. Commun.* **2013**, *8*, 1934578X1300800. [CrossRef]
39. Zhuravleva, O.I.; Kirichuk, N.N.; Denisenko, V.A.; Dmitrenok, P.S.; Yurchenko, E.A.; Min'ko, E.M.; Ivanets, E.V.; Afiyatullov, S.S. New Diorcinol J Produced by Co-Cultivation of Marine Fungi *Aspergillus sulphureus* and *Isaria felina*. *Chem. Nat. Compd.* **2016**, *52*, 227–230. [CrossRef]

40. Afiyatullov, S.S.; Zhuravleva, O.I.; Antonov, A.S.; Berdyshev, D.V.; Pivkin, M.V.; Denisenko, V.A.; Popov, R.S.; Gerasimenko, A.V.; von Amsberg, G.; Dyshlovoy, S.A.; et al. Prenylated Indole Alkaloids from Co-Culture of Marine-Derived Fungi *Aspergillus sulphureus* and *Isaria felina*. *J. Antibiot.* **2018**, *71*, 846–853. [CrossRef]
41. Ebada, S.S.; Fischer, T.; Hamacher, A.; Du, F.-Y.; Roth, Y.O.; Kassack, M.U.; Wang, B.-G.; Roth, E.H. Psychrophilin E, a New Cyclotripeptide, from Co-Fermentation of Two Marine Alga-Derived Fungi of the Genus *Aspergillus*. *Nat. Prod. Res.* **2014**, *28*, 776–781. [CrossRef]
42. Dalsgaard, P.W.; Blunt, J.W.; Munro, M.H.G.; Larsen, T.O.; Christophersen, C. Psychrophilin B and C: Cyclic Nitropeptides from the Psychrotolerant Fungus *Penicillium r Ivulum*. *J. Nat. Prod.* **2004**, *67*, 1950–1952. [CrossRef] [PubMed]
43. Dalsgaard, P.W.; Larsen, T.O.; Frydenvang, K.; Christophersen, C. Psychrophilin A and Cycloaspeptide D, Novel Cyclic Peptides from the Psychrotolerant Fungus *Penicillium r Ibeum*. *J. Nat. Prod.* **2004**, *67*, 878–881. [CrossRef] [PubMed]
44. Zhu, F.; Chen, G.; Chen, X.; Huang, M.; Wan, X. Aspergicin, a New Antibacterial Alkaloid Produced by Mixed Fermentation of Two Marine-Derived Mangrove Epiphytic Fungi. *Chem. Nat. Compd.* **2011**, *47*, 767–769. [CrossRef]
45. Ding, W.; Lu, Y.; Feng, Z.; Luo, S.; Li, C. A New Nonadride Derivative from the Co-Culture Broth of Two Mangrove Fungi. *Chem. Nat. Compd.* **2017**, *53*, 691–693. [CrossRef]
46. Li, C.-Y.; Ding, W.-J.; Shao, C.-L.; She, Z.-G.; Lin, Y.-C. A New Diimide Derivative from the Co-Culture Broth of Two Mangrove Fungi (Strain No. E33 and K38). *J. Asian Nat. Prod. Res.* **2010**, *12*, 809–813. [CrossRef] [PubMed]
47. Li, C.; Zhang, J.; Shao, C.; Ding, W.; She, Z.; Lin, Y. A New Xanthone Derivative from the Co-Culture Broth of Two Marine Fungi (Strain No. E33 and K38). *Chem. Nat. Compd.* **2011**, *47*, 382–384. [CrossRef]
48. Wang, J.; Ding, W.; Li, C.; Huang, S.; She, Z.; Lin, Y. A New Polysubstituted Benzaldehyde from the Co-Culture Broth of Two Marine Fungi (Strains Nos. E33 and K38). *Chem. Nat. Compd.* **2013**, *49*, 799–802. [CrossRef]
49. Huang, S.; Ding, W.; Li, C.; Cox, D.G. Two New Cyclopeptides from the Co-culture Broth of Two Marine Mangrove Fungi and Their Antifungal Activity. *Pharmacogn. Mag.* **2014**, *10*, 410.
50. Li, C.; Wang, J.; Luo, C.; Ding, W.; Cox, D.G. A New Cyclopeptide with Antifungal Activity from the Co-Culture Broth of Two Marine Mangrove Fungi. *Nat. Prod. Res.* **2014**, *28*, 616–621. [CrossRef]
51. Wang, J.; Huang, S.; Li, C.; Ding, W.; She, Z.; Li, C. A New Coumarin Produced by Mixed Fermentation of Two Marine Fungi. *Chem. Nat. Compd.* **2015**, *51*, 239–241. [CrossRef]
52. Chen, X.; Zheng, Y.; Shen, Y. Natural Products with Maleic Anhydride Structure: Nonadrides, Tautomycin, Chaetomellic Anhydride, and Other Compounds. *Chem. Rev.* **2007**, *107*, 1777–1830. [CrossRef] [PubMed]
53. Mandelare, P.E.; Adpressa, D.A.; Kaweesa, E.N.; Zakharov, L.N.; Loesgen, S. Co-culture of Two Developmental Stages of a Marine-Derived *Aspergillus alliaceus* Results in the Production of the Cytotoxic Bianthrone Allianthrone A. *J. Nat. Prod.* **2018**, *81*, 1014–1022. [CrossRef] [PubMed]
54. Lodhi, A.F.; Zhang, Y.; Adil, M.; Deng, Y. Antibiotic Discovery: Combining Isolation Chip (IChip) Technology and Co-Culture Technique. *Appl. Microbiol. Biotechnol.* **2018**, *102*, 7333–7341. [CrossRef] [PubMed]
55. MacIntyre, L.W.; Charles, M.J.; Haltli, B.A.; Marchbank, D.H.; Kerr, R.G. An Ichip-Domesticated Sponge Bacterium Produces an *N*-Acyltyrosine Bearing an α-Methyl Substituent. *Org. Lett.* **2019**, *21*, 7768–7771. [CrossRef] [PubMed]

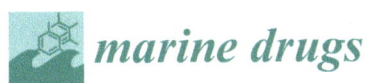

Review

Marine Microbial Fibrinolytic Enzymes: An Overview of Source, Production, Biochemical Properties and Thrombolytic Activity

Noora Barzkar [1,*], Saeid Tamadoni Jahromi [2,*] and Fabio Vianello [3]

1. Department of Marine Biology, Faculty of Marine Science and Technology, University of Hormozgan, Bandar Abbas 74576, Iran
2. Persian Gulf and Oman Sea Ecology Research Center, Iranian Fisheries Sciences Research Institute, Agricultural Research Education and Extension Organization (AREEO), Bandar Abbas 93165, Iran
3. Department of Comparative Biomedicine and Food Science, University of Padova, Viale dell'Università 16, 35020 Legnaro, Italy; fabio.vianello@unipd.it
* Correspondence: noora.barzkar@gmail.com (N.B.); stamadoni@gmail.com (S.T.J.)

Abstract: Cardiovascular diseases (CVDs) have emerged as a major threat to global health resulting in a decrease in life expectancy with respect to humans. Thrombosis is one of the foremost causes of CVDs, and it is characterized by the unwanted formation of fibrin clots. Recently, microbial fibrinolytic enzymes due to their specific features have gained much more attention than conventional thrombolytic agents for the treatment of thrombosis. Marine microorganisms including bacteria and microalgae have the significant ability to produce fibrinolytic enzymes with improved pharmacological properties and lesser side effects and, hence, are considered as prospective candidates for large scale production of these enzymes. There are no studies that have evaluated the fibrinolytic potential of marine fungal-derived enzymes. The current review presents an outline regarding isolation sources, production, features, and thrombolytic potential of fibrinolytic biocatalysts from marine microorganisms identified so far.

Keywords: cardiovascular diseases; fibrinolytic enzymes; marine microorganisms; thrombolytic activity

1. Introduction

Thrombosis is a major cause of cardiovascular diseases (CVDs) including acute myocardial infarction, ischemic heart disease, valvular heart disease, peripheral vascular disease, arrhythmias, high blood pressure and stroke, and it is a leading cause of death worldwide [1]. With population growth, aging and changing lifestyles, thrombotic diseases have become a more serious problem [2]. Thrombin catalyzes the conversion of fibrinogen to fibrin, which is a key component of blood clots or thrombi [3]. Public health data of CVDs is well documented by the World Health Organization (WHO). As for WHO, in 2016 alone, CVDs caused 17.9 million deaths globally [4], with a prediction that approximately 23.3 million people will be affected by 2030 [5]; hence, CVDs are emerging as a global health concern as well as economic burden [2]. Thrombosis is known as one of the foremost causes of CVDs and is characterized by the formation of fibrin clots. During normal physiological conditions, there is a homeostatic balance in the formation and degradation of fibrin; however, in some pathological disorders, it is unbalanced, resulting in aggregation of fibrin resulting in thrombosis [6,7]. The rapid dissolution of blood clots and the re-establishment of blood flow are critical for treating thrombotic diseases effectively.

Fibrinolytic enzymes are deemed as the most promising medication for the clinical treatment of thrombosis [6]. They can be grouped according to their function as plasminogen activators (e.g., tissue-type plasminogen activator t-PA, urokinase plasminogen activator u-PA, streptokinase and plasmin-like (e.g., nattokinase) and lumbrokinase fibrinolytic enzymes [8].

Plasminogen activators hydrolyze fibrin by the production of plasmin, and the latter can directly break down fibrin clots [9]. To date, a recombinant tissue-type plasminogen activator (rt-PA) is the only commercial thrombolytic agent with FDA approval. However, clinical data revealed its short time window along with its potential neurotoxicity, and hemorrhages resulted in the possible failure of t-PA treatment [10–12] in addition to its short half-life [13–15] and low effectiveness [16]. For instance, the high cost and undesirable side effects prompted investigators to explore the cost-effective and safer thrombolytic agents [17].

In the last decades, many fibrinolytic enzymes from natural resources, such as snakes [18], earthworms [19,20], insects [21], plants [22], mushrooms [23], microorganisms [24,25] and fermented foods such as Chungkook-jang [26] and Tempeh [27], have been identified and studied. Even though these enzymes have been characterized from a wide range of different sources, microbial fibrinolytic enzymes are considered attractive tools due to their features, such as enhanced specificity [8], low production cost [8], comparatively high yield [28] and the possibility to be genetically modified by recombinant DNA technology and protein engineering approaches [29]. Marine ecosystems serve as a reservoir of microorganisms producing important therapeutic metabolites, especially enzymes [30–39], but they remain largely unexplored to date. Due to the wide biodiversity of the marine environment, marine microorganisms can provide a diverse array of enzymes for biotechnological development, with possible improved pharmacological properties and lesser side effects [40]. Although many other research studies must be carried out to assess the toxicity of these enzymes, evidence showed minimal side effects upon their application to humans [40,41]. In this view, particular attention should be paid to possible allergenic properties of microbial fibrinolytic enzymes [42]. Hence, fibrinolytic enzymes from marine sources have gathered clinical interest during these decades.

The current review presents an overview regarding the resources, production, properties and thrombolytic activity of fibrinolytic enzymes from marine microbes identified so far.

2. Marine Microorganisms as Sources of Fibrinolytic Enzyme

Marine microorganisms are important resources of fibrinolytic enzymes. These enzymes possess potential efficacy for health augmentation and nutraceutical use, and their application could prevent cardiovascular diseases effectively [28]. Marine microorganisms producing fibrinolytic enzymes, including bacteria (*Streptomyces lusitanus* [43], *Streptomyces radiopugnans* VITSD8 [44], *Streptomyces violaceus* VI-TYGM [45], *Pseudomonas aeruginosa* KU1 [46,47], *Alteromonas piscicida* [48], *Pseudoalteromonas* sp. IND11 [49], bacterial strain GPJ3 [50], *Marinobacter aquaeolei* MS2-1 [51], *Bacillus flexus* [52], *Bacillus subtilis* [53], *Bacillus subtilis* HQS-3 [54], *Bacillus vallismortis* [55], *Bacillus subtilis* D21-8 [56], *Bacillus pumilus* BS15 [29], *Bacillus subtilis* WR350 [57], *Bacillus subtilis* JS2 [58], *Bacillus velezensis* BS2 [59], *Bacillus subtilis* ICTF-1 [41], *Shewanella* sp. IND20 [60], *Serratia rubidaea* KUAS001 [61] and *Serratia marcescens* subsp. *sakuensis* [62–64], *Arthrospira platensis* [65]) and microalgae (*Chlorella vulgaris* [66,67], *Dunaliella tertiolecta* [68] and *Tetraselmis subcordiformis* [69]), are summarized in Table 1. As shown in Table 1, marine microorganisms that are classified to the genus *Bacillus* are considered as the most valuable resources for the production of fibrinolytic enzymes, while there are no studies that have evaluated the fibrinolytic potential of marine fungal-derived enzymes. It should be noted that the catalytic activity of fibrinolytic enzymes can be improved by chemical modifications and mutant selection [70,71].

Table 1. Marine sources of fibrinolytic enzymes.

Isolated From	Microorganism	Enzyme	Reference
Marine sediment from Kovalam beach, Chennai, Tamil Nadu	*Streptomyces lusitanus*	-	[43]
Marine brown tube sponges *Agelas conifera*	*Streptomyces radiopugnans* VITSD8	-	[44]
Soil samples from South East Coast of India, Chennai	*Streptomyces rubiginosus* VITPSS1	-	[72]
Marine water sample	*Streptomyces venezuelae*	Thrombinase	[73]
Mangrove Sediments Pitchavaram, South East Coast of India	*Bacillus circulans*	-	[74]
Marine sediments of Ezhara beach, Kannur District, Kerala, India	*Pseudomonas aeruginosa* KU1	-	[46,47]
Mangrove sediments of Pulicat Lake, India	Bacterial strain GPJ3	-	[50]
South West Coast of India	*Bacillus flexus*	-	[52]
Mutagenesis of *B. subtilis* HQS-3	*Bacillus subtilis*	-	[53]
Surface seawater	*Bacillus vallismortis*	Bvsp	[55]
Fish scales, Kanyakumari, India	*Pseudoalteromonas* sp. IND11	-	[49]
Coast of Beihai prefecture of China	*Bacillus subtilis* HQS-3	-	[54]
Deep-sea sediment of Bay of Bengal	*Marinobacter aquaeolei* MS2-1	-	[51]
Jeotgal from gul (Oyster, *Crassostrea gigas*), korean fermented food	*Bacillus pumilus* BS15	AprEBS15	[29]
Marine niches covering 300 km of the western seacoast of Maharashtra, India	*Bacillus subtilis* ICTF-1	-	[41]
Oriyara beach in Kasargod district, Kerala, India	*Serratia rubidaea* KUAS001	-	[61]
Jeotgal from munggae (sea squirt), Korean fermented seafood	*Bacillus velezensis* BS2	AprEBS2	[59]
Sea mud	*Bacillus subtilis* WR350	-	[57]
Sea water collected from a depth of 10 m, 5 km away from Surathkal Coast in the Arabian Sea	*Serratia marcescens* subsp. *sakuensis* (KU296189.1)	-	[62–64,70]
Jeotgals from salted saeu (small shrimp), Korean fermented seafoods	*Bacillus subtilis* JS2	AprEJS2	[58]
Marine isolate	*Shewanella* sp. IND20	-	[60]
Jeotgal, Korean fermented seafood	*Bacillus licheniformis* KJ-31	BpKJ-31	[75]
Culture Collection of Algae, University of Texas, Austin	*Arthrospira* (*Spirulina*) *platensis*	-	[65]
University of Texas, Austin	*Chlorella vulgaris*	-	[66,67]
Dalian Institute of Chemical Physics, Chinese Academy of Sciences	*Tetraselmis subcordiformis*	-	[69]

3. Purification of Fibrinolytic Enzymes

The main purpose of purifying enzymes is to remove other contaminating proteins and other interfering biomolecules. Furthermore, enzyme purification allows the acquisition of insights about structural and functional features of the purified enzyme, as well as foretells its applications [76]. The required level of purity depends on the purpose for which the protein is to be used. If deemed for therapeutic use, the enzyme must have higher level purity and be processed through several subsequent purification steps.

Currently, several approaches have been used for separating and purifying fibrinolytic enzymes from marine microorganisms (Table 2). These approaches involved the extraction of bacteria with aqueous buffer solution as first step, followed by a concentration/precipitation step using acetone or ammonium sulfate and dialysis [41,43,44,52,62,65,66]. As shown in Table 2, the use of ammonium sulfate for protein precipitation is preferred, as it is a low-cost reagent, highly soluble in water and it is able to stabilize proteins and enzymes [41,43,44,47,52,62,65]. Further purification is carried out by employing different chromatographic steps (Table 2).

Several purification strategies are listed in Table 2, along with their efficiencies (enzyme specific activities obtained). For example, Barros and colleagues (2020) used ammonium sulfate precipitation (40–70%), acetone precipitation, DEAE-Sephadex (anion exchange) and Superdex 75 (size exclusion) chromatography to purify a fibrinolytic enzyme from *Arthrospira platensis*. The eluted enzyme showed a specific activity of 7,988 U/mg with 32.42-fold purification [65]. A fibrinolytic enzyme from *Bacillus subtilis* ICTF-1 was purified by a three-step procedure. As a first step, ammonium sulfate precipitation was adopted for providing suitable protein concentration, followed by UnoQ Sepharose Strong Anion Exchanger and Butyl Sepharose FF chromatography. The enzyme had a molecular mass of 72 kDa [41].

Table 2. Purification strategies for isolating fibrinolytic enzymes from marine microorganisms.

Source	Enzyme	Purification Methods	Total Protein (mg)	Specific Activity (U mg^{-1})	Purification (Fold)	Yield (%)	References
Bacillus flexus	-	Ammonium sulphate precipitation (20%, 40% and 60%), Sephadex G-75 chromatography	4.4	315.2	5.2	10.8	[52]
Bacillus pumilus BS15	AprEBS15	Affinity chromatography by HiTrap IMAC FF column	-	-	-	-	[29]
Bacillus velezensis BS2	AprEBS2	Affinity chromatography by HiTrap IMAC FF column	-	131.15 m	-	-	[59]
Bacillus subtilis HQS-3	-	Ammonium sulphate precipitation, alkaline solution treatment, membrane concentration, dialysis, ion exchange and gel filtration chromatography	12	62,745	30	13	[54]
Bacillus subtilis JS2	AprEJS2	Affinity chromatography by HiTrap IMAC FF column	-	-	-	-	[58]
Serratia marcescens subsp. sakuensi	-	Ammonium sulfate precipitation (40%), dialysis, Fast protein liquid chromatography	0.03	1033	21.08	19.38	[62]
Pseudomonas aeruginosa KU1	-	Ammonium sulphate precipitation (50–80%), DEAE Sepharose, Sepharose 6B chromatography	0.8 mg·mL^{-1}	1491.50	13.52	17.79	[47]
Bacillus licheniformis KJ-31	BpKJ-31	DEAE-Sepharose FF column and gel filtration chromatography (HiPrep 16/60 Sephacryl S-200 HR column)	3.2	242.8	19	0.2	[75]
Bacillus subtilis ICTF-1	-	Ammonium sulfate precipitation (0–60%), UnoQ Sepharose Strong Anion Exchanger, Butyl Sepharose FF chromatography	0.669	280	32.42	7.5	[41]
Streptomyces lusitanus	-	Ammonium sulfate precipitation (60%), dialysis, size exclusion gel filtration chromatography	-	-	-	-	[43]
Streptomyces radiopugnans VITSD8	-	Ammonium sulphate precipitation (0–85%), dialysis, ion-exchange chromatography, Size exclusion chromatography	1.1	3891	22.36	35	[44]
Arthrospira platensis	-	Ammonium sulfate precipitation (40–70%), anion exchange (DEAE-Sephadex), size exclusion (Superdex 75) chromatography	0.02 mg·mL^{-1}	7988	32.72	28.85	[65]
Chlorella vulgaris	-	Acetone precipitation, anion exchange chromatography HiTrapTM DEAE FF cloumn	2.0	1834.6	2	4.0	[66]

4. Biochemical Characterization of Marine Microbial Fibrinolytic Enzymes

4.1. Physicochemical Properties of Fibrinolytic Enzymes

4.1.1. Molecular Weight and Effect of pH, Temperature, Inhibitors and Ions

Table 3 provides a detailed overview of the significant physicochemical characteristics of marine microbial fibrinolytic enzymes, including molecular mass, optimal pH and temperature. The molecular mass of the purified marine microbial fibrinolytic enzymes varied significantly, ranging from as low as 21 kDa in an actinomycete (*Streptomyces lusitanus*) [43] to as high as 72 kDa in a cyanobacterium (*Arthrospira platensis*) [65]. Most marine microbial fibrinolytic enzymes have optimum pH fluctuating from neutral to alkaline values, ranging from 6 [65] to 7 [43,44,62] and from 8 [29,52,58–60] to 9 [41,75]. The optimal temperature of marine microbial fibrinolytic enzymes ranges between 33 °C (*Streptomyces radiopugnans* VITSD8) [44] to 60 °C (*Bacillus flexus*) [52].

Table 3. Some physicochemical characteristics of marine microbial fibrinolytic enzymes.

Source	Enzyme	Molecular Weight (kDa)	pH Opt.	Temp. Opt. (°C)	Activator/Co-Factor (Metal Ions)	Inhibitor	Class	References
Bacillus flexus	-	32	8	60	Mg^{2+}, Mn^{2+}	Zn^{2+}, Fe^{2+} and Hg^{2+}	-	[52]
Bacillus pumilus BS15	AprEBS15	27	8	40	K^+, Mg^{2+}, Zn^{2+}	Na^+, Fe^{3+}, Mn^{2+}, Co^{2+}, PMSF, SDS, EDTA and EGTA	Serine protease	[29]
Bacillus velezensis BS2	AprEBS2	27	8	37	Mg^{2+}, Ca^{2+}, Mn^{2+}	Fe^{3+}, Zn^{2+}, K^+, Co^{2+}, PMSF, EDTA, SDS	Serine protease	[59]
Bacillus licheniformis KJ-31	BpKJ-31	37	9	40	-	PMSF	Alkaline serine protease	[75]
Bacillus subtilis JS2	AprEJS2	24	8	40	K^+, Mn^{2+}, Mg^{2+}, Zn^{2+}	PMSF, EDTA, EGTA	Serine protease	[58]
Bacillus subtilis HQS-3	-	26	8	45–50	Mn^{2+}, Ca^{2+}, Mg^{2+}	PMSF, EDTA, Cu^{2+}, Zn^{2+} and Co^{2+}	Serine metallo-protease	[54]
Marinobacter aquaeolei MS2-1	-	39	8	50	DTT	PMSF	Thiol-dependent serine protease	[51]
Bacillus subtilis ICTF-1	-	28	9	50	Ca^{2+}	Zn^{2+}, Fe^{3+}, Hg^{2+} and PMSF	Serine protease	[41]
Bacillus vallismortis	Bvsp	34.4	6.5	54	Ca^{2+}, Zn^{2+} and Ba^{2+}	Na^+, K^+, NH_4^+ and Mg^{2+}, PMSF, AEBSF, SDS, Guanidine-HCL, Urea and Isopropyl alcohol	Alkaline serine protease	[55]
Serratia marcescens subsp. *sakuensi*	-	43	7	55	Mn^{2+}, Mg^{2+}, Zn^{2+}	PMSF, EDTA	Serine metallo-protease	[62]
Pseudomonas aeruginosa KU1	-	~50	-	-	Na^+, K^+ and Co^{2+}	Fe^{2+}, Mn^{2+} and Zn^{2+}	Metalloprotease	[47]
Shewanella sp. IND20	-	55.5	8	50	Ca^{2+} and Mg^{2+}	-	-	[60]
Streptomyces lusitanus	-	21	7	37	-	-	-	[43]
Streptomyces radiopugnans VITSD8	-	38	7	33	-	-	Serine endopeptidase	[44]
Streptomyces rubiginosus VITPSS1	-	45	-	-	-	-	-	[72]
Arthrospira platensis	-	72	6	40	Fe^{2+}	PMSF	Serine metallo-protease	[65]
Chlorella vulgaris	-	45	-	-	Fe^{2+}	PMSF, EDTA	Serine metallo-protease	[66]

Moreover, some studies have focused on the effect of chemical reagents and metal ions to delineate and characterize catalysis by these novel fibrinolytic enzymes. Table 3 summarizes the effect of metal ions as well as inhibitors on the fibrinolytic enzyme activities. Indeed, according to the specific chemical functionality in their active site, fibrinolytic enzymes can be classified as metalloproteases, serine proteases and serine metalloproteases. As shown in Table 3, the majority of fibrinolytic enzymes from *Bacillus* spp. belongs to serine proteases, and their activity is inhibited by PMSF (Phenyl Methyl Sulphonyl Fluoride). Proteolytic enzymes possessing an active group (OH) from serine amino acid in the catalytic site are recognized as serine proteases. During inhibition of catalytic activity, sulfonyl group of PMSF binds irreversibly to the serine OH group in the active site [77]. In addition, a metalloprotease from *Pseudomonas aeruginosa* KU1 is repressed by some metal ions, e.g., Mn^{2+}, Fe^{2+} and Zn^{2+} [47]. Similarly, the activities of fibrinolytic enzymes that belong to serine metalloprotease are dependent on divalent metal ions, such as Mn^{2+}, Mg^{2+} and Zn^{2+}, for enzymes from *Serratia marcescens* subsp. *sakuensi* [62], Fe^{2+} for enzymes from *Arthrospira platensis* [65] and *Chlorella vulgaris* [66]; thus, their catalyses were inhibited by chelating agents such as EDTA (ethylenediaminetetraacetic acid) and EGTA (ethylene glycol-bis(β-aminoethyl ether)-N,N,N′,N′-tetraacetic acid).

4.1.2. Fibrinogen Lytic Activity

The efficacy of fibrinolytic enzymes is determined by two different mechanisms: indirectly activating the plasminogen and directly acting on fibrins [78]. In Table 4, the activity of different fibrinolytic enzymes isolated from marine microbial sources reported in terms of direct or indirect fibrinogen lytic activity is listed. As shown in Table 4, marine *Bacillus* enzymes are generally directly acting on fibrin forming or fibrin degradation products. AprEBS2 isolated from *Bacillus velezensis* BS2 revealed high Aα fibrinolytic activity, followed by moderate Bβ and mild γ chains fibrinolysis [59]. Nevertheless, fibrinolytic enzymes from *Bacillus pumilus* BS15 [29] and *Bacillus subtilis* JS2 [58] displayed no γ-chain lysis. *Bacillus licheniformis* KJ-31 was one of the microorganisms that only produced fibrinolytic enzymes with high Aα fibrinogen lytic activity [75].

Table 4. Fibrino(ogen) lytic activity of various marine microbial enzymes.

Source	Enzyme	Reference	Mode of Action	References
Bacillus velezensis BS2	AprEBS2	Strong α-fibrinogenase and moderate β-fibrinogenase	Direct	[59]
Bacillus pumilus BS15	AprEBS15	Strong α-fibrinogenase and moderate β-fibrinogenase activities	Direct	[29]
Bacillus subtilis JS2	AprEJS2	Strong α-fibrinogenase and moderate β-fibrinogenase activities	Direct	[58]
Bacillus licheniformis KJ-31	BpKJ-31	Strong Aα and fibrino (geno) lytic activity	Direct	[75]
Bacillus subtilis HQS-3	-	Hydrolyzed α chain of fibrin, followed by the β chain and finally the γ–γ chain	Direct	[54]
Bacillus vallismortis	Bvsp	Digest Aα- and Bβ-chains readily, but the γ-chain of fibrinogen slowly	Direct	[55]

4.2. *Amidolytic and Kinetic Properties of Marine Microbial Fibrinolytic Enzymes*

Microbial fibrinolytic enzymes display amidolytic (or pro-coagulant) activity, which is assessed using different synthetic chromogenic substrates (Table 5). Most of the studied enzymes show high specificity towards N-Succ-Ala-Ala-Pro-Phe-pNA, classifying them as serine proteases [29,41,58,59,75]. In addition, kinetic parameters including the Michaelis constant [79], rate of reaction (V_{max}) and the turnover number (k_{cat}) help understand the specificity and affinity of an enzyme for a particular substrate [6]. Table 6 summarizes the kinetic properties of selected fibrinolytic enzymes isolated from marine microorganisms in different reaction conditions by using both natural and synthetic substrates.

Table 5. Kinetic properties of fibrinolytic enzymes.

Source	Enzyme	Substrate Specificity	V_{max}	K_m	k_{cat}	k_{cat}/K_m	Reference
Bacillus velezensis BS2	AprEBS2	N-Succ-Ala-Pro-Phe-pNA	39.68 µM min^{-1}	0.15 mM	18.14 s^{-1}	1.25×10^5 M^{-1}s^{-1}	[59]
Bacillus pumilus BS15	AprEBS15	N-succinyl-ala-pro-phe-pNA	21.88 µM min^{-1}	0.26 mM	10.02 s^{-1}	3.83×10^4 M^{-1}s^{-1}	[29]
Bacillus subtilis JS2	AprEJS2	N-Succ-Ala-Pro-Phe-pNA	16.71 µM min^{-1}	0.09 mM	7.66 s^{-1}	8.51×10^4 M^{-1}s^{-1}	[58]
Bacillus subtilis ICTF-1	-	N-Succ-Ala-Pro-Phe-pNA	-	-	-	-	[41]
Bacillus licheniformis KJ-31	BpKJ-31	N-Succ-Ala-Pro-Phe-pNA	-	-	-	-	[75]
Serratia marcescens subsp. sakuensis	-	Fibrin	15.873 µmol min^{-1}	0.66 mg mL^{-1}	12.21 min^{-1}	18.32 mL mg^{-1} min^{-1}	[62]
Bacillus subtilis	Fibase	-	0.03 mM min^{-1}	2.7 mmol L^{-1}	-	-	[71]
Bacillus vallismortis	Bvsp	Fibrin	49.8 g mL^{-1} min^{-1}	0.319 g mL^{-1}	4.35 min^{-1}	13.63 mL mg^{-1} min^{-1}	[55]

Table 6. Cloning and expression parameters used for fibrinolytic enzymes production.

Bacterial Strain	Gene	Primer	Cloning Host	Cloning Vector	Expression Host	Expression Vector	References
Bacillus velezensis BS2	aprEBS2	CH51-F (5′-AGGATCCCAAGAGAGCGATTGCGCTGTGTAC-3′, BamHI site underlined) CH51-R (5′-AGAATTCTTCAGAGGGAGCCACCCGTCGATCA-3′, EcoRI site underlined)	B. subtilis WB600	pHY300PLK	E. coli BL21 (DE3)	pETBS2	[59]
Bacillus subtilis JS2	aprEJS2	CH51-F (5′-AGGATCCCAAGAGAGCGATTGCGGCTGTGTAC-3′, BamHI site underlined) and CH51-R (5′-AGAATTCTTCAGAGGGAGCCACCCGTCGATCA-3′, EcoRI site underlined)	B. subtilis WB600	pHY300PLK	E. coli BL21 (DE3)	pHYJS2	[58]
Bacillus pumilus BS15	aprEBS15	CH51-F (5′-ACGATC CCAAGAGAGCGATTGCGCTGTGTAC-3′, BamHI site underlined) and CH51-R (5′-AGAATTCTTCAGAGG GAGCCACCCGTCGATCA-3′, EcoRI site underlined)	B. subtilis WB600	pHY300PLK	E. coli BL21 (DE3)	pHYBS15	[29]
Bacillus vallismortis	Bvsp	BVSPF (5′-CGCGGATCC-ATGCAAGGTGAAATTAGGTTAATTCCATATTT-3′) containing BamH I and BVSPR (5′-CCGCTCGAGTCAGCCAATCTGTCAAGTGGC-3′, Xho I sites (underlined)	-	-	E. coli BL21 (DE3)	pGEX-6P-bvsp	[55]
Marinobacter aquaeolei MS2-1	-	SPro F (5′-CCG GAT CCA TGG CGT TCA GCA AC-3′) and SPro R (5′-GGC TCG AGT TAG CGG GCA GGT GC-3′)	E. coli	pGEM-T	E. coli BL21 (DE3)	pET-28a-(+)	[51]
Tetraselmis subcordiformis	rt-PA	bar1F (5′-TCTGCACCATGTCAACCACTACA-3′), bar1R (5′-TCAAATCTCGTGACGGCAGAC-3′), rpa3F (5′-TCTTGGCAGAACATACC-3′) and rpa3R (5′-TCCCCTGAACCTGAAAC-3′)	-	-	E. coli Top10	pSVrPA/CaMVbar	[69]

5. Production of Marine Microbial Fibrinolytic Enzymes

5.1. Construction of Genetically Engineered Strains

Gene cloning, mutagenesis and recombinant DNA technology have also been employed for the overexpression of fibrinolytic enzymes in bacterial hosts and to engineer their catalytic properties. For example, Yao and colleagues (2018) achieved significantly higher fibrinolytic activity of the recombinant fibrinolytic enzyme from *Bacillus pumilus* BS15 [29]. In another example, Che and colleagues (2020), using gene dosage, codon optimization and process optimization, achieved high expression and secretion of a fibrinolytic enzyme (fibase) isolated from marine *Bacillus subtilis* [71]. Hence, a combination of culture media optimization and recombinant DNA technology has been effectively employed for augmenting the enzyme titer. Table 6 indicates some of the heterologously expressed fibrinolytic enzymes from marine microorganisms.

5.2. Fermentation Approach

The production cost of an enzyme is one of the challenging factors for the industrial sector. The commercial obtainability of microbial fibrinolytic enzymes needs high yield at the lowest possible costs [80]. Hence, fermentation approaches are highly remarkable in cutting down the cost of production for an enzyme. For instance, selected submerged fermentations can improve production yield and efficiency. Similarly, Anusree and colleagues (2020), by using submerged fermentation, were able to improve the expression of fibrinolytic enzyme from a bacterium *Serratia rubidaea* KUAS001 obtained from marine milieus [61]. In addition, Pan and colleagues (2019) showed the utilization of non-sterile submerged fermentation to minimize the production cost of enzymes from *Bacillus subtilis* D21-8 [56]. Moreover, several researchers showed that the use and application of diverse statistical tools, such as Box–Behnken design [46], two-level full factorial design (2^5) [49,52,60], response surface methodology [52,60,72,81], Plackett–Burman design [64,81], one-factor experiment [64], L_{18}-orthogonal array method [41] and central composite experimental design [49,67], are useful approaches for optimizing physico-chemical parameters for the production of fibrinolytic enzymes. For example, Farraj and colleagues (2020), applying a two-level full factorial design and response surface methodology, were able to increase the expression of the fibrinolytic enzyme isolated from *Bacillus flexus* using a solid state fermentation process. They demonstrated an enhanced production of fibrinolytic enzymes up to 3.5-fold [52].

6. Thrombolytic Activity of Marine Microbial Fibrinolytic Enzymes

The effective treatment of CVDs relies on thrombolysis agents, such as microbial fibrinolytic enzymes [82,83]. Microorganisms have been utilized to produce fibrinolytic enzymes since ancient times. In the last decades, researchers have intensively reported on the production of fibrinolytic enzymes from marine microorganisms. For example, a study carried out by Hwang et al. (2007) showed that BpKJ-31 is a promising candidate as a health-promoting biomaterial that does not induce bleeding [75]. Studies on in vitro lysis of clots by a purified fibrinolytic enzyme from the marine *Serratia marcescens* resulted in 38% clot lysis, which was significantly higher than that reported by streptokinase and heparin [62]. In addition, in the study carried by Gowthami and colleagues (2021), the fibrinolytic enzyme isolated from bacterial strain GPJ3 displayed digestion of blood clot completely under in vitro condition and exhibited potent activity on wound healing of macrophages [50]. The characteristics of the recombinant fibase from a marine *Bacillus subtilis* suggest its potential use for the treatment and/or prevention of thrombosis [71]. Moreover, purified PEKU1, a novel fibrinolytic protease from *Pseudomonas aeruginosa* KU1, has exceptional potential for being developed as a therapeutic agent to treat CVDs [47].

7. Conclusions

The scientific community already effectively utilizes all available information on fibrinolytic enzymes. As a future prospective, the community should focus on the exploration of novel sources of fibrinolytic enzymes, especially from the marine environment. Marine microbial fibrinolytic enzymes have immense therapeutic potential as target drugs to prevent or cure CVDs. Extensive studies on these enzymes promises to develop cost effective, safe and preventive solutions for the management of cardiac diseases. The new trend for developing and improving thrombolytic agents is to enhance its fibrin specificity and binding efficacy. Further optimization of production parameters is also required to design economical, effective and safe drugs. Thus, the use of marine microbial fibrinolytic enzymes as thrombolytic agents might be auspicious and a safe option in future.

Author Contributions: Conceptualization, writing and original draft preparation, N.B.; reviewing, S.T.J.; reviewing and funding acquisition, F.V. All authors have read and agreed to the published version of the manuscript.

Funding: This work was supported by Regione Veneto (Italy) POR FESR 2014–2020, "3S_4H-Safe, Smart, Sustainable Food for Health, 1.1.4. DGR n. 1139.

Acknowledgments: The authors gratefully acknowledge the excellence department project of the Italian Ministry of Education, University and Research (MIUR) "Excellence for Aquatic Animal Health—ECCE AQUA."

Conflicts of Interest: The authors declare that there are no conflicts of interest regarding the publication of this paper.

References

1. Raskob, G.; Angchaisuksiri, P.; Blanco, A.; Buller, H.; Gallus, A.; Hunt, B.; Hylek, E.; Kakkar, A.; Konstantinides, S.; McCumber, M. Isth steering committee for world thrombosis day. Thrombosis: A major contributor to global disease burden. *Arter. Thromb Vasc Biol.* **2014**, *34*, 2363–2371. [CrossRef]
2. Roth, G.A.; Mensah, G.A.; Johnson, C.O.; Addolorato, G.; Ammirati, E.; Baddour, L.M.; Barengo, N.C.; Beaton, A.Z.; Benjamin, E.J.; Benziger, C.P. Global burden of cardiovascular diseases and risk factors, 1990–2019: Update from the gbd 2019 study. *J. Am. Coll. Cardiol.* **2020**, *76*, 2982–3021. [CrossRef]
3. Winter, W.E.; Flax, S.D.; Harris, N.S. Coagulation testing in the core laboratory. *Lab. Med.* **2017**, *48*, 295–313. [CrossRef]
4. Roth, G.A.; Johnson, C.; Abajobir, A.; Abd-Allah, F.; Abera, S.F.; Abyu, G.; Ahmed, M.; Aksut, B.; Alam, T.; Alam, K. Global, regional, and national burden of cardiovascular diseases for 10 causes, 1990 to 2015. *J. Am. Coll. Cardiol.* **2017**, *70*, 1–25. [CrossRef] [PubMed]
5. World Health Organization (WHO). NCDs Mortality and Morbidity. 2016 [Updated 2016; Cited]. Available online: http://www.who.int/gho/ncd/mortality_morbidity/en/ (accessed on 20 November 2021).
6. Kotb, E. Activity assessment of microbial fibrinolytic enzymes. *Appl. Microbiol. Biotechnol.* **2013**, *97*, 6647–6665. [CrossRef] [PubMed]
7. Chapin, J.C.; Hajjar, K.A. Fibrinolysis and the control of blood coagulation. *Blood Rev.* **2015**, *29*, 17–24. [CrossRef]
8. Peng, Y.; Yang, X.; Zhang, Y. Microbial fibrinolytic enzymes: An overview of source, production, properties, and thrombolytic activity in vivo. *Appl. Microbiol. Biotechnol.* **2005**, *69*, 126–132. [CrossRef] [PubMed]
9. Chitte, R.R.; Deshmukh, S.V.; Kanekar, P.P. Production, purification, and biochemical characterization of a fibrinolytic enzyme from thermophilic *Streptomyces* sp. MCMB-379. *Appl. Biochem. Biotechnol.* **2011**, *165*, 1406–1413. [CrossRef]
10. Simoons, M.L.; de Jaegere, P.; van Domburg, R.; Boersma, E.; Maggioni, A.; Franzosi, M.; Leimberger, J.; Califf, R.; Schröder, R.; Knatterud, G. Individual risk assessment for intracranial haemorrhage during thrombolytic therapy. *Lancet* **1993**, *342*, 1523–1528. [CrossRef]
11. Fromm, R.E., Jr.; Hoskins, E.; Cronin, L.; Pratt, C.M.; Spencer, W.H., III; Roberts, R. Bleeding complications following initiation of thrombolytic therapy for acute myocardial infarction: A comparison of helicopter-transported and nontransported patients. *Ann. Emerg. Med.* **1991**, *20*, 892–895. [CrossRef]
12. Niego, B.e.; Freeman, R.; Puschmann, T.B.; Turnley, A.M.; Medcalf, R.L. t-PA–specific modulation of a human blood-brain barrier model involves plasmin-mediated activation of the Rho kinase pathway in astrocytes. *Blood J. Am. Soc. Hematol.* **2012**, *119*, 4752–4761. [CrossRef]
13. Eisenberg, P.R.; Sherman, L.A.; Tiefenbrunn, A.J.; Ludbrook, P.A.; Sobel, B.E.; Jaffe, A.S. Sustained fibrinolysis after administration of t-PA despite its short half-life in the circulation. *Thromb. Haemost.* **1987**, *57*, 035–040. [CrossRef]
14. Nilsson, T.; Wallén, P.; Mellbring, G. In vivo metabolism of human tissue-type plasminogen activator. *Scand. J. Haematol.* **1984**, *33*, 49–53. [CrossRef]
15. Tsikouris, J.P.; Tsikouris, A.P. A review of available fibrin-specific thrombolytic agents used in acute myocardial infarction. *Pharmacother. J. Hum. Pharmacol. Drug Ther.* **2001**, *21*, 207–217. [CrossRef]
16. Matsuo, O.; Rijken, D.; Collen, D. Comparison of the relative fibrinogenolytic, fibrinolytic and thrombolytic properties of tissue plasminogen activator and urokinase in vitro. *Thromb. Haemost.* **1981**, *45*, 225–229. [CrossRef]

17. Lu, F.; Lu, Z.; Bie, X.; Yao, Z.; Wang, Y.; Lu, Y.; Guo, Y. Purification and characterization of a novel anticoagulant and fibrinolytic enzyme produced by endophytic bacterium *Paenibacillus polymyxa* EJS-3. *Thromb. Res.* **2010**, *126*, e349–e355. [CrossRef] [PubMed]
18. Zhang, Y.; Wisner, A.; Xiong, Y.; Bon, C. A novel plasminogen activator from snake venom: Purification, characterization, and molecular cloning. *J. Biol. Chem.* **1995**, *270*, 10246–10255. [CrossRef] [PubMed]
19. Wu, J.X.; Zhao, X.Y.; Pan, R.; He, R.Q. Glycosylated trypsin-like proteases from earthworm *Eisenia fetida*. *Int. J. Biol. Macromol.* **2007**, *40*, 399–406. [CrossRef] [PubMed]
20. Iannucci, N.; Camperi, S.; Cascone, O. Purification of lumbrokinase from *Eisenia fetida* using aqueous two-phase systems and anion-exchange chromatography. *Sep. Purif. Technol.* **2008**, *64*, 131–134. [CrossRef]
21. Ahn, M.Y.; Hahn, B.-S.; Ryu, K.S.; Kim, J.W.; Kim, I.; Kim, Y.S. Purification and characterization of a serine protease with fibrinolytic activity from the dung beetles, *Catharsius molossus*. *Thromb. Res.* **2003**, *112*, 339–347. [CrossRef]
22. Chung, D.-M.; Choi, N.-S.; Maeng, P.J.; Chun, H.K.; Kim, S.-H. Purification and characterization of a novel fibrinolytic enzyme from chive (*Allium tuberosum*). *Food Sci. Biotechnol.* **2010**, *19*, 697–702. [CrossRef]
23. Katrolia, P.; Liu, X.; Zhao, Y.; Kopparapu, N.K.; Zheng, X. Gene cloning, expression and homology modeling of first fibrinolytic enzyme from mushroom (*Cordyceps militaris*). *Int. J. Biol. Macromol.* **2020**, *146*, 897–906. [CrossRef] [PubMed]
24. Lv, F.; Zhang, C.; Guo, F.; Lu, Y.; Bie, X.; Qian, H.; Lu, Z. Expression, purification, and characterization of a recombined fibrinolytic enzyme from endophytic *Paenibacillus polymyxa* EJS-3 in *Escherichia coli*. *Food Sci. Biotechnol.* **2015**, *24*, 125–131. [CrossRef]
25. Taneja, K.; Bajaj, B.K.; Kumar, S.; Dilbaghi, N. Production, purification and characterization of fibrinolytic enzyme from *Serratia* sp. KG-2-1 using optimized media. *3 Biotech* **2017**, *7*, 184. [CrossRef] [PubMed]
26. Kim, W.; Choi, K.; Kim, Y.; Park, H.; Choi, J.; Lee, Y.; Oh, H.; Kwon, I.; Lee, S. Purification and characterization of a fibrinolytic enzyme produced from *Bacillus* sp. strain ck 11-4 screened from Chungkook-Jang. *Appl. Environ. Microbiol.* **1996**, *62*, 2482–2488. [CrossRef] [PubMed]
27. Sugimoto, S.; Fujii, T.; Morimiya, T.; Johdo, O.; Nakamura, T. The fibrinolytic activity of a novel protease derived from a tempeh producing fungus, *Fusarium* sp. BLB. *Biosci. Biotechnol. Biochem.* **2007**, *71*, 2184–2189. [CrossRef]
28. Mine, Y.; Wong, A.H.K.; Jiang, B. Fibrinolytic enzymes in asian traditional fermented foods. *Food Res. Int.* **2005**, *38*, 243–250. [CrossRef]
29. Yao, Z.; Kim, J.A.; Kim, J.H. Gene cloning, expression, and properties of a fibrinolytic enzyme secreted by *Bacillus pumilus* bs15 isolated from gul (oyster) jeotgal. *Biotechnol. Bioprocess Eng.* **2018**, *23*, 293–301. [CrossRef]
30. Barzkar, N.; Sohail, M.; Jahromi, S.T.; Nahavandi, R.; Khodadadi, M. Marine microbial l-glutaminase: From pharmaceutical to food industry. *Appl. Microbiol. Biotechnol.* **2021**, *105*, 4453–4466. [CrossRef]
31. Barzkar, N.; Sohail, M.; Jahromi, S.T.; Gozari, M.; Poormozaffar, S.; Nahavandi, R.; Hafezieh, M. Marine bacterial esterases: Emerging biocatalysts for industrial applications. *Appl. Biochem. Biotechnol.* **2021**, *193*, 1187–1214. [CrossRef]
32. Barzkar, N.; Khan, Z.; Jahromi, S.T.; Poormozaffar, S.; Gozari, M.; Nahavandi, R. A critical review on marine serine protease and its inhibitors: A new wave of drugs? *Int. J. Biol. Macromol.* **2020**, *170*, 674–687. [CrossRef]
33. Barzkar, N.; Sohail, M. An overview on marine cellulolytic enzymes and their potential applications. *Appl. Microbiol. Biotechnol.* **2020**, *104*, 6873–6892. [CrossRef]
34. Barzkar, N. Marine microbial alkaline protease: An efficient and essential tool for various industrial applications. *Int. J. Biol. Macromol.* **2020**, *161*, 1216–1229. [CrossRef] [PubMed]
35. Barzkar, N.; Jahromi, S.T.; Poorsaheli, H.B.; Vianello, F. Metabolites from marine microorganisms, micro, and macroalgae: Immense scope for pharmacology. *Mar. Drugs* **2019**, *17*, 464. [CrossRef] [PubMed]
36. Jahromi, S.T.; Barzkar, N. Marine bacterial chitinase as sources of energy, eco-friendly agent, and industrial biocatalyst. *Int. J. Biol. Macromol.* **2018**, *120*, 2147–2154. [CrossRef] [PubMed]
37. Jahromi, S.T.; Barzkar, N. Future direction in marine bacterial agarases for industrial applications. *Appl. Microbiol. Biotechnol.* **2018**, *102*, 6847–6863. [CrossRef] [PubMed]
38. Barzkar, N.; Homaei, A.; Hemmati, R.; Patel, S. Thermostable marine microbial proteases for industrial applications: Scopes and risks. *Extremophiles* **2018**, *22*, 335–346. [CrossRef]
39. Izadpanah Qeshmi, F.; Javadpour, S.; Malekzadeh, K.; Tamadoni Jahromi, S.; Rahimzadeh, M. Persian gulf is a bioresource of potent l-asparaginase producing bacteria: Isolation & molecular differentiating. *Int. J. Environ. Res* **2014**, *8*, 813–818.
40. Sabu, A. Sources, properties and applications of microbial therapeutic enzymes. *Indian J. Biotechnol.* **2003**, *2*, 334–341.
41. Mahajan, P.M.; Nayak, S.; Lele, S.S. Fibrinolytic enzyme from newly isolated marine bacterium *Bacillus subtilis* ictf-1: Media optimization, purification and characterization. *J. Biosci. Bioeng.* **2012**, *113*, 307–314. [CrossRef]
42. Sharma, C.; Osmolovskiy, A.; Singh, R. Microbial fibrinolytic enzymes as anti-thrombotics: Production, characterisation and prodigious biopharmaceutical applications. *Pharmaceutics* **2021**, *13*, 1880. [CrossRef]
43. SudeshWarma, S.; Devi, C.S. *Production of Fibrinolytic Protease from Streptomyces Lusitanus Isolated from Marine Sediments*; IOP Conference Series: Materials Science and Engineering; IOP Publishing: Bristol, UK, 2017; p. 022048.
44. Dhamodharan, D. Novel fibrinolytic protease producing *Streptomyces radiopugnans* VITSD8 from marine sponges. *Mar. Drugs* **2019**, *17*, 164.
45. Mohanasrinivasan, V.; Yogesh, S.; Govindaraj, A.; Jemimah Naine, S.; Subathra Devi, C. In vitro thrombolytic potential of actinoprotease from marine *Streptomyces violaceus* VITYGM. *Cardiovasc. Hematol. Agents Med. Chem. (Former. Curr. Med. Chem.-Cardiovasc. Hematol. Agents)* **2016**, *14*, 120–124. [CrossRef] [PubMed]

46. Kumar, S.S.; Haridas, M.; Sabu, A. Process optimization for production of a fibrinolytic enzyme from newly isolated marine bacterium *Seudomonas aeruginosa* KU1. *Biocatal. Agric. Biotechnol.* **2018**, *14*, 33–39. [CrossRef]
47. Kumar, S.S.; Haridas, M.; Abdulhameed, S. A novel fibrinolytic enzyme from marine *Pseudomonas aeruginosa* KU1 and its rapid in vivo thrombolysis with little haemolysis. *Int. J. Biol. Macromol.* **2020**, *162*, 470–479. [CrossRef]
48. Demina, N.; Veslopolova, E.; Gaenko, G. The marine bacterium *Alteromonas piscicida*–a producer of enzymes with thrombolytic action. *Izv. Akad. Nauk SSSR. Seriia Biol.* **1990**, *3*, 415–419.
49. Vijayaraghavan, P.; Vincent, S.G.P. Statistical optimization of fibrinolytic enzyme production by *Pseudoalteromonas* sp. IND11 using cow dung substrate by response surface methodology. *SpringerPlus* **2014**, *3*, 60. [CrossRef] [PubMed]
50. Gowthami, K.; Madhuri, R.J. Optimization of cultural conditions for maximum production of fibrinolytic enzymes from the local marine bacterial isolates and evaluation of their wound healing and clot dissolving properties. *J. Pharm. Res. Int.* **2021**, *33*, 246–255. [CrossRef]
51. Masilamani, R.; Natarajan, S. Molecular cloning, overexpression and characterization of a new thiol-dependent, alkaline serine protease with destaining function and fibrinolytic potential from *Marinobacter aquaeolei* MS2-1. *Biologia* **2015**, *70*, 1143–1149. [CrossRef]
52. Al Farraj, D.A.; Kumar, T.S.J.; Vijayaraghavan, P.; Elshikh, M.S.; Alkufeidy, R.M.; Alkubaisi, N.A.; Alshammari, M.K. Enhanced production, purification and biochemical characterization of therapeutic potential fibrinolytic enzyme from a new *Bacillus flexus* from marine environment. *J. King Saud Univ.-Sci.* **2020**, *32*, 3174–3180. [CrossRef]
53. Pan, S.; Chen, G.; Zeng, J.; Cao, X.; Zheng, X.; Zeng, W.; Liang, Z. Fibrinolytic enzyme production from low-cost substrates by marine *Bacillus subtilis*: Process optimization and kinetic modeling. *Biochem. Eng. J.* **2019**, *141*, 268–277. [CrossRef]
54. Huang, S.; Pan, S.; Chen, G.; Huang, S.; Zhang, Z.; Li, Y.; Liang, Z. Biochemical characteristics of a fibrinolytic enzyme purified from a marine bacterium, *Bacillus subtilis* HQS-3. *Int. J. Biol. Macromol.* **2013**, *62*, 124–130. [CrossRef] [PubMed]
55. Cheng, Q.; Xu, F.; Hu, N.; Liu, X.; Liu, Z. A novel Ca^{2+}-dependent alkaline serine-protease (Bvsp) from *Bacillus* sp. With high fibrinolytic activity. *J. Mol. Catal. B Enzym.* **2015**, *117*, 69–74. [CrossRef]
56. Pan, S.; Chen, G.; Wu, R.; Cao, X.; Liang, Z. Non-sterile submerged fermentation of fibrinolytic enzyme by marine *Bacillus subtilis* harboring antibacterial activity with starvation strategy. *Front. Microbiol.* **2019**, *10*, 1025. [CrossRef]
57. Wu, R.; Chen, G.; Pan, S.; Zeng, J.; Liang, Z. Cost-effective fibrinolytic enzyme production by *Bacillus subtilis* WR350 using medium supplemented with corn steep powder and sucrose. *Sci. Rep.* **2019**, *9*, 6824. [CrossRef] [PubMed]
58. Yao, Z.; Kim, J.A.; Kim, J.H. Properties of a fibrinolytic enzyme secreted by *Bacillus subtilis* JS2 isolated from saeu (small shrimp) jeotgal. *Food Sci. Biotechnol.* **2018**, *27*, 765–772. [CrossRef]
59. Yao, Z.; Kim, J.A.; Kim, J.H. Characterization of a fibrinolytic enzyme secreted by *Bacillus velezensis* BS2 isolated from sea squirt jeotgal. *J. Microbiol. Biotechnol.* **2019**, *29*, 347–356. [CrossRef]
60. Vijayaraghavan, P.; Vincent, S.P. A low cost fermentation medium for potential fibrinolytic enzyme production by a newly isolated marine bacterium, *Shewanella* sp. IND20. *Biotechnol. Rep.* **2015**, *7*, 135–142. [CrossRef]
61. Anusree, M.; Swapna, K.; Aguilar, C.; Sabu, A. Optimization of process parameters for the enhanced production of fibrinolytic enzyme by a newly isolated marine bacterium. *Bioresour. Technol. Rep.* **2020**, *11*, 100436. [CrossRef]
62. Krishnamurthy, A.; Belur, P.D. A novel fibrinolytic serine metalloprotease from the marine *Serratia marcescens* subsp. *sakuensis*: Purification and characterization. *Int. J. Biol. Macromol.* **2018**, *112*, 110–118. [CrossRef]
63. Krishnamurthy, A.; Belur, P.D.; Rai, P. Studies on fibrinolytic enzyme from marine *Serratia marcescens* subsp. *sakuensis* (KU296189.1). *Int. J. Appl. Bioeng.* **2017**, *11*, 1–5.
64. Krishnamurthy, A.; Belur, P.D.; Rai, P.; Rekha, P.D. Production of fibrinolytic enzyme by the marine isolate *Serratia marcescens* subsp. *sakuensis* and its in-vitro anticoagulant and thrombolytic potential. *Pure Appl. Microbiol* **2017**, *11*, 1987–1998. [CrossRef]
65. de Barros, P.D.S.; e Silva, P.E.C.; Nascimento, T.P.; Costa, R.M.P.B.; Bezerra, R.P.; Porto, A.L.F. Fibrinolytic enzyme from *Arthrospira platensis* cultivated in medium culture supplemented with corn steep liquor. *Int. J. Biol. Macromol.* **2020**, *164*, 3446–3453. [CrossRef] [PubMed]
66. e Silva, P.E.d.C.; de Barros, R.C.; Albuquerque, W.W.C.; Brandão, R.M.P.; Bezerra, R.P.; Porto, A.L.F. In vitro thrombolytic activity of a purified fibrinolytic enzyme from *Chlorella vulgaris*. *J. Chromatogr. B* **2018**, *1092*, 524–529. [CrossRef]
67. Páblo, E.; de Souza, F.; de Barros, R.; Marques, D.; Porto, A.; Bezerra, R. Enhanced production of fibrinolytic protease from microalgae *Chlorella vulgaris* using glycerol and corn steep liquor as nutrient. *Ann. Microbiol. Res.* **2017**, *1*, 9–19.
68. Silva, T.; Barros, P.; Silva, P.; Bezerra, R.; Porto, A. Effects of Metal Ions and Proteases Inhibitors on Fibrinolytic. Available online: https://www.sbmicrobiologia.org.br/29cbm-anais/resumos/15/R0528-2.PDF (accessed on 20 November 2021).
69. Wu, C.; Zheng, C.; Wang, J.; Jiang, P. Recombinant expression of thrombolytic agent reteplase in marine microalga *Tetraselmis subcordiformis* (chlorodendrales, chlorophyta). *Mar. Drugs* **2021**, *19*, 315. [CrossRef] [PubMed]
70. Krishnamurthy, A.; Mundra, S.; Belur, P.D. Improving the catalytic efficiency of fibrinolytic enzyme from *Serratia marcescens* subsp. *sakuensis* by chemical modification. *Process Biochem.* **2018**, *72*, 79–85. [CrossRef]
71. Che, Z.; Cao, X.; Chen, G.; Liang, Z. An effective combination of codon optimization, gene dosage, and process optimization for high-level production of fibrinolytic enzyme in *Komagataella phaffii* (*Pichia pastoris*). *BMC Biotechnol.* **2020**, *20*, 63. [CrossRef]
72. Verma, P.; Chatterjee, S.; Keziah, M.S.; Devi, S.C. Fibrinolytic protease from marine *Streptomyces rubiginosus* VITPSS1. *Cardiovasc. Hematol. Agents Med. Chem. (Former. Curr. Med. Chem.-Cardiovasc. Hematol. Agents)* **2018**, *16*, 44–55. [CrossRef]

73. Naveena, B.; Gopinath, K.P.; Sakthiselvan, P.; Partha, N. Enhanced production of thrombinase by *Streptomyces venezuelae*: Kinetic studies on growth and enzyme production of mutant strain. *Bioresour. Technol.* **2012**, *111*, 417–424. [CrossRef]
74. Sadeesh Kumar, R.; Rajesh, R.; Gokulakrishnan, S.; Subramanian, J. Screening and characterization of fibrinolytic protease producing *Bacillus circulans* from mangrove sediments pitchavaram, South east coast of India. *Int. Lett. Nat. Sci.* **2015**, *28*, 10–16.
75. Hwang, K.-J.; Choi, K.-H.; Kim, M.-J.; Park, C.-S.; Cha, J.-H. Purification and characterization of a new fibrinolytic enzyme of *Bacillus licheniformis* KJ-31, isolated from korean traditional Jeot-gal. *J. Microbiol. Biotechnol.* **2007**, *17*, 1469–1476. [PubMed]
76. Bajpai, P. *Xylanolytic Enzymes*; Academic Press: Cambridge, MA, USA, 2014.
77. Koffman, B.; Modarress, K.; Bashirelahi, N. The effects of various serine protease inhibitors on estrogen receptor steroid binding. *J. Steroid Biochem. Mol. Biol.* **1991**, *38*, 569–574. [CrossRef]
78. Weisel, J.W.; Litvinov, R.I. Fibrin formation, structure and properties. *Fibrous Proteins: Struct. Mech.* **2017**, *82*, 405–456.
79. Lam, K.; Lloyd, G.; Neuteboom, S.; Palladino, M.; Sethna, K.; Spear, M.; Potts, B. *Natural Product Chemistry for Drug Discovery*; Buss, A.D., Butler, M.S., Eds.; Royal Society of Chemistry Cambridge: Cambridge, UK, 2010.
80. Silva, R.; Ferreira, H.; Little, C.; Cavaco-Paulo, A. Effect of ultrasound parameters for unilamellar liposome preparation. *Ultrason. Sonochemistry* **2010**, *17*, 628–632. [CrossRef]
81. Agrebi, R.; Haddar, A.; Hajji, M.; Frikha, F.; Manni, L.; Jellouli, K.; Nasri, M. Fibrinolytic enzymes from a newly isolated marine bacterium *Bacillus subtilis* A26: Characterization and statistical media optimization. *Can. J. Microbiol.* **2009**, *55*, 1049–1061. [CrossRef] [PubMed]
82. Jeong, Y.-k.; Kim, J.H.; Gal, S.-w.; Kim, J.-e.; Park, S.-s.; Chung, K.-t.; Kim, Y.-H.; Kim, B.-W.; Joo, W.-H. Molecular cloning and characterization of the gene encoding a fibrinolytic enzyme from *Bacillus subtilis* strain A1. *World J. Microbiol. Biotechnol.* **2004**, *20*, 711–717. [CrossRef]
83. Mukherjee, A.K.; Rai, S.K.; Thakur, R.; Chattopadhyay, P.; Kar, S.K. Bafibrinase: A non-toxic, non-hemorrhagic, direct-acting fibrinolytic serine protease from *Bacillus* sp. strain AS-S20-I exhibits in vivo anticoagulant activity and thrombolytic potency. *Biochimie* **2012**, *94*, 1300–1308. [CrossRef]

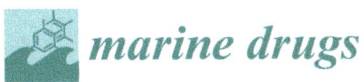

Communication

Apoptotic Activity of New Oxisterigmatocystin Derivatives from the Marine-Derived Fungus *Aspergillus nomius* NC06

Muh. Ade Artasasta [1,2], Yanwirasti Yanwirasti [3], Muhammad Taher [4], Akmal Djamaan [1], Ni Putu Ariantari [5], Ru Angelie Edrada-Ebel [6] and Dian Handayani [1,*]

1. Laboratory of Sumatran Biota, Faculty of Pharmacy, Andalas University, Padang 25163, Indonesia; muh.ade.artasasta.fmipa@um.ac.id (M.A.A.); akmaldjamaan@phar.unand.ac.id (A.D.)
2. Biotechnology Department, Faculty of Mathematics and Natural Sciences, Universitas Negeri Malang (UM), Malang 65145, Indonesia
3. Departement of Biomedical, Faculty of Medicine, Andalas University, Padang 25163, Indonesia; yanwirasti@yahoo.com
4. Faculty of Pharmacy, International Islamic University Malaysia, Kuantan 25200, Malaysia; mtaher@iium.edu.my
5. Department of Pharmacy, Faculty of Mathematics and Natural Sciences, Udayana University, Bali 80361, Indonesia; putu_ariantari@unud.ac.id
6. Strathclyde Institute of Pharmacy and Biomedical Sciences, University of Strathclyde, The John Arbuthnott Building, 161 Cathedral Street, Glasgow G4 0RE, UK; ruangelie.edrada-ebel@strath.ac.uk
* Correspondence: dianhandayani@phar.unand.ac.id; Tel.: +62-751-71682

Citation: Artasasta, M.A.; Yanwirasti, Y.; Taher, M.; Djamaan, A.; Ariantari, N.P.; Edrada-Ebel, R.A.; Handayani, D. Apoptotic Activity of New Oxisterigmatocystin Derivatives from the Marine-Derived Fungus *Aspergillus nomius* NC06. *Mar. Drugs* **2021**, *19*, 631. https://doi.org/10.3390/md19110631

Academic Editor: Bill J. Baker

Received: 5 October 2021
Accepted: 10 November 2021
Published: 11 November 2021

Publisher's Note: MDPI stays neutral with regard to jurisdictional claims in published maps and institutional affiliations.

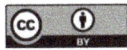

Copyright: © 2021 by the authors. Licensee MDPI, Basel, Switzerland. This article is an open access article distributed under the terms and conditions of the Creative Commons Attribution (CC BY) license (https://creativecommons.org/licenses/by/4.0/).

Abstract: Sponge-derived fungi have recently attracted attention as an important source of interesting bioactive compounds. *Aspergillus nomius* NC06 was isolated from the marine sponge *Neopetrosia chaliniformis*. This fungus was cultured on rice medium and yielded four compounds including three new oxisterigmatocystins, namely, J, K, and L (**1**, **2**, and **3**), and one known compound, aspergillicin A (**4**). Structures of the compounds were elucidated by 1D and 2D NMR spectroscopy and by high-resolution mass spectrometry. The isolated compounds were tested for cytotoxic activity against HT 29 colon cancer cells, where compounds **1**, **2**, and **4** exhibited IC$_{50}$ values of 6.28, 15.14, and 1.63 µM, respectively. Under the fluorescence microscope by using a double staining method, HT 29 cells were observed to be viable, apoptotic, and necrotic after treatment with the cytotoxic compounds **1**, **2**, and **4**. The result shows that compounds **1** and **2** were able to induce apoptosis and cell death in HT 29 cells.

Keywords: marine sponge-derived fungus; *Neopetrosia chaliniformis*; *Aspergillus nomius*; oxisterigmatocystin; cytotoxic activity; HT 29 colon cancer cells; apoptosis cells

1. Introduction

In recent years, sponge-derived fungi have drawn increasing attention as a rich source of interesting bioactive marine natural products [1–6]. Many fungi associated with marine sponges produce interesting secondary metabolites such as alkaloids, polyketides, and terpenoids [6–9]. This has encouraged many researchers to explore more bioactive compounds from marine sponge-derived fungi, potentially used as antimicrobials or as anticancer drugs and against other diseases [9–13]. The fungus *Aspergillus nomius* NC06 was isolated from the marine sponge *Neopetrosia chaliniformis*. The fungal ethyl acetate extract showed cytotoxic activity against WiDr and HCT 116 colon cancer cells. However, it was not toxic against the normal Vero cell line [14,15].

Extracts and secondary metabolites yielded by the fungal genus *Aspergillus* have been frequently reported in the literature for their potent cytotoxic activity [16,17]. One family of compounds described from this genus is the oxisterigmatocystins [18]. Oxisterigmatocystins A, B, and C, as well as 5-methoxysterigmatocystin, were isolated from *A. versicolor*.

5-Methoxysterigmatocystin exhibited moderate cytotoxicity against the A-549 and HL-60 cell lines, with IC$_{50}$s of 3.86 and 5.32 µM, respectively [18]. Oxisterigmatocystin D was also reported from *Aspergillus* sp. with an additional methoxyl group in C-4′ (δ_H 3.10; δ_C 54.5) [19]. Other derivatives (E, F, G, H) were isolated from the fungus *Botryotrichum piluliferum* [20], and oxisterigmatocystin I was isolated from the fungus *Aspergillus* sp. F40 derived from the sponge *Callyspongia* [21]. In our continuing study, new oxisterigmatocystin derivatives J, K, and L (**1**, **2**, and **3**) and one known compound, aspergillicin A (**4**) [22], were isolated from the ethyl acetate extract of *A. nomius* NC06.

2. Results and Discussion

Compound **1** was isolated as a yellow amorphous powder. Its molecular formula was determined as $C_{19}H_{14}O_7$ based on an HR-ESI-MS ion peak at *m/z* 355.0811 [M + H]$^+$ calculated at 355.0812 Da for $C_{19}H_{15}O_7$. The 1D NMR data of this compound (Table 1) contained resonances for one carbonyl group, nine quaternary carbons, five methine units (CH), two methoxys (O-CH$_3$), and one hydroxyl group (Figure 1). Analysis of 1D and 2D NMR showed that compound **1** was an oxisterigmatocystin derivative [18]. The isolated compound **1** had comparable ^{1}H NMR spectral data (Figures S3 and S4) to those of oxisterigmatocystin C [18] on the aromatic region with a singlet for H-2 at 6.62 ppm and a similar ABC system at δ_H 6.94, dd (8.5, 0.9); 7.65, t (8.4), and 7.08, dd (8.4, 0.9) for H-5, H-6, and H-7, respectively. In comparison to oxisterigmatocystin C, there was the loss of an exchangeable resonance at 13.4 ppm due to the methylation of the hydroxyl substituent on C-8 in compound **1**, which was replaced by a methoxy singlet at δ_H 3.85 with the corresponding ^{13}C signal at 56.1 ppm. The major structural difference between compound **1** and the earlier described oxisterigmatocystin derivatives was the demethylation of the hydroxyl substituent at C-4′ in compound **1** and the additional olefinic methine signal for C-3′ at δ_H 6.77, d (*J* = 2.8 Hz) and δ_C 148.3 that was established by HSQC (Figure S5). Moreover, the existence of a double bond between the shielded quaternary C-2′ at δ_C 89.2 and C-3′ in compound **1** could be confirmed by the COSY and HMBC correlations with the hydroxylated methine unit on C-4′ at δ_H 5.71, d (*J* = 2.8 Hz) and δ_C 107.0, as well as with the C-4′OH singlet at 6.50 ppm, as shown in Figure 2 (Figures S4 and S6).

Table 1. ^{1}H (600 MHz) and ^{13}C (150 MHz) NMR data for compounds **1–3** in DMSO-d_6.

Position	1		2		3	
	δ_C, Type	δ_H (*J* in Hz)	δ_C, Type	δ_H (*J* in Hz)	δ_C, Type	δ_H (*J* in Hz)
1	162.5, C		161.9, C		162.1, C	
2	91.0, CH	6.62, s	90.3, CH	6.50, s	90.3, CH	6.55, s
3	163.5, C		163.0, C		162.9, C	
4	108.3, C		107.0, C		107.9, C	
5	106.8, CH	6.94, dd (8.5, 0.9)	108.9, CH	7.02, dd (8.4, 0.9)	108.7, CH	7.04, d (8.3)
6	134.3, CH	7.65, t (8.4)	134.1, CH	7.61, t (8.3)	133.9, CH	7.62, t (8.4)
7	109.1, CH	7.08, dd (8.4, 0.9)	106.8, CH	6.93, dd (8.4, 0.9)	106.6, CH	6.93, d (8.3)
8	155.9, C		159.6, C		159.6, C	
9	173.0, C		173.2, C		173.1, C	
10	159.6, C		156.0, C		155.8, C	
11	113.9, C		112.9, C		113.1, C	
12	108.2, C		107.5, C		106.0, C	
13	152.7, C		152.2, C		152.7, C	
1′	117.3, CH	6.41, s	113.3, CH	6.56, d (6.1)	111.0, CH	6.48, d (5.9)
2′	89.2, C		42.0, CH	4.19, dd (9.3, 6.2)	41.8, CH	4.24, ddd (9.2, 5.9, 3.4)
3′	148.3, CH	6.77, d (2.8)	36.7, CH$_2$	2.39, ddd (13.4, 9.5, 5.2); 2.23, d (13.3)	36.0, CH$_2$	2.35, dd (13.2, 4.8, 3.4); 2.25, ddd (13.5, 9.0, 5.3)
4′	107.0, CH	5.71, d (2.8)	106.3, CH	5.25, d (5.0)	106.1, CH	5.17, t (5.0)
1-OMe	56.5, CH$_3$	3.84, s	56.3, CH$_3$	3.81, s	56.1, CH$_3$	3.82, s
8-OMe	56.1, CH$_3$	3.85, s	56.1, CH$_3$	3.85, s	55.8, CH$_3$	3.85, s
4′-OH		6.50, s				
4′-OMe			54.5, CH$_3$	3.09, s	55.7, CH$_3$	3.36, s

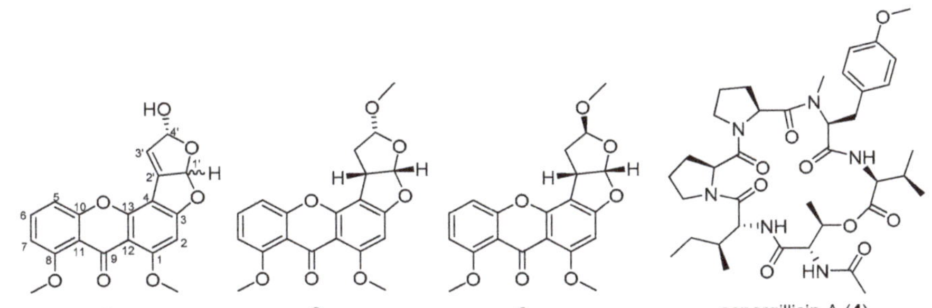

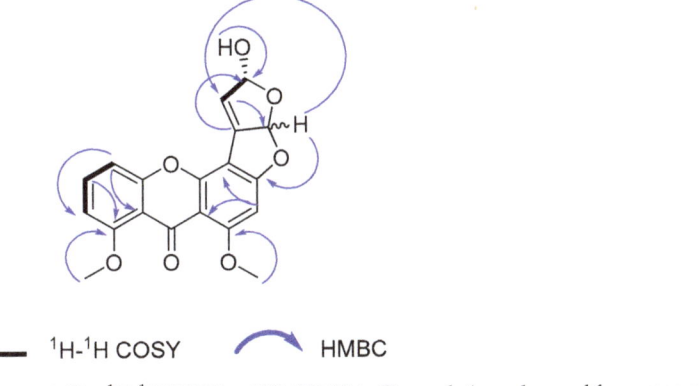

Figure 1. Structures of isolated compounds **1**–**4**. Stereochemistry shown for compounds **2** and **3** is relative.

Figure 2. Key ^{1}H-^{1}H COSY and HMBC (H to C) correlations observed for compound **1**.

By modifying the Mosher method [23], the absolute stereochemistry on C-4′ was established to have the *R* configuration (Figure S7). Compound **1** was derivatized with chiral reagents *R*- and *S*-methoxy-α-(trifluoromethyl)phenylacetyl chloride (MTPA-Cl). The ^{1}H-NMR spectrum for both congeners was measured, and the differences ($\Delta^{\delta(S)-\delta(R)}$) in chemical shifts for H-1′ and H-3′ in the respective spectra of the derivatized components were recorded. The ^{1}H assignments for the MTPA esters were verified by COSY. H-1′ and H-3′ afforded a $\Delta\delta^{S-R}$ of >0 and <0, respectively. The Mosher results apparently assigned the respective positions of H-1′ and H-3′ at the right and left sides of the *R*-hydroxyl stereocenter on C-4′, while the stereochemistry at position C-1′ remained undetermined. The observed nOe was inconclusive because in both cases, whether H-1′ has the *R* or *S* configuration, the through-space distances between H-1′ and H-4′ are 3.814 and 3.448Å, respectively, which are both less than the internuclear separation of 5Å that is the minimum requirement to identify spatially close pairs of nuclei. These through-space distances were determined by MM2 calculation at a minimum energy of 84.5646 and 81.4504 kcal/mol, respectively, using PerkinElmer's 3D ChemDraw v 18.2. We assigned compound **1** the trivial name oxisterigmatocystin J.

Compounds **2** and **3** were also isolated as yellow amorphous powders. The molecular formulae for both compounds were established by HR-ESI-MS as $C_{20}H_{18}O_7$ affording molecular ion peaks at [M + H]$^+$, *m/z* 371.1127 and 371.1128, respectively, which were both calculated for $C_{20}H_{19}O_7$ at 371.1125 Da. The aromatic regions of the ^{1}H NMR spectral data of both **2** and **3** were comparable to those of the isolated compound **1** and oxisterigmatocystin C (Table 1). A methine singlet for H-2 was observed at 6.50 and 6.55 ppm for compounds **2** and **3**, respectively, while, again, a similar ABC system was observed for H-5, H-6, and H-7 in both congeners **2** and **3** at δ_H 7.02/7.04 (d, *J* = 8.4/8.3 Hz), 7.61/7.62 (t, *J* = 8.3/8.4 Hz), and 6.93 (d, *J* = 8.4/8.3 Hz), respectively, with differences in chemical shifts between ±0.01 and 0.02 ppm between the two isolated derivatives. As in compound **1**, C-1- and C-8-O*H* were methylated (Figures S10, S11, S16, and S17) as observed at 3.82 and 3.85 ppm, respectively. The ^{13}C NMR spectral data of the xanthone moiety for the congeners **1**, **2**, and **3** were comparable, with an average chemical shift difference of 0.74 ppm, as shown in Table 1. This resulted in almost superimposable 2D NMR spectral data for HSQC and HMBC (Figures S4, S6, S12, S13, S18, and S19) for the compounds' xanthone unit.

Structural differences between compounds **2** and **3** were evident at the 4′-methoxyhexahydrofuro [2,3-*b*]furan ring. The relative configurations of compounds **2** and **3** were resolved by comparison of their coupling constants, optical rotations, and conformational analysis with known congeners described in the literature [18]. The coupling constant between H-1′ and H-2′ of compounds **2** and **3** was at 6 Hz (with actual values at 6.1 and 5.9 Hz, respectively) that implied the *cis* configuration for the two vicinal protons and indicated a 1′*S*, 2′*S* stereochemistry [18].

Compound **2** afforded similar ^{13}C and ^{1}H NMR spectral data, which diverged at less than 0.1 and 0.5 ppm to those of oxisterigmatocystin C, respectively, while the coupling constants were also comparable at a maximum difference of 0.4 Hz between both derivatives, which indicated an identical spatial conformation. The β-configuration of the methoxy unit on C-4′ of compound **2** was similar to that found in oxisterigmatocystins A and C [18], which was based on the coupling pattern observed for an α-hemiacetal sterigmatocystin [18,24]. The coupling constant between H-2′ at 4.19 ppm and H-3′A at 2.39 ppm gave 9 Hz (with actual values at 9.3 and 9.5 Hz, respectively) for a dihedral angle of about 20° [24]. Albeit there was no observable coupling between H-3′B and H-2′, their dihedral angle must be between 80° and 100° as earlier described [24]. Furthermore, H-3′A displayed a geminal coupling of 13.3 Hz and a vicinal coupling of 5.0 Hz with H-4′ at 5.25 ppm for an expected dihedral angle of about 40°. The relative configurations for compound **2** were determined as 1′*S*, 2′*S*, and 4′*R* as in oxisterigmatocystin C [18,21]. We named compound **2** oxisterigmatocystin K, which is the 8-methoxy derivative of oxisterigmatocystin C [18].

On the other hand, the relative configuration of 4′-OMe in compound **3** was compatible with a β-hemiacetal sterigmatocystin [24] that is identical to oxisterigmatocystins B [18] and I [21], as evidenced by their comparable ^{13}C and ^{1}H NMR spectral data. The coupling constant between H-1′ at 6.48 and H-2′ at 4.24 ppm was 5.9 Hz. Moreover, H-2′ to H-3′A and H-3′B at 2.35 and 2.25 ppm coupled at 3.4 and 9.2 Hz, which would imply a dihedral angle of 20° and 120°, respectively, while H-3′A and H-3′B coupled with H-4′ at 5.17 ppm coupled at 5.0 Hz, which are not larger than 120° but both nearer to 60°. From the Noesy cross-peaks (Figure S20), correlations were observed between H-1′and H-2′, establishing the *cis* fusion for the bisfuran unit, as well as between H-2′ and 4-′OMe. Therefore, as with oxisterigmatocystin B, the relative configurations for compound **3** were inferred as 1′*S*, 2′*S*, and 4′*S*. Consecutively, compound **3** was assigned the trivial name oxisterigmatocystin L, which is an 8-methoxy congener of oxisterigmatocystin I [21] that is a 5-demothoxylated derivative of oxisterigmatocystin B [18].

The structural diversity of the fungal metabolites oxisterigmatocystins has been predominantly based on the configuration of the hydroxyl or methoxy substituent on C-4′ [18,20,21,24]. When the C-4′ substituent has the β-configuration as in an α-hemiacetal sterigmatocystin, the bisfuran ring (C-1′ to C-4′) has an envelope conformation, and H-4′ is observed as a doublet. However, when the C-4′ substituent has the α-configuration for a β-hemiacetal sterigmatocystin, the bisfuran ring has a half-chair conformation, while H-4′ emerges as a triplet or a doublet of a doublet.

In this study, all four isolated compounds were tested for their cytotoxic activity (IC_{50}) against HT 29 colon cancer cells (Table 2). Oxisterigmatocystins J and K along with the peptide aspergillicin A were found to be active, while oxisterigmatocystin L was inactive. The three oxisterigmatocystin congeners (J, K, and L) mainly differed on the hydroxyhexahydrofuro [2,3-*b*]furan moiety. The difference in the activity of the three sterigmatocystin derivatives was probably due to a change in spatial conformation on the hydrofuro [2,3-*b*]furan ring. There was a total loss of cytotoxicity in compound **3** with its β-configuration. Compounds **1** and **2** were bioactive, with IC$_{50}$ values below 15 µg/mL. Alternatively, compound **2** had an α-configuration, which could be essential to the bioactivity of oxisterigmatocystins. However, as reported by Cai et al. 2011, the change in the spatial conformation of the methoxy substituent at C-4′ did not affect the cytotoxicity of the compounds as both α and β congeners were found to be inactive. Instead, as earlier proposed, the presence of a double bond on the methoxy furan ring (C-3′ and C-4′) was suspected to be the main cause of its cytotoxic activity against cancer cell lines A-549 and HL-60. In the case of oxisterigmatocystin J, in this study, the double bond on C-2′ and C-3′ could have been the basis of its cytotoxicity. It could also be further hypothesized that the cytotoxicity of oxisterigmatocystins must be specific to certain cancer cell lines.

Table 2. Cytotoxic activity of all compounds against HT29 colon cancer cells.

Compound No	Compound Name	IC50 (µM)
1	oxisterigmatocystin J	6.28
2	oxisterigmatocystin K	15.14
3	oxisterigmatocystin L	988.05
4	aspergillicin A	1.63
	Taxol	0.48

All compounds did not show antibacterial activity against *E. coli* and *S. aureus*. This activity was influenced by bacterial resistance, susceptibility, persistence, and tolerance, the host factor, and the concentration of the compound [25].

Analysis of HT 29 cell death upon treatment with cytotoxic compounds **1**, **2**, and **4** was performed by a double staining method to determine the mechanism of cell death either by apoptosis or necrosis. The process of cell death in this test is expected to occur by apoptosis or programmed cell death due to the induction of the cytotoxic compounds. HT 29 cells were stained with acridine orange (AO) and propidium iodide (PI) to identify and quantify the viable cells versus cell death by apoptosis and necrosis and then observed under a fluorescence microscope after 24 h of exposure with the compounds. AO intercalates into DNA which gives a green fluorescence to the viable cells, while PI is only taken up by nonvisible cells which intercalate into the DNA and give an orange fluorescence. Apoptotic cells have an orange to red nucleus with condensed or fragmented chromatin. Necrotic cells display a uniform red nucleus with a condensed structure [26–28].

As shown in Figure 3, an intact nucleus and membrane for untreated HT 29 cells were observed with a bright green fluorescence at 24 h. The fluorescence produced from HT 29 cells after the addition of AO–PI was generally of a uniform bright green color. The uniform bright green fluorescence in the nucleus is possessed by living cells that still have intact cell membranes. The treated HT 29 cells showed a non-uniform fluorescence color, a mixture of green with yellow fluorescence, which indicated apoptosis, and reddish-orange fluorescence for cells undergoing necrosis [26].

The apoptotic cells were quantified (as shown in Table 3) by calculating the percentage of viable cells, apoptotic cells, and necrotic cells from a total of 200 cells observed under the fluorescence microscope. The quantification of apoptotic cells is described as the percentage of apoptotic cells within the overall cell population. Compound **1** was able to induce the apoptosis of HT 29 with an apoptotic percentage of 30.65%, while the necrotic percentage was only 4.81%. In parallel, compound **2** exhibited an apoptotic and necrotic percentage of 59.38 and 4.12%. However, in contrast, compound **4** showed a higher percentage of necrotic cells at 69.85% than the percentage of apoptotic cells at 4.80%. The observed difference between the percentage of apoptotic and necrotic cells was significant at $p < 0.05$. The tests results carried out on HT 29 cells with oxisterigmatocystins J (**1**) and K (**2**), which both contained a xanthone nucleus and bisfuran structure, indicated the activation of apoptosis. On the other hand, aspergicillin A (**4**), which is a peptide, could not stimulate apoptosis. Based on these structural differences, it can be concluded that the xanthones and bisfuran nuclei were essential structural moieties capable of activating programmed cell death.

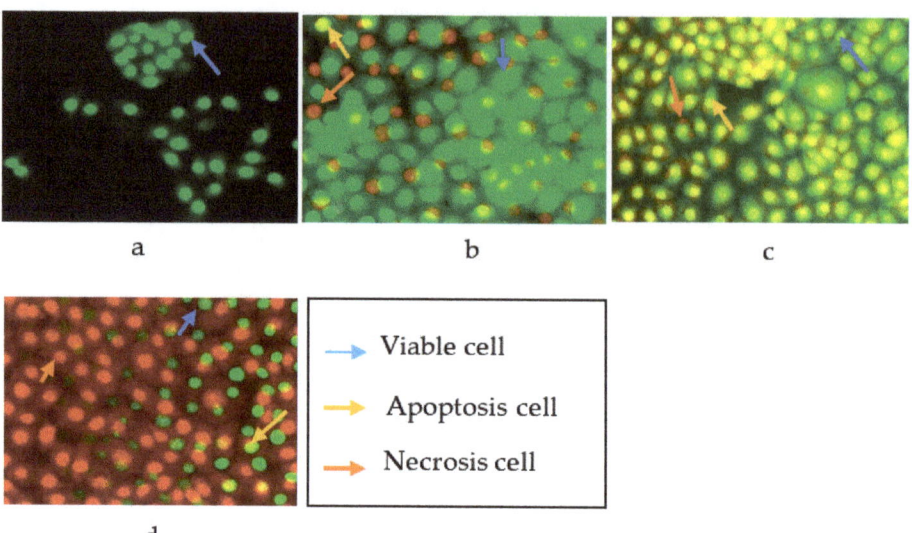

Figure 3. Cells after staining with AO–PI: (**a**) untreated HT 29 cells; (**b**) HT 29 cells treated with compound 1; (**c**) HT 29 cells treated with compound 2; (**d**) HT 29 cells treated with compound 4.

Table 3. Percentages of viable, apoptotic, and necrotic cells after treatment for 24 h.

Cytotoxic Compound	Viable Cell (%)	Apoptotic Cell (%)	Necrotic Cell (%)
1	64.53 ± 3.05	30.65 ± 3.22	4.81 ± 1.02
2	36.49 ± 4.08	59.38 ± 4.88	4.12 ± 1.37
4	25.24 ± 4.21	4.80 ± 0.98	69.95 ± 4.16

Data are shown as mean ± standard error (n = 3).

Some studies have reported that fungal cytotoxic compounds such as those explored by Yeh et al. (2009) from *Antrodia camphonata*, which included methyl antcinate, zhankuic acid A, and zhankuic acid C, promoted apoptosis of HT 29 cells at 41.7%, 32.7%, and 29.5%, respectively. Moreover, Schmelz et al. (1997) reported fumonisin B1 from *Fusarium moniliforme* that was able to activate the apoptosis of HT 29 cells at only 16% [29,30].

3. Conclusions

Chemical investigation of the EtOAc extract of the marine sponge-derived fungus *Aspergillus nomius* NC06 from Mandeh Island, West Sumatra, Indonesia, yielded four compounds, including three new oxisterigmatocystin congeners, namely, J (**1**), K (**2**), and L (**3**), along with one known compound, aspergillicin A (**4**). The bifuroxanthenone derivatives **1** and **2** with the peptide compound **4** were found to exhibit significant cytotoxicity against HT 29 colon cancer cell lines, with IC$_{50}$ values of 6.28, 15.14, and 1.63 µM, respectively. The difference in the activity of the three sterigmatocystin derivatives was probably due to a change in spatial conformation and/or the presence of a double bond on the bisfuran ring. There was a total loss of cytotoxicity in compound **3** with its β-configuration. However, the xanthones and bisfuran nuclei in compounds **1** and **2** were thought to play a vital role in inducing cell apoptosis, as demonstrated through a double staining method. In summary, this study reveals the cytotoxic activity of secondary metabolites from the marine-derived fungus *A. nomius* NC06.

4. Materials and Methods

4.1. General Procedures

The isolation of compounds from *A. nomius* NC06 involved several instruments including chromatographic methods consisting of both analytical and semipreparative HPLC, NMR spectroscopy, and ESIMS. HPLC analysis was carried out on a Dionex Ultimate 3000 system with a C_{18} column, 4.6 × 150 mm, 5 μm, mobile phase A: H_2O with 0.1% TFA; B: methanol, flow rate: 1 mL/min. Gradient elution from 0 to 35 min was 10–100% B, then washed at 100% B from 35 to 45 min and equilibrated back to 10% B from 46 to 60 min. Semipreparative HPLC was carried out with a Merck Hitachi Chromaster HPLC system. The chromatography method was conducted with silica gel 60 M for VLC and Sephadex LH-20 for column chromatography. The purity of the isolated compound was monitored by TLC using silica gel 60 F_{254} by using DCM and 5% MeOH as mobile phase. The 1D and 2D NMR spectra were recorded on a Bruker AVANCE DMX 600 NMR spectrometer. The chemical shifts (δ) were referenced to the residual solvent signals (DMSO-d_6: $δ_H$ 2.50/$δ_C$ 39.5). ESIMS spectra were acquired on a Finnigan LCQ Deca mass spectrometer. HRESIMS spectra were measured with a UHR-QTOF maXis 4G (Bruker Daltonics) mass spectrometer.

4.2. Fungal Isolation, Identification, and Cultivation

The fungus *A. nomius* NC06 was isolated from the marine sponge *N. chaliniformis*. The sponge was collected in December 2015 from Mandeh Island, West Sumatra, Indonesia. The fungal strain was characterized by molecular identification of the 18S rRNA region. The sequence data were submitted to the GenBank with accession no MN242781. The fungal strain was deposited in the Laboratory of Biota Sumatra, Andalas University, Padang, Indonesia. Fermentation of the strain was carried out in 20 Erlenmeyer flasks, each containing 100 g of sterile rice media. The culture was kept under static conditions for 4–8 weeks or until the fungal mycelia fully grew on top of media.

4.3. Extraction and Isolation

Overgrown *A. nomius* NC06 on rice was extracted with 300 mL ethyl acetate (EtOAc). The EtOAc extract was evaporated in vacuo to obtain the crude extract (25.7 g). The crude extract was subjected to liquid–liquid partitioning between n-hexane and aqueous MeOH containing 10% of H_2O. The MeOH extract (19.7 g) was subjected to vacuum liquid chromatography (VLC) on silica gel 60 by step gradient elution employing n-hexane, EtOAc, CH_2Cl_2, and MeOH to afford five fractions (F1 to F5). All fractions were screened for their cytotoxic activity against human colorectal adenocarcinoma (HT29) cells. Among the tested fractions, F3 eluted at EtOAc:DCM (1:1) showed the highest activity with an IC_{50} value of 2.59 μg/mL. F3 (3.95 g) was further chromatographed on silica gel 60 (VLC) by step gradient elution with n-hexane, EtOAc, CH_2Cl_2, and MeOH to yield 13 more subfractions (F3V1–F3V13). Compound **1** (7.23 mg) was obtained following the chromatographic purification of subfraction F3V7 on the Sephadex LH-20 column, which was eluted with CH_2Cl_2-MeOH (1:1 v/v), and final purification was achieved by semipreparative HPLC employing gradient elution with MeOH-H_2O from 35% to 100% MeOH. Similarly, compound **2** (7.72 mg) and compound **3** (3.13 mg) were also purified using the same mobile phase. Furthermore, F4 was chromatographed on a silica column by gradient elution using CH_2Cl_2 and MeOH to afford 9 fractions. Subfraction F4V9 (112 mg) was subjected to semipreparative HPLC employing MeOH-H_2O (from 35% to 100% MeOH) as a mobile phase to give compound **4** (52 mg). The structure of aspergillicin A was deduced by comparison of its spectral data from those found in the literature [31,32].

Oxisterigmatocystin J (1). Yellow amorphous solid; [α]20 °C—185 (*c* 0.05, CHCl$_3$); UV (MeOH, PDA): $λ_{max}$ 241.5 and 313.9 nm; ^{1}H and ^{13}C NMR data, see Table 1; HRESIMS *m/z* 355.0811 [M + H]$^+$ (calc. for $C_{19}H_{15}O_7$, 355.0812).

Oxisterigmatocystin K (2). Yellow amorphous solid; [α]20 °C—314 (*c* 0.05, CHCl$_3$); UV (MeOH, PDA): $λ_{max}$ 203.4, 237.5 and 314.3 nm; ^{1}H and ^{13}C NMR data, see Table 1; HRESIMS *m/z* 371.1127 [M + H]$^+$ (calc. for $C_{20}H_{19}O_7$, 371.1125).

Oxisterigmatocystin L (3). Yellow amorphous solid; [α]20 °C—181 (c 0.05, CHCl$_3$); UV (MeOH, PDA): λ$_{max}$ 202.9, 237.4 and 312.0 nm; ^{1}H and ^{13}C NMR data, see Table 1; HRESIMS m/z 371.1128 [M + H]$^+$ (calc. for C$_{20}$H$_{19}$O$_7$, 371.1125).

4.4. Mosher Ester Analysis of 1

Mosher's method for compound **1** was adopted from a previously described procedure [28]. Two vials each containing (1.0 mg, 2.8 µmol) of compound **1** were each dissolved in 100 µL pyridine-d5. Each solution was transferred to an NMR tube. To the first solution, 10 µL (R)-MTPA-Cl (53.4 µmol) was added, while 10 µL (S)-MTPA-Cl (53.4 µmol) was added to the second solution. Both solutions were kept at room temperature for 3 h. Afterward, 500 µL of pyridine-d5 was added to each solution. ^{1}H NMR spectra for both (S)- and (R)-MTPA ester derivatives were measured.

4.5. Cytotoxic Assay

All isolated compounds were tested against the HT29 colon cancer cell line by using the MTT method. This cell line was obtained from the Laboratory of Biotechnology and Cell Culture Pharmacy Faculty, International Islamic University Malaysia. HT29 was cultured by using DMEM Gibco^{TM} (high glucose). Cells were seeded in 96-well plates (density: 6×10^3 cells/well) and incubated at 37 °C, 98% relative humidity, with 5% CO$_2$, for 3 days. After cells were confluent in each well (70–80% confluent), compounds **1–4** were added to their respective wells with a concentration of 100, 10, 1, and 0.1 µg/mL. Then, 100 µL MTT (5 mg/mL) was added to each well and incubated for 4 h. Tecan Microplate was used for measuring the absorbance of the cells at 560 nm after treatment with all isolated compounds. DMSO was used for negative control and taxol was used for positive control.

4.6. Antibacterial Activity

Antibacterial activity was assessed by following the prototype of Balouiri et al. (2016) [32]. *E. coli* ATCC 25,922 and *S. aureus* ATCC 2592 were used as bacterial pathogens. Briefly, a paper disk (6 mm) was soaked with 10 µg/mL of all isolated compounds, **1–4**. Meanwhile, DMSO was used as negative control and 30 µg/disc chloramphenicol was used as a positive control. The diameter of the zone (mm) of inhibition was measured after incubation for 24 h.

4.7. Apoptotic Cells Using AO–PI Double Staining

Acridine orange (AO) and propidium iodide (PI) were used for quantifying viable, apoptotic, and necrotic cells of HT 29. The double staining method was a standard procedure and examined under a fluorescence microscope. As many as 1×10^5 cells in 4 mL were seeded in a T25 cm^3 flask. After 24 h of incubation, the medium in each well was removed and replaced with the IC$_{50}$ concentrations of compounds **1–2** and **4** (6.28, 15.14, 1.63 µg/mL) as treated cells, and untreated cells were cells without any treatment. Once the cytotoxic compound was added to the medium, the cells were incubated at 37 °C, 98% relative humidity, with 5% CO$_2$, for 24 h. After 24 h incubation, the cells were washed with 1 mL PBS. The cells were then trypsinized and centrifuged at 1000× *g* rpm for 5 min. The AO–PI double stain was dissolved with PBS and then added to the cell pellet for the staining step. The suspension (50 µL) of stained cells was dropped onto a glass slide and covered with a coverslip. The observation was conducted with a fluorescence microscope at 400 magnification within 30 min before the fluorescence faded. Viable, apoptotic, and necrotic cells were quantified in a population of 200 cells. The results were expressed as a proportion of the total number of the cells examined [26].

Supplementary Materials: The following are available online at https://www.mdpi.com/article/10.3390/md19110631/s1, Figures S1–S22: EIMS, and 1D and 2D NMR for compounds **1–4**; Figure S23: Phylogenetic tree of strain MN242781.1.

Author Contributions: Conceptualization, M.A.A., Y.Y., A.D. and D.H.; methodology, M.A.A., Y.Y., A.D. and D.H.; software, M.A.A., D.H., M.T. and N.P.A.; validation, M.A.A., Y.Y., A.D., D.H., M.T., N.P.A. and R.A.E.-E.; formal analysis, M.A.A., Y.Y., A.D., D.H. and N.P.A.; investigation, M.A.A., D.H., M.T. and N.P.A.; resources, D.H., M.T. and R.A.E.-E., data curation, M.A.A. and D.H.; writing—original draft preparation, M.A.A., D.H. and N.P.A.; writing—review and editing, M.A.A., D.H., N.P.A. and R.A.E.-E.; visualization, M.A.A., M.T. and N.P.A.; supervision, D.H., Y.Y., A.D. and R.A.E.-E.; project administration, M.A.A. and D.H.; funding acquisition, D.H. All authors have read and agreed to the published version of the manuscript.

Funding: This research was funded by The Ministry of Research and Technology, Indonesia, through PMDSU Research, 059/SP2H/LT/DRPM/IV/2016-2018, and the Directorate General of Higher Education, Ministry of Education and Culture, Indonesia, with project name Fundamental Research, number T/20/UN.16.17/PT.01.03/AMD/PD-Kesehatan/2020.

Institutional Review Board Statement: Not applicable.

Informed Consent Statement: Not applicable.

Data Availability Statement: Data are contained within the article or Supplementary Material.

Acknowledgments: Muh. Ade Artasasta and Dian Handayani acknowledge the help of the Institute of Pharmaceutical Biology and Biotechnology, Heinrich-Heine University, for purification and structure elucidation of compounds 1–4. Muh. Ade Artasasta and Dian Handayani wish to express their sincere gratitude to their supervisor, Peter Proksch, for his invaluable trust and support.

Conflicts of Interest: The authors declare no conflict of interest.

References

1. Liu, S.; Wang, H.; Su, M.; Hwang, G.J.; Hong, J.; Jung, J.H. New metabolites from the sponge-derived fungus *Aspergillus sydowii* J05B-7F-4. *Nat. Prod. Res.* **2017**, *31*, 1682–1686. [CrossRef]
2. Pang, X.; Lin, X.; Tian, Y.; Liang, R.; Wang, J.; Yang, B.; Zhou, X.; Kaliyaperumal, K.; Luo, X.; Tu, Z.; et al. Three new polyketides from the marine sponge-derived fungus *Trichoderma* sp. SCSIO41004. *Nat. Prod. Res.* **2018**, *32*, 105–111. [CrossRef] [PubMed]
3. Jia, Q.; Du, Y.; Wang, C.; Wang, Y.; Zhu, T.; Zhu, W. Azaphilones from the Marine Sponge-Derived Fungus *Penicillium sclerotiorum* OUCMDZ-3839. *Mar. Drugs* **2019**, *17*, 260. [CrossRef] [PubMed]
4. Sun, Y.; Liu, J.; Li, L.; Gong, C.; Wang, S.; Yang, F.; Hua, H.; Lin, H. New butenolide derivatives from the marine sponge-derived fungus *Aspergillus terreus*. *Bioorg. Med. Chem. Lett.* **2018**, *28*, 315–318. [CrossRef] [PubMed]
5. Yamada, T.; Fujii, A.; Kikuchi, T. New Diterpenes with a Fused 6-5-6-6 Ring System Isolated from the Marine Sponge-Derived Fungus *Trichoderma harzianum*. *Mar. Drugs* **2019**, *17*, 480. [CrossRef]
6. Pang, X.; Cai, G.; Lin, X.; Salendra, L.; Zhou, X.; Yang, B.; Wang, J.; Wang, J.; Xu, S.; Liu, Y. New Alkaloids and Polyketides from the Marine Sponge-Derived Fungus *Penicillium* sp. SCSIO41015. *Mar. Drugs* **2019**, *17*, 398. [CrossRef]
7. Elissawy, A.M.; Ebada, S.S.; Ashour, M.L.; Özkaya, F.C.; Ebrahim, W.; Singab, A.B.; Proksch, P. Spiroarthrinols a and B, two novel meroterpenoids isolated from the sponge-derived fungus *Arthrinium* sp. *Phytochem. Lett.* **2017**, *20*, 246–251. [CrossRef]
8. Ma, H.G.; Liu, Q.; Zhu, G.L.; Liu, H.S.; Zhu, W.M. Marine natural products sourced from marine-derived *Penicillium* fungi. *J. Asian Nat. Prod. Res.* **2016**, *18*, 92–115. [CrossRef]
9. Lei, H.; Lei, J.; Zhou, X.; Hu, M.; Niu, H.; Song, C.; Chen, S.; Liu, Y.; Zhang, D. Cytotoxic Polyketides from the Marine Sponge-Derived Fungus *Pestalotiopsis heterocornis* XWS03F09. *Molecules* **2019**, *24*, 2655. [CrossRef]
10. Li, Y.; Liu, D.; Cheng, Z.; Proksch, P.; Lin, W. Cytotoxic trichothecene-type sesquiterpenes from the sponge-derived fungus *Stachybotrys chartarum* with tyrosine kinase inhibition. *RSC Adv.* **2017**, *7*, 7259–7267. [CrossRef]
11. Shah, M.; Sun, C.; Sun, Z.; Zhang, G.; Che, Q.; Gu, Q.; Zhu, T.; Li, D. Antibacterial Polyketides from Antarctica Sponge-Derived Fungus *Penicillium* sp. HDN151272. *Mar. Drugs* **2020**, *18*, 71. [CrossRef]
12. Zhang, L.; Qiu, P.; Ding, L.; Li, Q.; Song, J.; Han, Z.; He, S. A New Antibacterial Chlorinated Amino Acid Derivative from the Sponge-Derived Fungus *Aspergillus* sp. LS53. *Chem. Nat. Compd.* **2020**, *56*, 109–111. [CrossRef]
13. Liu, Y.; Ding, L.; Fang, F.; He, S. Penicillilactone A, a novel antibacterial 7-membered lactone derivative from the sponge-associated fungus *Penicillium* sp. LS54. *Nat. Prod. Res.* **2019**, *33*, 2466–2470. [CrossRef]
14. Artasasta, M.A.; Taher, M.; Djamaan, A.; Handayani, D. Cytotoxic and Antibacterial Activities of Marine Sponge-Derived Fungus *Aspergillus Nomius* NC06. *Rasayan J. Chem.* **2019**, *12*, 1463–1469. [CrossRef]
15. Artasasta, M.A.; Djamaan, A.; Handayani, D. Cytotoxic activity screening of ethyl acetate fungal extracts derived from the marine sponge *Neopetrosia chaliniformis* AR-01. *J. Appl. Pharm. Sci.* **2017**, *7*, 174–178. [CrossRef]
16. Lee, Y.M.; Li, H.; Hong, J.; Cho, H.Y.; Bae, K.S.; Kim, M.A.; Kim, D.K.; Jung, J.H. Bioactive metabolites from the sponge-derived fungus *Aspergillus versicolor*. *Arch. Pharm. Res.* **2010**, *33*, 231–235. [CrossRef]
17. Tian, Y.Q.; Lin, X.P.; Wang, Z.; Zhou, X.F.; Qin, X.C.; Kaliyaperumal, K.; Zhang, T.Y.; Tu, Z.C.; Liu, Y. Asteltoxins with Antiviral Activities from the Marine Sponge-Derived Fungus *Aspergillus* sp. SCSIO XWS02F40. *Molecules* **2015**, *21*, 34. [CrossRef]

18. Cai, S.; Zhu, T.; Du, L.; Zhao, B.; Li, D.; Gu, Q. Sterigmatocystins from the deep-sea-derived fungus *Aspergillus versicolor*. *J. Antibiot.* **2011**, *64*, 193–196. [CrossRef]
19. Zhao, H.; Wang, G.-Q.; Tong, X.-P.; Chen, G.-D.; Huang, Y.-F.; Cui, J.-Y.; Kong, M.-Z.; Guo, L.-D.; Zheng, Y.-Z.; Yao, X.-S.; et al. Diphenyl ethers from *Aspergillus* sp. and their anti-Aβ42 aggregation activities. *Fitoterapia* **2014**, *98*, 77–83. [CrossRef] [PubMed]
20. Rajachan, O.A.; Kanokmedhakul, K.; Soytong, K.; Kanokmedhakul, S. Mycotoxins from the Fungus *Botryotrichum piluliferum*. *J. Agric. Food Chem.* **2017**, *65*, 1337–1341. [CrossRef] [PubMed]
21. Tian, Y.-Q.; Lin, S.-T.; Kumaravel, K.; Zhou, H.; Wang, S.-Y.; Liu, Y.-H. Polyketide-derived metabolites from the sponge-derived fungus Aspergillus sp. F40. *Phytochem. Lett.* **2018**, *27*, 74–77. [CrossRef]
22. Capon, R.J.; Skene, C.; Stewart, M.; Ford, J.; O'Hair, R.A.J.; Williams, L.; Lacey, E.; Gill, J.H.; Heiland, K.; Friedel, T. Aspergillicins A–E: Five novel depsipeptides from the marine-derived fungus *Aspergillus carneus*. *Org. Biomol. Chem.* **2003**, *1*, 1856–1862. [CrossRef]
23. Gouda, H.; Sunazuka, T.; Ui, H.; Handa, M.; Sakoh, Y.; Iwai, Y.; Hirono, S.; Omura, S. Stereostructure of luminamicin, an anaerobic antibiotic, via molecular dynamics, NMR spectroscopy, and the modified Mosher method. *Proc. Natl. Acad. Sci. USA* **2005**, *102*, 18286–18291. [CrossRef] [PubMed]
24. Ashley, D.L.; Orti, D.L.; Hill, R.H. Proton nuclear magnetic resonance evidence for two configurations of the hemiacetals of aflatoxin B1 and sterigmatocystin. *J. Agric. Food Chem.* **1987**, *35*, 782–785. [CrossRef]
25. Li, J.; Xie, S.; Ahmed, S.; Wang, F.; Gu, Y.; Zhang, C.; Chai, X.; Wu, Y.; Cai, J.; Cheng, G. Antimicrobial Activity and Resistance: Influencing Factors. *Front. Pharm.* **2017**, *8*, 364. [CrossRef] [PubMed]
26. Baharuddin, A.A.; Roosli, R.A.J.; Zakaria, Z.A.; Md Tohid, S.F. Dicranopteris linearis extract inhibits the proliferation of human breast cancer cell line (MDA-MB-231) via induction of S-phase arrest and apoptosis. *Pharm. Biol.* **2018**, *56*, 422–432. [CrossRef]
27. Gerl, R.; Vaux, D.L. Apoptosis in the development and treatment of cancer. *Carcinogenesis* **2005**, *26*, 263–270. [CrossRef] [PubMed]
28. Alabsi, A.M.; Ali, R.; Ali, A.M.; Al-Dubai, S.A.; Harun, H.; Abu Kasim, N.H.; Alsalahi, A. Apoptosis induction, cell cycle arrest and in vitro anticancer activity of gonothalamin in a cancer cell lines. *Asian Pac. J. Cancer Prev.* **2012**, *13*, 5131–5136. [CrossRef]
29. Yeh, C.T.; Rao, Y.K.; Yao, C.J.; Yeh, C.F.; Li, C.H.; Chuang, S.E.; Luong, J.H.; Lai, G.M.; Tzeng, Y.M. Cytotoxic triterpenes from *Antrodia camphorata* and their mode of action in HT-29 human colon cancer cells. *Cancer Lett.* **2009**, *285*, 73–79. [CrossRef]
30. Schmelz, E.M.; Dombrink-Kurtzman, M.A.; Roberts, P.C.; Kozutsumi, Y.; Kawasaki, T.; Merrill, A.H., Jr. Induction of apoptosis by fumonisin B1 in HT29 cells is mediated by the accumulation of endogenous free sphingoid bases. *Toxicol. Appl. Pharmacol.* **1998**, *148*, 252–260. [CrossRef]
31. Kikuchi, H.; Hoshikawa, T.; Fujimura, S.; Sakata, N.; Kurata, S.; Katou, Y.; Oshima, Y. Isolation of a Cyclic Depsipetide, Aspergillicin F, and Synthesis of Aspergillicins with Innate Immune-Modulating Activity. *J. Nat. Prod.* **2015**, *78*, 1949–1956. [CrossRef] [PubMed]
32. Balouiri, M.; Sadiki, M.; Ibnsouda, S.K. Methods for in vitro evaluating antimicrobial activity: A review. *J. Pharm. Anal.* **2016**, *6*, 71–79. [CrossRef] [PubMed]

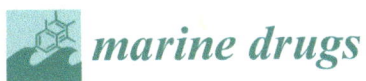

Article

Chemical Constituents of the Deep-Sea-Derived *Penicillium solitum*

Zhi-Hui He [1,†], Jia Wu [2,†], Lin Xu [1], Man-Yi Hu [1], Ming-Ming Xie [1], You-Jia Hao [1], Shu-Jin Li [1], Zong-Ze Shao [1] and Xian-Wen Yang [1,*]

[1] Key Laboratory of Marine Biogenetic Resources, Third Institute of Oceanography, Ministry of Natural Resources, 184 Daxue Road, Xiamen 361005, China; hezhihui@tio.org.cn (Z.-H.H.); xulin@tio.org.cn (L.X.); humanyi@tio.org.cn (M.-Y.H.); xiemingmin@tio.org.cn (M.-M.X.); haoyoujia888@163.com (Y.-J.H.); lishujin98@163.com (S.-J.L.); shaozongze@tio.org.cn (Z.-Z.S.)

[2] Yanjing Medical College, Capital Medical University, 4 Dadong Road, Beijing 101300, China; wujia@ccmu.edu.cn

* Correspondence: yangxianwen@tio.org.cn; Tel.: +86-592-219-5319

† These authors contributed equally to this work.

Abstract: A systematic chemical investigation of the deep-sea-derived fungus *Penicillium solitum* MCCC 3A00215 resulted in the isolation of one novel polyketide (**1**), two new alkaloids (**2** and **3**), and 22 known (**4–25**) compounds. The structures of the new compounds were established mainly on the basis of exhaustive analysis of 1D and 2D NMR data. Viridicatol (**13**) displayed moderate anti-tumor activities against PANC-1, Hela, and A549 cells with IC_{50} values of around 20 µM. Moreover, **13** displayed potent in vitro anti-food allergic activity with an IC_{50} value of 13 µM, compared to that of 92 µM for the positive control, loratadine, while indole-3-acetic acid methyl ester (**9**) and penicopeptide A (**10**) showed moderate effects (IC_{50} = 50 and 58 µM, respectively).

Keywords: deep-sea; fungus; *Penicillium solitum*; anti-tumor; anti-food allergy

1. Introduction

Penicillium solitum is a filamentous fungus associated with the decay of pomaceous fruits during storage [1]. As a matter of fact, it can infect fruit through wounds and cause significant economic losses [2]. Besides pome fruits such as apples and pears, this fungus was also isolated from other foods, including cheeses and processed meats [3,4]. Surprisingly, it can also be found under extremophilic circumstances: in the Berkeley Pit Lake (pH 2.7) [5] and the maritime Antarctic [6]. Chemical investigation of this fungus provided a broad spectrum of secondary metabolites, including compactin (known as mevastatin or ML-236B, which is utilized for the production of an important cholesterol-lowering drug, pravastatin) [7] and its analogues [8,9], in addition to sesquiterpenoids [5], alkaloids [10], and polyketides etc. [11].

Penicillium solitum MCCC 3A00215 is a deep-sea-derived fungus from the Northwest Atlantic Ocean (−3034 m). A previous study on this strain provided a unique 6/6/6/6/5-pentacyclic steroid [12]. In order to discover more novel compounds, a further chemical investigation was conducted. As a result, three new (**1–3**) and 22 known (**4–25**) compounds (Figure 1) were obtained. By comparison of the NMR and MS data with those published in the literature, the known compounds were determined to be (−)-solitumidines D (**4**) [10], ML-236A (**5**) [13], solitumidine A (**6**) [10], methyl-2-([2-(1H-indol-3-yl)-ethyl]carbamoyl)acetate (**7**) [14], solitumine A (**8**) [10], indole-3-acetic acid methyl ester (**9**) [15], penicopeptide A (**10**) [16], (2′S)-7-hydroxy-2-(2-hydroxypropyl)-5-methylchromone (**11**) [17], hydroxypropan-2′,3′-diol orsellinate (**12**) [18], viridicatol (**13**) [19], viridicatin (**14**) [19], (−)-cyclopenol (**15**) [20], cyclopenin (**16**) [21], 3-benzylidene-3,4-dihydro-4-methyl-1H-1,4-benzodiazepine-2,5-dione (**17**) [16], β-sitosterol-3-O-β-D-glucopyranoside (**18**) [22], cerebrosides C (**19**) [23], methyl-2,4-dihydroxy-3,5,6-trimethylbenzoate (**20**) [24], felinone

A (**21**) [25], xylariphilone (**22**) [26], 5,6-dihydroxy-2,3,6-trimethylcyclohex-2-enone (**23**) [27], (*R*)-mevalonolactone (**24**) [28], and 3-methyl-2-penten-5-olide (**25**) [29]. Here, we report the isolation, structure, and bioactivities of these 25 compounds.

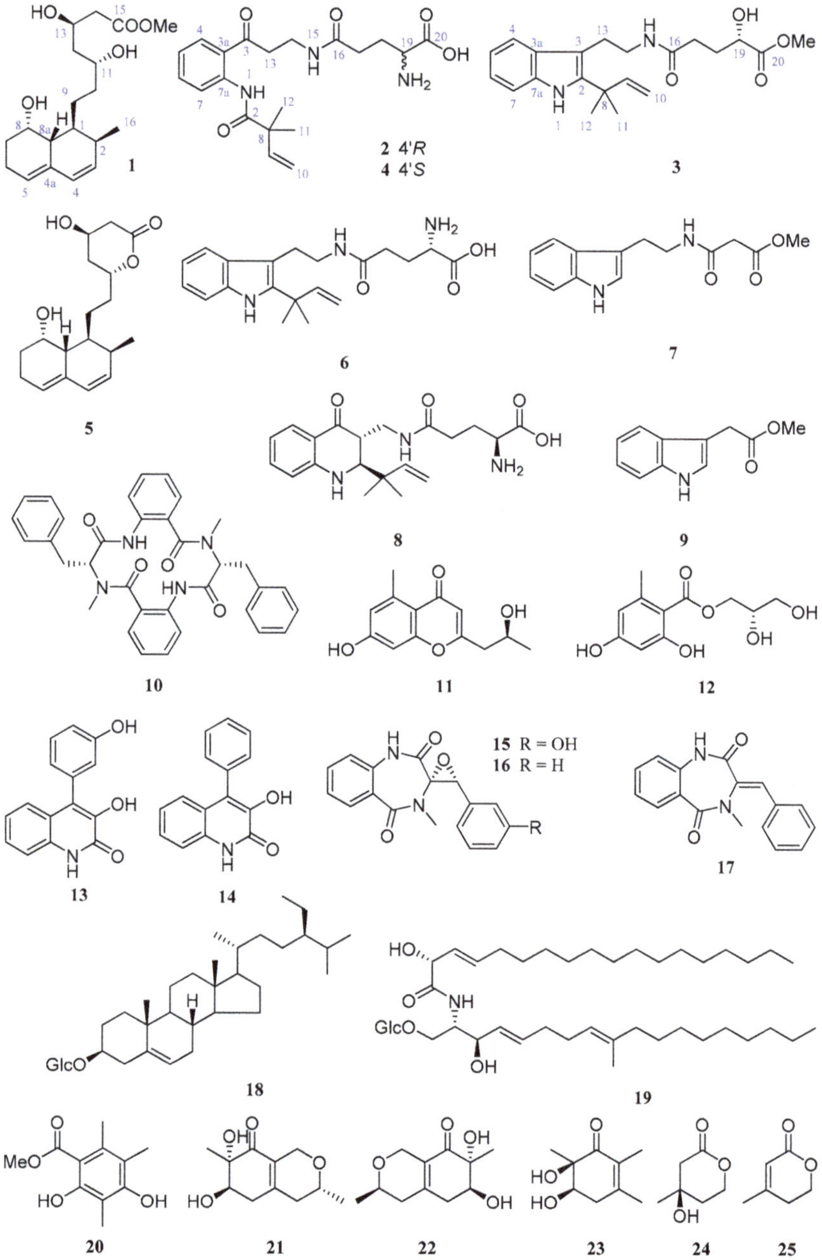

Figure 1. Compounds **1–25** from *Penicillium solitum* MCCC 3A00215.

2. Results and Discussion

Compound **1** had a molecular formula $C_{19}H_{30}O_5$, as established by its positive HRES-IMS at m/z 361.1989 [M + Na]$^+$, requiring five degrees of unsaturation. The ^{1}H and ^{13}C NMR spectroscopic data (Figures S1 and S2 from the Supplementary Materials, Table 1) revealed the presence of one methyl doublet [δ_H 0.89 (d, J = 6.8 Hz, H$_3$-16); δ_C 14.3 (q, C-16)], one methoxyl [δ_H 3.70 (s, OMe); δ_C 52.1 (q, OMe)], six sp^3 methylenes, nine methines including three aliphatic [δ_H 1.77 (m, H-1), 2.19 (brd, J = 11.8 Hz, H-8a), 2.37 (m, H-2); δ_C 32.1 (d, C-2), 37.8 (d, C-1), 40.0 (d, C-8a)], three olefinic [δ_H 5.47 (brs, H-5), 5.69 (dd, J = 9.4, 6.1 Hz, H-3), 5.91 (d, J = 9.4 Hz, H-4); δ_C 124.5 (d, C-5), 129.9 (d, C-4), 133.6 (d, C-3)] and three oxygenated [δ_H 3.80 (m, H-11), 4.19 (m, H-13), 4.22 (m, H-8); δ_C 65.2 (d, C-8), 68.1 (d, C-13), 71.1 (d, C-11)] ones, and two non-protonated carbons with one olefinic [δ_C 135.1 (s, C-4a)] and one carbonyl [δ_C 173.9 (s, C-15)] group. Altogether, the ^{1}H and ^{13}C NMR spectra provided 19 carbons, categorized as one methyl, one methoxyl, six methylenes, nine methines, and two quaternary carbons.

Table 1. ^{1}H (400 Hz) and ^{13}C (100 Hz) NMR data of **1–3** (δ in ppm, J in Hz within parentheses).

No.	1 [a] δ_C	1 [a] δ_H	2 [b] δ_C	2 [b] δ_H	3 [a] δ_C	3 [a] δ_H
1	37.8 CH	1.77 m		11.5 s		
2	32.1 CH	2.37 m	174.8 C		141.3 C	
3	133.6 CH	5.69 (dd, 9.4, 6.1)	203.2 C		108.4 C	
3a			139.9 C		130.8 C	
4	129.9 CH	5.91 (d, 9.4)	131.4 CH	8.04 (d, 7.8)	118.7 CH	7.49 (d, 7.9)
4a	135.1 C					
5	124.5 CH	5.47 (brs)	122.8 CH	7.19 (t, 7.8)	119.5 CH	6.95 (t, 7.9)
6	21.6 CH$_2$	2.09 m, 2.33 m	134.5 CH	7.60 (t, 7.8)	121.7 CH	7.01 (t, 7.9)
7	30.6 CH$_2$	1.68 m, 1.96 m	120.1 CH	8.54 (d, 7.8)	111.6 CH	7.28 (d, 7.9)
7a			122.6 C		136.4 C	
8	65.2 CH	4.22 m	46.2 C		40.1 C	
8a	40.0 CH	2.19 (brd, 11.8)				
9	25.0 CH$_2$	1.33 m, 1.83 m	142.4 CH	6.08 (dd, 17.4, 10.6)	147.8 CH	6.18 (dd, 17.4, 10.6)
10	35.5 CH$_2$	1.41 m; 1.54 m	114.6 CH$_2$	5.25 (d, 17.4); 5.29 (d, 10.6)	111.7 CH$_2$	5.06 (dd, 17.4, 1.5); 5.09 (dd, 10.6, 1.5)
11	71.1 CH	3.80 m	24.5 CH$_3$	1.32 s	28.5 CH$_3$	1.54 s
12	44.8 CH$_2$	1.64 m	24.5 CH$_3$	1.32 s	28.5 CH$_3$	1.54 s
13	68.1 CH	4.19 m	39.3 CH$_2$	3.22 (t, 6.6)	26.3 CH$_2$	2.99 (dd, 8.2, 7.6)
14	43.1 CH$_2$	2.46 m, 2.57 m	34.6 CH$_2$	3.37 m	41.6 CH$_2$	3.36 (dd, 9.9, 7.6)
15	173.9 C			8.16 (t, 4.9)		
16	14.3 CH$_3$	0.89 (d, 6.8)	172.1 C		175.1 C	
17			31.8 CH$_2$	2.23 m	32.6 CH$_2$	2.27 (ddd, 11.0, 8.5, 8.0) 2.29 (ddd, 11.0, 6.4, 4.4)
18			27.0 CH$_2$	1.77–1.95 m	31.2 CH$_2$	1.88 (ddt, 14.3, 8.5, 6.4) 2.06 (ddt, 14.3, 8.0, 4.4)
19			53.7 CH	3.19 m	71.0 CH	4.16 (dd, 8.0, 4.4)
20			169.6 C		176.0 C	
OMe	52.1 CH$_3$	3.70 s			52.5 CH$_3$	3.73 s

[a] Recorded in CD$_3$OD. [b] Recorded in DMSO-d_6.

In the COSY spectrum, correlations were observed for H-5/H$_2$-6/H$_2$-7/H-8/H-8a/H-1/H$_2$-9/H$_2$-10/H-11/H$_2$-12/H-13/H$_2$-14 and H-1/H-2/H$_3$-16/H-3/H-4, which constructed a long chain of C-5/C-6/C-7/C-8/C-8a/C-1/C-9/C-10/C-11/C-12/C-13/C-14 and C-1 via C-2 to C-16/C-3/C-4 (Figure 2). The segment and the methoxyl moiety could be connected on the basis of the HMBC correlations of H-4 to C-8a/C-4a/C-5, H$_2$-14 and 15-OMe to C-15 (Figure 2). Therefore, the planar structure of **1** was established as a methyl ester of acyclic form of ML-236A (**5**) [13], which was previously prepared in the lab by the saponification of ML-236A in 0.1 N NaOH at 50 °C for 2 h [30].

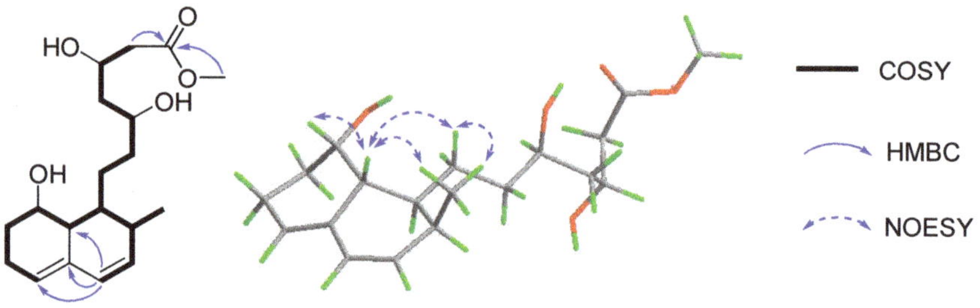

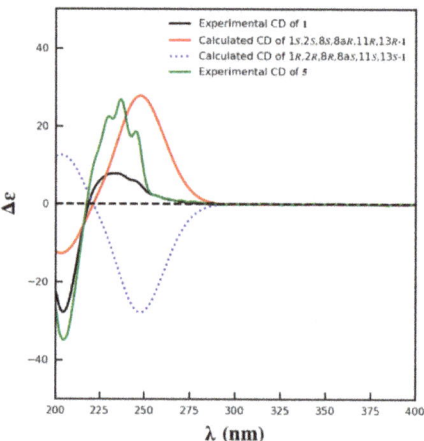

Figure 2. The key COSY, HMBC, and NOESY correlations of **1**.

The relative configuration of **1** was supposed to be the same as that of **5**, according to the NOESY correlations of H-8a to H-8/H-9a/H$_3$-16 and H$_3$-16 to H$_2$-9. On the basis of the similar optical rotation values of **1** (+62.7) and **5** (+73.3), and further by comparison of their electronic circular dichroism (ECD) spectrum (Figure 3), **1** was then established to be 15-*O*-methyl ML-236A.

Figure 3. The calculated ECD spectrum of **1** and the experimental ECD spectra of **1** and **5**.

Compound **2** was assigned the molecular formula $C_{20}H_{27}N_3O_5$ on the basis of the [M − H]$^-$ ionic peak at *m/z* 388.2821 in its negative HRESIMS spectrum, suggesting nine degrees of unsaturation. The ^{1}H and ^{13}C NMR spectroscopic data, by the aide of the HSQC and ^{1}H–^{1}H COSY spectra, showed characteristics of a 1,2-disubsituted benzoic unit [$δ_H$ 7.19 (t, *J* = 7.8 Hz, H-5), 7.60 (t, *J* = 7.8 Hz, H-6), 8.04 (t, *J* = 7.8 Hz, H-4), 8.54 (t, *J* = 7.8 Hz, H-7); $δ_C$ 120.1 (d, C-7), 122.6 (s, C-7a), 122.8 (d, C-5), 131.4 (d, C-4), 134.5 (d, C-6), 139.9 (s, C-3a)], an isoprene [$δ_H$ 1.32 (s × 2, C-11, 12), 5.25 (d, *J* = 17.4 Hz, H-10a), 5.29 (d, *J* = 10.6 Hz, H-10b), 6.08 (d, *J* = 17.4, 10.6 Hz); $δ_C$ 24.5 (q × 2, C-11, 12), 46.2 (s, C-8), 114.6 (t, C-10), 142.4 (d, C-9)], glutamic acid [$δ_H$ 1.77−1.95 (m, H$_2$-18), 2.23 (m, H$_2$-17), 3.19 (m, H-19); $δ_C$ 27.0 (t, C-18), 31.8 (t, C-17), 53.7 (d, C-19), 169.6 (s, C-20), 172.1 (s, C-16)], β-aminopropanone [$δ_H$ 3.22 (t, *J* = 6.6 Hz, H$_2$-13), 3.37 (m, H$_2$-14), 8.16 (t, *J* = 4.9 Hz, H-15); $δ_C$ 34.6 (t, C-14), 39.3 (t, C-13), 203.2 (s, C-3)], and one acylamide [$δ_H$ 11.5 (s, H-1); $δ_C$ 174.8 (s, C-2)]. These five fragments could be connected by the HMBC correlations of H$_3$-11/H$_3$-12 to C-2, H-1 to C-2/C-3a/C-7/C-7a, H$_2$-4 to C-3, and H-14 to C-16 to construct the planar structure of **2** (Figure 4), the same as solitumidine D [10], namely **4**, which was simultaneously obtained along with **2** by HPLC using the A4-5 chiral column. Since the specific optical rotation of **2** was +6, opposite to that of **4** (−7) in the same concentration of MeOH (*c* 0.10), **2** was then deduced to be the enantiomer of **4**. Accordingly, **2** was determined as (+)-solitumidine D.

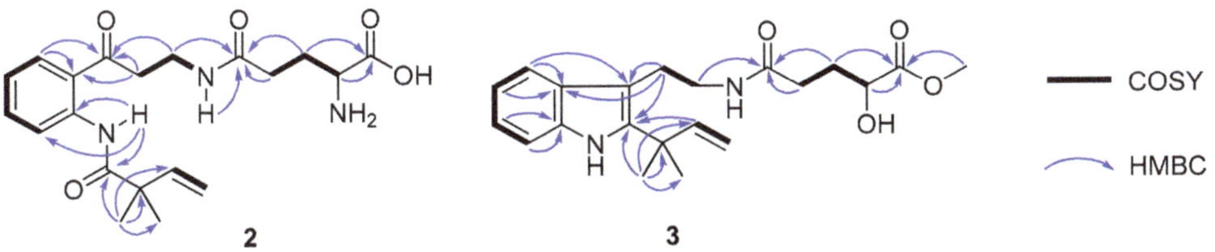

Figure 4. Key ^{1}H–^{1}H COSY and HMBC correlations of **2** and **3**.

Compound **3** presented its molecular formula as $C_{21}H_{28}N_2O_4$ by the positive HRESIMS at m/z 395.1947 [M + Na]$^+$. The ^{1}H and ^{13}C NMR spectra consisted of signals almost the same as those of solitumidine B [10] except for an additional methoxyl unit. This was confirmed by the HMBC correlation of 20-OMe (δ_H 3.73, s) to C-20 (δ_C 176.0, s). Furthermore, by extensive analysis of the COSY and HMBC NMR spectra (Figure 4), **3** was determined as 20-O-methyl solitumidine B. Since the optical rotation value for solitumidine B was −55 in MeOH, while it was 0 for **3** in the same solvent, **3** was supposed to be a racemic mixture. As such, it was subjected to further isolation by HPLC with chiral columns. Yet, **3** seemed to be inseparable as it exhibited only one peak using several different mobile phases in A3-5 and A4-5 chiral columns, the latter of which was utilized to successfully isolate **2** from its enantiomer, **4**. On the basis of the above evidence, **3** was then named as (±)-solitumidine E.

All isolates were tested for antiproliferative effect against 17 human tumor cell lines of A431, A549, MB231, MCF-7, PANC1, HepG2, HCT116, H460, H1299, QGY-7701, BGC823, SKGT4, A375, U2OS, HL-60, K562, and KYSE450 under the concentration of 20 µM and were tested for anti-food allergic activity under the concentration of 50 µM. Notably, viridicatol (**13**) showed significant cytotoxic activities against PANC1, Hela and A549 cells with IC$_{50}$ values of 18, 19, and 24 µM, respectively.

Moreover, compounds **1–25** were also tested in vitro for anti-food allergic activity. Indole-3-acetic acid methyl ester (**9**) and penicopeptide A (**10**) showed modest activity (IC$_{50}$ = 50 and 58 µM, respectively), while **13** displayed a potent effect with an IC$_{50}$ value of 13 µM, compared to that of 92 µM for loratadine, an anti-food allergic medicine in clinic. In fact, viridicatol isolated from another deep-sea-derived fungus, *Penicillium griseofulvum* MCCC 3A00225, showed a significant anti-food allergic effect in the RBL-2H3 cell model and the ovalbumin-induced food allergy mouse [31]. Therefore, it may represent a novel therapeutic for allergic diseases.

3. Materials and Methods

3.1. General Experimental Procedures

NMR spectra were recorded on a Bruker 400 MHz spectrometer. The HRESIMS spectra were recorded on a Waters Q-TOF mass spectrometer (Xevo G2). Optical rotations were obtained with an Anton Paar polarimeter (MCP100). ECD spectra were measured on a Chirascan spectrometer. The semi-preparative HPLC was conducted on an Agilent instrument (1260) with different kinds of columns (COSMOSIL 5 C18-MS-II, Nacalai Tesque, Japan; ColumnTek^{TM} Chiral A3-5 and A4-5). Column chromatography was performed on silica gel, Sephadex LH-20, and ODS.

3.2. Fungal Identification, Fermentation, and Extract

The fungus *Penicillium solitum* MCCC 3A00215 was isolated from a sediment sample of the Northwest Atlantic Ocean (−3034 m, W 44.9801°, N 14.7532°). For the large-scale fermentation procedure, see our recently published literature [12]. The crude extract (200 g) was subjected to column chromatography on silica gel using petroleum ether (PE), CH_2Cl_2, EtOAc to provide a CH_2Cl_2-soluble extract (11 g) and a EtOAc-soluble extract (114.5 g), respectively.

3.3. Isolation and Purification

The CH$_2$Cl$_2$ crude extract was separated into six fractions (Fr.A−Fr.F) via medium pressure liquid chromatography (MPLC, 460 mm × 36 mm) with gradient PE-EtOAc (5:1→1:5). Subfractions Fr.B-Fr.F were subsequently purified by column chromatography (CC) over Sephadex LH-20 (1.5 m × 3 cm; CH$_2$Cl$_2$-MeOH, 1:1) followed by semi-preparative HPLC with MeOH-H$_2$O (40%→100%) to provide **10** (280 mg), **11** (2 mg), **17** (57 mg), **20** (3 mg), **21** (2 mg), **22** (1.5 mg), **23** (2 mg), and **25** (4.4 mg).

The EtOAc part was subjected to MPLC (460 mm × 46 mm) on silica gel with gradient CH$_2$Cl$_2$-MeOH (100%→50%) to obtain five fractions (Fr.1−Fr.5). Fraction Fr.1 (1 g) was separated by CC over Sephadex LH-20 (1.5 m × 3 cm, CH$_2$Cl$_2$-MeOH, 1:1) and subsequently purified by recrystallization to give **14** (60 mg). Fraction Fr.2 (4 g) was separated by CC over ODS (310 mm × 5 mm; MeOH-H$_2$O, 10%→100%) and Sephadex LH-20 (1.5 m × 2 cm, MeOH), followed by semi-prep. HPLC (MeOH-H$_2$O, 40%→100%) afforded **1** (22 mg), **3** (3 mg), **5** (6 mg), **7** (2 mg), **9** (12 mg), **12** (2 mg), **13** (1.4 g), **15** (3 mg), **16** (10 mg), **18** (3 mg), and **19** (50 mg), while **2** (4 mg), **4** (2 mg), **6** (30 mg), **8** (27 mg), and **24** (5 mg) were isolated from Fr.4 (8 g) by CC on ODS (310 mm × 5 mm; MeOH-H$_2$O, 10%→100%) and Sephadex LH-20 (1.5 m × 2 cm, MeOH), followed by semi-prep. HPLC with chiral column A4-5 (MeOH-H$_2$O, 40%→80%).

15-*O*-methyl ML-236A (**1**): colorless oil; [α]$^{20}_D$ +62.7 (*c* 0.30, MeOH); UV (MeOH) λmax (logε) 237 (3.08) nm; CD (MeOH) (Δε) 204 (−1.90), 233 (+0.53), 236 (+0.53), 245 (+0.40) nm; ^{1}H and ^{13}C NMR data, see Table 1; HRESIMS *m/z* 361.1989 [M + Na]$^+$ (calcd for C$_{19}$H$_{30}$O$_5$Na, 361.1991).

(+)-solitumidine D (**2**): white amorphous solid; [α]$^{20}_D$ +6 (*c* 0.10, MeOH); UV (MeOH) λmax (logε) 231 (4.73) nm, 261 (4.25) nm, 325 (3.85) nm; CD (MeOH) (Δε) 203 (+2.62) nm; ^{1}H and ^{13}C NMR data, see Table 1; HRESIMS *m/z* 388.1877 [M−H]$^-$ (calcd for C$_{20}$H$_{26}$N$_3$O$_5$, 388.1872).

(±)-Solitumidine E (**3**): white amorphous power; [α]$^{20}_D$ 0 (*c* 0.44, MeOH); UV (MeOH) λmax (logε) 222 (4.10) nm, 261 (3.70) nm, 291 (3.52) nm; CD (MeOH) (Δε) 203 (−0.48), 299 (−0.04) nm; ^{1}H and ^{13}C NMR data, see Table 1; HRESIMS *m/z* 395.1945 [M + Na]$^+$ (calcd for C$_{21}$H$_{28}$N$_2$O$_4$Na, 395.1947).

3.4. ECD Calculation

Conformational analysis was performed by the Sybyl-X 2.0 using the MMFF94S force field as reported [32]. Predominant conformers were relocated and confirmed at the B3LYP/6-31G(d) level. The theoretical ECD spectra were calculated with the time-dependent density functional theory (TD-DFT) in acetonitrile. The ECD spectrum was obtained by averaging each conformer using the Boltzmann distribution theory.

3.5. Cell Proliferation Assay

Cytotoxic activities of all isolates were conducted on 17 human tumor cell lines of A431, A549, MB231, MCF-7, PANC1, HepG2, HCT116, H460, H1299, QGY-7701, BGC823, SKGT4, A375, U2OS, HL-60, K562, and KYSE450 by the MTT method [33]. Paclitaxel was used as a positive control, and DMSO was used as a negative control. Different cancer cells were incubated on 96-well cell plates and cultured for 24 h. Thereafter, the cells were treated with different concentrations of tested compounds and controls. After 48 h, MTT (20 μL) was added to incubate for another 4 h. The supernatant was discarded softly, and the deposited formazan formed in the cells was dissolved with DMSO (100 μL). The absorbencies were measured at 490 nm.

3.6. Anti-Allergic Bioassay

The in vitro anti-food allergic experiment was performed as previously reported [32]. In brief, rat basophilic leukemia 2H3 (RBL-2H3) cells were incubated with dinitrophenyl (DNP)–immunoglobulin E (IgE) overnight. Then, the IgE-sensitized RBL-2H3 cells were pretreated with tested compounds and stimulated with DNP–bovine serum albumin (BSA).

The bioactivity was quantified by measuring the fluorescence intensity of the hydrolyzed substrate in a fluorometer. Loratadine, a commercially available antiallergic medicine, was used as a positive control.

4. Conclusions

One new compactin analogue (**1**) and two previously unreported alkaloids (**2** and **3**), together with 22 known compounds (**4–25**), were isolated from the deep-sea-derived *Penicillium solitum* MCCC 3A00215. Viridicatol (**13**) exhibited weak cytotoxic activities against PANC-1, Hela, and A549 cells with IC_{50} values of 18, 19, and 24, respectively, while it showed remarkable anti-food allergic activity, with an IC_{50} value of 13 μM.

Supplementary Materials: The following are available online at https://www.mdpi.com/article/10.3390/md19100580/s1, Table S1 and Table S2, Figure S1–S65: One-dimensional and two-dimensional NMR spectra of all compounds.

Author Contributions: X.-W.Y. designed the project; Z.-H.H., L.X., M.-Y.H. and S.-J.L. isolated and purified all compounds. J.W. conducted the cytotoxic experiments. M.-M.X. and Y.-J.H. performed the fermentation. Z.-Z.S. provided the strain. Z.-H.H. and X.-W.Y. analyzed the data and wrote the paper, while critical revision of the publication was performed by all authors. All authors have read and agreed to the published version of the manuscript.

Funding: The work was supported by the National Natural Science Foundation of China (21877022) and the COMRA program (DY135-B2-08).

Institutional Review Board Statement: Not applicable.

Acknowledgments: The authors wish to thank Guangming Liu of the Jimei University for the anti-food allergic tests.

Conflicts of Interest: The authors declare no conflict of interest.

References

1. Pitt, J.I.; Spotts, R.A.; Holmes, R.J.; Cruickshank, R.H. *Penicillium solitum* revived, and its role as a pathogen of pomaceous fruits. *Phytopathology* **1991**, *81*, 1108–1112. [CrossRef]
2. Jurick, W.M., 2nd; Vico, I.; Gaskins, V.L.; Whitaker, B.D.; Garrett, W.M.; Janisiewicz, W.J.; Conway, W.S. *Penicillium solitum* produces a polygalacturonase isozyme in decayed Anjou pear fruit capable of macerating host tissue in vitro. *Mycologia* **2012**, *104*, 604–612. [CrossRef] [PubMed]
3. Lund, F.; Filtenborg, O.; Frisvad, J.C. Associated mycoflora of cheese. *Food Microbiol.* **1995**, *12*, 173–180. [CrossRef]
4. Sørensen, L.M.; Jacobsen, T.; Nielsen, P.V.; Frisvad, J.C.; Koch, A.G. Mycobiota in the processing areas of two different meat products. *Int. J. Food Microbiol.* **2008**, *124*, 58–64. [CrossRef]
5. Stierle, D.B.; Stierle, A.A.; Girtsman, T.; McIntyre, K.; Nichols, J. Caspase-1 and -3 inhibiting drimane sesquiterpenoids from the extremophilic fungus *Penicillium solitum*. *J. Nat. Prod.* **2012**, *75*, 262–266. [CrossRef] [PubMed]
6. Gonçalves, V.N.; Campos, L.S.; Melo, I.S.; Pellizari, V.H.; Rosa, C.A.; Rosa, L.H. *Penicillium solitum*: A mesophilic, psychrotolerant fungus present in marine sediments from Antarctica. *Polar Biol.* **2013**, *36*, 1823–1831. [CrossRef]
7. Boruta, T.; Przerywacz, P.; Ryngajllo, M.; Bizukojc, M. Bioprocess-related, morphological and bioinformatic perspectives on the biosynthesis of secondary metabolites produced by *Penicillium solitum*. *Process Biochem.* **2018**, *68*, 12–21. [CrossRef]
8. Larsen, T.O.; Lange, L.; Schnorr, K.; Stender, S.; Frisvad, J.C. Solistatinol, a novel phenolic compactin analogue from *Penicillium solitum*. *Tetrahedron Lett.* **2007**, *48*, 1261–1264. [CrossRef]
9. Sørensen, D.; Larsen, T.O.; Christophersen, C.; Nielsen, P.H.; Anthoni, U. Solistatin, an aromatic compactin analogue from *Penicillium solitum*. *Phytochemistry* **1999**, *51*, 1027–1029. [CrossRef]
10. Rodriguez, J.P.G.; Bernardi, D.I.; Gubiani, J.R.; de Oliveira, J.M.; Morais-Urano, R.P.; Bertonha, A.F.; Bandeira, K.F.; Bulla, J.I.Q.; Sette, L.D.; Ferreira, A.G.; et al. Water-soluble glutamic acid derivatives produced in culture by *Penicillium solitum* IS1-A from King George Island, Maritime Antarctica. *J. Nat. Prod.* **2020**, *83*, 55–65. [CrossRef]
11. Guo, W.; Kong, X.; Zhu, T.; Gu, Q.; Li, D. Penipyrols A–B and peniamidones A–D from the mangrove derived *Penicillium solitum* GWQ-143. *Arch. Pharmacal Res.* **2015**, *38*, 1449–1454. [CrossRef]
12. He, Z.H.; Xie, C.L.; Hao, Y.J.; Xu, L.; Wang, C.F.; Hu, M.Y.; Li, S.J.; Zhong, T.H.; Yang, X.W. Solitumergosterol A, a unique 6/6/6/6/5 steroid from the deep-sea-derived *Penicillium solitum* MCCC 3A00215. *Org. Biomol. Chem.* **2021**. [CrossRef]
13. Endo, A.; Kuroda, M.; Tsujita, Y. ML-236A, ML-236B, and ML-236C, new inhibitors of cholesterogenesis produced by *Penicillium citrinium*. *J. Antibiot.* **1976**, *29*, 1346–1348. [CrossRef] [PubMed]

14. Shaala, L.A.; Youssef, D.T. Identification and bioactivity of compounds from the fungus *Penicillium* sp. CYE-87 isolated from a marine tunicate. *Mar. Drugs* **2015**, *13*, 1698–1709. [CrossRef] [PubMed]
15. Evidente, A.; Iacobellis, N.S.; Sisto, A. Isolation of indole-3-acetic acid methyl ester, a metabolite of indole-3-acetic acid from *Pseudomonas amygdali*. *Experientia* **1993**, *49*, 182–183. [CrossRef]
16. Sun, W.; Chen, X.; Tong, Q.; Zhu, H.; He, Y.; Lei, L.; Xue, Y.; Yao, G.; Luo, Z.; Wang, J.; et al. Novel small molecule 11beta-HSD1 inhibitor from the endophytic fungus *Penicillium commune*. *Sci. Rep.* **2016**, *6*, 26418. [CrossRef] [PubMed]
17. Kashiwada, Y.; Nonaka, G.; Nishioka, I. Studies on *Rhubarb* (*Rhei Rhizoma*). V. isolation and characterization of chromone and chromanone derivatives. *Chem. Pharm. Bull.* **1984**, *32*, 3493–3500. [CrossRef]
18. Talontsi, F.M.; Facey, P.; Tatong, M.D.; Islam, M.T.; Frauendorf, H.; Draeger, S.; Tiedemann, A.; Laatsch, H. Zoosporicidal metabolites from an endophytic fungus *Cryptosporiopsis* sp. of *Zanthoxylum leprieurii*. *Phytochemistry* **2012**, *83*, 87–94. [CrossRef] [PubMed]
19. Kobayashi, Y.; Harayama, T. A concise and versatile synthesis of Viridicatin alkaloids from cyanoacetanilides. *Org. Lett.* **2009**, *11*, 1603–1606. [CrossRef]
20. Fremlin, L.J.; Piggott, A.M.; Lacey, E.; Capon, R.J. Cottoquinazoline A and cotteslosins A and B, metabolites from an Australian marine-derived strain of *Aspergillus Wersicolor*. *J. Nat. Prod.* **2009**, *72*, 666–670. [CrossRef] [PubMed]
21. Hodge, R.P.; Harris, C.M.; Harris, T.M. Verrucofortine, a major metabolite of *Penicillium verrucosum var. Cyclopium*, the fungus that produces the Mycotoxin Verrucosidin. *J. Nat. Prod.* **1988**, *51*, 66–73. [CrossRef] [PubMed]
22. Mizushina, Y.; Nakanishi, R.; Kuriyama, I.; Kamiya, K.; Satake, T.; Shimazaki, N.; Koiwai, O.; Uchiyama, Y.; Yonezawa, Y.; Takemura, M.; et al. β-sitosterol-3-O-β-D-glucopyranoside: A eukaryotic DNA polymerase lambda inhibitor. *J. Steroid Biochem. Mol. Biol.* **2006**, *99*, 100–107. [CrossRef]
23. Koga, J.; Yamauchi, T.; Shimura, M.; Ogawa, N.; Oshima, K.; Umemura, K.; Kikuchi, M.; Ogasawara, N. Cerebrosides A and C, sphingolipid elicitors of hypersensitive cell death and phytoalexin accumulation in rice plants. *J. Biol. Chem.* **1998**, *273*, 31985–31991. [CrossRef]
24. Soman, A.G.; Gloer, J.B.; Wicklow, D.T. Antifungal and antibacterial metabolites from a sclerotium-colonizing isolate of *Mortierella vinacea*. *J. Nat. Prod.* **1999**, *62*, 386–388. [CrossRef]
25. Du, F.Y.; Li, X.M.; Zhang, P.; Li, C.S.; Wang, B.G. Cyclodepsipeptides and other O-containing heterocyclic metabolites from *Beauveria felina* EN-135, a marine-derived entomopathogenic fungus. *Mar. Drugs* **2014**, *12*, 2816–2826. [CrossRef]
26. Arunpanichlert, J.; Rukachaisirikul, V.; Phongpaichit, S.; Supaphon, O.; Sakayaroj, J. Xylariphilone: A new azaphilone derivative from the seagrass-derived fungus *Xylariales* sp. PSU-ES163. *Nat. Prod. Res.* **2016**, *30*, 46–51. [CrossRef]
27. Sommart, U.; Rukachaisirikul, V.; Sukpondma, Y.; Phongpaichit, S.; Towatana, N.H.; Graidist, P.; Hajiwangoh, Z.; Sakayaroj, J. A cyclohexenone derivative from *Diaporthaceous* fungus PSU-H2. *Arch. Pharmacal Res.* **2009**, *32*, 1227–1231. [CrossRef]
28. Kishida, M.; Yamauchi, N.; Sawada, K.; Ohashi, Y.; Eguchi, T.; Kakinuma, K. Diacetone-glucose architecture as a chirality template. Part 9.1 enantioselective synthesis of (R)-mevalonolactone and (R)-[2H9]mevalonolactone on carbohydrate template. *J. Chem. Soc. Perkin Trans.* **1997**, *1*, 891–896. [CrossRef]
29. Shimomura, H.; Sashida, Y.; Mimaki, Y.; Adachi, T.; Yoshinari, K. A new mevalonolactone glucoside derivative from the bark of *Prunus buergeriana*. *Chem. Pharm. Bull.* **1989**, *37*, 829–830. [CrossRef]
30. Endo, A.; Kuroda, M.; Tanzawa, K. Competitive inhibition of 3-hydroxy-3-methylglutaryl coenzyme A reductase by ML-236A and ML-236B fungal metabolites, having hypocholesterolemic activity. *FEBS Lett.* **1976**, *72*, 323–326. [CrossRef]
31. Shu, Z.; Liu, Q.; Xing, C.; Zhang, Y.; Zhou, Y.; Zhang, J.; Liu, H.; Cao, M.; Yang, X.; Liu, G. Viridicatol isolated from deep-sea *Penicillium griseofulvum* alleviates anaphylaxis and repairs the intestinal barrier in mice by suppressing mast cell activation. *Mar. Drugs* **2020**, *18*, 517. [CrossRef] [PubMed]
32. Xie, C.L.; Liu, Q.; He, Z.H.; Gai, Y.B.; Zou, Z.B.; Shao, Z.Z.; Liu, G.M.; Chen, H.F.; Yang, X.W. Discovery of andrastones from the deep-sea-derived *Penicillium allii-sativi* MCCC 3A00580 by OSMAC strategy. *Bioorg. Chem.* **2021**, *108*, 104671. [CrossRef] [PubMed]
33. Wang, C.F.; Huang, X.F.; Xiao, H.X.; Hao, Y.J.; Xu, L.; Yan, Q.X.; Zou, Z.B.; Xie, C.L.; Xu, Y.Q.; Yang, X.W. Chemical constituents of the marine fungus *Penicillium* sp. MCCC 3A00228. *Chem. Biodivers.* **2021**, *18*, e2100697.

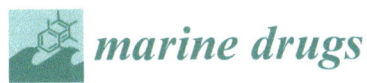

Article

Secondary Metabolites with α-Glucosidase Inhibitory Activity from Mangrove Endophytic Fungus *Talaromyces* sp. CY-3

Wencong Yang [1], Qi Tan [1], Yihao Yin [1], Yan Chen [1,2], Yi Zhang [3], Jianying Wu [1], Leyao Gao [1], Bo Wang [1,*] and Zhigang She [1,*]

[1] School of Chemistry, Sun Yat-Sen University, Guangzhou 510275, China; yangwc6@mail2.sysu.edu.cn (W.Y.); tanq27@mail2.sysu.edu.cn (Q.T.); yinyh6@mail2.sysu.edu.cn (Y.Y.); chenyan27@mail2.sysu.edu.cn (Y.C.); wujy89@mail2.sysu.edu.cn (J.W.); gaoly6@mail2.sysu.edu.cn (L.G.)

[2] National R & D Center for Edible Fungus Processing Technology, Henan University, Kaifeng 475004, China

[3] Research Institute for Marine Drugs and Nutrition, College of Food Science and Technology, Guangdong Ocean University, Zhanjiang 524088, China; hubeizhangyi@163.com

* Correspondence: ceswb@mail.sysu.edu.cn (B.W.); cesshzhg@mail.sysu.edu.cn (Z.S.)

Abstract: Eight new compounds, including two sambutoxin derivatives (**1–2**), two highly oxygenated cyclopentenones (**7–8**), four highly oxygenated cyclohexenones (**9–12**), together with four known sambutoxin derivatives (**3–6**), were isolated from semimangrove endophytic fungus *Talaromyces* sp. CY-3, under the guidance of molecular networking. The structures of new isolates were elucidated by analysis of detailed spectroscopic data, ECD spectra, chemical hydrolysis, ^{13}C NMR calculation, and DP4+ analysis. In bioassays, compounds **1–5** displayed better α-glucosidase inhibitory activity than the positive control 1-deoxynojirimycin (IC$_{50}$ = 80.8 ± 0.3 μM), and the IC$_{50}$ value was in the range of 12.6 ± 0.9 to 57.3 ± 1.3 μM.

Keywords: *Talaromyces* sp.; molecular networking; sambutoxin; polyketides; α-glucosidase

1. Introduction

According to the WHO forecast, the number of diabetes patients will reach 693 million in 2045. Type II diabetes accounts for 90%, and α-glucosidase inhibitors originating from natural products, such as acarbose, miglitol, and voglibose, are used to treat type II diabetes [1]. However, most clinical antidiabetic drugs cause side effects [2]. Therefore, there is an urgent need to find and discover new antidiabetic drugs.

Mangrove endophytic fungi are an important resource to provide a large number of structurally unique secondary metabolites [3,4] with good biological activities, such as α-glucosidase inhibitory activities [5], antibacterial [6], antifungal [7], anti-insect [8], antitumor [9], antiviral [10], antioxidant [11], and anti-inflammatory activities [12]. As part of our ongoing search for new compounds with α-glucosidase inhibitory activities from mangrove-derived fungi [5,12–14], secondary metabolites of fungus *Talaromyces* sp. CY-3, collected from the fresh leaves of the semimangrove *Hibiscus tiliaceus* in Zhanjiang, were studied.

Recently, the advent of visual molecular network technology has led to a new perspective in the research of natural products [15]. Global Natural Product Social (GNPS) can establish a molecular network to classify compounds with the same LC–MS/MS ion fragments into similar clusters. Moreover, it can rapidly discover novel compounds through accurate MS data and database comparison [16].

Extracts of CY-3 were analyzed by LC–MS/MS, and a visible molecular network was generated (Figure 1). Guided by MS/MS-based molecular networking through the GNPS platform, small clusters of compounds were tracked for isolation with *m/z* 492 [M+K]$^+$, 336 [M+H]$^+$, 438 [M+H]$^+$, 474 [M+Na]$^+$, 201 [M+H]$^+$, and 187 [M+H]$^+$. Two new sambutoxin derivatives (**1–2**), six highly oxygenated new polyketides (**7–12**), and four known sambutoxin derivatives (**3–6**) were isolated (Figure 2). Herein, the isolation, structure elucidation, and α-glucosidase inhibitory activity of all compounds are presented.

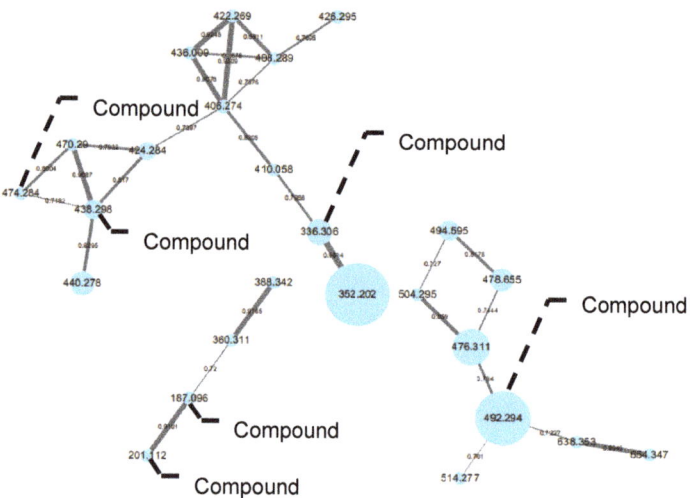

Figure 1. Clusters of nodes from *Talaromyces* sp. for compounds **1–3**, **5**, **8**, and **10–12**.

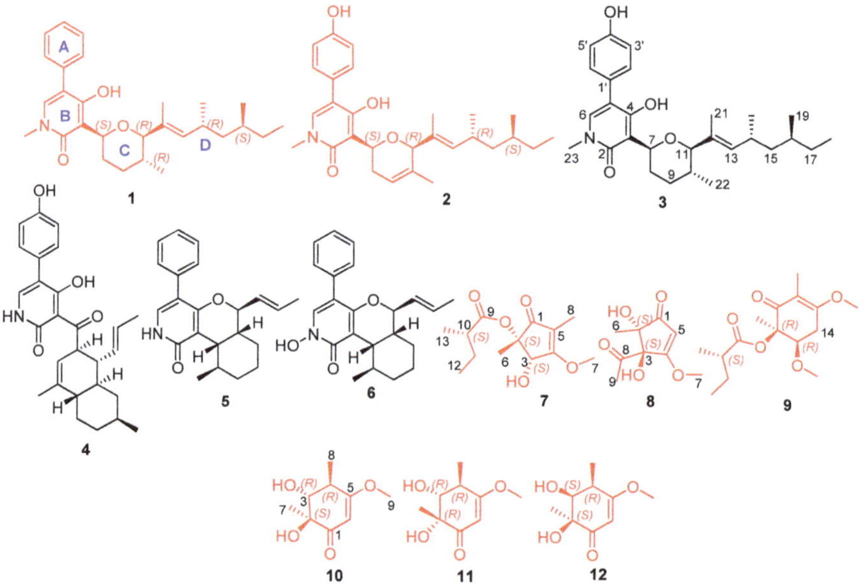

Figure 2. Structure of compounds **1–12**.

2. Results

2.1. Structure Identification

Sambutoxin A (**1**), obtained as a light-yellow oil, was displayed to have a molecular formula of $C_{28}H_{37}NO_4$ with 10 degrees of unsaturation at m/z 438.2999 [M+H]$^+$ (calcd. 438.3002), as shown by a positive HR–ESI–MS spectrum. The ^{1}H NMR of **1** showed six methyls (δ_H 0.74, 0.82, 0.83, 0.90, 1.61, and 3.50), four methylenes (δ_H 1.03, 1.19, 1.34, 1.44, 1.64, 1.91, and 2.09), five methines (δ_H 1.30, 1.69, 2.45, 3.53, and 5.02), seven unsaturated protons (δ_H 5.18, 7.14, 7.32, 7.39, and 7.42), and one exchangeable hydrogen atom (δ_H 9.99). Its ^{13}C NMR displayed a total of 28 carbons resonances, six methyls (δ_c 11.3, 11.7, 17.8, 19.7, 20.8, and 37.2), four methylenes (δ_c 29.0, 30.8, 32.2, and 44.8), five methines (δ_c 29.7, 32.1, 32.5, 78.0, and 92.7), seven carbons with unsaturated protons (δ_c 127.5, 128.4, 129.3, 136.4, and 138.1), and six quaternary carbons (δ_c 110.4, 115.2, 130.4, 134.2, 161.5, and 162.0). The HMBC from H-13 to C-12, from H-21 to C-13, together with the ^{1}H-^{1}H COSY H-13/H-14(/H-20)/H-15/H-16(/H-19)/H-17/H-18 formed the side chain D. HMBC from H-11 to C-7, together with ^{1}H-^{1}H COSY H-7/H-8/H-9/H-10(/H-22)/H-11, established the ring C moiety. HMBC from H-6 to C-2, C-4, and C-5 and from H-23 to C-2 and C-6, constructed a ring B moiety. ^{1}H-^{1}H COSY H-2'/H-3'/H-4'/H-5'/H-6', together with HMBC from H-2' to C-1' and from H-6' to C-1', constructed ring A. Finally, rings A, B, C, and side chain D were connected by the HMBCs from H-6' to C-5, H-7 to C-2, C-3, and C-4, and H-21 to C-11. The 1D and 2D NMR data were similar to those of **3** (Table 1). The only difference between them was that the 4'-OH (δ_C 156.5) is reduced to a hydrogen atom (δ_H 7.29–7.34, δ_C 127.5). Thus, the planar structure of **1** was shown (Figure 3).

Table 1. ^{1}H NMR and ^{13}C NMR of **1–3**.

NO.	1 (CDCl$_3$)		2 (CDCl$_3$)		3 (CDCl$_3$)	
	δ_C, Type	δ_H(J in Hz)	δ_C, Type	δ_H(J in Hz)	δ_C, Type	δ_H(J in Hz)
2	161.5, C		161.7, C		162.7, C	
3	110.4, C		110.1, C		110.4, C	
4	162.0, C		162.5, C		162.4, C	
5	115.2, C		115.4, C		115.9, C	
6	136.4, CH	7.14, s	136.2, CH	7.11, s	136.0, CH	7.12, s
7	78.0, CH	5.02, d, (9.1)	73.7, CH	5.17, dd, (10.5, 3.1)	77.8, CH	5.02, d, (9.0)
8	30.8, CH$_2$	1.64–1.69, m, 2.09, d, (11.4)	29.9, CH$_2$	1.25–1.31, m, 2.25–2.35, m	30.9, CH$_2$	1.64–1.70, m, 2.09, d, (11.4)
9	32.3, CH$_2$	1.44, d, (10.1) 1.91, d, (13.1)	121.9, CH	5.72, d, (5.2)	32.2, CH$_2$	1.44, d, (10.1) 1.91, d, (13.1)
10	32.5, CH	1.64–1.69, m	132.9, C		32.1, CH	1.64–1.70, m
11	92.7, CH	3.53, s	86.9, CH	4.56, s	92.7, CH	3.53, s
12	130.4, C		130.2, C		130.3, C	
13	138.1, CH	5.18, d, (9.5)	139.7, CH	5.29, d, (9.6)	138.1, CH	5.18, d, (9.5)
14	29.7, CH	2.42–2.49, m	30.0, CH	2.40–2.50, m	29.7, CH	2.42–2.49, m
15	44.8, CH$_2$	1.01–1.07, m 1.16–1.21, m	44.8, CH$_2$	1.01–1.04, m, 1.25–1.31, m	44.8, CH$_2$	1.01–1.07, m 1.16–1.21, m
16	32.1, CH	1.29–1.35, m	32.2, CH	1.25–1.31, m	32.4, CH	1.29–1.34, m
17	29.0, CH$_2$	1.01–1.07, m 1.29–1.35, m	29.0, CH$_2$	1.01–1.04, m, 1.25–1.31, m	29.0, CH$_2$	1.01–1.07, m 1.29–1.34, m
18	11.3, CH$_3$	0.83, s	11.0, CH$_3$	1.53, d, (1.3)	11.3, CH$_3$	0.83, s
19	19.7, CH$_3$	0.82, d, (6.5)	20.8, CH$_3$	0.90, d, (6.6)	19.7, CH$_3$	0.82, d, (6.5)
20	20.8, CH$_3$	0.90, d, (6.6)	19.7, CH$_3$	0.82, d, (6.4)	20.8, CH$_3$	0.90, d, (6.6)
21	11.7, CH$_3$	1.61, s	11.3, CH$_3$	1.49, s	11.7, CH$_3$	1.61, s
22	17.8, CH$_3$	0.74, d, (6.5)	19.1, CH$_3$	0.81, s	17.7, CH$_3$	0.74, d, (6.5)
23	37.2, CH$_3$	3.50, s	37.3, CH$_3$	3.50, s	37.4, CH$_3$	3.50, s
1'	134.2, C		125.9, C		125.2, C	
2'	129.3, CH	7.35–7.44, m	130.6, CH	7.26, d, (9.0)	130.5, CH	7.26, d, (9.0)
3'	128.4, CH	7.35–7.44, m	115.5, CH	6.87, d, (8.1)	115.6, CH	6.92, d, (8.1)
4'	127.5, CH	7.29–7.34, m	155.8, C		156.5, C	
5'	128.4, CH	7.35–7.44, m	115.5, CH	6.87, d, (8.1)	115.6, CH	6.92, d, (8.1)
6'	129.3, CH	7.35–7.44, m	130.6, CH	7.26, d, (9.0)	130.5, CH	7.26, d, (9.0)
4'-OH		9.99, s		9.83, s		9.83, s

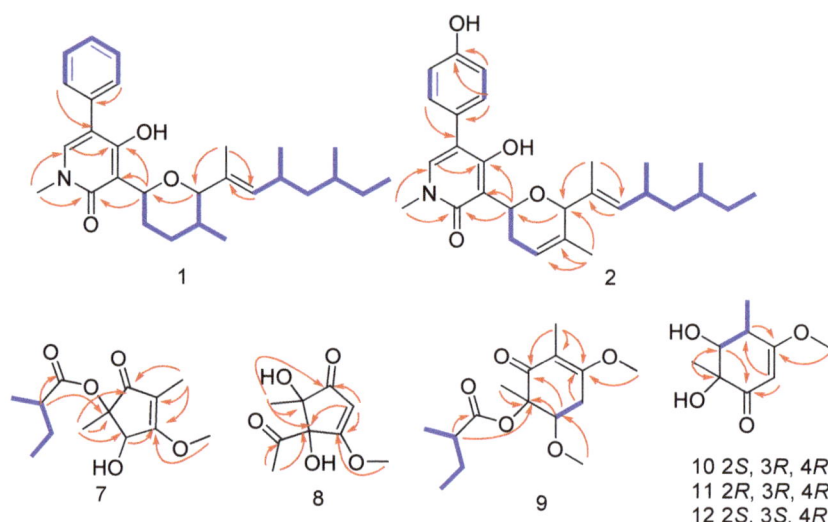

Figure 3. HMBC (red arrow) and key COSY (blue bold line) of **1–2** and **7–12**.

The relative configuration of ring C and the double bond between C-12 and C-13 of compound **1** were defined by the NOESY spectrum. The correlations of H-22/H-7/H-11 and H-14/H-21 were also observed in the NOESY spectrum (Figure 4), which means H-22, H-7, and H-11 were on the same side, as were H-14 and H-21. Therefore, the relative configuration of C-7, C-10, and C-11 in ring C was deduced to be (7S*, 10R*, 11R*), and the double bond between C-12 and C-13 was assigned to be (E). In the present work, assigning the configurations at C-14 and C-16 in the aliphatic side chains of **1** was a challenging task due to the high conformational flexibility of fatty chains. As described in the literature, the absolute side-chain configurations for C-14 and C-16 were also determined by ^{13}C NMR calculation and DP4+ analysis [17,18]. (14R, 16S)-**1** was assigned with a 100% probability (Figures S68 and S69). Consequently, the side-chain configurations of C-14 and C-16 of **1** were assigned to be 14R, 16S. The absolute configuration of **1** was determined by comparing the calculated ECD spectra (7S, 10R, 11R, 14R, 16S)-**1** and (7R, 10S, 11S, 14R, 16S)-**1** with the experimental one. The calculated ECD curves (7S, 10R, 11R, 14R, 16S)-**1** showed better agreement with the experimental one (Figure 5A). Thus, the absolute configuration of **1** was assigned to be 7S, 10R, 11R, 13E, 14R, 16S. Compounds **1** and **3** share a common biosynthetic pathway for sambutoxin derivatives, which is consistent with the configuration reported in the literature [19,20].

Sambutoxin B (**2**), also isolated as a light-yellow oil, displayed a molecular formula of $C_{28}H_{37}NO_4$ with 11 degrees of unsaturation at m/z 452.2794 [M+H]$^+$ (calcd. 452.2795) by positive HR–ESI–MS spectrum. Its 1D and 2D NMR were similar to **3**. The only difference between them was that the single bond between C-9 (δ_H 1.44, 1.97, δ_C 32.2) and C-10 (δ_H 1.64–1.70, δ_C 32.1) was converted to a double bond (δ_H 5.72, δ_C 121.9, 132.9). Thus, the planar structure of **2** was as shown in Figure 3. The correlations of H-7/H-11 and H-14/H-21 were observed in the NOESY spectrum (Figure 4). Thus, the double bond between C-12 and C-13 was assigned to be (E), and the relative configuration was deduced to be (7S*, 11R*). The calculated ECD spectra of (7S, 11R)-**2** and (7R, 11S)-**2** were compared to the measured one, and the calculated ECD curve of (7S, 11R)-**2** was showed a good agreement with the experimental one (Figure 5B). The stereochemistry of C-14 and C-16 was biogenetically established as 14R, 16S. Moreover, they were also verified by ^{13}C NMR calculation and DP4+ probability (Figures S70 and S71). Thus, the absolute configuration of **2** was determined as 7S, 11R, 13E, 14R, 16S.

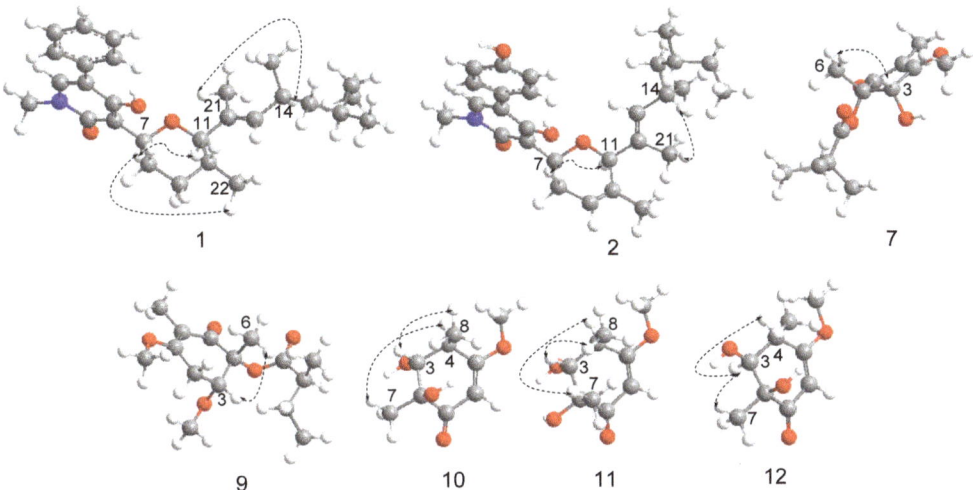

Figure 4. NOESY correlations of **1–2** and **7–12**.

Talaketides A(**7**) was isolated as a yellow oil, and its molecular formula was determined as $C_{13}H_{20}O_5$ by the HR–ESI–MS data at m/z 279.1197 [M+Na]$^+$ (calcd. 279.1203). The ^{1}H NMR of **7** displayed four methyls, one methylene, two methines, and one methoxy (Table 2). Its ^{13}C NMR showed a total of 13 carbons resonances, including four methyls, one methylene, two methines, one methoxy, one ester carboxyl, one carbonyl, two olefinic carbons, and one quaternary carbon (Table 3). The HMBC from H-3 to C-4, H-6 to C-1, C-2, and C-3, H-7 to C-4, H-8 to C-1, C-4, and C-5, H-10 to C-2 and C-9, together with the ^{1}H-^{1}H COSY correlation from H-13/H-10/H-11/H-12, formed the planar structure. In order to determine the absolute ring configuration of **7**, the ECD of (2*S*, 3*S*)-**7**, (2*R*, 3*R*)-**7**, (2*S*, 3*R*)-**7**, and (2*R*, 3*S*)-**7** was compared with the measured one. (2*S*, 3*S*)-**7** showed a good agreement with the experimental one (Figure 5C). Furthermore, the side chain of **7** was hydrolysis in 1M NaOH solution and compared to the standard of (*S*)-2-methylbutanoic acid and (*R*)-2-methylbutanoic acid through a chiral column by HPLC (Figure 6 and Figure S72). The retention time of hydrolyzate matched with (*S*)-2-methylbutanoic acid. Thus, the absolute configuration of **7** was determined as 2*S*, 3*S*, 10*S*.

Talaketides C (**9**) was isolated as a yellow oil, and its molecular formula was determined as $C_{15}H_{24}O_5$ by the HR–ESI–MS data at m/z 307.1517 [M+Na]$^+$ (calcd. 307.1516). The 1D and 2D NMR were also similar to **7**, and the only difference between them was compound **9** had one more methoxy group (δ_H 3.16, δ_C 51.8) and one more methylene group (δ_H 2.82, 3.03, δ_C 31.2) than compound **7**. According to the HMBCs, the methylene group was connected oxymethine (δ_H 5.10, δ_C 71.7) and a quaternary carbon (δ_C 188.2), and methoxy was connected to oxymethine (δ_H 5.10, δ_C 71.7), thus the planar structure of **9** was established (Figure 3). The NOESY correlation of H-5 to H-12 was observed (Figure 4), and the ECD curves of (2*R*, 3*R*) and (2*S*, 3*S*) were compared to the measured one. The calculated ECD of (2*R*, 3*R*) showed a good agreement with the experimental one (Figure 5E), and the side-chain stereostructure of C-10 was also determined as 10*S* through chemical hydrolysis. (Figure 6 and Figure S72). Therefore, the absolute configuration of **9** was determined as 2*R*, 3*R*, 10*S*.

Talaketides D (**10**) was isolated as a light-yellow oil, and its molecular formula was determined as $C_9H_{14}O_4$ by the HR–ESI–MS data at m/z 209.0783 [M+Na]$^+$ (calcd. 209.0784). Analysis of the 1D and 2D NMR spectrum found compound **10** to be similar to the known compound phomaligol D [21]. The only difference between them was the departure of hydroxyl at C-4 (δ_C 73.1 changed to δ_H 2.55, δ_C 41.5). Thus, the planar structure of **10** was determined (Figure 3), which was dehydroxylated phomaligol D. H-3/H-8 and H-4/H-7 correlations were observed in the NOESY spectrum, which indicated that the relative configuration of **10** was (2S^*, 3R^*, 4R^*) (Figure 4). In order to determine its absolution configuration, the ECD spectra of (2S, 3R, 4R)-**10** and (2R, 3S, 4S)-**10** were compared with the measured one. The calculated CD curve of (2S, 3R, 4R) showed a good agreement with the experimental one (Figure 5F). Therefore, the absolution configuration of **10** was deduced to be (2S, 3R, 4R) and named Talaketides D.

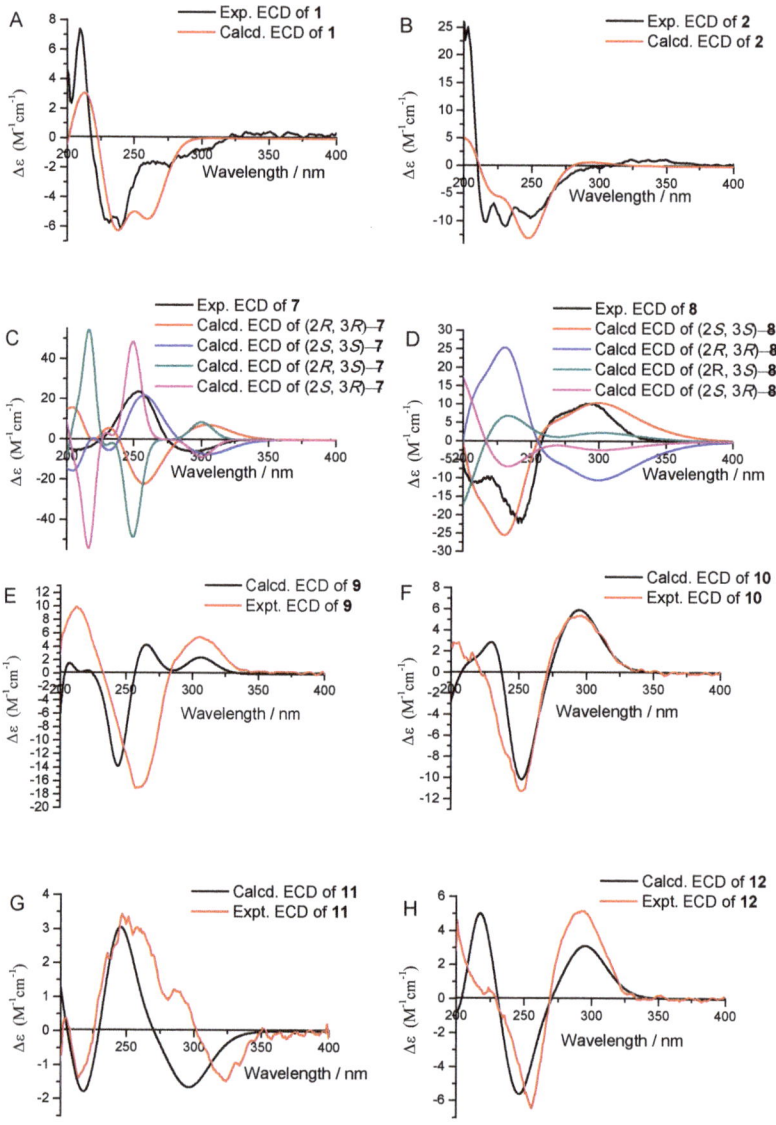

Figure 5. ECD spectra of compounds **1** (**A**), **2** (**B**), **7** (**C**), **8** (**D**), **9** (**E**), **10** (**F**), **11** (**G**) and **12** (**H**) in CH$_3$OH.

Table 2. ^{1}H NMR of **7–12**.

Position	7	8	9	10	11	12
3	4.98, s		5.10, q, (6.3)	3.51, d, (9.5)	3.40, d, (7.2)	3.80, d, (3.2)
4				2.55, dqd, (11.3, 6.8, 1.7)	2.77–2.83, m	3.02, qdd, (7.1, 3.2, 1.9)
5		5.55, s				
6	1.30, s	1.42, s	1.29, d, (6.4)	5.30, d, (1.7)	5.33, d, (1.2)	5.34, d, (1.9)
7	4.16, s	3.98, s	4.10, s	1.28, d, (6.8)	1.30, d, (7.2)	1.27, d, (7.1)
8	1.67, s		1.56, t, (1.8)	1.22, s	1.34, s	1.30, s
9		2.20, s		3.75, s	3.76, s	3.75, s
10	2.37, q, (7.0)		2.19–2.28, m			
11	1.44–1.50, m		1.34–1.40, m			
	1.58–1.65, m		1.44–1.50, m			
12	0.94, t, (7.5)		0.80, t, (7.5)			
13	1.12, d, (7.0)		1.02, d, (7.0)			
14			2.82, dq, (18.2, 1.8) 3.03, dq, (18.2, 1.8)			
15			3.16, s			

Table 3. ^{13}C NMR of **7–12**.

Position	7	8	9	10	11	12
1	202.0	200.6	205.0	203.0	200.9	203.3
2	86.4	80.4	84.3	78.4	75.5	77.7
3	73.5	92.5	71.7	78.1	78.7	79.0
4	179.7	192.4	188.2	41.5	40.1	39.0
5	115.6	103.3	117.5	180.1	180.5	178.9
6	19.5	23.5	14.9	99.5	99.6	99.0
7	59.1	60.1	58.2	14.0	14.2	13.4
8	6.08	207.2	5.6	19.2	21.4	23.6
9	177.5	27.5	176.4	57.2	57.0	57.1
10	42.0		42.4			
11	27.8		27.8			
12	11.8		11.7			
13	16.8		16.6			
14			31.2			
15			51.8			

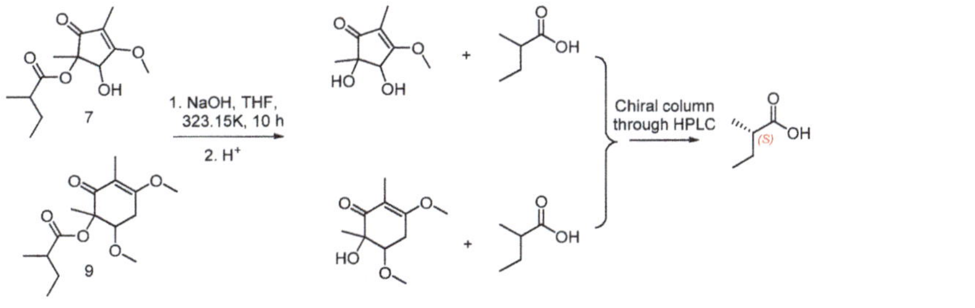

Figure 6. Confirmation for C-10 of compounds **7** and **9** through chemical hydrolysis.

Talaketides E (**11**) and Talaketides F (**12**), were also isolated as a light-yellow oil. Similarities in 1D and 2D NMR and HR–ESI–MS indicated that they shared the same planar structure (Figure 3), but the observed correlations were different: one was H-3/H-7/H-8, and the other was H-3/H-4/H-7 in the NOESY spectrum (Figure 4). This phenomenon indicated that their relative configuration was assigned to be (2R*, 3R*, 4R*) and (2S*, 3S*,

4R*), respectively. Their stereostructures were also determined by ECD calculation and comparison, and the absolution configuration of **11** and **12** was confirmed as (2R, 3R, 4R) and (2S, 3S, 4R), respectively (Figure 5G).

The structures of compounds **3–6** were identified as (−)-sambutoxin (**3**) [19], ilicicolin H (**4**) [22], deoxyleporin B (**5**) [23], and leporine B (**6**) [24], respectively, by comparison of their NMR data, MS, CD, and optical rotation with those in the literature.

2.2. Proposed Biosynthesis Pathway

A hypothetical biosynthetic pathway for compounds **1–2** and **7–12** was proposed (Figure 7) [25,26]. Compounds **1–2** are the PKS-NRPS biosynthetic pathway. Starting from one L-Phe molecule, one acetyl-CoA molecule, six malonyl-CoA molecules, and four SAM molecules through the PKS pathway formed intermediate i. Then, the formation of **1** was constructed by rearranging and reducing. The formation of **2** was similar to **1**, and the only difference between them was that L-Phe was replaced by L-Tyr (Figure 7A).

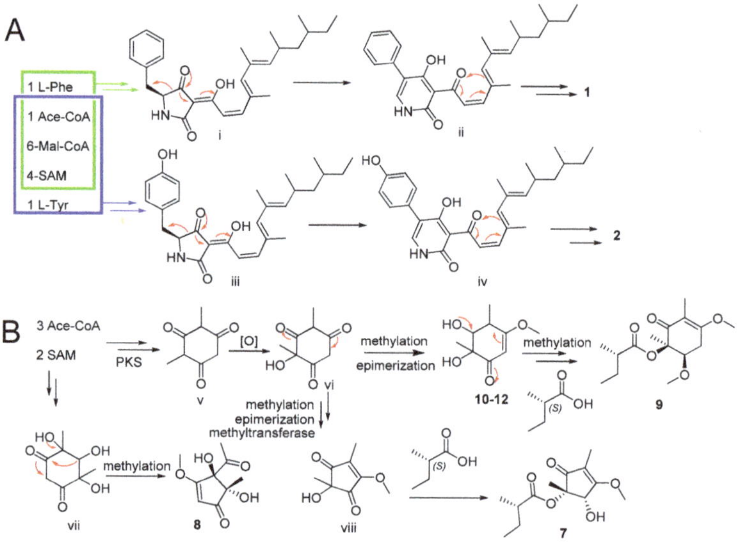

Figure 7. Proposed biogenetic pathways of **1–2** (**A**) and **7–12** (**B**).

The remaining compounds **7–12** are considered to be the origin of biosynthetic polyketides. The key intermediate vi was obtained through the PKS pathway, oxidation, and formed **10–12** by electron transfer, methylation, and epimerization. Further electron transfer, methylation, and esterification to form **9**. **7** was formed through electron transfer, methylation, epimerization, methyltransferase, and esterification. Together, compound **8** started from two SAM molecules and three acetyl-CoA molecules through the PKS pathway and further rearranging and methylating (Figure 7B).

2.3. α-Glucosidase Inhibitory Activity

Compounds **1–12** were tested for their α-glucosidase inhibitory activity (Table 4). Compounds **1–5** displayed better α-glucosidase inhibitory activity with an IC_{50} value in the range of 12.6 ± 0.9 to 57.3 ± 1.3 μM compared to the positive control 1-deoxynojirimycin (IC_{50} = 80.8 ± 0.3 μM).

The IC_{50} value of compound **2** is 37.4 ± 1.4 μM, lower than that of compound **1** (12.6 ± 0.9 μM) and compound **3** (16.9 ± 0.6 μM), which illustrates that the double bond formed between C-9 and C-10 reduced the α-glucosidase inhibitory activity. Different from compounds **1–3**, compound **5** presented a much bigger IC_{50} value of 57.3 ± 1.3 μM, and the IC$_{50}$ of compound **6** was even bigger than 100 μM. Therefore, it can be considered that the branch chain attached to ring C contributes a lot to the inhibitory activity. Compound **4** showed relatively higher inhibitory activity (IC$_{50}$ = 16.5 ± 0.7 μM), which may be due to its different structure from the other five.

Table 4. α-glucosidase inhibitory activity for **1–12**.

Compounds	IC$_{50}$/μM	Compounds	IC$_{50}$/μM
1	12.6 ± 0.9	7	>100
2	37.4 ± 1.4	8	>100
3	16.9 ± 0.6	9	>100
4	16.5 ± 0.7	10	>100
5	57.3 ± 1.3	11	>100
6	>100	12	>100
1-deoxynojirimycin	80.8 ± 0.3		

2.4. Molecular Docking Study

To explain the difference in inhibitory activity of compounds **1–5** to α-glucosidase, molecular docking between them and α-glucosidase was carried out using Autodock. The interaction energies of compounds **1–5** with α-glucosidase were 8.25, 7.99, 8.85, 9.19, and 7.96 kcal/mol, respectively, which is consistent with the change in IC$_{50}$ value. Compound **1** mainly formed a hydrogen bond with Glu-411 with a bond length of 2.85 Å (Figure 8A), **2** formed a hydrogen bond with Ser-241 with a bond length of 3.06 Å (Figure 8B), and **3** formed two hydrogen bonds with Asp-215 and Glu-411 with bond lengths of 3.06 and 2.85 Å, respectively. Moreover, compound **4** also formed two hydrogen bonds with Asp-242 and Thr-310 with bond lengths of 3.31 and 2.88 Å, respectively, while **5** only formed a hydrogen bond with Lys-156 with a bond length of 2.77 Å. In general, **1**, **3**, and **4** possess higher interaction energy and stronger interaction with amino acid residue than **2** and **5**, which explains their significant activity.

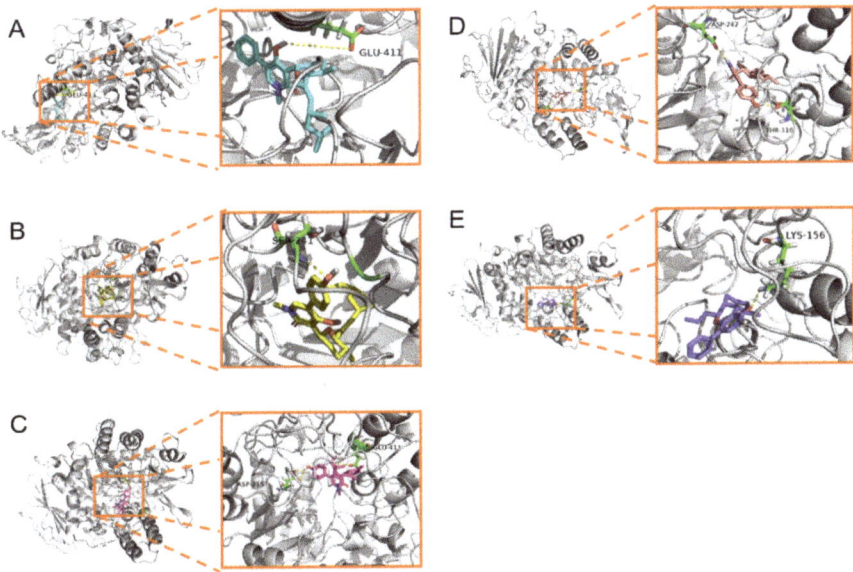

Figure 8. Binding mode of sambutoxins **1** (**A**), **2** (**B**), **3** (**C**), **4** (**D**), and **5** (**E**) with α-glucosidase.

3. Experimental Section

3.1. General Experimental Procedures

The 1D and 2D NMR were recorded on a Bruker Avance 400 MHz spectrometer (Karlsruhe, Germany) at room temperature. HR–ESI–MS spectra of all test compounds were acquired on a ThermoFisher LTQ–Orbitrap–LC–MS spectrometer (Palo Alto, CA, USA). UV–vis spectra were measured on a Shimadzu UV–2600 spectrophotometer (Kyoto, Japan). Optical rotations were acquired on an Anton–Paar MCP500 automatic polarimeter at 25 °C (Graz, Austria). CD curves were recorded on an Applied Photophysics Chirascan spectropolarimeter (Surrey, UK). All spectrophotometric measurements used a 96-well Bio-Rad microplate reader (Hercules, CA, USA). Solvent was removed by a Heidolph rotavapor with a vacuum pump. Semipreparative HPLC chromatography was used on a U3000 separation module coupled with a DAD detector manufactured by ThermoFisher and a chiral semipreparative column (Nu-Analytical Solutions Co., LTD-packed chiral INB, 5 μm, 4.6 × 250 mm) was used for separation. Column chromatography (CC) used silica gel (200–300 mesh (Qingdao Marine Chemical Factory)) and Sephadex LH-20 (Amersham Pharmacia, Stockholm, Sweden). Precoated silica gel plates (Qingdao Huang Hai Chemical Group Co., G60, F-254) were used for TLC analysis. LC–MS analysis was performed on a Q-TOF manufactured by Waters and a Waters Acquity UPLC BEH C18 column (1.7 μm, 2.1 × 100 mm) was used for analysis.

3.2. Fungal Material

Fungus CY-3 was isolated from the fresh leaves of the semimangrove *Hibiscus tiliaceus* (collected in June 2020 from Zhanjiang Mangrove National Nature Reserve in Guangdong Province, China). It was identified as *Talaromyces* sp. using ITS gene sequencing. The ITS rDNA gene sequence data of the fungi were deposited to GenBank (Accession No. MZ614621), and fungus CY-3 was deposited at Sun Yat-Sen University, China.

3.3. Fermentation

CY-3 was activated on a potato dextrose agar (PDA) Petri dish at 28 °C, then cultured in potato dextrose broth (PDB) in 6 × 500 mL Erlenmeyer flasks at 28 °C for 3 days in a shaker to obtain spore inoculum. The routine-scale fermentation was performed in 60 × 1 L Erlenmeyer flasks, each containing 50 mL of 2% saline and 50 g of rice. The Erlenmeyer flask containing the culture medium was autoclaved at 121 °C for 25 min. After cooling to room temperature, 10 mL of CY-3 inoculum was inoculated in each bottle and incubated at room temperature for 30 days.

3.4. Extraction and Purification

After fermentation, the mycelium and medium were extracted three times with EA (3 × 20 L). Then, the extracts were condensed under 50 °C in vacuo and combined to obtain a crude extract (31 g). The residue was separated by a silica gel column, eluting with a gradient of PE/EA (1:0–0:1) to afford 9 fractions (Frs. 1–8). Fr. 3 (2.4 g) was subjected to Sephadex LH-20 (methanol) to yield five sub-fractions (SFrs. 3.1–3.5). SFrs. 3–1 (352 mg) was applied to silica gel CC (DCM/MeOH v/v, 200:1) to give compounds **1** (5.3 mg), **2** (4.9 mg), and **3** (27.1 mg). Compounds **10** (6.3 mg, t_R = 7.3 min), **11** (5.7 mg, t_R = 9.1 min), and **12** (4.5 mg, t_R = 14.3 min) were obtained from SFr3-4 (298 mg) using chiral ND (the gradient was hexane/2-propanol v/v, 19:1, flow rate: 1 mL/min). Fr. 4 (2.5 g) was subjected to Sephadex LH-20 (ethanol) to yield three sub-fractions (SFrs. 4.1–4.3). Compounds **4** (8.7 mg), **5** (3.1 mg), and **6** (2.9 mg) were obtained from SFr4-1 (792 mg) using silica gel CC (DCM/MeOH v/v, 200:1). Fr. 6 (4.7 g) was subjected to Sephadex LH-20 (methanol) to yield three subfractions (SFrs. 6.1–6.3). Compounds **7** (50.1 mg), **8** (6.2 mg), and **9** (4.6 mg) were obtained from SFr6-3 (503 mg) using silica gel CC. (DCM/MeOH v/v, 50:1).

Sambutoxin A (**1**): $C_{28}H_{39}NO_3$; yellow oil; $[\alpha]_D^{25}$ − 30.75° (c 0.74 MeOH); UV (MeOH) λ_{max} (log ε) 240 (1.95) nm; ECD (MeOH) λ_{max} (Δε) 210 (+2.65), 230 (−2.04), 243 (−2.03),

279 (−0.59) nm; ^{1}H (400 MHz, CDCl$_3$) and ^{13}C NMR (100 MHz, CDCl$_3$) data, see Table 1; HR–ESI–MS: m/z 438.2999 [M+H]$^+$ (calcd. for C$_{28}$H$_{40}$NO$_3$, 438.3002).

Sambutoxin B (**2**): C$_{28}$H$_{37}$NO$_4$; yellow oil; $[\alpha]_D^{25}$ − 10.54° (c 1.05, MeOH); UV (MeOH) λ_{max} (log ε) 238 (2.86) nm; ECD (MeOH) λ_{max} (Δε) 217 (−3.45), 230 (−3.74), 259 (−3.16) nm; ^{1}H (400 MHz, CDCl$_3$) and ^{13}C NMR (100 MHz, CDCl$_3$) data, see Table 1; HR–ESI–MS: m/z 452.2794 [M+H]$^+$ (calcd. for C$_{28}$H$_{38}$NO$_4$, 452.2795).

Talaketides A (**7**): C$_{13}$H$_{20}$O$_5$; yellow oil; $[\alpha]_D^{25}$ − 14.09° (c 0.26, MeOH); UV (MeOH) λ_{max} (log ε) 252 (2.70) nm; ECD (MeOH) λ_{max} (Δε) 211 (−1.52), 251 (+6.85), 301 (−2.68) nm; ^{1}H (400 MHz, CDCl$_3$) and ^{13}C NMR (100 MHz, CDCl$_3$) data, see Tables 2 and 3; HR–ESI–MS: m/z 279.1197 [M+Na]$^+$ (calcd. for C$_{13}$H$_{20}$O$_5$Na, 279.1203).

Talaketides B (**8**): C$_9$H$_{12}$O$_5$; yellow oil; $[\alpha]_D^{25}$ + 3.69° (c 0.24, MeOH); UV (MeOH) λ_{max} (log ε) 240 (3.28), 295 (2.53) nm; ECD (MeOH) λ_{max} (Δε) 208 (−2.95), 241 (−5.73), 294 (+2.65) nm; ^{1}H (400 MHz, CDCl$_3$) and ^{13}C NMR (100 MHz, CDCl$_3$) data, see Tables 2 and 3; HR–ESI–MS: m/z 223.0574 [M+Na]$^+$ (calcd. for C$_9$H$_{12}$O$_5$Na, 233.0577).

Talaketides C (**9**): C$_{15}$H$_{24}$O$_5$; yellow oil; $[\alpha]_D^{25}$ + 2.96° (c 1.12, MeOH); UV (MeOH) λ_{max} (log ε) 261 (2.94) nm; ECD (MeOH) λ_{max} (Δε) 205 (+0.36), 243 (−3.35), 262 (+0.97), 307 (+0.60) nm; ^{1}H (400 MHz, CDCl$_3$) and ^{13}C NMR (100 MHz, CDCl$_3$) data, see Tables 2 and 3; HR–ESI–MS: m/z 307.1517 [M+Na]$^+$ (calcd. for C$_{15}$H$_{24}$O$_5$Na, 307.1516).

Talaketides D (**10**): C$_9$H$_{14}$O$_4$; yellow oil; $[\alpha]_D^{25}$ + 16.04° (c 0.24, MeOH); UV (MeOH) λ_{max} (log ε) 251 (2.84) nm; ECD (MeOH) λ_{max} (Δε) 205 (+0.52), 252 (−2.08), 296 (+1.02) nm; ^{1}H (400 MHz, CDCl$_3$) and ^{13}C NMR (100 MHz, CDCl$_3$) data, see Tables 2 and 3; HR–ESI–MS: m/z 209.0783 [M+Na]$^+$ (calcd. for C$_9$H$_{14}$O$_4$Na, 209.0784).

Talaketides E (**11**): C$_9$H$_{14}$O$_4$; yellow oil; $[\alpha]_D^{25}$ − 11.35° (c 0.25, MeOH); UV (MeOH) λ_{max} (log ε) 252 (2.81) nm; ECD (MeOH) λ_{max} (Δε) 216 (−0.23), 249 (+0.60), 323 (−0.26) nm; ^{1}H (400 MHz, CDCl$_3$) and ^{13}C NMR (100 MHz, CDCl$_3$) data, see Tables 2 and 3; HR–ESI–MS: m/z 209.0784 [M+Na]$^+$ (calcd. for C$_{23}$H$_{33}$O$_6$, 209.0784).

Talaketides F (**12**): C$_{19}$H$_{25}$ClO$_5$; yellow oil; $[\alpha]_D^{25}$ + 49.14° (c 0.19, MeOH); UV (MeOH) λ_{max} (log ε) 252 (2.91) nm; ECD (MeOH) λ_{max} (Δε) 201 (+1.09), 256 (−1.52), 294 (+1.24) nm; ^{1}H (400 MHz, CDCl$_3$) and ^{13}C NMR (100 MHz, CDCl$_3$) data, see Tables 2 and 3; HR–ESI–MS: m/z 369.1468 [M+H]$^+$ (calcd. for C$_{19}$H$_{26}$ClO$_5$, 369.1468).

3.5. Molecular Networking

The crude extract of CY-3 was analyzed by LC–MS/MS (LTQ Velos Pro-Orbitrap, Waltham, MA, USA) and a C$_{18}$ column (Thermo Fisher Scientific-packed Hypersil GOLD, 1.9 μm, 2.1 × 100 mm). Samples were dissolved in MeCN at 1 mg/mL. A 10 μL of sample was injected and eluted with a gradient of H$_2$O containing 0.1% HCOOH and MeCN containing 0.1% HCOOH with a gradient method as follows: 10% MeCN/H$_2$O for 1 min, 10% MeCN/H$_2$O to 60% in 9 min, 60% MeCN/H$_2$O to 90% in 3 min, held at 90% MeCN/H$_2$O for 3 min, then 90% MeCN/H$_2$O to 10% MeCN/H$_2$O in 0.2 min, and finally held at 10% MeCN/H$_2$O for 3.8 min with the flow rate of 0.3 mL/min. Mass spectra were recorded in positive ESI mode (m/z 200–2000) and with an automated fully dependent MS/MS scan enabled. The molecular networking were made as described previously [27,28].

3.6. ECD and ^{13}C NMR Calculations

ECD calculations and 13C NMR calculations were performed by the Gaussian 09 program and Spartan'14. The conformation with a Boltzmann population greater than 5% was selected for optimization and calculation in methanol at B3LYP/6-31+G (d, p). The ECD spectra were generated by the program SpecDis 1.6 (University of Würzburg, Würzburg, Germany) and drawn by OriginPro 8.0 (OriginLab, Ltd., Northampton, MA, USA) from dipole-length rotational strengths by applying Gaussian band shapes with sigma = 0.30 eV [29,30].

3.7. Bioassay

Compounds **1–12** were evaluated for α-glucosidase inhibitory activity, as described previously [31]. Three parallel concentrations of 1-deoxynojirimycin were taken as positive controls. DMSO was used as blank controls.

3.8. Molecular Docking

Because the crystal structure of glucosidase from *Saccharomyces cerevisiae* cannot be obtained, the α-glucosidase homology model (PDB:3AXH) provided by SWISSMODEL Repository was used, and the model quality was evaluated [29]. The α-glucosidase homology model (PDB:3AXH) with compounds **1–5** was performed on Autodock, as described previously [31–34].

4. Conclusions

In summary, two new sambutoxin derivatives (**1–2**) and six new highly oxygenated polyketides derivatives (**7–12**), together with four known compounds (**3–6**), were obtained using guidance through molecular networking from semimangrove endophytic fungus *Talaromyces* sp. CY-3. The structures of new isolates were elucidated by 1D and 2D NMR, HR–ESI–MS, ECD spectra, ^{13}C NMR calculation, and DP4+ analysis, as well as chemical hydrolysis. The absolute configuration of sambutoxin derivatives (**1–2**) was determined through ^{13}C NMR calculation and DP4+ analysis for the first time. In bioassays, compounds **1–5** displayed better α-glucosidase inhibitory activity with IC$_{50}$ values in the range of 12.6 ± 0.9 to 57.3 ± 1.3 μM compared to the positive control 1-deoxynojirimycin (IC$_{50}$ = 80.8 ± 0.3 μM).

Supplementary Materials: The following are available online at https://www.mdpi.com/article/10.3390/md19090492/s1, Figure S1 LC-MS/MS of CY-3. Figure S2 ^{1}H NMR of **1**. Figure S3 ^{13}C NMR of **1**. Figure S4 DEPT 135 of **1**. Figure S5 HSQC spectrum of **1**. Figure S6 HMBC spectrum of **1**. Figure S7 COSY spectrum of **1**. Figure S8 NOESY spectrum of **1**. Figure S9 HR–ESI–MS spectrum of **1**. Figure S10 UV spectrum of **1**. Figure S11 ^{1}H NMR of **2**. Figure S12 ^{13}C NMR of **2**. Figure S13 DEPT 135 of **2**. Figure S14 HSQC spectrum of **2**. Figure S15 HMBC spectrum of **2**. Figure S16 COSY spectrum of **2**. Figure S17 NOESY spectrum of **2**. Figure S18 HR–ESI–MS spectrum of **2**. Figure S19 UV spectrum of **2**. Figure S20 ^{1}H NMR of **7**. Figure S21 ^{13}C NMR of **7**. Figure S22 HSQC spectrum of **7**. Figure S23 HMBC spectrum of **7**. Figure S24 COSY spectrum of **7**. Figure S25 NOESY spectrum of **7**. Figure S26 HR–ESI–MS spectrum of **7**. Figure S27 UV spectrum of **7**. Figure S28 ^{1}H NMR of **8**. Figure S29 ^{13}C NMR of **8**. Figure S30 HSQC spectrum of **8**. Figure S31 HMBC spectrum of **8**. Figure S32 COSY spectrum of **8**. Figure S33 NOESY spectrum of **8**. Figure S34 HR–ESI–MS spectrum of **8**. Figure S35 UV spectrum of **8**. Figure S36 ^{1}H NMR of **9**. Figure S37 ^{13}C NMR of **9**. Figure S38 HSQC spectrum of **9**. Figure S39 HMBC spectrum of **9**. Figure S40 COSY spectrum of **9**. Figure S41 NOESY spectrum of **9**. Figure S42 HR–ESI–MS spectrum of **9**. Figure S43 UV spectrum of **9**. Figure S44 ^{1}H NMR of **10**. Figure S45 ^{13}C NMR of **10**. Figure S46 HSQC spectrum of **10**. Figure S47 HMBC spectrum of **10**. Figure S48 COSY spectrum of **10**. Figure S49 NOESY spectrum of **10**. Figure S50 HR–ESI–MS spectrum of **10**. Figure S51 UV spectrum of **10**. Figure S52 ^{1}H NMR of **11**. Figure S53 ^{13}C NMR of **11**. Figure S54 HSQC spectrum of **11**. Figure S55 HMBC spectrum of **11**. Figure S56 COSY spectrum of **11**. Figure S57 NOESY spectrum of **11**. Figure S58 HR–ESI–MS spectrum of **11**. Figure S59 UV of **11**. Figure S60 ^{1}H NMR of **12**. Figure S61 ^{13}C NMR of **12**. Figure S62 HSQC spectrum of **12**. Figure S63 HMBC spectrum of **12**. Figure S64 COSY spectrum of **12**. Figure S65 NOESY spectrum of **12**. Figure S66 HR–ESI–MS spectrum of **12**. Figure S67 UV spectrum of **12**. Figure S68 Comparison of the experimental ^{13}C NMR data of the 2,4,6-trimethyloct-2-ene side chain for compound **1** and the calculated chemical shifts for four 2,4,6-trimethyloct-2-ene side-chain diastereomers (14*R*,16*S*-1, 14*R*,16*R*-1 14*S*,16*R*-1, and 14*S*, 16*S*-1). Figure S69 DP4+ analysis of **1**. Figure S70 Comparison of the experimental ^{13}C NMR data of the 2,4,6-trimethyloct-2-ene side chain for compound **2** and the calculated chemical shifts for four 2,4,6-trimethyloct-2-ene side-chain diastereomers (14*R*,16*S*-2, 14*R*,16*R*-2 14*S*,16*R*-2, and 14*S*, 16*S*-2). Figure S71 DP4+ analysis of **2**. Figure S72 Hydrolysis of **7** and **9** compared with the standard through HPLC chiral column.

Author Contributions: W.Y. performed the large-scale fermentation and isolated all compounds. W.Y. and Y.C. carried out the structure elucidation and edited the manuscript. J.W. carried out the biological assays. Q.T., Y.Y., Y.Z. and L.G. participated in the experiments. B.W. and Z.S. designed and supervised this research. All authors have read and agreed to the published version of the manuscript.

Funding: This research was funded by the National Natural Science Foundation of China (U20A2001, 21877133), the Key-Area Research and Development Program of Guangdong Province (2020B1111030005), the National Key R&D Program of China (2019YFC0312501), the Key Project of Natural Science Foundation of Guangdong Province (2016A030311026) and the Fundamental Research Funds for the Central Universities (No. 20ykjc04) for generous support.

Institutional Review Board Statement: Not applicable.

Data Availability Statement: Data are contained within the article and Supplementary Material.

Acknowledgments: We acknowledge the IARC, SYSU for support towards LC–MS equipment. We also thank SCSIO for the generous support towards ECD equipment.

Conflicts of Interest: The authors declare no conflict of interest.

References

1. Dhameja, M.; Gupta, P. Synthetic heterocyclic candidates as promising α-glucosidase inhibitors: An overview. *Eur. J. Med. Chem.* **2019**, *176*, 343–377. [CrossRef] [PubMed]
2. Rajalakshmi, R.; Lalitha, P.; Sharma, S.C.; Rajiv, A.; Chithambharan, A.; Ponnusamy, A. In Silico studies: Physicochemical properties, drug score, toxicity predictions and molecular docking of organosulphur compounds against *Diabetes mellitus*. *J. Mol. Recognit.* **2021**, e2925. [CrossRef]
3. Carroll, A.R.; Coop, B.R.; Davis, R.A.; Keyzers, R.A.; Prinsep, M.R. Marine natural products. *Nat. Prod. Rep.* **2021**, *38*, 362–413. [CrossRef] [PubMed]
4. Blunt, J.W.; Carroll, A.R.; Coop, B.R.; Davis, R.A.; Keyzers, R.A.; Prinsep, M.R. Marine natural products. *Nat. Prod. Rep.* **2018**, *16*, 319–349. [CrossRef] [PubMed]
5. Liu, Y.Y.; Yang, Q.; Xia, G.P.; Huang, H.B.; Li, H.X.; Ma, L.; Lu, Y.J.; He, L.; Xia, X.K.; She, Z.G. Polyketides with α-glucosidase inhibitory activity from a mangrove endophytic fungus, *Penicillium* sp. HN29-3B1. *J. Nat. Prod.* **2015**, *78*, 1816–1822. [CrossRef] [PubMed]
6. Chen, S.H.; Chen, D.N.; Cai, R.L.; Cui, H.; Long, Y.H.; Lu, Y.J.; Li, C.Y.; She, Z.G. Cytotoxic and antibacterial preussomerins from the mangrove endophytic fungus *Lasiodiplodia theobromae* ZJ-HQ1. *J. Nat. Prod.* **2016**, *79*, 2397–2402. [CrossRef]
7. Liang, Z.Y.; Shen, N.X.; Zheng, Y.Y.; Wu, J.T.; Miao, L.; Fu, X.M.; Chen, M.; Wang, C.Y. Two new unsaturated fatty acids from the mangrove rhizosphere soil-derived fungus *Penicillium javanicum* HK1-22. *Bioorg. Chem.* **2019**, *93*, 103331. [CrossRef]
8. An, C.Y.; Li, X.M.; Li, C.S.; Wang, M.H.; Xu, G.M.; Wang, B.G. Aniquinazolines A-D, four new quinazolinone alkaloids from marine-derived endophytic fungus *Aspergillus nidulans*. *Mar. Drugs* **2013**, *11*, 2682–2694. [CrossRef]
9. Chen, Y.; Liu, Z.M.; Huang, Y.; Liu, L.; He, J.G.; Wang, L.; Yuan, J.; She, Z.G. Ascomylactams A–C, cytotoxic 12- or 13-membered-ring macrocyclic alkaloids isolated from the mangrove endophytic fungus *Didymella* sp. CYSK-4, and structure eevisions of phomapyrrolidones A and C. *J. Nat. Prod.* **2019**, *82*, 1752–1758. [CrossRef]
10. Peng, J.X.; Lin, T.; Wang, W.; Xin, Z.H.; Zhu, T.J.; Gu, Q.Q.; Li, D.H. Antiviral alkaloids produced by the mangrove-derived fungus *Cladosporium* sp. PJX-41. *J. Nat. Prod.* **2013**, *76*, 1133–1140. [CrossRef]
11. Zou, G.; Tan, Q.; Chen, Y.; Yang, W.C.; Zang, Z.M.; Jiang, H.M.; Chen, S.Y.; Wang, B.; She, Z.G. Furobenzotropolones A, B and 3-hydroxyepicoccone B with antioxidative activity from mangrove endophytic fungus *Epicoccum nigrum* MLY-3. *Mar. Drugs* **2021**, *19*, 395. [CrossRef]
12. Chen, Y.; Yang, W.C.; Zou, G.; Yan, Z.Y.; Qiu, P.; Long, Y.H.; She, Z.G. Metabolites with anti-inflammatory and alpha-glucosidase inhibitory activities from the mangrove endophytic fungus *Phoma* sp. SYSU-SK-7. *Tetrahedron Lett.* **2020**, *61*, 152578. [CrossRef]
13. Cai, R.L.; Wu, Y.N.; Chen, S.H.; Cui, H.; Liu, Z.M.; Li, C.Y.; She, Z.G. Peniisocoumarins A–J: Isocoumarins from *Penicillium commune* QQF-3, an endophytic fungus of the mangrove plant *Kandelia candel*. *J. Nat. Prod.* **2018**, *81*, 1376–1383. [CrossRef]
14. Wu, Y.N.; Chen, Y.; Huang, X.S.; Pan, Y.H.; Liu, Z.M.; Yan, T.; Cao, W.H.; She, Z.G. α-Glucosidase inhibitors: Diphenyl ethers and phenolic bisabolane sesquiterpenoids from the mangrove endophytic fungus *Aspergillus flavus* QQSG-3. *Mar. Drugs* **2018**, *16*, 307. [CrossRef]
15. Allard, P.M.; Péresse, T.; Bisson, J.; Gindro, K.; Marcourt, L.; Pham, V.C.; Roussi, F.; Litaudon, M.; Wolfender, J.L. Integration of molecular networking and in-silico MS/MS fragmentation for natural products dereplication. *Anal. Chem.* **2016**, *88*, 3317–3323. [CrossRef]
16. Nie, Y.Y.; Yang, W.C.; Liu, Y.Y.; Yang, J.M.; Lei, X.L.; Gerwick, W.H.; Zhang, Y. Acetylcholinesterase inhibitors and antioxidants mining from marine fungi: Bioassays, bioactivity coupled LC–MS/MS analyses and molecular networking. *Mar. Life Sci. Technol.* **2020**, *2*, 386–397. [CrossRef]

17. Gu, B.; Wu, Y.; Tang, J.; Jiao, W.; Li, L.; Sun, F.; Wang, S.; Yang, F.; Lin, H. Azaphilone and isocoumarin derivatives from the sponge-derived fungus *Eupenicillium* sp. 6A-9. *Tetrahedron Lett.* **2018**, *59*, 3345–3348. [CrossRef]
18. Huo, C.; Lu, X.; Zheng, Z.; Li, Y.; Xu, Y.; Zheng, H.; Niu, Y. Azaphilones with protein tyrosine phosphatase inhibitory activity isolated from the fungus *Aspergillus deflectus*. *Phytochemistry* **2020**, *170*, 112224. [CrossRef]
19. Kim, J.C.; Lee, Y.W.; Tamura, H.; Yoshizawa, T. Sambutoxin: A new mycotoxin isolated from *Fusarium sambucinum*. *Tetrahedron Lett.* **1995**, *36*, 1047–1050. [CrossRef]
20. Williams, D.R.; Turske, R.A. Construction of 4-hydroxy-2-pyridinones. Total synthesis of (+)-sambutoxin. *Org. Lett.* **2000**, *2*, 3217–3220. [CrossRef] [PubMed]
21. Chunyu, W.X.; Zhao, J.Y.; Ding, Z.G.; Han, X.L.; Wang, Y.X.; Ding, J.H.; Wang, F.; Li, M.G.; Wen, M.L. A new cyclohexenone from the tin mine tailingsderived fungus *Aspergillus flavus* YIM DT 10012. *Nat. Prod. Res.* **2019**, *33*, 113–116. [CrossRef]
22. Matsumoto, M.; Minato, H. Structure of ilicicolin H, an antifungal antibiotic. *Tetrahedron Lett.* **1976**, *42*, 3827–3830. [CrossRef]
23. Sinder, B.B.; Lu, Q. Total synthesis of (±)-leporin A. *J. Org. Chem.* **1996**, *61*, 2839–2844. [CrossRef]
24. Zhang, C.; Jin, L.; Mondie, B.; Mitchell, S.S.; Castelhano, A.L.; Cai, W.; Bergenhem, N. Leporin B: A novel hexokinase II gene inducing agent from an unidentified fungus. *Bioorg. Med. Chem. Lett.* **2003**, *13*, 1433–1435. [CrossRef]
25. Zhang, Z.; Jamieson, C.S.; Zhao, Y.; Li, D.; Ohashi, M.; Houk, K.N.; Tang, Y. Enzyme-catalyzed inverse-electron demand Diels-Alder reaction in the biosynthesis of antifungal ilicicolin H. *J. Am. Chem. Soc.* **2019**, *141*, 5659–5663. [CrossRef]
26. Millot, M.; Dieu, A.; Tomosi, S. Dibenzofurans and derivatives from lichens and ascomycetes. *Nat. Prod. Rep.* **2016**, *33*, 801–811. [CrossRef] [PubMed]
27. Wang, M.; Carver, J.J.; Phelan, V.V.; Sanchez, L.M.; Garg, N.; Peng, Y.; Nguyen, D.D.; Watrous, J.; Kapono, C.A.; Luzzatto-Knaan, T.; et al. Sharing and community curation of mass spectrometry data with Global Natural Products Social Molecular Networking. *Nat. Biotechnol.* **2016**, *34*, 828–837. [CrossRef] [PubMed]
28. Li, Y.; Yu, H.B.; Zhang, Y.; Leao, T.; Glukhov, E.; Pierce, M.L.; Zhang, C.; Kim, H.; Mao, H.H.; Fang, F.; et al. Pagoamide A, a cyclic depsipeptide isolated from a cultured marine chlorophyte, *Derbesia* sp., using MS/MS-based molecular networking. *J. Nat. Prod.* **2020**, *83*, 617–625. [CrossRef] [PubMed]
29. Cui, H.; Liu, Y.N.; Li, J.; Huang, X.S.; Yan, T.; Cao, W.H.; Liu, H.J.; Long, Y.H.; She, Z.G. Diaporindenes A–D: Four unusual 2,3-dihydro-1H-indene analogues with anti-inflammatory activities from the mangrove endophytic fungus *Diaporthe* sp. SYSU. *J. Org. Chem.* **2018**, *83*, 11804–11813. [CrossRef]
30. Frisch, M.J.; Trucks, G.W.; Schlegel, H.B.; Scuseria, G.E.; Robb, M.A.; Cheeseman, J.R.; Scalmani, G.; Barone, V.; Mennucci, B.; Petersson, G.A.; et al. *Gaussian 09*; Gaussian, Inc.: Wallingford, UK, 2016.
31. Ye, G.J.; Lan, T.; Huang, Z.X.; Cheng, X.N.; Cai, C.Y.; Ding, S.M.; Xie, M.L.; Wang, B. Design and synthesis of novel xanthone-triazole derivatives aspotential antidiabetic agents:α-glucosidase inhibition and glucoseuptake promotion. *Eur. J. Med. Chem.* **2019**, *177*, 362–373. [CrossRef]
32. Chen, T.; Huang, Y.; Hong, J.; Wei, X.; Zeng, F.; Li, J.; Ye, G.; Yuan, J.; Long, Y. Preparation, COX-2 inhibition and anticancer activity of sclerotiorin derivatives. *Mar. Drugs* **2021**, *19*, 12. [CrossRef] [PubMed]
33. DeLano, W.L. The PyMOL Molecular Graphics System. 2002. Available online: http://www.pymol.org (accessed on 30 August 2020).
34. Wallace, A.C.; Laskowski, R.A.; Thornton, J.M. LIGPLOT: A program to generate schematic diagrams of protein-ligand interactions. *Protein Eng.* **1995**, *8*, 127–134. [CrossRef] [PubMed]

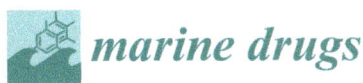

Review

Marine Power on Cancer: Drugs, Lead Compounds, and Mechanisms

Lichuan Wu [1], Ke Ye [2], Sheng Jiang [2,*] and Guangbiao Zhou [3,*]

1. Medical College, Guangxi University, Nanning 530004, China; richard_wu@gxu.edu.cn
2. School of Pharmacy, China Pharmaceutical University, Nanjing 211198, China; yekecpu@163.com
3. State Key Laboratory of Molecular Oncology, National Cancer Center/National Clinical Research Center for Cancer/Cancer Hospital, Chinese Academy of Medical Sciences and Peking Union Medical College, Beijing 100021, China
* Correspondence: jiangsh9@gmail.com (S.J.); gbzhou@cicams.ac.cn (G.Z.)

Abstract: Worldwide, 19.3 million new cancer cases and almost 10.0 million cancer deaths occur each year. Recently, much attention has been paid to the ocean, the largest biosphere of the earth that harbors a great many different organisms and natural products, to identify novel drugs and drug candidates to fight against malignant neoplasms. The marine compounds show potent anticancer activity in vitro and in vivo, and relatively few drugs have been approved by the U.S. Food and Drug Administration for the treatment of metastatic malignant lymphoma, breast cancer, or Hodgkin's disease. This review provides a summary of the anticancer effects and mechanisms of action of selected marine compounds, including cytarabine, eribulin, marizomib, plitidepsin, trabectedin, zalypsis, adcetris, and OKI-179. The future development of anticancer marine drugs requires innovative biochemical biology approaches and introduction of novel therapeutic targets, as well as efficient isolation and synthesis of marine-derived natural compounds and derivatives.

Keywords: marine environment drug; natural compounds; anticancer; mechanisms of action

1. Introduction

With its great biodiversity and unique chemical diversity, the marine environment is a huge treasury of medicinal resources [1–3]. There are 17 clinically available drugs that were based on marine natural products or their derivatives, and 28 drugs that are currently being tested in phase I–III clinical trials [4,5]. Cancer has been the second leading cause of mortality worldwide, causing approximately 10 million deaths in 2020 [6]. In the past decades, substantial efforts have been made to unveil the pathogenesis of cancers and new anticancer drugs have been developed [7–10]. Here, we review the original resources, anticancer effects, mechanisms, and clinical applications of selected marine-derived compounds including cytarabine (the first approved marine-derived anticancer drug), eribulin (a microtubule-depolymerizing drug), marizomib (a proteasome inhibitor), plitidepsin (a DNA synthesis inhibitor), trabectedin (a nucleotide drug), adcetris (an antibody drug conjugate), zalypsis (a new DNA binding alkaloid), and the largazole analogue OKI-179 (an HDAC inhibitor) (Table 1).

Citation: Wu, L.; Ye, K.; Jiang, S.; Zhou, G. Marine Power on Cancer: Drugs, Lead Compounds, and Mechanisms. *Mar. Drugs* **2021**, *19*, 488. https://doi.org/10.3390/md19090488

Academic Editors: RuAngelie Edrada-Ebel, Chang-Yun Wang and Bin-Gui Wang

Received: 19 July 2021
Accepted: 24 August 2021
Published: 27 August 2021

Publisher's Note: MDPI stays neutral with regard to jurisdictional claims in published maps and institutional affiliations.

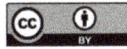

Copyright: © 2021 by the authors. Licensee MDPI, Basel, Switzerland. This article is an open access article distributed under the terms and conditions of the Creative Commons Attribution (CC BY) license (https://creativecommons.org/licenses/by/4.0/).

Table 1. Selected marine natural compounds or derivatives that have been approved or entered into clinical trials in the past decades.

Compound	Source	Indications	Mechanisms	Clinical Trial
Cytarabine	*Cryptotethia crypta*	AML	DNA synthesis inhibition	Approved
Eribulin	*Halichondria okadai*	Breast cancer, liposarcoma	Prevention the formation of spindles and EMT, apoptosis induction	Approved
Marizomib	*Salinispora tropica*	MM	Selectively inhibiting 20S proteasome	Approved
Plitidepsin	*Aplidium albican*	Solid tumor, MM	Cell cycle arrest, apoptosis induction	Approved
Trabectedin	*Ecteinascidia turbinata*	Liposarcoma, leiomyosarcoma	Binding to guanine residues in the DNA groove to form protein adducts	Approved
Adcetris	*Dolabella auricularia*	Hodgkin's lymphoma	Inhibiting tubulin formation, apoptosis induction	Approved
Zalypsis	*Joruna funebris*	Urothelial carcinoma, cervical carcinoma, MM	rendering DNA double strand breaks, cell cycle arrest, apoptosis induction	Phase II
OKI-179	*Cyanobacterium, Symploca*	Advanced solid tumors	Class I HDAC inhibition	Phase I

Abbreviations: HDAC: Histone Deacetylase; AML: Acute Myeloid Leukemia; EMT: Epithelial-Mesenchymal Transition; MM: Multiple Myeloma; MMPs: Matrix Metalloproteinases.

2. Cytarabine/Ara-C

Cytarabine (Figure 1), based on a lead compound from marine sponge was synthesized in 1959 by Walwick at the University of California, Berkeley. Cytarabine was the first clinically used marine anticancer drug to be approved in 1969 by the US Food and Drug Administration (FDA), mainly for treating acute leukemia [11,12]. Cytarabine is a cytosine base-containing pyrimidine nucleoside. It is converted from 1-β-d-arabinofuranosyluracil through the acylation of its hydroxyl group and conversion of the 4-carbonyl group in the pyrimidine ring into a thiocarbonyl group. Subsequently, the thiol group was replaced by an amino group and the acetyl group was hydrolyzed to obtain the final pyrimidine structure. The difference between the synthetic cytarabine and the naturally occurring cytarabine is that in the latter, there is a hydroxyl group in the 2'-β configuration of the sugar moiety. The resulting arabinose binds to the replicating DNA chain and inhibits the initiation and extension of the chain, resulting in the production of erroneous DNA.

Cytarabine is metabolized in vivo and transformed into its active form "ara-CTP". The entire process involves three steps [13]. First, cytarabine is converted to the inactive form arabinouridine (Ara-U) after deamination and only small amount of cytarabine subsequently enters into the cell. Cytarabine is catalyzed into Ara-CMP via deoxycytidine kinase (DCK) in the cytoplasm. Second, Ara-CMP is transformed into Ara-CDP by pyrimidine nucleoside kinase. Third, the Ara-CDP is metabolized into Ara-CTP. Ara-CTP may be incorporated into the nucleotide chain of ribonucleic acid (DNA), which prevents chain elongation and causes chain breaks. By affecting the replication of the chain, the drug inhibits the proliferation of tumor cells. Studies have shown that Ara-CTP can bind to the topoisomerase complex limiting its activity by inhibiting DNA synthesis (Figure 1) [14].

The anticancer effect of cytarabine depends on the dosage. When cytarabine at low dosage enters into the structure of oligonucleotides, it reduces the binding capacity of transcription factors with their respective DNA binding elements and the transduction of new messenger RNA. At high doses, it exhibits a significant antitumor effect by inducing cell cycle arrest at the G0 and G1 phases. While cytarabine at medium and small doses can induce S phase cell cycle arrest. DNA fragmentation analysis shows that cytarabine induces cellular apoptosis in a dose-dependent manner (Figure 1) [15].

In the clinic, high and medium dosages of cytarabine are usually applied to treat acute myeloid leukemia (AML) [15]. However, serious side effects, such as bone marrow suppression, which will lead to anemia, leukopenia, thrombocytopenia, infection, and musculoskeletal and connective tissue abnormalities have limited its clinical use [16–18]. Therefore, combination medication becomes an alternative which can avoid serious adverse effects. Although decitabine combined with low-dose of Ara-C has a higher risk of bone marrow suppression and infection in the initial stage of treatment, patients can tolerate it and with the extension of the treatment course, the adverse reactions gradually decreased [19].

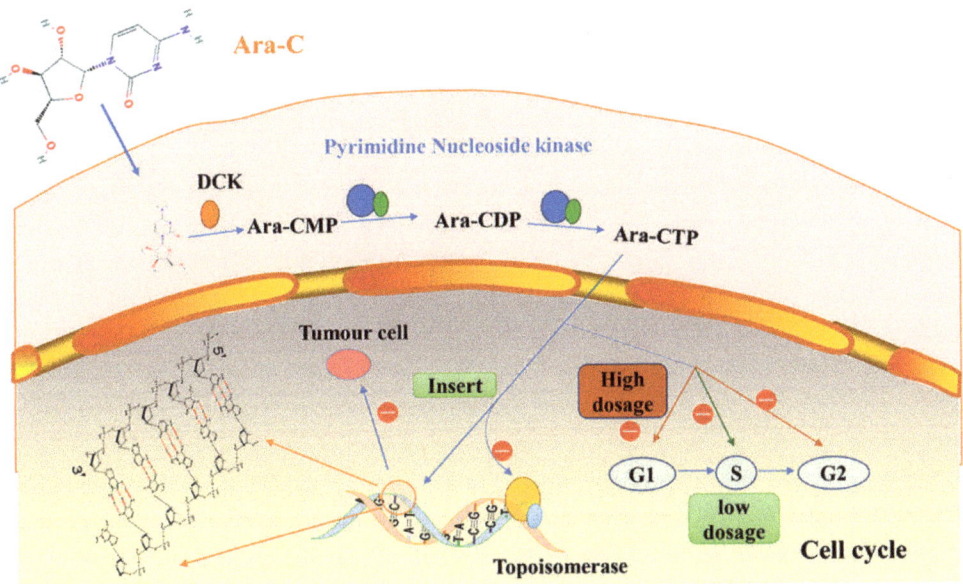

Figure 1. Cytarabine exhibits anticancer effects by inhibiting DNA synthesis and inducing cell cycle arrest.

Drug resistance has always been a major problem in the clinical application of cytarabine. In recent years, research on drug resistance of cytarabine has gradually increased and studies have shown that drug resistance is related to biological factors, proteins, and gene mutations [20,21]. Cytarabine induces apoptosis of HL60 cells and activates nuclear factor-κB (NF-κB), which may cause early resistance of leukemia cells to cytarabine. It has been reported that NF-κB plays an important role in anti-apoptosis [22–25]. Deoxycytidine kinase (DCK) protein, one of the most critical proteins identified in research reports, is the key rate-limiting enzyme for the phosphorylation of cytarabine in the body. It has been found that DCK is down-regulated and mutated in drug-resistant mouse AML cell lines. As a result, the first phosphorylation of cytarabine in the body is restricted, affecting the activation and the therapeutic effect of cytarabine in the body [26].

3. Eribulin/E7389

Eribulin (Figure 2) is a derivative of halichondrin B which was isolated from *Halichondria okadai* [27,28]. Eribulin was approved by FDA for treatment of breast cancer and liposarcoma in 2010 and 2016, respectively [29]. The synthesis of eribulin is complicated and difficult [30]. Eribulin is a microtubule-depolymerizing drug, which interferes with the mitotic phase of cell cycle. Eribulin mainly binds with high affinity to the ends of positive microtubules, preventing the polymerization of tubulin. Eribulin can also bind to soluble α- or β-tubulin, decreasing the effectiveness of subunit polymerization and inducing cell cycle arrest at the G2/M phase and apoptosis through mitochondrial obstruction (Figure 2) [31]. In preclinical studies, eribulin has shown antitumor activity in various types of cancer, including colon cancer, glioblastoma, head and neck cancer, melanoma, non-small cell lung cancer (NSCLC), ovarian cancer, pancreatic cancer, and small cell lung cancer [32].

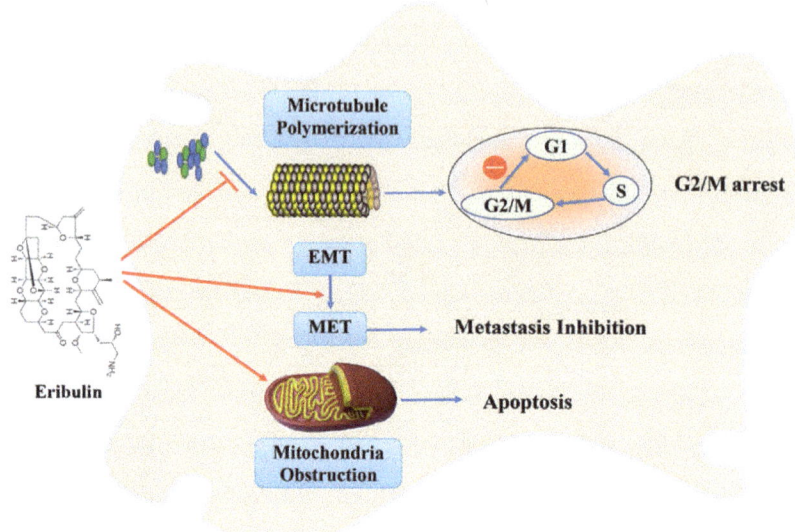

Figure 2. Eribulin exerts its anticancer effects by inducing cell cycle arrest, apoptosis, and tumor metastasis inhibition.

Eribulin can inhibit tumor metastasis by inhibiting epithelial-mesenchymal transition (EMT) and inducing mesenchymal-epithelial transition (MET). Yoshida et al. found that treatment of triple negative breast cancer (TNBC) cells with eribulin led to MET [33]. Eribulin treatment decreases expression of mesenchymal marker genes and increases the expression of epithelial markers. Funahashi et al. reported that eribulin remodels tumor vasculature in human breast cancer xenograft models by increasing microvessel density and decreasing mean vascular areas and branched vessels in tumor tissues [34]. Further, the authors reported that eribulin affects the expression of genes involved in the angiogenesis signaling pathway and the EMT pathway, and was posited to be related to the decrease in hypoxia. Clinical studies support the use of eribulin in the treatment of advanced or metastatic breast cancer, and also indicate that eribulin may treat solid tumors that are resistant to other types of microtubule kinetic inhibitors. In addition, the combination of eribulin and paclitaxel exerts a synergistic anti-proliferative effect on TNBC cells by increasing the expression of E-cadherin and decreasing the expression of cell mesenchymal markers [35].

4. Marizomib/NPI-0052

Proteasome degradation plays a critical role in the survival of malignant tumor cells. The increase of proteasome has been observed in various types of tumor cells, indicating that the survival and growth of tumor cells rely on the proteasome [36]. In the late stage of plasma cell differentiation, proteasome activity decreases with the accumulation of immunoglobulin, leading to the accumulation of ubiquitinated protein [37]. Marizomib (NPI-0052), a natural compound isolated from marine *Salinispora tropica* [38], possessing a γ-lactam-β-lactone fragment is a proteasome inhibitor. Studies have shown that marizomib induces loss of mitochondrial membrane potential, increases ROS production, cytochrome C/Smac release and activation of caspases, leading to multiple myeloma cell apoptosis [39]. Marizomib may also exert antitumor activity through the inner mitochondrial apoptotic pathway and death receptor pathway (Figure 3) [40–42]. Inhibition of the proteasome by marizomib is generally considered to be the result of inhibiting the NF-κB pathway. Proteasome inhibition increases the level of IκBα, thereby inhibiting the NF-κB pathway, resulting in a decrease in the production of anti-apoptotic factors, angiogenic factors and inhibition of apoptosis [43]. Proteasome inhibition leads to an imbalance in the self-regulation of cyclins, cyclin-dependent kinases and other cell cycle regulatory proteins and this can disrupt cell division.

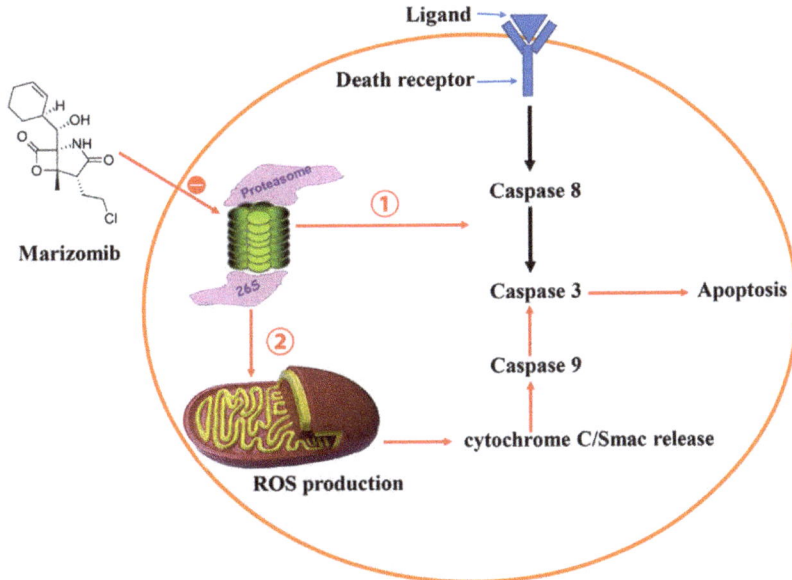

Figure 3. Marizomib exerts its anticancer effects by inducing mitochondria and death receptor pathways.

Chauhan et al. found that intravenous injection of single or multiple doses of marizomib (0.15 mg/kg) into mice can inhibit proteasome activity in peripheral organs, but not in the brain [39]. Marizomib is rapidly distributed to various organs and tumors from the vascular compartment, and clearly inhibits the caspase-like, trypsin-like, and chymotrypsin-like activity of proteasomes. Marizomib synergizes with the immunosuppressive agent pomalidomide in treatment of multiple myeloma by inducing apoptosis by activation of caspases and downregulation of CRBN, MYC, IRF4, and MCL1 [44].

Clinical studies have shown that Marizomib is effective in treating neoplastic malignancies including multiple myeloma, brain tumor, and glioma, and was approved by FDA in 2013 and the European Medicines Agency (EMA) in 2014 for treatment of multiple myeloma [45–47]. Marizomib is well tolerated, and adverse events include nausea, neutropenia, pneumonia, anemia, thrombocytopenia, and febrile neutropenia. Marizomib also causes central nervous system toxicity, such as cognitive changes, expressive aphasia, visual or auditory hallucinations, disorientation, and unstable gait, which can be relieved after ceasing the drug [48].

5. Plitidepsin/Aplidine

Plitidepsin (aplidine), a natural compound isolated from *Aplidium albican* [49], is a cyclic depsipeptide whose structure is similar to that of bisbenzophenone [50]. Plitidepsin has strong antitumor activity with low toxicity and was approved by FDA in 2004 to treat multiple myeloma [51].

The mechanism of plitidepsin in treating multiple tumors has been thoroughly investigated. Plitidepsin exhibits anticancer effects by inhibiting tumor cell proliferation and inducing cell apoptosis in multiple myeloma (MM), plasmacytoma, prostate cancer, pancreatic cancer, and ovarian cancer [52,53]. Plitidepsin treatment resulted in oxidative stress, rapid activation of Rac1 GTPase, and continuous activation of c-Jun N-terminal kinase (JNK) and p38 mitogen-activated protein kinase (p38/MAPK), leading to caspase activation and cell apoptosis (Figure 4) [54]. Recent studies have found that the translation elongation factor eEF1A2 is the primary target of plitidepsin, which can bind to eEF1A2 at the interface between domains 1 and 2 of this protein in the GTP conformation [51,55,56]. It has been further reported that plitidepsin also inhibits the activation and subsequent destruction of aggregates in lysosomes, which accumulate excessive misfolded proteins in cells, thereby triggering apoptosis. In chronic lymphocytic leukemia (CLL), plitidepsin affects the viability of leukemic cells through direct and indirect pathways. It inhibits the malignant B-CLL clone directly and restrains tumor growth by indirect modification of the micro-environment [53]. A recent study showed that plitidepsin analogs PM01215 and PM02781 inhibit angiogenesis in vitro and in vivo [57].

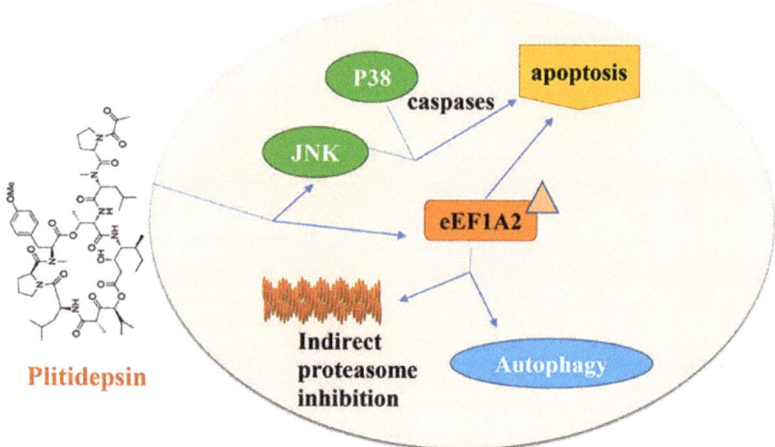

Figure 4. Plitidepsin displays anticancer effects by inducing cell apoptosis and autophagy.

6. Trabectedin/ET-743

Trabectedin (ET-743) is a tetrahydroisoquinoline alkaloid derivative which was approved to treat liposarcoma and leiomyosarcoma by EMA and FDA in 2007 and 2015, respectively [58,59]. Trabectedin is isolated from extracts of *Ecteinascidia turbinata* and described as able to prevent oncogenic transcription factors from binding to the target promoters [60]. Trabectedin contains three fused tetrahydroisoquinoline rings (A, B, and C rings) [61]. The A and B rings form a rigid five-ring skeleton, which is connected to the C ring through a 10-membered lactone bridge. Ring A and B insert into deoxyribonucleic acid (DNA) by interacting with DNA minor grooves through hydrogen bonds and Van der Waals forces to promote the alkylation of adjacent nucleotides in the same or opposite strands of DNA [62]. The N2 of guanine in the 5′-CGG, TGG, GGC, AGC sequence is the alkylation site [63]. In addition, protonated amines are involved in the production of reactive imine ions (N2) that catalyze DNA binding [64]. The carbon ring protrudes from the deoxyribonucleic acid backbone and interferes with the deoxyribonucleic acid binding protein, while traditional alkylating agent drugs usually bind at the N-terminal or O-terminal. In addition, trabectedin inhibits transcription by binding to transcription RNA polymerase II (Pol II) and blocking its activity [65], leading to degradation of Pol II enzyme (Figure 5) [66].

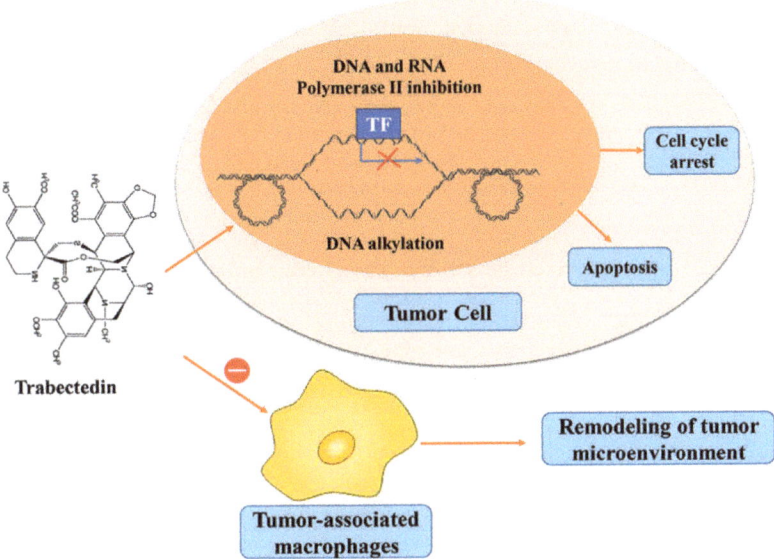

Figure 5. Trabectedin displays anticancer effects through inducing cell cycle arrest, apoptosis, and remodeling of tumor microenvironment. (TF: transcription factor).

Studies in vivo and in vitro have shown that trabectedin can reduce tumor growth and regulate the tumor micro-environment. In addition to the approved treatment of soft tissue sarcoma and ovarian cancer, trabectedin is undergoing clinical evaluation with other cancer types, including breast cancer, bone cancer, and prostate cancer [60]. Trabectedin inhibits transcription by reducing the transactivation ability of the chimeric protein, achieving some success in myxoid liposarcoma and Ewing's sarcoma and other sarcoma subtypes, and ultimately leading to adipocyte differentiation and apoptosis [67]. The clinical application of trabectedin was first applied to soft tissue sarcoma (STS). A number of clinical phase I studies have found that it has a good effect on ovarian cancer when used alone or in combination with other chemotherapeutic drugs, such as cisplatin [68–70]. Phase II and III clinical studies have shown that trabectedin alone or in combination with other anticancer drugs is effective in soft tissue tumors, especially liposarcoma and leiomyosarcoma, and prolongs the survival time of the patients [30,71–73].

Clinical application of trabectedin is gradually expanding. It is reported that trabectedin could regulate the tumor micro-environment (TME) by decreasing the concentration of immune cells, such as monocytes and tumor-associated macrophages, and indirectly reducing the production of inflammatory mediators, such as interleukin-6, interleukin-8 and vascular endothelial growth factor, and affecting the expression of extracellular matrix-related genes [74]. Trabectedin could also inhibit genes and pathways related to the phenotype of cancer stem cells [75,76]. Moreover, trabectedin-induced DNA damage in an RNA-DNA hybrid-dependent manner in Hela cells has been observed. This RNA-DNA hybrid is also called R-loop, and high level of R-loops sensitizes tumor cells to trabectedin. [77].

7. Adcetris/Brentuximab Vedotin

Adcetris, or Brentuximab Vedotin is an antibody drug conjugate which couples a CD30 antibody and a tubulin targeted compound, monomethyl auristatin E (MMAE). Compound MMAE is a derivative of natural compound dolastatin 10 isolated from *Dolabella auricularia* [78–80]. Adcetris was approved in 2011 to treat Hodgkin's lymphoma (HL) and systemic anaplastic large cell lymphoma (ALCL) [81]. Adcetris consists of three parts: a monoclonal antibody with a targeting function, which can guide adcetris to its target cells; an effective cytotoxic compound called the payload or warhead, which has the pharmacological effect of killing tumor cells; and a central part composed of hexanoic acid and maleimide that has a linking function. It can covalently connect the first two parts and be further responsible for releasing payloads and linkers in the target cells [82–85]. Brentuximab is a monoclonal antibody that locates tumor cells by searching for the tumor marker CD30 membrane protein. Vedotin is the second part of the conjugate, including the linker and the cytotoxic principle MMAE. To meet the requirements, the main ingredient of linker in adcetris is cathepsin-cleavable valine-citrulline, which can be cut precisely to release a cytotoxic compound. Adcetris exerts its anticancer activity in a few steps in vivo. First, the recognition of brentuximab antibody by CD30 protein leads to the decomposition of adcetris. Then, the selective proteolytic cleavage of adcetris promoted by lysosomal cysteine protease releases vedotin. Second, vedotin releases MMAE in cytoplasm. When free MMAE reaches its goal, it prevents cell division in G2/M by disrupting microtubule dynamics, and ultimately induces cell death (Figure 6) [85,86].

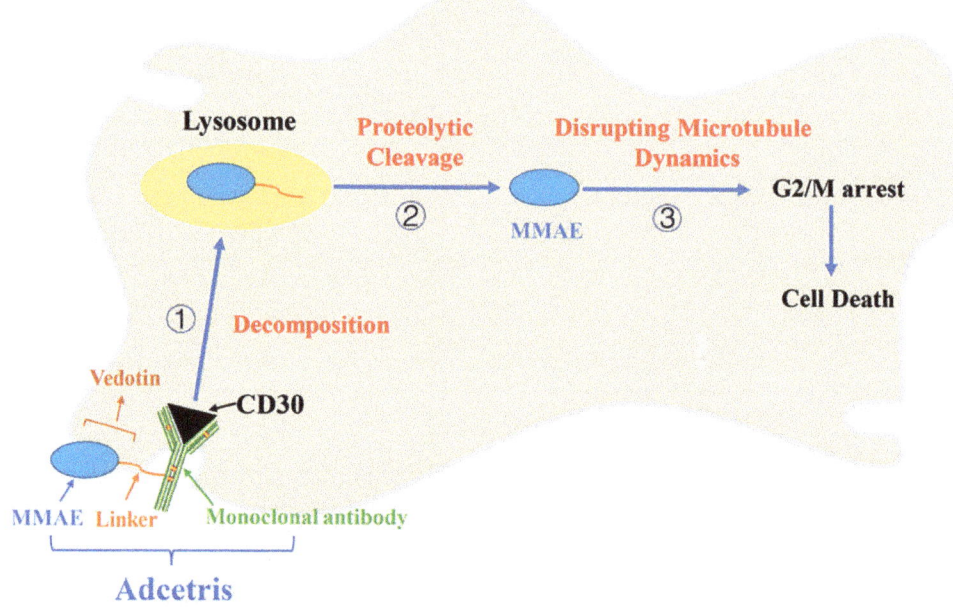

Figure 6. The action model of adcetris targeting CD30 positive tumor cells.

Adcetris is used in the clinic as a consolidation therapy after autologous stem cell transplantation (ASCT). Some studies have evaluated the efficacy of adcetris as a consolidation therapy for adult patients with Hodgkin's lymphoma at risk of relapse or progression after receiving ASCT through a randomized, double-blind, Phase 3 trial [87]. During the 30-month follow-up, in the main independent retrospective analysis, treatment with adcetris, compared with placebo, significantly prolonged progression-free survival (PFS; 42.9 months vs. 24.1 months). Adcetris has a certain effect on other CD30-positive lymphomas. The efficacy of adcetris on B-cell lymphoma was evaluated in a phase II trial. The study included 65 patients with CD30-positive relapsed or refractory B-cell lymphoma who were given 1.8 mg/kg of adcetris. Among 48 evaluable basal cell carcinoma patients, eight and thirteen patients achieved complete and partial remission, respectively [88].

Adcetris has attracted great attention because of its excellent antitumor activity and its acceptable side effects. The successful development of adcetris indicates that CD30 can be used as a therapeutic target for HL and ALCL, which leads to the development of more CD30-targeting agents. Currently, more than 80 active phase I–III clinical trials have been carried out to evaluate the efficacies of adcetris in cancers, but drug resistance has been reported in patients treated with adcetris. Strategies to overcome drug resistance and combinatory regimens to achieve maximal efficacy are being tested in lymphoma [89].

8. Zalypsis/M00104

Zalypsis, an alkaloid newly isolated from *Joruna funebris*, is a tetrahydroisoquinolone alkaloid that is structurally similar to ascidianin and nephromycin [90]. It binds covalently to guanine residues in for example, the AGG, GGC, AGC, CGG, and TGG groups to form a DNA-zalypsis adduct, leading to early transcription inhibition and a double-stranded DNA break, affecting cell proliferation and development (Figure 7) [91,92]. Zalypsis shows antitumor activity against cell lines of bladder cancer, gastric cancer, liver cancer, prostate cancer, pancreatic cancer, thyroid cancer, sarcoma, leukemia, and lymphoma [91,93–96]. In multiple myeloma, zalypsis in combination with bortezomib and dexamethasone exerts enhanced efficacy with acceptable toxicity in vitro and in vivo [97]. Phase II and Phase III clinical trials have shown that zalypsis is effective in treating Ewing's sarcoma, urothelial cancer, multiple myeloma, endometrial cancer, and cervical cancer [91,98].

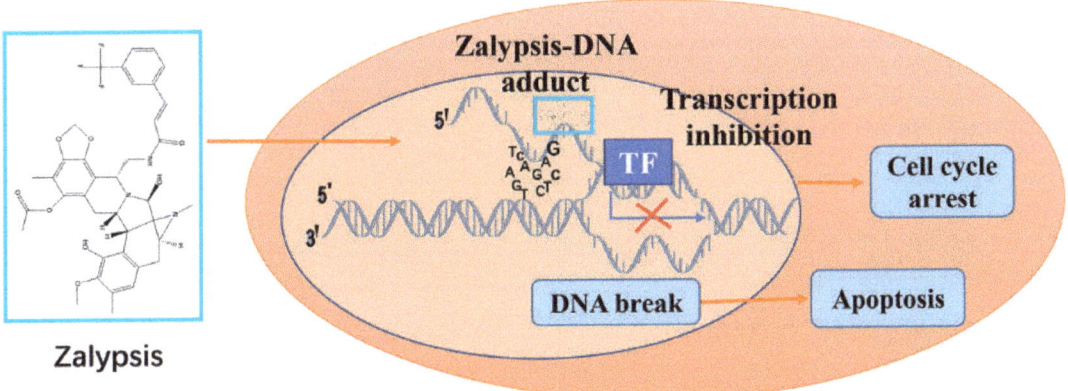

Figure 7. Zalypsis forms a DNA-drug adduct which induces cell cycle arrest and apoptosis.

9. Largazole and Its Analogues

HDACs are responsible for the deacetylation of lysine residues in histone and non-histone proteins, leading to chromatin condensation and transcriptional repression [99]. To date, eighteen human HDACs have been identified, and they are divided into four classes (I–IV). HDACs, especially class I HDACs, are overexpressed in various cancer cell types [100,101] and contribute to tumor development and progression [102,103]. Thus, HDACs have been validated as valuable anticancer targets, and four HDAC inhibitors, including vorinostat, romidepsin, belinostat, and panobinostat, have been approved by FDA for the treatment of hematologic malignancies including T-cell lymphoma and multiple myeloma. Selective HDAC inhibitors are highly desirable since they can not only serve as pharmacological tools to help elucidate the biological roles of specific HDAC class or isoforms, but also as therapeutic agents with potentially reduced side effects commonly existing in the pan-HDAC inhibitors [104,105].

Largazole, **1**, a cyclic depsipeptide, was isolated from marine *cyanobacterium Symploca sp.* in 2008 by Luesch et al. [106]. This research group firstly revealed the robust potency of largazole against HDAC1 in the low nanomolar range and with selectivity over HDAC6 [107,108]. Subsequently, largazole was found to strongly inhibit HDAC1, HDAC2 and HDAC3 in the picomolar range in a biological assay developed by Williams et al. [109]. Studies suggests that largazole possesses a wide range of pharmacological activities, such as anti-inflammation [110], anti-liver fibrosis [111], anti-virus [112], osteogenic activity [113], and anticancer activity [114]. Largazole has received much attention due to its potent anti-proliferative activity against various cancer cells and substantial potency as a class I histone deacetylase (HDAC1) inhibitor. Wu et al. reported that largazole could potently and selectively suppress lung cancer cell proliferation and colony formation activity with no obvious cytotoxicity against normal bronchial epithelial cells [115]. Largazole induce a G1 cell cycle arrest via upregulation of p21 and down-regulation of E2F1. Liu et al. found that largazole showed stronger inhibition of colon cancer cell lines than of other type of cancer cells by screening the National Cancer Institute's 60 cancer cell lines [116]. Largazole exerted its anti-colon cancer effects by inducing cell cycle arrest, cell apoptosis, and down-regulation of insulin receptor substrate 1 in vitro and in vivo [116]. Law et al. reported that largazole and glucocorticoid dexamethasone cooperate to induce E-cadherin (E-cad) localization to the plasma membrane of triple-negative breast cancer cells, leading to inhibition of cell invasion [117]. Michelle et al. designed a multidimensional screening platform and found largazole was an inhibitor of oncogenic Kirsten ras (KRAS) and the hypoxia inducible factor (HIF) pathway which could inhibit colon cancer proliferation and angiogenesis [118]. Gilson et al. performed RNA sequencing to identify altered gene expression upon largazole treatment [119]. Their results demonstrated that largazole could particularly decrease RNA polymerase II accumulation at super-enhancers and inhibit oncogene activities in cancer cells induced by super-enhancers. Recently, largazole was also found to inhibit proliferation of glioblastoma multiforme (GBM) cell lines in vitro at nanomolar concentrations [120]. More importantly, it was shown to be highly brain-penetrant and, therefore, could achieve therapeutically relevant doses in mouse brain which led to upregulation of neuroprotective genes, including Bdnf and Pax6. Wang et al. revealed that largazole markedly suppressed cell proliferation and induced apoptosis in non-small cell lung cancer (NSCLC) and chronic myeloid leukemia (CML) by decreasing the expression of oncogenic protein Musashi-2 (MSI2) [121]. The anticancer mechanisms of largazole are summarized in Figure 8.

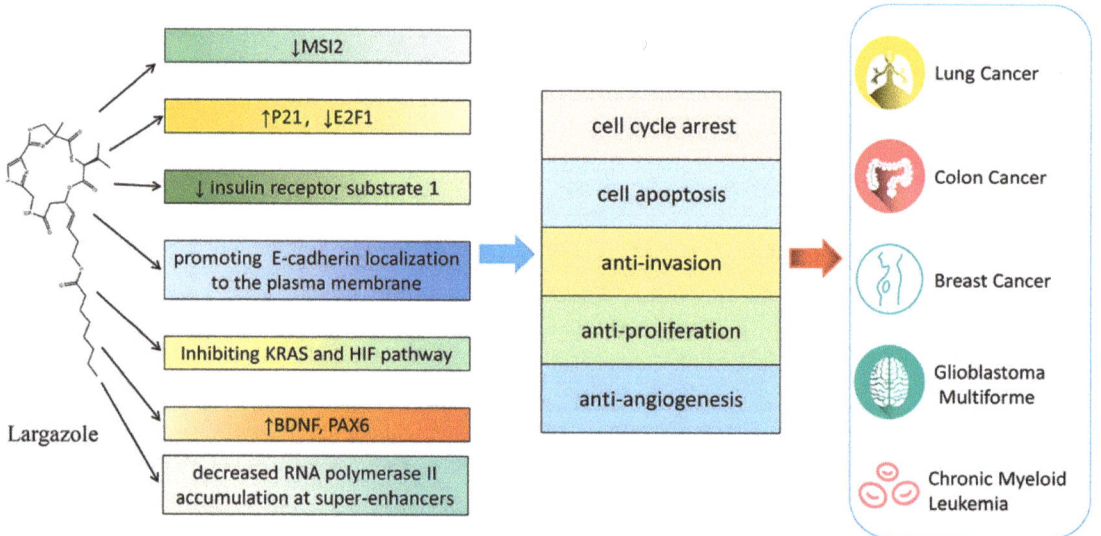

Figure 8. Anticancer mechanism of largazole.

These excellent properties of largazole have prompted extensive structural modifications and structure-activity relationship (SAR) studies with the aim of searching for more potent and selective HDAC inhibitors [122–124]. Structurally, largazole is a prodrug which can be converted to the free thiol form (**2**) through removal of the octanoyl group by esterases or lipases [109]. As is shown in the co-crystal structure of HDAC8 complexed with largazole thiol (**2**), the free sulfhydryl group of **2** as a warhead chelates Zn^{2+} in the active site of the HDACs [125]. The octanoyl group makes largazole more cell-permeant and allows facile liberation of the free thiol within the cell [109]. The 16-membered depsipeptide ring system acts as a surface recognition group which interacts with the surrounding hydrophobic residues on the outer rim of the enzyme, contributing to enzyme potency and selectivity. The four-atom length of linker connecting the Zn^{2+}-binding group (ZBG) to the depsipeptide ring occupies the narrow hydrophobic channel [125]. The structural modifications of largazole are mainly focused on the linker, ZBG and depsipeptide ring system (mainly focusing on the L-valine residue and the 4-methylthiazoline–thiazole subunit).

Initial SAR studies suggested that largazole analogues with a four-atom linker, a *trans*-form alkene attached to the macrocyclic ring and an *S*-configured C-17 are critical for HDAC inhibitory activity and antiproliferative effect against cancer cells [108,126,127]. Introduction of an aromatic group in the linker region results in complete loss of HDAC inhibitory activity [128]. In order to fully ascertain the role of the metal-binding domain in HDAC inhibition, a series of largazole analogues with various ZBGs were prepared. Analogues **3** and **4** with an α-thioamide or mercaptosulfide, respectively, and analogues **5** and **6** which added a second heteroatom for multiple heteroatomic chelation with Zn^{2+} showed reduced inhibitory activity (Figure 9). However, these compounds conferred selectivity inhibition on HDAC6 or HDAC10 over HDAC1 [129–131]. In addition, our group identified an analogue **7** with an octyldisulfide side chain which confers a significant selectivity on HDAC1 over HDAC7 [132]. Together, these studies indicated that ZBGs have profound effects on HDAC inhibitory potency and isoform selectivity.

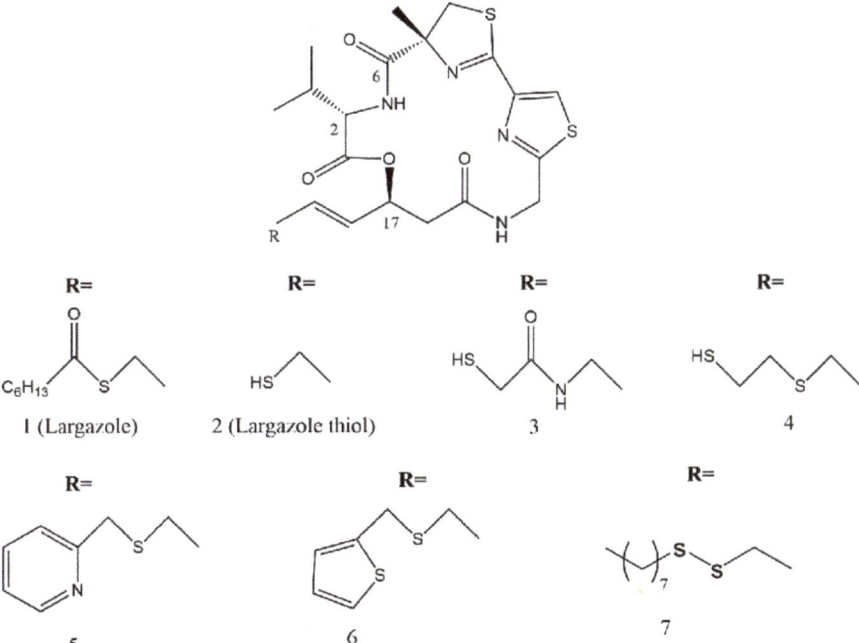

Figure 9. Largazole, largazole thiol, and largazole analogues with different ZBGs.

Many largazole analogues with a modified L-valine unit have been reported. Different amino acid residues, such as Ala, Gly, Phe, Tyr, Asp, His, Leu, 1-naphthylmethylglycine, and 1-allylglycine were introduced into largazole at the C2 position and these modifications were well tolerated, albeit with a minimal loss in inhibitory activity or isoform selectivity [108,127,128,133,134]. Recently, Lei et al. reported a promising analogue (**8**) (Figure 10) that had an S-Me L-cysteine (MeS) substitution at the C2 position [135]. This compound showed a more potent inhibitory activity on HDAC1 than largazole thiol (**2**), and exhibited a comparable selectivity for HDAC1 over HDAC6.

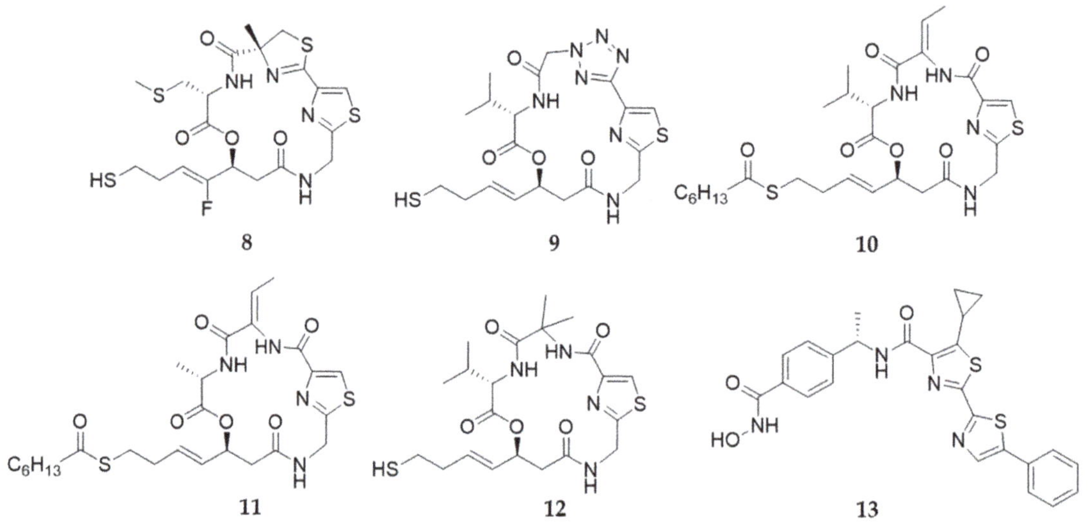

Figure 10. Largazole analogues with a modified depsipeptide ring.

A few largazole analogues with modified thiazole-thiazoline groups have been reported. The elimination or replacement of the methyl group of 4-methylthiazoline with an ethyl or a benzyl group is tolerated, indicating that 4-methylthiazoline moiety is not necessary for HDAC inhibition [136,137]. Based on this assumption, our group reported the largazole analogue (**9**) with a more hydrophobic tetrazole group in place of the 4-methylthiazoline, which showed potent inhibition of HDAC1, HDAC2, and HDAC3 (HDAC1, IC_{50} = 100 nM; HDAC2, IC_{50} = 224 nM; and HDAC3, IC_{50} = 31 nM) and better selectivity for HDAC1 over HDAC9 than largazole [138]. Based on the largazole analogue (**10**) discovered by our group, which contains an unsaturated dehydrobutyrine (Dhb) in place of 4-methylthiazoline, we replaced the L-valine region of **10** with different amino acid residues, such as glycine, butyrine, leucine, t-butylglycine and methionine [139,140]. Among these, compound **11** with L-alanine in place of L-valine showed the most potent and selective inhibitory effects on HDAC1-3 (HDAC1, IC_{50} = 1.3 nM; HDAC2, IC_{50} = 1.6 nM; and HDAC3, IC_{50} = 3.2 nM), and promising anti-proliferative activity against cancer cell lines Molt-4 and A549 (Molt-4, GI_{50} = 2.1 nM; A549, GI_{50} = 7.5 nM). This compound showed desirable antitumor efficacy in a PC3 xenograft model with no apparent toxicity [140].

Analogue **12** was obtained by replacing the 4-methylthiazoline group with a simplified α-aminoisobutyric acid residue, which showed a 20-fold reduced nanomolar HDAC inhibition compared to largazole thiol [133]. Recently, Nan and coworkers identified a bisthiazole-based HDAC inhibitor (**13**) through structural simplification of largazole skeleton. This compound exhibited potent nanomolar HDAC inhibition (HDAC1, IC_{50} = 3.64 nM; HDAC2, IC_{50} = 3.02 nM; and HDAC3, IC_{50} = 4.96 nM) and strong antiproliferative activity against NCI-N87 (IC_{50} = 28 nM) and T47D cells (IC_{50} = 40 nM). Furthermore, **13** showed good antitumor efficacy in the HT-29 xenograft model with good oral bioavailability and safety profile [124,141].

Among these largazole analogues, a compound named OKI-179 was identified as a candidate drug which has entered phase I clinical study to treat advanced solid tumors [142,143]. OKI-179 was discovered by Liu et al. who were aiming to improve the physiochemical properties and simplify the synthesis of largazole [144]. The results of in vitro enzyme activities assay indicated that OKI-179 displays significant inhibition towards class I, IIb, and IV HDACs. Wang et al. reported that compound OKI-179 could sensitize PD1 blockade-resistant B cell lymphomas to PD1 antibody treatment [145]. Treatment with OKI-179 leads to cell-cycle arrest, apoptosis, and growth inhibition in tumors. According to the mechanism of action of OKI-179, MHC proteins are downregulated in PD1 blockade-resistant B cell lymphomas (G1XP lymphomas). Upon OKI-179 treatment, MHCs including class I and II are up-regulated. Furthermore, MHC knockout attenuates OKI-179 induced tumor growth inhibition. OKI-179 and OKI-179/anti-PD1 treatment activates tumor-infiltrating lymphocytes (TILs) in G1XP lymphomas. These results displayed that OKI-179 sensitizes lymphomas to PD1-blockade by enhancing tumor immunogenicity.

10. Conclusions and Prospect

Terrestrial animals and plants have always been important sources of natural products. Humans began to extract active ingredients from terrestrial plants and animals to treat diseases thousands of years ago. With the progress of drug discovery, it is increasingly difficult to develop new molecular entity drugs from terrestrial animals and plants, which cannot cope with the increasing threat to human life and health. Therefore, "asking for drugs from the sea" has become a key to find new drug sources. The continuous innovation of deep-sea mining technology, extraction and separation technology, molecular modification technology, genetic engineering technology, and organic synthesis technology provide hope and new opportunities for the development of marine anticancer drugs.

Author Contributions: G.Z. conceived, designed, and supervised the manuscript; L.W., K.Y. and S.J. collected the literature, analyzed the data, and wrote the manuscript. All authors have read and agreed to the published version of the manuscript.

Funding: This work was supported by the National Key Research and Development Program of China (Nos. 2020YFA0803300), the Guangxi Natural Science Foundation (2017GXNSFBA198240, 2018GXNSFAA050055, and 2021GXNSFAA075038), the Key Project of the National Natural Science Foundation of China (81830093), the CAMS Innovation Fund for Medical Sciences (CIFMS; 2019-I2M-1-003), and the National Natural Science Foundation of China (81672765, 81802796, and 82073092).

Data Availability Statement: No new data were created or analyzed in this study. Data sharing is not applicable to this article.

Conflicts of Interest: The authors declare no conflict of interest.

References

1. Blunt, J.W.; Carroll, A.R.; Copp, B.R.; Davis, R.A.; Keyzers, R.A.; Prinsep, M.R. Marine natural products. *Nat. Prod. Rep.* **2018**, *35*, 8–53. [CrossRef]
2. Carroll, A.R.; Copp, B.R.; Davis, R.A.; Keyzers, R.A.; Prinsep, M.R. Marine natural products. *Nat. Prod. Rep.* **2019**, *36*, 122–173. [CrossRef]
3. Jimenez, C. Marine Natural Products in Medicinal Chemistry. *ACS Med. Chem. Lett.* **2018**, *9*, 959–961. [CrossRef] [PubMed]
4. Khalifa, S.A.M.; Elias, N.; Farag, M.A.; Chen, L.; Saeed, A.; Hegazy, M.F.; Moustafa, M.S.; Abd El-Wahed, A.; Al-Mousawi, S.M.; Musharraf, S.G.; et al. Marine Natural Products: A Source of Novel Anticancer Drugs. *Mar. Drugs* **2019**, *17*, 491. [CrossRef] [PubMed]
5. Shinde, P.; Banerjee, P.; Mandhare, A. Marine natural products as source of new drugs: A patent review (2015–2018). *Expert. Opin. Pat.* **2019**, *29*, 283–309. [CrossRef] [PubMed]
6. Siegel, R.L.; Miller, K.D.; Fuchs, H.E.; Jemal, A. Cancer Statistics, 2021. *CA Cancer J. Clin.* **2021**, *71*, 7–33. [CrossRef] [PubMed]
7. Spano, V.; Venturini, A.; Genovese, M.; Barreca, M.; Raimondi, M.V.; Montalbano, A.; Galietta, L.J.V.; Barraja, P. Current development of CFTR potentiators in the last decade. *Eur. J. Med. Chem.* **2020**, *204*, 112631. [CrossRef] [PubMed]

8. Barreca, M.; Spanò, V.; Montalbano, A.; Cueto, M.; Bertoni, F. Marine Anticancer Agents: An Overview with a Particular Focus on Their Chemical Classes. *Mar. Drugs* **2020**, *18*, 619. [CrossRef]
9. Spanò, V.; Rocca, R.; Barreca, M.; Giallombardo, D.; Barraja, P. Pyrrolo[2′,3′:3,4]cyclohepta[1,2-d][1,2]oxazoles, a New Class of Antimitotic Agents Active against Multiple Malignant Cell Types. *J. Med. Chem.* **2020**, *63*, 12023–12042. [CrossRef]
10. Spanò, V.; Pennati, M.; Parrino, B.; Carbone, A.; Montalbano, A.; Cilibrasi, V.; Zuco, V.; Lopergolo, A.; Cominetti, D.; Diana, P. Preclinical Activity of New [1,2]Oxazolo[5,4-e]isoindole Derivatives in Diffuse Malignant Peritoneal Mesothelioma. *J. Med. Chem.* **2016**, *59*, 7223–7238. [CrossRef]
11. Sippel, T.R.; White, J.; Nag, K.; Tsvankin, V.; Klaassen, M.; Kleinschmidt-DeMasters, B.K.; Waziri, A. Neutrophil Degranulation and Immunosuppression in Patients with GBM: Restoration of Cellular Immune Function by Targeting Arginase I. *Clin. Cancer Res.* **2011**, *17*, 6992–7002. [CrossRef] [PubMed]
12. Dombret, H.; Gardin, C. An update of current treatments for adult acute myeloid leukemia. *Blood* **2016**, *127*, 53–61. [CrossRef]
13. Schwartsmann, G.; da Rocha, A.B.; Berlinck, R.G.S.; Jimeno, J. Marine organisms as a source of new anticancer agents. *Lancet Oncol.* **2001**, *2*, 221–225. [CrossRef]
14. Pourquier, P.; Takebayashi, Y.; Urasaki, Y.; Gioffre, C.; Kohlhagen, G.; Pommier, Y. Induction of topoisomerase I cleavage complexes by 1-beta-D-arabinofuranosylcytosine (ara-C) in vitro and in ara-C-treated cells. *Proc. Natl. Acad. Sci. USA* **2000**, *97*, 1885–1890. [CrossRef] [PubMed]
15. Nakayama, T.; Sakamoto, S.; Sassa, S.; Suzuki, S.; Kudo, H.; Nagasawa, H. Paradoxical effect of cytosine arabinoside on mouse leukemia cell line L-1210 cells. *Anticancer Res.* **2005**, *25*, 157–160. [PubMed]
16. Herzig, R.H.; Wolff, S.N.; Lazarus, H.M.; Phillips, G.L.; Karanes, C.; Herzig, G.P. High-dose cytosine arabinoside therapy for refractory leukemia. *Blood* **1983**, *62*, 361–369. [CrossRef]
17. Peters, W.G.; Colly, L.P.; Willemze, R. High-dose cytosine arabinoside: Pharmacological and clinical aspects. *Blut* **1988**, *56*, 1–11. [CrossRef]
18. Carden, P.A.; Mitchell, S.L.; Waters, K.D.; Tiedemann, K.; Ekert, H. Prevention of cyclophosphamide/cytarabine-induced emesis with ondansetron in children with leukemia. *J. Clin.* **1990**, *8*, 1531–1535. [CrossRef]
19. Lv, S.Q.; Li, A.H.; Wu, H.J.; Wang, X.L. Observation of clinical efficacy and toxic and side effects of pirarubicin combined with cytarabine on acute myeloid leukemia. *Oncol. Lett.* **2019**, *17*, 3411–3417. [CrossRef]
20. Drenberg, C.D.; Hu, S.; Li, L.; Buelow, D.R.; Orwick, S.J.; Gibson, A.A.; Schuetz, J.D.; Sparreboom, A.; Baker, S.D. ABCC4 Is a Determinant of Cytarabine-Induced Cytotoxicity and Myelosuppression. *Clin. Transl. Sci.* **2016**, *9*, 51–59. [CrossRef]
21. Adema, A.D.; Floor, K.; Smid, K.; Honeywell, R.J.; Scheffer, G.L.; Jansen, G.; Peters, G.J. Overexpression of MRP4 (ABCC4) and MRP5 (ABCC5) confer resistance to the nucleoside analogs cytarabine and troxacitabine, but not gemcitabine. *Springerplus* **2014**, *3*, 732. [CrossRef] [PubMed]
22. Waddick, K.G.; Uckun, F.M. Innovative treatment programs against cancer: II. Nuclear factor-kappaB (NF-kappaB) as a molecular target. *Biochem. Pharmacol.* **1999**, *57*, 9–17. [CrossRef]
23. Wang, C.Y.; Cusack, J.C., Jr.; Liu, R.; Baldwin, A.S., Jr. Control of inducible chemoresistance: Enhanced antitumor therapy through increased apoptosis by inhibition of NF-kappaB. *Nat. Med.* **1999**, *5*, 412–417. [CrossRef] [PubMed]
24. Berenson, J.R.; Ma, H.M.; Vescio, R. The role of nuclear factor-kappaB in the biology and treatment of multiple myeloma. *Semin. Oncol.* **2001**, *28*, 626–633. [CrossRef]
25. Cusack, J.C., Jr.; Liu, R.; Houston, M.; Abendroth, K.; Elliott, P.J.; Adams, J.; Baldwin, A.S., Jr. Enhanced chemosensitivity to CPT-11 with proteasome inhibitor PS-341: Implications for systemic nuclear factor-kappaB inhibition. *Cancer Res.* **2001**, *61*, 3535–3540.
26. Rathe, S.K.; Moriarity, B.S.; Stoltenberg, C.B.; Kurata, M.; Aumann, N.K.; Rahrmann, E.P.; Bailey, N.J.; Melrose, E.G.; Beckmann, D.A.; Liska, C.R.; et al. Using RNA-seq and targeted nucleases to identify mechanisms of drug resistance in acute myeloid leukemia. *Sci. Rep.* **2014**, *4*, 6048. [CrossRef]
27. Hirata, Y.; Uemura, D. Halichondrins—Antitumor polyether macrolides from a marine sponge. *Pure Appl. Chem.* **1986**, *58*, 701–710. [CrossRef]
28. Seletsky, B.M.; Wang, Y.; Hawkins, L.D.; Palme, M.H.; Habgood, G.J.; DiPietro, L.V.; Towle, M.J.; Salvato, K.A.; Wels, B.F.; Aalfs, K.K.; et al. Structurally simplified macrolactone analogues of halichondrin B. *Bioorganic Med. Chem. Lett.* **2004**, *14*, 5547–5550. [CrossRef]
29. In, G.K.; Hu, J.S.; Tseng, W.W. Treatment of advanced, metastatic soft tissue sarcoma: Latest evidence and clinical considerations. *Ther. Adv. Med. Oncol.* **2017**, *9*, 533–550. [CrossRef]
30. Jimenez, P.C.; Wilke, D.V.; Branco, P.C.; Bauermeister, A.; Rezende-Teixeira, P.; Gaudencio, S.P.; Costa-Lotufo, L.V. Enriching cancer pharmacology with drugs of marine origin. *Br. J. Pharmacol.* **2020**, *177*, 3–27. [CrossRef]
31. Eslamian, G.; Wilson, C.; Young, R.J. Efficacy of eribulin in breast cancer: A short report on the emerging new data. *OncoTargets Ther.* **2017**, *10*, 773–779. [CrossRef] [PubMed]
32. Towle, M.J.; Nomoto, K.; Asano, M.; Kishi, Y.; Yu, M.J.; Littlefield, B.A. Broad spectrum preclinical antitumor activity of eribulin (Halaven(R)): Optimal effectiveness under intermittent dosing conditions. *Anticancer Res.* **2012**, *32*, 1611–1619.
33. Yoshida, T.; Ozawa, Y.; Kimura, T.; Sato, Y.; Kuznetsov, G.; Xu, S.; Uesugi, M.; Agoulnik, S.; Taylor, N.; Funahashi, Y.; et al. Eribulin mesilate suppresses experimental metastasis of breast cancer cells by reversing phenotype from epithelial-mesenchymal transition (EMT) to mesenchymal-epithelial transition (MET) states. *Br. J. Cancer* **2014**, *110*, 1497–1505. [CrossRef]

34. Funahashi, Y.; Okamoto, K.; Adachi, Y.; Semba, T.; Uesugi, M.; Ozawa, Y.; Tohyama, O.; Uehara, T.; Kimura, T.; Watanabe, H.; et al. Eribulin mesylate reduces tumor microenvironment abnormality by vascular remodeling in preclinical human breast cancer models. *Cancer Sci.* **2014**, *105*, 1334–1342. [CrossRef]
35. Oba, T.; Ito, K.I. Combination of two anti-tubulin agents, eribulin and paclitaxel, enhances antitumor effects on triple-negative breast cancer through mesenchymal-epithelial transition. *Oncotarget* **2018**, *9*, 22986–23002. [CrossRef]
36. Manasanch, E.E.; Orlowski, R.Z. Proteasome inhibitors in cancer therapy. *Nat. Rev. Clin. Oncol.* **2017**, *14*, 417–433. [CrossRef]
37. Cenci, S.; Mezghrani, A.; Cascio, P.; Bianchi, G.; Cerruti, F.; Fra, A.; Lelouard, H.; Masciarelli, S.; Mattioli, L.; Oliva, L.; et al. Progressively impaired proteasomal capacity during terminal plasma cell differentiation. *EMBO J.* **2006**, *25*, 1104–1113. [CrossRef] [PubMed]
38. Fenical, W.; Jensen, P.R.; Palladino, M.A.; Lam, K.S.; Lloyd, G.K.; Potts, B.C. Discovery and development of the anticancer agent salinosporamide A (NPI-0052). *Bioorganic Med. Chem.* **2009**, *17*, 2175–2180. [CrossRef] [PubMed]
39. Chauhan, D.; Hideshima, T.; Anderson, K.C. A novel proteasome inhibitor NPI-0052 as an anticancer therapy. *Br. J. Cancer* **2006**, *95*, 961–965. [CrossRef]
40. Baritaki, S.; Suzuki, E.; Umezawa, K.; Spandidos, D.; Berenson, J.; Daniels, T.; Penichet, M.; Jazirehi, A.; Palladino, M.; Bonavida, B. Inhibition of Yin Yang 1-dependent repressor activity of DR5 transcription and expression by the novel proteasome inhibitor NPI-0052 contributes to its TRAIL-enhanced apoptosis in cancer cells. *J. Immunol.* **2008**, *180*, 6199–6210. [CrossRef]
41. Chauhan, D.; Catley, L.; Li, G.; Podar, K.; Hideshima, T.; Velankar, M.; Mitsiades, C.; Mitsiades, N.; Yasui, H.; Letai, A.; et al. A novel orally active proteasome inhibitor induces apoptosis in multiple myeloma cells with mechanisms distinct from Bortezomib. *Cancer Cell* **2005**, *8*, 407–419. [CrossRef]
42. Delic, J.; Masdehors, P.; Omura, S.; Cosset, J.M.; Dumont, J.; Binet, J.L.; Magdelenat, H. The proteasome inhibitor lactacystin induces apoptosis and sensitizes chemo- and radioresistant human chronic lymphocytic leukaemia lymphocytes to TNF-alpha-initiated apoptosis. *Br. J. Cancer* **1998**, *77*, 1103–1107. [CrossRef]
43. Nencioni, A.; Grunebach, F.; Patrone, F.; Ballestrero, A.; Brossart, P. Proteasome inhibitors: Antitumor effects and beyond. *Leukemia* **2007**, *21*, 30–36. [CrossRef]
44. Das, D.S.; Ray, A.; Song, Y.; Richardson, P.; Trikha, M.; Chauhan, D.; Anderson, K.C. Synergistic anti-myeloma activity of the proteasome inhibitor marizomib and the IMiD immunomodulatory drug pomalidomide. *Br. J. Haematol.* **2015**, *171*, 798–812. [CrossRef] [PubMed]
45. Mateos, M.; Ocio, E.; San Miguel, J. Novel generation of agents with proven clinical activity in multiple myeloma. *Semin. Oncol.* **2013**, *40*, 618–633. [CrossRef] [PubMed]
46. Zhang, J.; Wu, P.; Hu, Y. Clinical and marketed proteasome inhibitors for cancer treatment. *Curr. Med. Chem.* **2013**, *20*, 2537–2551. [CrossRef] [PubMed]
47. Allegra, A.; Alonci, A.; Gerace, D.; Russo, S.; Innao, V.; Calabrò, L.; Musolino, C. New orally active proteasome inhibitors in multiple myeloma. *Leuk. Res.* **2014**, *38*, 1–9. [CrossRef] [PubMed]
48. Wang, H.; Guan, F.; Chen, D.; Dou, Q.; Yang, H. An analysis of the safety profile of proteasome inhibitors for treating various cancers. *Expert Opin. Drug Saf.* **2014**, *13*, 1043–1054. [CrossRef] [PubMed]
49. Urdiales, J.L.; Morata, P.; Nunez De Castro, I.; Sanchez-Jimenez, F. Antiproliferative effect of dehydrodidemnin B (DDB), a depsipeptide isolated from Mediterranean tunicates. *Cancer Lett.* **1996**, *102*, 31–37. [CrossRef]
50. Sakai, R.; Rinehart, K.L.; Kishore, V.; Kundu, B.; Faircloth, G.; Gloer, J.B.; Carney, J.R.; Namikoshi, M.; Sun, F.; Hughes, R.G., Jr.; et al. Structure–activity relationships of the didemnins. *J. Med. Chem.* **1996**, *39*, 2819–2834. [CrossRef]
51. Gomes, N.G.M.; Valentao, P.; Andrade, P.B.; Pereira, R.B. Plitidepsin to treat multiple myeloma. *Drugs Today* **2020**, *56*, 337–347. [CrossRef] [PubMed]
52. Gonzalez-Santiago, L.; Suarez, Y.; Zarich, N.; Munoz-Alonso, M.J.; Cuadrado, A.; Martinez, T.; Goya, L.; Iradi, A.; Saez-Tormo, G.; Maier, J.V.; et al. Aplidin induces JNK-dependent apoptosis in human breast cancer cells via alteration of glutathione homeostasis, Rac1 GTPase activation, and MKP-1 phosphatase downregulation. *Cell Death Differ.* **2006**, *13*, 1968–1981. [CrossRef]
53. Morande, P.E.; Zanetti, S.R.; Borge, M.; Nannini, P.; Jancic, C.; Bezares, R.F.; Bitsmans, A.; Gonzalez, M.; Rodriguez, A.L.; Galmarini, C.M.; et al. The cytotoxic activity of Aplidin in chronic lymphocytic leukemia (CLL) is mediated by a direct effect on leukemic cells and an indirect effect on monocyte-derived cells. *Investig. New Drugs* **2012**, *30*, 1830–1840. [CrossRef]
54. Garcia-Fernandez, L.F.; Losada, A.; Alcaide, V.; Alvarez, A.M.; Cuadrado, A.; Gonzalez, L.; Nakayama, K.; Nakayama, K.I.; Fernandez-Sousa, J.M.; Munoz, A.; et al. Aplidin induces the mitochondrial apoptotic pathway via oxidative stress-mediated JNK and p38 activation and protein kinase C delta. *Oncogene* **2002**, *21*, 7533–7544. [CrossRef]
55. Losada, A.; Lopez-Oliva, J.M.; Sanchez-Puelles, J.M.; Garcia-Fernandez, L.F. Establishment and characterisation of a human carcinoma cell line with acquired resistance to Aplidin. *Br. J. Cancer* **2004**, *91*, 1405–1413. [CrossRef] [PubMed]
56. Losada, A.; Muñoz-Alonso, M.; García, C.; Sánchez-Murcia, P.; Martínez-Leal, J.; Domínguez, J.; Lillo, M.; Gago, F.; Galmarini, C. Translation Elongation Factor eEF1A2 is a Novel Anticancer Target for the Marine Natural Product Plitidepsin. *Sci. Rep.* **2016**, *6*, 35100. [CrossRef] [PubMed]
57. Borjan, B.; Steiner, N.; Karbon, S.; Kern, J.; Francesch, A.; Hermann, M.; Willenbacher, W.; Gunsilius, E.; Untergasser, G. The Aplidin analogs PM01215 and PM02781 inhibit angiogenesis in vitro and in vivo. *BMC Cancer* **2015**, *15*, 738. [CrossRef] [PubMed]

58. Grosso, F.; Jones, R.L.; Demetri, G.D.; Judson, I.R.; Blay, J.-Y.; Le Cesne, A.; Sanfilippo, R.; Casieri, P.; Collini, P.; Dileo, P.; et al. Efficacy of trabectedin (ecteinascidin-743) in advanced pretreated myxoid liposarcomas: A retrospective study. *Lancet Oncol.* **2007**, *8*, 595–602. [CrossRef]
59. Pautier, P.; Floquet, A.; Chevreau, C.; Penel, N.; Guillemet, C.; Delcambre, C.; Cupissol, D.; Selle, F.; Isambert, N.; Piperno-Neumann, S.; et al. Trabectedin in combination with doxorubicin for first-line treatment of advanced uterine or soft-tissue leiomyosarcoma (LMS-02): A non-randomised, multicentre, phase 2 trial. *Lancet Oncol.* **2015**, *16*, 457–464. [CrossRef]
60. D'Incalci, M.; Galmarini, C.M. A review of trabectedin (ET-743): A unique mechanism of action. *Mol. Cancer Ther.* **2010**, *9*, 2157–2163. [CrossRef] [PubMed]
61. Rinehart, K.L.; Holt, T.G.; Fregeau, N.L.; Stroh, J.G.; Martin, D.G. Ecteinascidins 729, 743, 745, 759A, 759B, and 770: Potent antitumor agents from the Caribbean tunicate Ecteinascidia turbinata. *J. Org. Chem.* **1990**, *55*, 4512–4515. [CrossRef]
62. Wright, A.; Forleo, D.A.; Gunawardana, G.P.; Gunasekera, S.P.; Koehn, F.E.; Mcconnell, O.J. Antitumor tetrahydroisoquinoline alkaloids from the colonial ascidian Ecteinascidia turbinata. *J. Org. Chem.* **1990**, *55*, 4508–4512. [CrossRef]
63. Seaman, F.C.; Hurley, L.H. Molecular Basis for the DNA Sequence Selectivity of Ecteinascidin 736 and 743: Evidence for the Dominant Role of Direct Readout via Hydrogen Bonding. *J. Am. Chem. Soc.* **1998**, *120*, 13028–13041. [CrossRef]
64. Moore, B.M.; Seaman, F.C.; Wheelhouse, R.T.; Hurley, L.H. Mechanism for the Catalytic Activation of Ecteinascidin 743 and Its Subsequent Alkylation of Guanine N2. *J. Am. Chem. Soc.* **1998**, *120*, 2490–2491. [CrossRef]
65. Feuerhahn, S.; Giraudon, C.; Martinez-Diez, M.; Bueren-Calabuig, J.A.; Galmarini, C.M.; Gago, F.; Egly, J.M. XPF-dependent DNA breaks and RNA polymerase II arrest induced by antitumor DNA interstrand crosslinking-mimetic alkaloids. *Chem. Biol.* **2011**, *18*, 988–999. [CrossRef]
66. Aune, G.J.; Takagi, K.; Sordet, O.; Guirouilh-Barbat, J.; Antony, S.; Bohr, V.A.; Pommier, Y. Von Hippel-Lindau-coupled and transcription-coupled nucleotide excision repair-dependent degradation of RNA polymerase II in response to trabectedin. *Clin. Cancer Res.* **2008**, *14*, 6449–6455. [CrossRef]
67. Forni, C.; Minuzzo, M.; Virdis, E.; Tamborini, E.; Simone, M.; Tavecchio, M.; Erba, E.; Grosso, F.; Gronchi, A.; Aman, P.; et al. Trabectedin (ET-743) promotes differentiation in myxoid liposarcoma tumors. *Mol. Cancer Ther.* **2009**, *8*, 449–457. [CrossRef] [PubMed]
68. Evangelisti, G.; Barra, F.; D'Alessandro, G.; Tantari, M.; Stigliani, S.; Corte, L.D.; Bifulco, G.; Ferrero, S. Trabectedin for the therapy of ovarian cancer. *Drugs Today* **2020**, *56*, 669–688. [CrossRef]
69. Jones, R.; Herzog, T.; Patel, S.; von Mehren, M.; Schuetze, S.; Van Tine, B.; Coleman, R.; Knoblauch, R.; Triantos, S.; Hu, P.; et al. Cardiac safety of trabectedin monotherapy or in combination with pegylated liposomal doxorubicin in patients with sarcomas and ovarian cancer. *Cancer Med.* **2021**, *10*, 3565–3574. [CrossRef] [PubMed]
70. Pignata, S.; Scambia, G.; Villanucci, A.; Naglieri, E.; Ibarbia, M.; Brusa, F.; Bourgeois, H.; Sorio, R.; Casado, A.; Reichert, D.; et al. A European, Observational, Prospective Trial of Trabectedin Plus Pegylated Liposomal Doxorubicin in Patients with Platinum-Sensitive Ovarian Cancer. *Oncologist* **2021**, *26*, e658–e668. [CrossRef]
71. Palmerini, E.; Sanfilippo, R.; Grignani, G.; Buonadonna, A.; Romanini, A.; Badalamenti, G.; Ferraresi, V.; Vincenzi, B.; Comandone, A.; Pizzolorusso, A.; et al. Trabectedin for Patients with Advanced Soft Tissue Sarcoma: A Non-Interventional, Retrospective, Multicenter Study of the Italian Sarcoma Group. *Cancers* **2021**, *13*, 1053. [CrossRef]
72. Grosso, F.; D'Ambrosio, L.; Zucchetti, M.; Ibrahim, T.; Tamberi, S.; Matteo, C.; Rulli, E.; Comandini, D.; Palmerini, E.; Baldi, G.; et al. Pharmacokinetics, safety, and activity of trabectedin as first-line treatment in elderly patients who are affected by advanced sarcoma and are unfit to receive standard chemotherapy: A phase 2 study (TR1US study) from the Italian Sarcoma Group. *Cancer* **2020**, *126*, 4726–4734. [CrossRef]
73. Gronchi, A.; Palmerini, E.; Quagliuolo, V.; Martin Broto, J.; Lopez Pousa, A.; Grignani, G.; Brunello, A.; Blay, J.; Tendero, O.; Beveridge, R.D.; et al. Neoadjuvant Chemotherapy in High-Risk Soft Tissue Sarcomas: Final Results of a Randomized Trial From Italian (ISG), Spanish (GEIS), French (FSG), and Polish (PSG) Sarcoma Groups. *J. Clin. Oncol.* **2020**, *38*, 2178–2186. [CrossRef]
74. Carlos, G.; Maurizio, D.; Paola, A. Trabectedin and Plitidepsin: Drugs from the Sea that Strike the Tumor Microenvironment. *Mar. Drugs* **2014**, *12*, 719–733.
75. Martinez-Cruzado, L.; Tornin, J.; Rodriguez, A.; Santos, L.; Allonca, E.; Fernandez-Garcia, M.; Astudillo, A.; Garcia-Pedrero, J.; Rodriguez, R. Trabectedin and Campthotecin Synergistically Eliminate Cancer Stem Cells in Cell-of-Origin Sarcoma Models. *Neoplasia* **2017**, *19*, 460–470. [CrossRef] [PubMed]
76. Acikgoz, E.; Guven, U.; Duzagac, F.; Uslu, R.; Kara, M.; Soner, B.; Oktem, G. Enhanced G2/M Arrest, Caspase Related Apoptosis and Reduced E-Cadherin Dependent Intercellular Adhesion by Trabectedin in Prostate Cancer Stem Cells. *PLoS ONE* **2015**, *10*, e0141090. [CrossRef] [PubMed]
77. Tumini, E.; Herrera-Moyano, E.; San Martín-Alonso, M.; Barroso, S.; Galmarini, C.; Aguilera, A. The Antitumor Drugs Trabectedin and Lurbinectedin Induce Transcription-Dependent Replication Stress and Genome Instability. *Mol. Cancer Res.* **2019**, *17*, 773–782. [CrossRef]
78. Dosio, F.; Brusa, P.; Cattel, L. Immunotoxins and anticancer drug conjugate assemblies: The role of the linkage between components. *Toxins* **2011**, *3*, 848–883. [CrossRef]
79. Martino, M.; Festuccia, M.; Fedele, R.; Console, G.; Cimminiello, M.; Gavarotti, P.; Bruno, B. Salvage treatment for relapsed/refractory Hodgkin lymphoma: Role of allografting, brentuximab vedotin and newer agents. *Expert Opin. Biol. Ther.* **2016**, *16*, 347–364. [CrossRef]

80. Alperovich, A.; Younes, A. Targeting CD30 Using Brentuximab Vedotin in the Treatment of Hodgkin Lymphoma. *Cancer J.* **2016**, *22*, 23–26. [CrossRef]
81. Andrade-Gonzalez, X.; Ansell, S. Novel Therapies in the Treatment of Hodgkin Lymphoma. *Curr. Treat. Options Oncol.* **2021**, *22*, 42. [CrossRef]
82. Wahl, A.F.; Klussman, K.; Thompson, J.D.; Chen, J.H.; Francisco, L.V.; Risdon, G.; Chace, D.F.; Siegall, C.B.; Francisco, J.A. The anti-CD30 monoclonal antibody SGN-30 promotes growth arrest and DNA fragmentation in vitro and affects antitumor activity in models of Hodgkin's disease. *Cancer Res.* **2002**, *62*, 3736–3742.
83. Ducry, L.; Stump, B. Antibody-drug conjugates: Linking cytotoxic payloads to monoclonal antibodies. *Bioconjugate Chem.* **2010**, *21*, 5–13. [CrossRef] [PubMed]
84. Younes, A. CD30-targeted antibody therapy. *Curr. Opin. Oncol.* **2011**, *23*, 587–593. [CrossRef]
85. Doronina, S.O.; Toki, B.E.; Torgov, M.Y.; Mendelsohn, B.A.; Cerveny, C.G.; Chace, D.F.; DeBlanc, R.L.; Gearing, R.P.; Bovee, T.D.; Siegall, C.B.; et al. Development of potent monoclonal antibody auristatin conjugates for cancer therapy. *Nat. Biotechnol.* **2003**, *21*, 778–784. [CrossRef]
86. Senter, P.D.; Sievers, E.L. The discovery and development of brentuximab vedotin for use in relapsed Hodgkin lymphoma and systemic anaplastic large cell lymphoma. *Nat. Biotechnol.* **2012**, *30*, 631–637. [CrossRef] [PubMed]
87. Moskowitz, C.H.; Nademanee, A.; Masszi, T.; Agura, E.; Holowiecki, J.; Abidi, M.H.; Chen, A.I.; Stiff, P.; Gianni, A.M.; Carella, A.; et al. Brentuximab vedotin as consolidation therapy after autologous stem-cell transplantation in patients with Hodgkin's lymphoma at risk of relapse or progression (AETHERA): A randomised, double-blind, placebo-controlled, phase 3 trial. *Lancet* **2015**, *385*, 1853–1862. [CrossRef]
88. Yi, J.H.; Kim, S.J.; Kim, W.S. Brentuximab vedotin: Clinical updates and practical guidance. *Blood Res.* **2017**, *52*, 243–253. [CrossRef]
89. Barreca, M.; Stathis, A.; Barraja, P.; Bertoni, F. An overview on anti-tubulin agents for the treatment of lymphoma patients. *Pharmacol. Ther.* **2020**, *211*, 107552. [CrossRef]
90. Petek, B.J.; Jones, R.L. PM00104 (Zalypsis(R)): A marine derived alkylating agent. *Molecules* **2014**, *19*, 12328–12335. [CrossRef]
91. Leal, J.F.; Garcia-Hernandez, V.; Moneo, V.; Domingo, A.; Bueren-Calabuig, J.A.; Negri, A.; Gago, F.; Guillen-Navarro, M.J.; Aviles, P.; Cuevas, C.; et al. Molecular pharmacology and antitumor activity of Zalypsis in several human cancer cell lines. *Biochem. Pharmacol.* **2009**, *78*, 162–170. [CrossRef] [PubMed]
92. Ocio, E.M.; Maiso, P.; Chen, X.; Garayoa, M.; Pandiella, A. Zalypsis: A novel marine-derived compound with potent antimyeloma activity that reveals high sensitivity of malignant plasma cells to DNA double-strand breaks. *Blood* **2009**, *113*, 3781. [CrossRef] [PubMed]
93. Elices, M.; Sasak, H.; Caylor, T.; Grant, W.; Guillen, M.J.; Martin, J.; Cuevas, C.; Aviles, P.; Faircloth, G. Antitumor activity of the novel investigational compound PM00104. *Cancer Res.* **2005**, *65*, 1384.
94. Lepage, D.; Sasak, H.; Guillen, M.J.; Grant, W.; Cuevas, C.; Aviles, P. Antitumor activity of Zalypsis® (PM00104) in experimental models of bladder, gastric and liver cancer. *Mol. Cancer Ther.* **2007**, *6*, C62.
95. Elices, M.; Grant, W.; Harper, C.; Guillen, M.J.; Cuevas, C.; Faircloth, G.; Aviles, P. The novel compound PM00104 exhibits significant in vivo activity against breast tumors. PM00104 exhibits significant in vivo activity against breast tumors. *Cancer Res.* **2005**, *65*, 147.
96. Greiner, T.; Maier, A.; Bausch, N.; Fiebig, H.; Lepage, D.; Guillen, M.J.; Cuevas, C.; Aviles, P. Preclinical evaluation of PM00104 to support the selection of tumor indications for clinical development. *Mol. Cancer Ther.* **2007**, *6*, 3545S–3546S.
97. Guirouilh-Barbat, J.; Antony, S.; Pommier, Y. Zalypsis (PM00104) is a potent inducer of gamma-H2AX foci and reveals the importance of the C ring of trabectedin for transcription-coupled repair inhibition. *Mol. Cancer Ther.* **2009**, *8*, 2007–2014. [CrossRef]
98. Colado, E.; Paino, T.; Maiso, P.; Ocio, E.M.; Chen, X.; Alvarez-Fernandez, S.; Gutierrez, N.C.; Martin-Sanchez, J.; Flores-Montero, J.; San Segundo, L.; et al. Zalypsis has in vitro activity in acute myeloid blasts and leukemic progenitor cells through the induction of a DNA damage response. *Haematologica* **2011**, *96*, 687–695. [CrossRef] [PubMed]
99. Falkenberg, K.J.; Johnstone, R.W. Histone deacetylases and their inhibitors in cancer, neurological diseases and immune disorders. *Nat. Rev. Drug Discov.* **2014**, *13*, 673–691. [CrossRef]
100. Stojanovic, N.; Hassan, Z.; Wirth, M.; Wenzel, P.; Beyer, M.; Schäfer, C.; Brand, P.; Kroemer, A.; Stauber, R.H.; Schmid, R.M.; et al. HDAC1 and HDAC2 integrate the expression of p53 mutants in pancreatic cancer. *Oncogene* **2017**, *36*, 1804–1815. [CrossRef]
101. McLeod, A.B.; Stice, J.P.; Wardell, S.E.; Alley, H.M.; Chang, C.Y.; McDonnell, D.P. Validation of histone deacetylase 3 as a therapeutic target in castration-resistant prostate cancer. *Prostate* **2018**, *78*, 266–277. [CrossRef] [PubMed]
102. Maiti, A.; Qi, Q.; Peng, X.; Yan, L.; Takabe, K.; Hait, N.C. Class I histone deacetylase inhibitor suppresses vasculogenic mimicry by enhancing the expression of tumor suppressor and anti-angiogenesis genes in aggressive human TNBC cells. *Int. J. Oncol.* **2019**, *55*, 116–130. [CrossRef]
103. von Tresckow, B.; Sayehli, C.; Aulitzky, W.E.; Goebeler, M.E.; Schwab, M.; Braz, E.; Krauss, B.; Krauss, R.; Hermann, F.; Bartz, R. Phase I study of domatinostat (4SC-202), a class I histone deacetylase inhibitor in patients with advanced hematological malignancies. *Eur. J. Haematol.* **2019**, *102*, 163–173. [CrossRef] [PubMed]
104. Zhang, Y.; Xu, W. Isoform-selective histone deacetylase inhibitors: The trend and promise of disease treatment. *Epigenomics* **2015**, *7*, 5–7. [CrossRef]

105. Bieliauskas, A.V.; Pflum, M.K. Isoform-selective histone deacetylase inhibitors. *Chem. Soc. Rev.* **2008**, *37*, 1402–1413. [CrossRef] [PubMed]
106. Kuphal, S.; Wallner, S.; Bosserhoff, A.K. Loss of nephronectin promotes tumor progression in malignant melanoma. *Cancer Sci.* **2008**, *99*, 229–233. [CrossRef] [PubMed]
107. Ying, Y.; Taori, K.; Kim, H.; Hong, J.; Luesch, H. Total synthesis and molecular target of largazole, a histone deacetylase inhibitor. *J. Am. Chem. Soc.* **2008**, *130*, 8455–8459. [CrossRef] [PubMed]
108. Ying, Y.; Liu, Y.; Byeon, S.R.; Kim, H.; Luesch, H.; Hong, J. Synthesis and activity of largazole analogues with linker and macrocycle modification. *Org. Lett.* **2008**, *10*, 4021–4024. [CrossRef] [PubMed]
109. Bowers, A.; West, N.; Taunton, J.; Schreiber, S.L.; Bradner, J.E.; Williams, R.M. Total synthesis and biological mode of action of largazole: A potent class I histone deacetylase inhibitor. *J. Am. Chem. Soc.* **2008**, *130*, 11219–11222. [CrossRef]
110. Zhou, H.; Jiang, S.; Chen, J.; Ren, X.; Jin, J.; Su, S.B. Largazole, an inhibitor of class I histone deacetylases, attenuates inflammatory corneal neovascularization. *Eur. J. Pharmacol.* **2014**, *740*, 619–626. [CrossRef]
111. Liu, Y.; Wang, Z.; Wang, J.; Lam, W.; Kwong, S.; Li, F.; Friedman, S.L.; Zhou, S.; Ren, Q.; Xu, Z.; et al. A histone deacetylase inhibitor, largazole, decreases liver fibrosis and angiogenesis by inhibiting transforming growth factor-beta and vascular endothelial growth factor signalling. *Liver Int.* **2013**, *33*, 504–515. [CrossRef]
112. Ghosh, S.K.; Perrine, S.P.; Williams, R.M.; Faller, D.V. Histone deacetylase inhibitors are potent inducers of gene expression in latent EBV and sensitize lymphoma cells to nucleoside antiviral agents. *Blood* **2012**, *119*, 1008–1017. [CrossRef]
113. Lee, S.U.; Kwak, H.B.; Pi, S.H.; You, H.K.; Byeon, S.R.; Ying, Y.; Luesch, H.; Hong, J.; Kim, S.H. In Vitro and In Vivo Osteogenic Activity of Largazole. *ACS Med. Chem. Lett.* **2011**, *2*, 248–251. [CrossRef] [PubMed]
114. Newman, D.J.; Giddings, L.-A. Natural products as leads to antitumor drugs. *Phytochem. Rev.* **2013**, *13*, 123–137. [CrossRef]
115. Wu, L.C.; Wen, Z.S.; Qiu, Y.T.; Chen, X.Q.; Chen, H.B.; Wei, M.M.; Liu, Z.; Jiang, S.; Zhou, G.B. Largazole Arrests Cell Cycle at G1 Phase and Triggers Proteasomal Degradation of E2F1 in Lung Cancer Cells. *ACS Med. Chem. Lett.* **2013**, *4*, 921–926. [CrossRef] [PubMed]
116. Liu, Y.; Salvador, L.A.; Byeon, S.; Ying, Y.; Kwan, J.C.; Law, B.K.; Hong, J.; Luesch, H. Anticolon cancer activity of largazole, a marine-derived tunable histone deacetylase inhibitor. *J. Pharmacol. Exp. Ther.* **2010**, *335*, 351–361. [CrossRef] [PubMed]
117. Law, M.E.; Corsino, P.E.; Jahn, S.C.; Davis, B.J.; Chen, S.; Patel, B.; Pham, K.; Lu, J.; Sheppard, B.; Norgaard, P.; et al. Glucocorticoids and histone deacetylase inhibitors cooperate to block the invasiveness of basal-like breast cancer cells through novel mechanisms. *Oncogene* **2013**, *32*, 1316–1329. [CrossRef] [PubMed]
118. Bousquet, M.S.; Ma, J.J.; Ratnayake, R.; Havre, P.A.; Yao, J.; Dang, N.H.; Paul, V.J.; Carney, T.J.; Dang, L.H.; Luesch, H. Multidimensional Screening Platform for Simultaneously Targeting Oncogenic KRAS and Hypoxia-Inducible Factors Pathways in Colorectal Cancer. *ACS Chem. Biol.* **2016**, *11*, 1322–1331. [CrossRef]
119. Sanchez, G.J.; Richmond, P.A.; Bunker, E.N.; Karman, S.S.; Azofeifa, J.; Garnett, A.T.; Xu, Q.; Wheeler, G.E.; Toomey, C.M.; Zhang, Q.; et al. Genome-wide dose-dependent inhibition of histone deacetylases studies reveal their roles in enhancer remodeling and suppression of oncogenic super-enhancers. *Nucleic Acids Res.* **2018**, *46*, 1756–1776. [CrossRef]
120. Al-Awadhi, F.H.; Salvador-Reyes, L.A.; Elsadek, L.A.; Ratnayake, R.; Chen, Q.Y.; Luesch, H. Largazole is a Brain-Penetrant Class I HDAC Inhibitor with Extended Applicability to Glioblastoma and CNS Diseases. *ACS Chem. Neurosci.* **2020**, *11*, 1937–1943. [CrossRef]
121. Min, W.; Xiao-Yan, S.; Yong-Chun, Z.; Kuo-Jun, Z.; Yong-Zhi, L.; Jinsong, L.; Yun-Chao, H.; Gui-Zhen, W.; Sheng, J.; Guang-Biao, Z. Suppression of Musashi-2 by the small compound largazole exerts inhibitory effects on malignant cells. *Int. J. Oncol.* **2020**, *56*, 1274–1283.
122. Clausen, D.J.; Smith, W.B.; Haines, B.E.; Wiest, O.; Bradner, J.E.; Williams, R.M. Modular synthesis and biological activity of pyridyl-based analogs of the potent Class I Histone Deacetylase Inhibitor Largazole. *Bioorganic Med. Chem.* **2015**, *23*, 5061–5074. [CrossRef]
123. Almaliti, J.; Al-Hamashi, A.A.; Negmeldin, A.T.; Hanigan, C.L.; Perera, L.; Pflum, M.K.; Casero, R.A., Jr.; Tillekeratne, L.M. Largazole Analogues Embodying Radical Changes in the Depsipeptide Ring: Development of a More Selective and Highly Potent Analogue. *J. Med. Chem.* **2016**, *59*, 10642–10660. [CrossRef] [PubMed]
124. Chen, F.; Chai, H.; Su, M.B.; Zhang, Y.M.; Li, J.; Xie, X.; Nan, F.J. Potent and orally efficacious bisthiazole-based histone deacetylase inhibitors. *ACS Med. Chem. Lett.* **2014**, *5*, 628–633. [CrossRef]
125. Cole, K.E.; Dowling, D.P.; Boone, M.A.; Phillips, A.J.; Christianson, D.W. Structural Basis of the Antiproliferative Activity of Largazole, a Depsipeptide Inhibitor of the Histone Deacetylases. *J. Am. Chem. Soc.* **2011**, *133*, 12474–12477. [CrossRef] [PubMed]
126. Seiser, T.; Kamena, F.; Cramer, N. Synthesis and biological activity of largazole and derivatives. *Angew. Chem. Int. Ed.* **2008**, *47*, 6483–6485. [CrossRef] [PubMed]
127. Zeng, X.; Yin, B.; Hu, Z.; Liao, C.; Liu, J.; Li, S.; Li, Z.; Nicklaus, M.C.; Zhou, G.; Jiang, S. Total synthesis and biological evaluation of largazole and derivatives with promising selectivity for cancers cells. *Org. Lett.* **2010**, *12*, 1368–1371. [CrossRef] [PubMed]
128. Kim, B.; Park, H.; Salvador, L.A.; Serrano, P.E.; Kwan, J.C.; Zeller, S.L.; Chen, Q.-Y.; Ryu, S.; Liu, Y.; Byeon, S.; et al. Evaluation of class I HDAC isoform selectivity of largazole analogues. *Bioorganic Med. Chem. Lett.* **2014**, *24*, 3728–3731. [CrossRef] [PubMed]
129. Bowers, A.A.; West, N.; Newkirk, T.L.; Troutman-Youngman, A.E.; Schreiber, S.L.; Wiest, O.; Bradner, J.E.; Williams, R.M. Synthesis and histone deacetylase inhibitory activity of largazole analogs: Alteration of the zinc-binding domain and macrocyclic scaffold. *Org. Lett.* **2009**, *11*, 1301–1304. [CrossRef] [PubMed]

130. Kim, B.; Ratnayake, R.; Lee, H.; Shi, G.; Zeller, S.L.; Li, C.; Luesch, H.; Hong, J. Synthesis and biological evaluation of largazole zinc-binding group analogs. *Bioorganic Med. Chem.* **2017**, *25*, 3077–3086. [CrossRef] [PubMed]
131. Bhansali, P.; Hanigan, C.L.; Casero, R.A.; Tillekeratne, L.M. Largazole and analogues with modified metal-binding motifs targeting histone deacetylases: Synthesis and biological evaluation. *J. Med. Chem.* **2011**, *54*, 7453–7463. [CrossRef]
132. Su, J.; Qiu, Y.; Ma, K.; Yao, Y.; Wang, Z.; Li, X.; Zhang, D.; Tu, Z.; Jiang, S. Design, synthesis, and biological evaluation of largazole derivatives: Alteration of the zinc-binding domain. *Tetrahedron* **2014**, *70*, 7763–7769. [CrossRef]
133. Benelkebir, H.; Marie, S.; Hayden, A.L.; Lyle, J.; Loadman, P.M.; Crabb, S.J.; Packham, G.; Ganesan, A. Total synthesis of largazole and analogues: HDAC inhibition, antiproliferative activity and metabolic stability. *Bioorganic Med. Chem.* **2011**, *19*, 3650–3658. [CrossRef] [PubMed]
134. Bhansali, P.; Hanigan, C.L.; Perera, L.; Casero, R.A.; Tillekeratne, L.M.V. Synthesis and biological evaluation of largazole analogues with modified surface recognition cap groups. *Eur. J. Med. Chem.* **2014**, *86*, 528–541. [CrossRef]
135. Zhang, B.; Ruan, Z.W.; Luo, D.; Zhu, Y.; Ding, T.; Sui, Q.; Lei, X. Unexpected Enhancement of HDACs Inhibition by MeS Substitution at C-2 Position of Fluoro Largazole. *Mar. Drugs* **2020**, *18*, 344. [CrossRef] [PubMed]
136. Chen, F.; Gao, A.-H.; Li, J.; Nan, F.-J. Synthesis and Biological Evaluation of C7-Demethyl Largazole Analogues. *ChemMedChem* **2009**, *4*, 1269–1272. [CrossRef]
137. Souto, J.A.; Vaz, E.; Lepore, I.; Pöppler, A.-C.; Franci, G.; Álvarez, R.; Altucci, L.; de Lera, Á.R. Synthesis and Biological Characterization of the Histone Deacetylase Inhibitor Largazole and C7- Modified Analogues. *J. Med. Chem.* **2010**, *53*, 4654–4667. [CrossRef] [PubMed]
138. Li, X.; Tu, Z.; Li, H.; Liu, C.; Li, Z.; Sun, Q.; Yao, Y.; Liu, J.; Jiang, S. Biological evaluation of new largazole analogues: Alteration of macrocyclic scaffold with click chemistry. *ACS Med. Chem. Lett.* **2013**, *4*, 132–136. [CrossRef]
139. Yao, Y.; Tu, Z.; Liao, C.; Wang, Z.; Li, S.; Yao, H.; Li, Z.; Jiang, S. Discovery of Novel Class I Histone Deacetylase Inhibitors with Promising in Vitro and in Vivo Antitumor Activities. *J. Med. Chem.* **2015**, *58*, 7672–7680. [CrossRef]
140. Zhang, K.; Yao, Y.; Tu, Z.; Liao, C.; Wang, Z.; Qiu, Y.; Chen, D.; Hamilton, D.J.; Li, Z.; Jiang, S. Discovery of class I histone deacetylase inhibitors based on romidpesin with promising selectivity for cancer cells. *Futur. Med. Chem.* **2020**, *12*, 311–323. [CrossRef]
141. Zhang, S.-W.; Gong, C.-J.; Su, M.-B.; Chen, F.; He, T.; Zhang, Y.-M.; Shen, Q.-Q.; Su, Y.; Ding, J.; Li, J.; et al. Synthesis and in Vitro and in Vivo Biological Evaluation of Tissue-Specific Bisthiazole Histone Deacetylase (HDAC) Inhibitors. *J. Med. Chem.* **2020**, *63*, 804–815. [CrossRef] [PubMed]
142. Diamond, J.R.; Kagihara, J.A.; Liu, X.; Gordon, G.; Heim, A.M.; Winkler, J.; DeMattei, J.A.; Piscopio, A.D.; Eckhardt, S.G. OKI-179 is a novel, oral, class I specific histone deacetylase inhibitor in phase 1 clinical trials. In Proceedings of the AACR-NCI-EORTC International Conference on Molecular Targets and Cancer Therapeutics, Boston, MA, USA, 26–30 October 2019; pp. 26–30.
143. Diamond, J.; Gordon, G.; Kagihara, J.; Corr, B.; Piscopio, A. Initial results from a phase 1 trial of OKI-179, an oral Class 1-selective depsipeptide HDAC inhibitor, in patients with advanced solid tumors. *Eur. J. Cancer* **2020**, *138*, S12. [CrossRef]
144. Liu, X.; Phillips, A.J.; Ungermannova, D.; Nasveschuk, C.G.; Zhang, G. Macrocyclic Compounds Useful as Inhibitors of Histone Deacetylases. U.S. Patent 9,422,340, 23 August 2016.
145. Wang, X.; Waschke, B.C.; Woolaver, R.A.; Chen, Z.; Zhang, G.; Piscopio, A.D.; Liu, X.; Wang, J.H. Histone Deacetylase Inhibition Sensitizes PD1 Blockade-Resistant B-cell Lymphomas. *Cancer Immunol. Res.* **2019**, *7*, 1318–1331. [CrossRef] [PubMed]

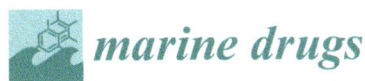

Article

Anthraquinones, Diphenyl Ethers, and Their Derivatives from the Culture of the Marine Sponge-Associated Fungus *Neosartorya spinosa* KUFA 1047 †

Joana D. M. de Sá [1], José A. Pereira [2,3], Tida Dethoup [4], Honorina Cidade [1,3], Maria Emília Sousa [1,3], Inês C. Rodrigues [2], Paulo M. Costa [2,3], Sharad Mistry [5], Artur M. S. Silva [6] and Anake Kijjoa [2,3,*]

[1] Laboratório de Química Orgânica, Departamento de Ciências Químicas, Faculdade de Farmácia, Universidade do Porto, Rua de Jorge Viterbo Ferreira, 228, 4050-313 Porto, Portugal; joanadmsa2703@gmail.com (J.D.M.d.S.); hcidade@ff.up.pt (H.C.); esousa@ff.up.pt (M.E.S.)

[2] ICBAS—Instituto de Ciências Biomédicas Abel Salazar, Rua de Jorge Viterbo Ferreira, 228, 4050-313 Porto, Portugal; jpereira@icbas.up.pt (J.A.P.); inescoutorodrigues@gmail.com (I.C.R.); pmcosta@icbas.up.pt (P.M.C.)

[3] Interdisciplinary Centre of Marine and Environmental Research (CIIMAR), Terminal de Cruzeiros do Porto de Leixões, Av. General Norton de Matos s/n, 4450-208 Matosinhos, Portugal

[4] Department of Plant Pathology, Faculty of Agriculture, Kasetsart University, Bangkok 10240, Thailand; tdethoup@yahoo.com

[5] Department of Chemistry, University of Leicester, University Road, Leicester LE 7RH, UK; scm11@leicester.ac.uk

[6] Departamento de Química & QOPNA, Universidade de Aveiro, 3810-193 Aveiro, Portugal; artur.silva@ua.pt

* Correspondence: ankijjoa@icbas.up.pt; Tel.: +351-22-042-8331; Fax: +351-22-206-2232

† Dedicated to Prof. Peter Proksch, one of the pioneers of marine natural products research in Europe.

Abstract: Previously unreported anthraquinone, acetylpenipurdin A (**4**), biphenyl ether, neospinosic acid (**6**), dibenzodioxepinone, and spinolactone (**7**) were isolated, together with (*R*)-6-hydroxymellein (**1**), penipurdin A (**2**), acetylquestinol (**3**), tenellic acid C (**5**), and vermixocin A (**8**) from the culture of a marine sponge-associated fungus *Neosartorya spinosa* KUFA1047. The structures of the previously unreported compounds were established based on an extensive analysis of 1D and 2D NMR spectra as well as HRMS data. The absolute configurations of the stereogenic centers of **5** and **7** were established unambiguously by comparing their calculated and experimental electronic circular dichroism (ECD) spectra. Compounds **2** and **5**–**8** were tested for their in vitro acetylcholinesterase and tyrosinase inhibitory activities as well as their antibacterial activity against Gram-positive and Gram-negative reference, and multidrug-resistant strains isolated from the environment. The tested compounds were also evaluated for their capacity to inhibit biofilm formation in the reference strains.

Keywords: *Neosartorya spinosa*; Trichocomaceae; marine sponge-associated fungus; anthraquinones; biphenyl ethers; anti-tyrosinase; antibacterial activity; antibiofilm activity

1. Introduction

Fungi are among organisms that have a remarkable capacity to produce different classes of structurally diverse secondary metabolites with relevant biological and pharmacological activities. This capability may be due to their necessity to produce highly bioactive molecules for their communications or inhibition of the growth of antagonistic neighbor microorganisms with which they cohabit in the same ecological niches [1]. Although secondary metabolites of terrestrial fungi have been extensively investigated for many decades due to their importance in pharmaceutical research [2], only in the past two decades that marine-derived fungi started to gain more attention from researchers [3]. Marine-derived fungi have become one of the most important sources of bioactive compounds not only because they are among the world's most important resources for unprecedented chemodiversity but also because they can produce quantity of compounds with potential for drug development, clinical trials, and even marketing [4].

In our research program with an objective to search for new bioactive compounds from marine-derived fungi, we investigated several members of the genus *Neosartorya* (Trichocomaceae) isolated from different marine organisms such as sponges, coral, and algae. Many different chemical classes of secondary metabolites, such as polyketides, isocoumarins, ergosterol derivatives, meroditerpenes, pyripyropenes, benzoic acid derivatives, prenylated indole derivatives, tryptoquivalines, fiscalins, phenylalanine-derived alkaloids, and cyclopeptides, have been isolated and investigated for their anticancer and antibacterial activities [5–7]. Therefore, in our ongoing search for new natural antibiotics from marine-derived fungi, we investigated secondary metabolites from the culture of *N. spinosa* KUFA 1047, isolated from a marine sponge *Mycale* sp., which was collected from the Samae San Island in the Gulf of Thailand. Although the soil-derived *N. spinosa* has already been investigated for its secondary metabolites [8], this is the first study of the secondary metabolites from a marine-derived *N. spinosa*.

Fractionation of the ethyl acetate extract of the culture of *N. spinosa* KUFA 1047 by column chromatography of silica gel, followed by purification by preparative TLC, Sephadex LH-20 column, and crystallization led to the isolation of undescribed acetylpenipurdin A (**4**), neospinosic acid (**6**), and spinolactone (**7**), as well as the previously reported (*R*)-6-hydroxymellein (**1**) [9,10], penipurdin A (**2**) [11], acetylquestinol (**3**) [12], tenellic acid C (**5**) [13], and vermixocin A (**8**) [14–16] (Figure 1). The structures of the undescribed compounds were established based on an extensive analysis of their 1D and 2D NMR as well as HRMS spectra. In the case of **5** and **7**, the absolute configurations of their stereogenic carbons were established by comparison of their experimental and calculated electronic circular dichroism (ECD) spectra.

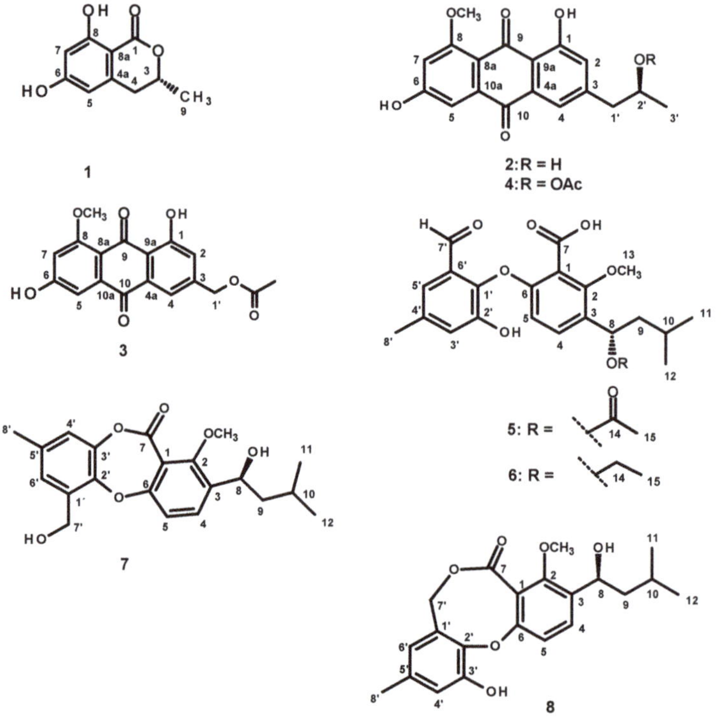

Figure 1. Structures of (*R*)-6-hydroxymellein (**1**), penipurdin A (**2**), acetylquestinol (**3**), acetylpenipurdin A (**4**), tenellic acid C (**5**), neospinosic acid (**6**), spinolactone (**7**), and vermixocin A (**8**).

Compounds **2** and **5–8** were tested for their in vitro acetylcholinesterase and tyrosinase inhibitory activities, as well as their antibacterial activity against Gram-negative and Gram-positive bacteria by disk diffusion and by determination of the minimum inhibitory concentration (MIC) and minimal bactericidal concentration (MBC) of several reference strains and environmental multidrug-resistant isolates. The tested compounds were also evaluated for their potential synergy with clinically relevant antibiotics on the multidrug-resistant isolates, by a disk diffusion method and by the checkerboard assay, as well as their capacity to prevent biofilm formation in all four reference strains, by measuring a total biomass using the crystal violet assay.

2. Results and Discussion

The structures of (*R*)-6-hydroxymellein (**1**) [9,10], penipurdin A (**2**) [11], acetylquestinol (**3**) [12], tenellic acid C (**5**) [13], and vermixocin A (**8**) [14–16] (Figure 1) were elucidated by analysis of their 1D and 2D NMR spectra as well as HRMS data, and also by comparison of their spectral data and signs of optical rotations (Figures S1–S25 and S38–S43, Tables S1–S5) with those reported in the literature.

Compounds **3** and **4** were isolated as a 1:3 mixture (estimated by the integration of protons in the ^{1}H NMR spectrum). The molecular formula of the minor compound (**3**) was determined as $C_{18}H_{14}O_7$ on the basis of its (+)-HRESIMS *m/z* 343.0809 [M + H]$^+$ (calculated for $C_{18}H_{15}O_7$, 343.0818), while the molecular formula of the major compound (**4**) was established as $C_{20}H_{18}O_7$ on the basis of (+)-HRESIMS *m/z* 371.1124 [M + H]$^+$ (calculated for $C_{20}H_{19}O_7$, 371.1131) (Figures S18 and S19). The ^{1}H and ^{13}C signals as well as correlations observed in the COSY, HSQC, and HMBC spectra of a minor component (Table S3, Figures S13–S17) revealed its identity as acetylquestinol, previously reported from the culture of *Eurotium chevalieri* KUFA0006 [12].

The ^{13}C NMR spectrum (Table 1, Figure S14) of the major compound (**4**) showed 20 carbon signals, which, in combination with DEPT and HSQC spectra (Figure S16), can be categorized as two conjugated ketone carbonyls (δ_C 186.4 and 183.0), one ester carbonyl (δ_C 170.2), three oxygen-bearing sp^2 (δ_C 166.6, 164.1, 162.1), five non-protonated sp^2 (δ_C 146.6, 137.2, 132.6, 115.6, 112.2), four protonated sp^2 (δ_C 125.1, 119.6, 108.3, 105.5), one oxygen-bearing methine sp^3 (δ_C 70.7), one methoxy (δ_C 56.7), one methylene sp^2 (δ_C 41.5), and two methyl (δ_C 21.4 and 20.0) carbons. The ^{1}H NMR spectrum (Figure S13), in conjunction with COSY and HMBC spectra (Table 1, Figures S15 and S17), showed the following proton signals: a singlet of a hydrogen-bonded phenolic hydroxyl proton at δ_H 13.40, two pairs of *meta*-coupled aromatic protons at δ_H 7.15, d (*J* = 1.5 Hz, δ_C 125.1)/δ_H 7.47, d (*J* = 1.5 Hz, δ_C 119.6) and δ_H 7.16, d (*J* = 2.2 Hz, δ_C 108.3)/δ_H 6.78, d (*J* = 2.2 Hz, δ_C 105.5), a multiplet at δ_H 5.06 (δ_C 70.7), a methoxyl singlet at δ_H 3.89 (δ_C 56.7), a multiplet at δ_H 2.92 (δ_C 41.5), a methyl singlet at δ_H 1.94 (δ_C 21.4), and a methyl doublet at δ_H 1.20, d (*J* = 6.3 Hz, δ_C 20.0). The general feature of the ^{1}H and ^{13}C NMR spectra of **4** resembled those of **2** [11], except for the presence of the ester carbonyl at δ_C 170.2 and a methyl singlet at δ_H 1.94 (δ_C 21.4), characteristic of an acetyl group. That the substituent on C-3 was 2-acetoxypropyl instead of 2-hydroxylpropyl in **2** was evidenced by the COSY correlations from H$_2$-1' (δ_H 2.92, m/δ_C 41.5) to H-2' (δ_H 5.06/δ_C 70.7), and from H-2' to H$_3$-3' (δ_H 1.20, *d*, *J* = 6.3 Hz/δ_C 20.0) as well as by HMBC correlations from H-2' and a methyl singlet at δ_H 1.94 (δ_C 21.1) to the carbonyl at δ_C 170.2, H-1' to C-2, C-3 (δ_C 146.6), C-4, and from H-2' to C-3.

Table 1. ^{1}H and ^{13}C NMR (DMSO-d_6, 500 and 125 MHz) and HMBC assignment for **4**.

Position	δ_C, Type	δ_H, J in Hz	COSY	HMBC
1	162.1, C			
2	125.1, CH	7.15, d (1.5)	H-4	C-1, 1′, 4, 9a
3	146.6, C			
4	119.6, CH	7.47, d (1.5)	H-2	C-1′, 2, 9a, 10
4a	132.6, C			
5	108.3, CH	7.16, d (2.2)	H-7	C-7, 8a, 10
6	166.6, C			
7	105.5, CH	6.78, d (2.2)	H-5	C-5, 6, 8a
8	164.1, C			
8a	112.2, C			
9	186.4, CO			
9a	115.6, C			
10	183.0, CO			
10a	137.2, C			
OMe-8	56.7, CH$_3$	3.89, s		C-8
1′	41.5, CH$_2$	2.92, m	H-2′	C-2, 3, 4
2′	70.7, CH	5.06, m	H$_2$-1′, H$_3$-3′	C-3, CO (Ac)
3′	20.0, CH$_3$	1.20, d (6.3)	H-2′	C-1′, 2′
CO (Ac)	170.2, CO			
Me (Ac)	21.4, CH$_3$	1.94, s		
OH-1′	-	13.40, s		C-1, 2, 9a

The optical rotation of a mixture of **3** and **4** is dextrorotatory, with $[\alpha]^{20}_D$ + 142.8 (c 0.035, MeOH). Since **3** is not a chiral molecule, only **4** is responsible for the optical activity. The structure of **4** corresponds to an acetylated derivative of **2** ($[\alpha]^{20}_D$ + 35.7 (c 0.033, MeOH; Lit. + 33 (c 1.14, MeOH)) and is, therefore, named acetylpenipurdin A. Based on the biogenetic consideration, the absolute configuration of C-2′ in **4** should be the same as that of C-2′ in **2**, i.e., (*S*). Additionally, this hypothesis was supported by the same sign of their optical rotations (dextrorotatory), which is based on the report by Singh et al. [17], that 1,3,8-trihydroxy-6-(2′-acetoxyptopyl) anthracene-9,10-dione, isolated from the marine crinoid *Pterometra venusta*, ($[\alpha]^{25}_D$ + 40, c 0.05, MeOH) and its deacetylated product ($[\alpha]^{25}_D$ + 37, c 0.05, MeOH) were both dextrorotatory. Literature search revealed that **4** has never been previously reported.

The (+)-HRESIMS, ^{1}H and ^{13}C NMR data (Table S4, Figures S20 and S21) of **5** ($[\alpha]^{20}_D$−7.8 (c 0.079, MeOH)) are compatible with those of tenellic acid C ($[\alpha]^{25}_D$−7.4 (c 0.13 g/dL, MeOH)), a biphenyl ether derivative isolated from the aquatic fungus *Dendrospora tenella* [13]; however, the absolute configuration of C-8 was not established. To determine the absolute configuration of C-8, the experimental ECD spectrum of **5** was measured and then compared with a quantum-mechanically simulated spectrum derived from the most significant computational models of (*S*)-**5** (Figure 2, please see the Experimental section for details). Figure 3 shows the visual match between experimental and calculated ECD spectra, with the spectrum of the (8*S*) configuration mostly in phase with the experimental spectrum, while the spectrum of (8*R*) configuration is mostly out of phase, leading to an unambiguous conclusion that the absolute configuration of C-8 is (*S*).

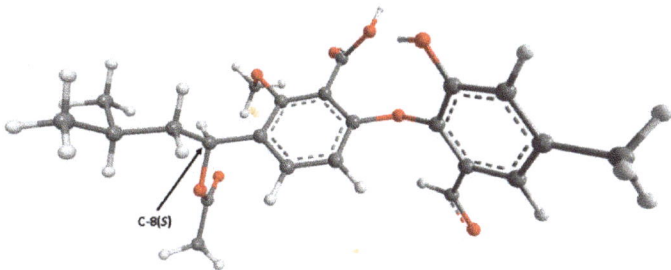

Figure 2. Model of one of the most abundant conformations of **5** (lowest B3LYP/6-31G/methanol energy conformer) in its ECD assigned (8*S*) configuration. Many other conformations have very similar energies to this one.

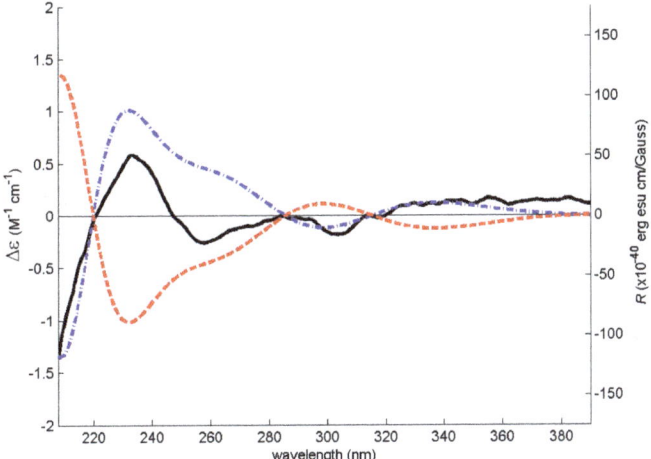

Figure 3. Experimental methanol ECD spectrum of **5** (solid black line) and theoretical ECD spectra of its (*S*) (dot–dashed blue line) and (*R*) (dashed red line) computational conformers.

Compound **6** was isolated as an amorphous yellow solid, and its molecular formula $C_{23}H_{28}O_7$ was established based on the (+)-HRESIMS *m/z* 417.1915 [M + H]$^+$ (calculated for $C_{23}H_{29}O_7$, 417.1913) (Figure S31), requiring 10 degrees of unsaturation. The general feature of the ^{1}H and ^{13}C NMR spectra of **6** resembled those of **5**. The ^{13}C NMR spectrum (Table 2, Figure S27) exhibited 23 carbon signals, which can be categorized, according to DEPT and HSQC spectra (Figure S29), as one aldehyde carbonyl (δ_C 189.8), one conjugated carboxy carbonyl (δ_C 167.2), four oxygen-bearing sp^2 (δ_C 155.1, 154.8, 150.9, and 142.3), four non-protonated sp^2 (δ_C 136.7, 130.5, 129.8, and 119.3), four protonated sp^2 (δ_C 128.5, 124.2, 118.4, and 110.3), one oxymethine sp^3 (δ_C 73.1), one oxymethylene sp^3 (δ_C 63.9), one methoxy (δ_C 62.8), one methylene sp^3 (δ_C 47.1), one methine sp^3 (δ_C 24.9), and four methyl (δ_C 23.7, 22.2, 21.0, and 15.7) carbons. The ^{1}H NMR spectrum (Figure S26), in combination with the COSY spectrum (Table 2, Figure S28), displayed a singlet of an aldehyde proton at δ_H 10.15, the signals of two *ortho*-coupled aromatic protons at δ_H 7.25, d (*J* = 8.7 Hz) and 6.32, d (*J* = 8.7 Hz), two *meta*-coupled aromatic protons at δ_H 7.14, d (*J* = 2.0 Hz) and 7.11, d (*J* = 2.0 Hz), a double doublet at δ_H 4.58 (*J* = 9.2, 3.8 Hz), a methoxy singlet at δ_H 3.83, a quartet at δ_H 3.25 (*J* = 7.0 Hz), two double of double doublets of two geminally coupled methylene protons at δ_H 1.57 (*J* = 13.8, 9.1, 5.0 Hz) and 1.27 (*J* = 13.8, 8.9, 3.9 Hz), a multiplet at δ_H 1.71, one methyl singlet at δ_H 2.31, one methyl triplet at δ_H 1.06 (*J* = 7.0 Hz), and two methyl doublets at δ_H 0.88 (*J* = 6.6 Hz) and 0.92 (*J* = 6.6 Hz). The ^{13}C and ^{1}H chemical shift values and multiplicities of the proton signals revealed that **6** is also a biphenyl ether derivative. Like **5**, one of the benzene ring is 1,2,3,5-tetrasubstituted and another is 1,2,3,4-tetrasubstituted. That the 1,2,3,5-tetrasubstituted benzene ring has a formyl group on C-1′, a hydroxyl group on C-3′, and a methyl group on C-5′ was corroborated by COSY correlations from the doublet at δ_H 7.14 (*J* = 2.0 Hz, H-4′/δ_C 124.2) to the doublet at δ_H 7.11 (*J* = 2.0 Hz, H-6′/δ_C 118.4) and the methyl singlet at δ_H 2.31 (Me-8′/δ_C 21.0), from Me-8′ to H-4′ and H-6′ as well as HMBC correlations (Figure S30) from H-4′ to C-6′, C-8′, C-2′ (δ_C 142.3), and C-3′(δ_C150.9), H-6′ to C-2′, C-7′ (δ_C 189.8), and C-8′, Me-8′ to C-4′, C-5′ (δ_C 136.7), and C-6′, H-7′ (δ_H 10.15, s) to C-1′ (δ_C 129.8) C-5′ and C-6′. That another benzene ring has a carboxyl substituent on C-1, a methoxyl group on C-2, and an alkyl sidechain on C-3 was substantiated by COSY correlations from H-4 (δ_H 7.25, d, *J* = 8.7 Hz/δ_C 128.5) to H-5 (δ_H 6.32, d, *J* = 8.7 Hz/δ_C 110.3) as well as HMBC correlations from H-4 to C-2 (δ_C 155.1), C-6 (δ_C 154.8) and C-8 (δ_C 73.1), H-5 to C-1(δ_C 119.3), C-3 (δ_C 130.5), C-6 and C-7 (δ_C 167.2), the methoxyl singlet at δ_H 3.83 (δ_C 62.8) to C-2. That the substituent on C-3 is 1-ethoxy-3-methylbutyl is corroborated by COSY correlations from H-8 (δ_H 4.58, dd, *J* = 9.2, 3.8 Hz/δ_C 73.1) to H$_2$-9 (δ_H 1.57, ddd, *J* = 13.8, 9.1, 5.0 Hz and 1.27, ddd, *J* = 13.8, 8.9, 3.9 Hz/δ_C 47.1), H$_2$-9 to H-10 (δ_H 1.71, m/δ_C 24.9), H-10 to Me-11 (δ_H 0.88, d, *J* = 6.6 Hz/δ_C 23.7) and Me-12 (δ_H 0.92, d, *J* = 6.6 Hz/δ_C 22.2), and H-14 (δ_H 3.25, q, *J* = 7.0 Hz/δ_C 63.9) to Me-15 (δ_H 1.06, t, *J* = 7.0 Hz/δ_C 15.7). This was supported by HMBC correlations from H-8 to C-9, C-14 and C-3, H-14 to C-8, Me-15, H-9 to C-8, C-11, Me-11 to C-9, C-10, C-12, and Me-12 to C-9, C-10 and C-11.

Table 2. ^{1}H and ^{13}C NMR (DMSO-*d*6, 300 and 75 MHz) and HMBC assignment for **6**.

Position	δ_C, Type	δ_H, (*J* in Hz)	COSY	HMBC
1	119.3, C	-		
2	155.1, C	-		
3	130.5, C			
4	128.5, CH	7.25, d (8.7)	H-5	C-2, 6, 8
5	110.3, CH	6.32, d (8.7)	H-4	C-1, 3, 6, 7 (w)
6	154.8, C	-		
7	167.2, CO	-		
8	73.1, CH	4.58, dd (9.2, 3.8)	H-9a, 9b	C-3, 9, 14
9a, b	47.1, CH$_2$	1.57, ddd (13.8, 9.2, 5.0) 1.27, ddd (13.8, 8.9, 3.9)		C-8, 9, 11, 12
10	24.9, CH	1.71, m	H-9a, 9b, 11, 12	
11	23.7, CH$_3$	0.88, d (6.6)	H-10	C-9, 10, 12
12	22.2, CH$_3$	0.92, d (6.6)	H-10	C.9, 10, 11
13	62.8, OMe	3.83, s		
14	63.9, CH$_2$	3.25, q (7.0)	H-15	C-8, 15
15	15.7, CH$_3$	1.06, t (7.0)	H-14	C-14
1′	129.8, C	-		
2′	142.3, C	-		
3′	150.9, C	-		
4′	124.2, CH	7.14, d (2.0)	H-6′, 8′	C-2′, 3′, 6′, 8′
5′	136.7, C	-		
6′	118.4, CH	7.11, d (2.0)	H-4′, 6′	C-2′, 3′ (w), 7′, 8′
7′	189.8, CHO	10.15, s		C-1′, 5′ (w), 6′
8′	21.0, CH$_3$	2.31, s	H-4′, 6′	

w = weak.

Taking together the molecular formula and the partial structures, the two substituted benzene rings must be connected by an ether bridge through C-6 and C-2′, forming a biphenyl ether derivative. The only difference between the structure of **6** and that of **5** is that the acetoxy group on C-8 in **5** was replaced by the ethoxy group in **6**. Since **6** cannot be obtained as a suitable crystal for X-ray analysis, we attempted to determine the absolute configuration of C-8 of **6** by comparing the experimental and calculated ECD spectra.

Unfortunately, **6** does not produce an ECD spectrum at a concentration that normally gives a visible spectrum for other compounds of this series. Therefore, based on the biogenic consideration, we presume that the absolute configuration of C-8 in **6** is the same as that in **5**. Moreover, this hypothesis is supported by the fact that both **5** and **6** are levorotatory. Thus, the absolute configuration of C-8 in **6** was proposed as (*S*). Since **6** has not been previously reported, it was named neospinosic acid.

Compound **7** was isolated as a yellow viscous oil, and its molecular formula was established as $C_{21}H_{24}O_6$ on the basis of (+)-HRESIMS *m/z* 373.1652 [M + H]$^+$ (calculated for $C_{21}H_{25}O_6$, 373.1651) (Figure S37), corresponding to 10 degrees of unsaturation. The ^{13}C NMR spectrum (Table 3, Figure S33) displayed 21 carbon signals, which, in combination with DEPT and HSQC spectra (Figure S35), can be categorized as nine non-protonated sp^2 (δ_C 161.6, 160.2, 157.9, 145.9, 143.4, 138.3, 136.3, 135.6, and 114.3), four protonated sp^2 (δ_C 132.8, 125.9, 119.9, and 115.6), one methoxy (δ_C 63.1), one oxymethine sp^3 (δ_C 64.4), one methine sp^3 (δ_C 24.8), one oxymethylene sp^3 (δ_C 57.9), one methylene sp^3 (δ_C 48.3), and three methyl (δ_C 23.9, 22.1, and 20.9) carbons. The ^1H NMR spectrum (Figure S32), in combination with the COSY spectrum (Table 3, Figure S34), showed two *ortho*-coupled aromatic protons at δ_H 7.67, d (*J* = 8.6 Hz) and 7.21, d (*J* = 8.6 Hz), two *meta*-coupled aromatic protons at δ_H 7.12, d (*J* = 0.5 Hz) and 7.11, brs, one triplet at δ_H 5.34 (*J* = 5.8 Hz), one double of double doublet at δ_H 4.87 (*J* = 9.2, 4.9, 4.2 Hz), two doublet at δ_H 4.72 (*J* = 5.7 Hz) and 5.13 (*J* = 4.9 Hz), a methoxy singlet at δ_H 3.76, two geminally coupled double of double doublets at δ_H 1.24 (*J* = 13.7, 9.2, 4.2 Hz) and δ_H 1.44 (*J* = 13.7, 9.2, 4.9 Hz), a multiplet at δ_H 1.72, one methyl singlet at δ_H 2.28, and two methyl doublets at δ_H 0.86 (*J* = 6.7 Hz) and 0.90 (*J* = 6.7 Hz). The ^1H and ^{13}C chemical shift values and multiplicities of the aromatic proton signals suggested the presence of two substituted benzene rings in the molecule. That one of the benzene ring is 1,2,3,4-tetrasubstituted, with a methoxyl group on C-2 and an oxygenated substituent on C-6, was evidenced by the COSY correlations (Table 3) from the doublet at δ_H 7.67 (*J* = 8.6 Hz, H-4/δ_C 132.8) to another doublet at δ_H 7.21 (*J* = 8.6 Hz, H-5/δ_C 115.6) as well as by HMBC correlations (Table 3, Figure S36) from H-4 to the carbons at δ_C 160.2 (C-6), 157.9 (C-2) and the oxymethine sp^3 carbon at δ_C 64.4, H-5 to the carbons at δ_C 114.3 (C-1), 138.3 (C-3), C-6, a methoxyl singlet at δ_H 3.76 (δ_C 63.1) to C-2. The chemical shift value of C-1 suggested that it was substituted by a carbonyl group. That the substituent on C-3 is 1-hydroxy-3-methylbutyl was substantiated by COSY correlations (Table 3) from H-8 (δ_H 4.87, ddd, *J* = 9.2, 4.9, 4.2 Hz/δ_C 64.4) to the double of double doublet at δ_H 1.44 (*J* = 13.7, 9.2, 4.9 Hz, H-9b/δ_C 48.3) and a doublet at δ_H 5.13 (*J* = 4.9 Hz, OH-8), and HMBC correlations (Table 3) from H-9b to C-8, OH-8 to C-9, the methyl doublet at δ_H 0.86 (*J* = 6.7 Hz/δ_C 23.9; Me-11) to the carbon at δ_C 48.3 (C-9), 24.8 (C-10), 22.1 (Me-12), the doublet at 0.90 (*J* = 6.7 Hz/δ_C 22.1; Me-12) to C-9, C-10 and Me-11.

That another benzene ring is 1,2,3,5-tetrasubstituted, with a methyl substituent on C-5′ and a hydroxymethyl group on C-1′, was substantiated by a COSY correlation (Table 3) from the triplet at δ_H 5.34 (*J* = 5.8 Hz, OH-7′) to a doublet at δ_H 4.72 (*J* = 5.8 Hz, H$_2$-7′/δ_C 57.9) and HMBC correlations (Table 3) from H$_2$-7′ to the carbons at δ_C 125.9 (C-6′), 135.6 (C-1′), 145.9 (C-2′), the methyl singlet at δ_H 2.28 (Me-8′/δ_C 20.9) to the carbons at δ_C 119.9 (C-4′), 136.3 (C-5′), and C-6′, a doublet at δ_H 7.12 (*J* = 0.5 Hz, H-6′/δ_C 125.9) to C-4′, C-2′ (δ_C 145.9), C-7′ and Me-8′, and from a broad singlet at δ_H 7.11 (H-4′/δ_C 119.9) to C-2′, C-3′ (δ_C 143.4) and C-6′. The chemical shift values of C-2′ and C-3′ suggested that they are oxygen-bearing aromatic carbons.

Considering the ^1H and ^{13}C chemical shift values and the molecular formula, the two substituted benzene rings must be connected by an ether bridge between C-2′ and C-6 as well as between the oxygen atom on C-3′ and the carbonyl on C-1, thus forming a 5*H*-1,4-dioxepin-5-one ring. Therefore, the carbon at δ_C 161.6 was assigned to C-7.

Table 3. ^{1}H and ^{13}C NMR (DMSO-d_6, 500 and 125 MHz) and HMBC assignment for **7**.

Position	δ_C, Type	δ_H, (J in Hz)	COSY	HMBC
1	114.3, C	-		
2	157.9, C	-		
3	138.3, C	-		
4	132.8, CH	7.67, d (8.6)	H-5	C-1, 3, 6
5	115.6, CH	7.21, d (8.6)	H-4	C-2, 6, 8
6	160.2, C	-		
7	161.6, CO	-		
8	64.4, CH	4.87, ddd (9.2, 4.9, 4.2)	H-9a, 9b, OH-8	
9a, b	48.3, CH$_2$	1.24, ddd (13.7, 9.2, 4.2) 1.44, ddd (13.7, 9.2, 4.9)	H-8, 9b, 10 H-8, 9a, 10	
10	24.8, CH	1.72, m	H-9a, b, Me-11, 12	
11	23.9, CH$_3$	0.86, d (6.7)	H-10	C-9, 12
12	22.1, CH$_3$	0.90, d (6.7)	H-10	C-9, 11
13	63.1, OMe	3.76, s		C-2
1'	135.6, C	-		
2'	145.9, C	-		
3'	143.4, C	-		
4'	119.9, CH	7.11, brs		C-2', 3', 6'
5'	136.3, C	-		
6'	125.9, CH	7.12, d (0.5)		C-2', 4', 7',8'
7'	57.9, CH$_2$	4.72, d (5.8)	OH-7'	C-1', 2', 6'
8'	20.9, CH$_3$	2.28, s		C-4', 5', 6'
OH-7'		5.34, t (5.8)	H-7'	C-7'
OH-8		5.13, d (4.9)	H-8	C-9

Since **7** has one stereogenic carbon (C-8), it is necessary to determine its absolute configuration. Compound **7** was isolated as a viscous oil, which was not able to determine the absolute configuration of C-8 by X-ray crystallography. Therefore, the absolute configuration of C-8 in **7** was determined by ECD. For this effect, the experimental ECD spectrum of **7** was measured and then compared with a quantum-mechanically simulated spectrum derived from the most significant computational models of (S)-**7** (Figure 4; please see Experimental section for details). Figure 5 shows a good match between experimental and calculated ECD spectra, with the two spectra in phase, leading to a conclusion that the absolute configuration of C-8 is (S).

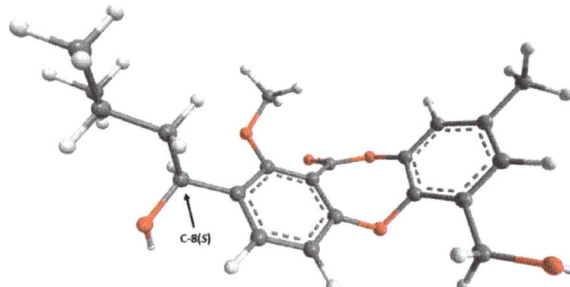

Figure 4. Model of the most abundant conformation of **7** (lowest B3LYP/6-31G/acetonitrile energy conformer) accounting for 48% of conformer population) in its ECD assigned (8S) configuration.

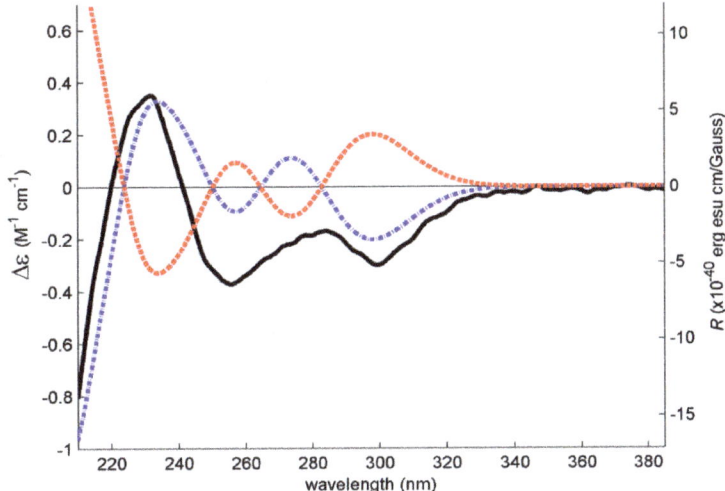

Figure 5. Experimental ECD spectrum of **7** in acetonitrile (solid black line) and theoretical ECD spectra of its (*S*) (dot–dashed blue line) and (*R*) (dashed red line) computational models.

Literature search through SciFinder revealed that **7** has never been previously described, and, therefore, was named spinolactone.

Interestingly, Nishida et al. [18] reported the structure of a similar compound containing a 11*H*-dibenzo[b,e][1,4]dioxepin-11-one scaffold, named purpactin C' which was obtained by conversion of purpactin C, isolated from a fermentation broth of *Penicillium purpurogenum* FO-608. However, the authors only presented its HREI-MS, ^{1}H and ^{13}C NMR data (CDCl$_3$, 300 and 75 MHz) of purpactin C'. Later on, Chen et al. isolated purpactin C' from a gorgonian-derived *Talaromyces* sp. [19], whereas Daengrot et al. also described the isolation of the same compound from a soil-derived *Penicillium aculeatum* PSU-RSPG105 [16]. In both cases, the authors reported neither its NMR data nor absolute configuration of the stereogenic carbon in the side chain but only referred to the work of Nishida et al. [18].

Since the two benzene rings of **5–8** possess the same substitution patterns, it is clearly that they share the same biosynthetic origin and route. Condensation of acetyl CoA (**I**) and malonyl CoA (**II**) gives an octaketide **III**, which undergoes a cyclization to give an intermediate **IV**. However, instead of enolization, one of the ketone carbonyl in ring C undergoes a reduction to form a secondary alcohol, which, after oxidation of the methylene group in ring B, gives rise to **VI**. Decarboxylation of ring A and dehydration of the secondary alcohol in ring C of **VI** gives rise to the anthraquinone **VII**. Prenylation on the activated carbon in **VII** by dimethylallyl pyrophosphate (DMAPP) gives rise to a prenyl intermediate **VIII**, followed by enolization to give an intermediate **IX**. Methylation of the phenolic hydroxyl group, *ortho* to the prenyl group, by SAM, leads to the formation of **X**. Oxidative cleavage of the anthraquinone ring gives rise to **XI**. Rotation of the bond between the benzene ring (A) and the carbonyl group in **XI** to **XII** allows a nucleophilic substitution of the hydroxyl group to give an intermediate **XIII**. Oxidation of the aldehyde to a carboxylic acid and oxidation of the double bond of the prenyl side chain lead to an intermediate **XIV**, which, after dehydration, gives **XV**. Regiospecific hydration of the double bond of the side chain of **XV** gives **XVI**, which, after reduction of one of the carboxylic acid group to aldehyde, results in a formation of **XVII**. Acetylation of the hydroxyl group of the side chain leads to the formation of **5**, which, after reduction of the carbonyl carbon of the acetyl group, gives rise to **6** (Figure 6).

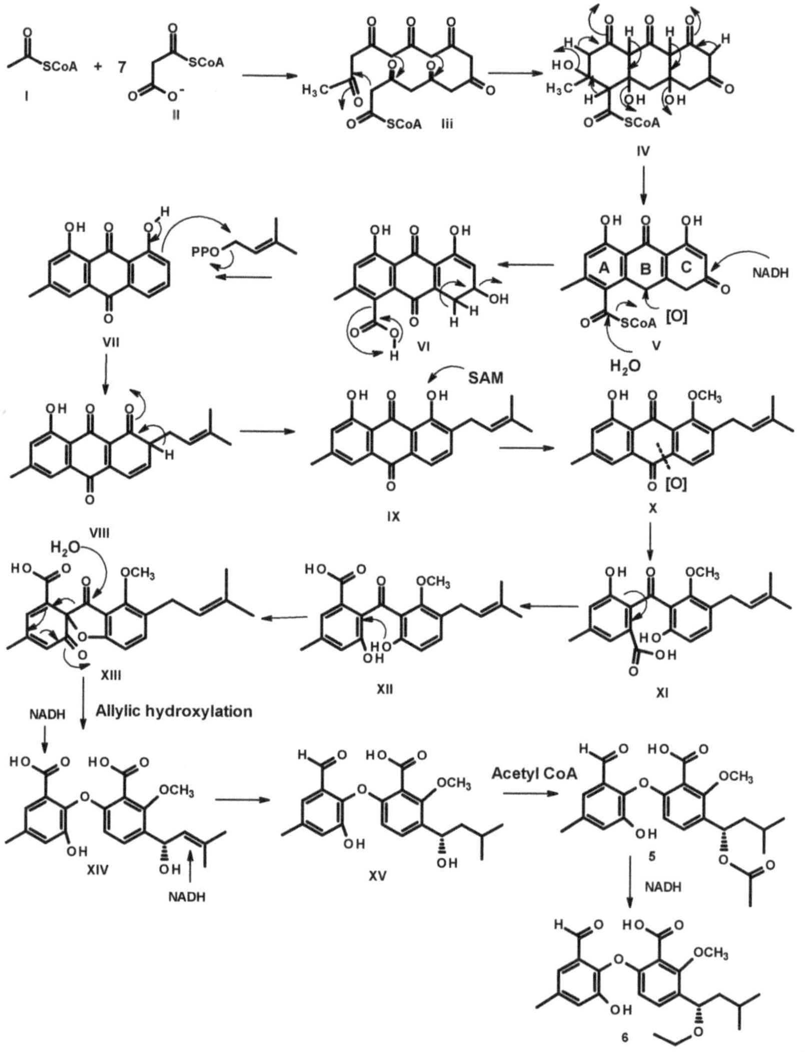

Figure 6. Proposed biogenesis of **5** and **6**.

Reduction of the aldehyde group on ring A of **XVII** to a primary alcohol in **XVIII** or **XIX**, followed by esterification of the carboxyl group by the phenolic hydroxyl group (in **XIX**) or by a hydroxyl group of the primary alcohol (in **XVIII**) leads to the formation of **7** and **8**, respectively (Figure 7).

The antimicrobial activity of **2** and **5–8** was evaluated against several reference bacterial species and multidrug-resistant isolates (Table 4); however, only **7** exhibited antibacterial activity against *Enterococcus faecalis* B3/101 with a MIC value of 64 µg/mL (Table 4). The MBC was more than one-fold higher than the MIC, suggesting a bacteriostatic effect.

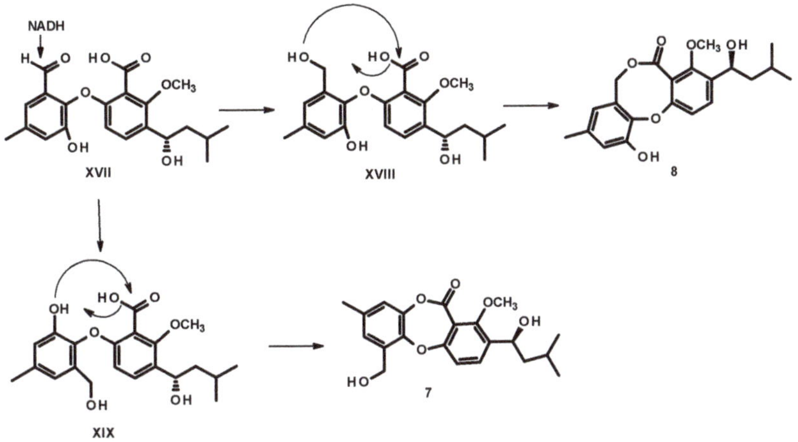

Figure 7. Proposed biogenesis of **7** and **8**.

Table 4. Antibacterial activity of **2** and **5–8** against Gram-positive reference and multidrug-resistant strains. MIC is expressed in µg/mL. Ceftazidime and kanamycin were used as positive controls.

Compound	E. faecalis ATCC 29212	E. faecalis B3/101 (VRE)	S. aureus ATCC 29213	S. aureus 66/1 (MRSA)
2	>64	>64	>64	>64
5	>64	>64	>64	>64
6	>64	>64	>64	>64
7	>64	64	>64	>64
8	>64	>64	>64	>64
CAZ	-	-	8	-
KAN	32	-	-	-

MIC, minimal inhibitory concentration. CAZ, ceftazidime. KAN, kanamycin.

Although **5** and **6** did not exhibit antibacterial activity, they were able to significantly inhibit biofilm formation in three of the four reference strains used in this study (Table 5): *Escherichia coli* ATCC 25922 (both **5** and **6**), *Staphylococcus aureus* ATCC 29213 (both **5** and **6**), and *E. faecalis* ATCC 29212 (**5**). A more extensive effect was found for **6**, which displayed the strongest inhibitory activity (56.00 ± 0.06) (mean ± SD) in *S. aureus* ATCC 29213.

Table 5. Percentage of biofilm formation for compounds that showed antibiofilm activity after 24 h incubation.

Compound	Concentration (µg/mL)	Biofilm Biomass (% of Control)		
		E. coli ATCC 25922	E. faecalis ATCC 29212	S. aureus ATCC 29213
5	64	88.39 ± 0.09 ***	75.89 ± 0.10 ***	84.46 ± 0.10 ***
6	64	83.89 ± 0.19 ***	-	56.00 ± 0.06 ***

Data are shown as mean ± SD of three independent experiments. One-sample t-test: *** $p < 0.001$ significantly different from 100%. MIC, minimal inhibitory concentration.

This result led us to investigate the influence of **6** in both biofilm viability (Figure 8) and its matrix spatial arrangement (Figure 9). After 8 h of incubation, the viability of the biofilm of *S. aureus* ATCC 29213 was significantly affected by **6**, exhibiting a percentage of control of 1.80 ± 0.0014, representing a viability reduction of 98%. On the contrary, after 24 h of incubation, the percentage of control increased to 89.65 ± 0.0021, showing only a

10% viability reduction. Although the results herein presented suggest a sublethal effect of **6** on a specific molecular or structural target of *S. aureus*, that could be reversed over time due to genetic and phenotypic adaptability of bacteria; however, it cannot be ruled out that the compound may undergo some degradation or biodegradation. Further studies are warranted to shed more light on this subject.

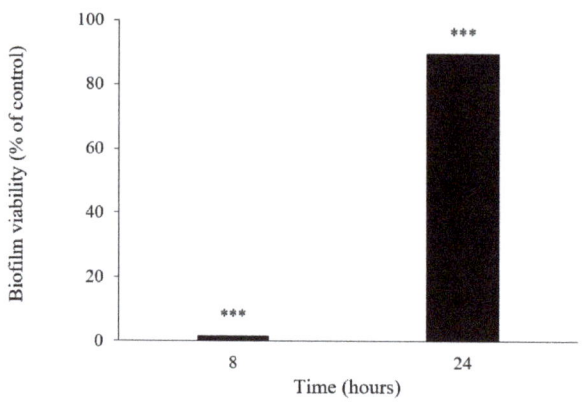

Figure 8. Biofilm viability effect in *S. aureus* ATCC 29213 in the presence of **6** after 8 and 24 h of incubation. Where *** represent statistical significance of data as $p < 0.001$.

Regarding the effect on biofilm extracellular polymeric substances, **6** caused an increased number of channels, homogeneously distributed by the biofilm, after 8 h of incubation (Figure 9). However, after 24 h of incubation, this biofilm did not maintain its structure, appearing quite similar to the control (data not shown). In fact, *S. aureus* ATCC 29213 typically produces a dense biofilm structure with lower number of observed channels. Biofilm interstitial voids (channels) are physiologically relevant for diffusion and circulation of nutrients, oxygen and essential substances. Factors such as cell-to-cell communication and alterations in attachment of bacterial cell to surfaces can influence the dynamic of biofilm, namely the evolution of the channels. Formation of channels was shown to be affected by molecules like surfactants, which have the ability to modulate gene expression and to maintain open channels [20,21]. Nonetheless, the present study highlights the promising results of **6** in *S. aureus* biofilm early development. Understanding the antibiofilm dynamic in the presence of **6** and its stability is essential to evaluate its activity, especially within the first 8 h of incubation. Compound **5** was also investigated for its potential synergy with clinically relevant antibiotics on the multidrug-resistant isolates, by both disk diffusion method and checkerboard assay; however, no interactions were observed.

Compounds **2** and **5–8** were also tested for their in vitro acetylcholinesterase (AChE) inhibitory activity by a modified Ellman's method [22]; however, none of the tested compounds showed inhibition of the enzyme at concentrations as high as 80 µM (a positive control galantamine showed a percentage inhibition of 94.82% at 80 µM, and an IC_{50} value of 16.76 µM). Additionally, **2** and **5–8** were also evaluated for their anti-tyrosinase activity at the maximum concentration of 200 µM by using a modified microplate assay as described previously [23]. All the tested compounds, except **6**, inhibited tyrosinase activity. However, as **8** showed a percentage of inhibition higher than 50% at 200 µM, its IC_{50} value (177.03 ± 8.17 µM) was obtained at lower doses (i.e., 150 and 100 µM), indicating its moderate anti-tyrosinase activity. On the contrary, **2, 5, 7** showed weak inhibitory effects. Table 6 shows percent inhibition at 200 µM and IC_{50} values (µM) of the tested compounds.

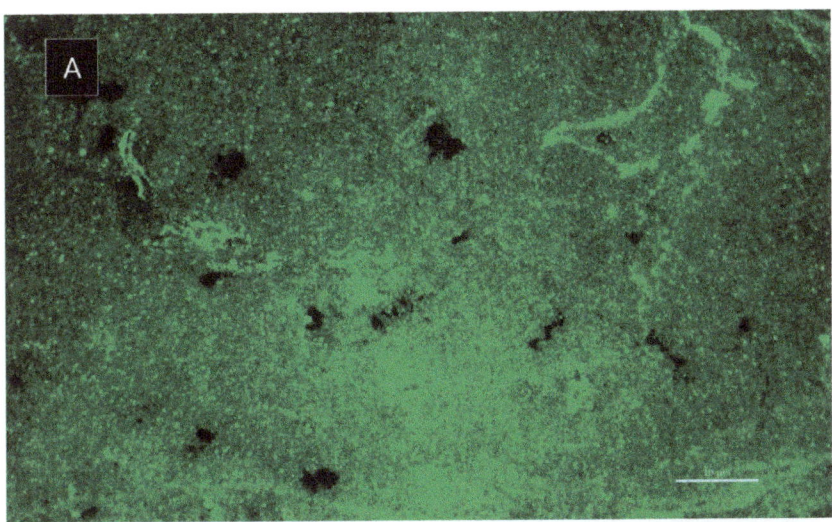
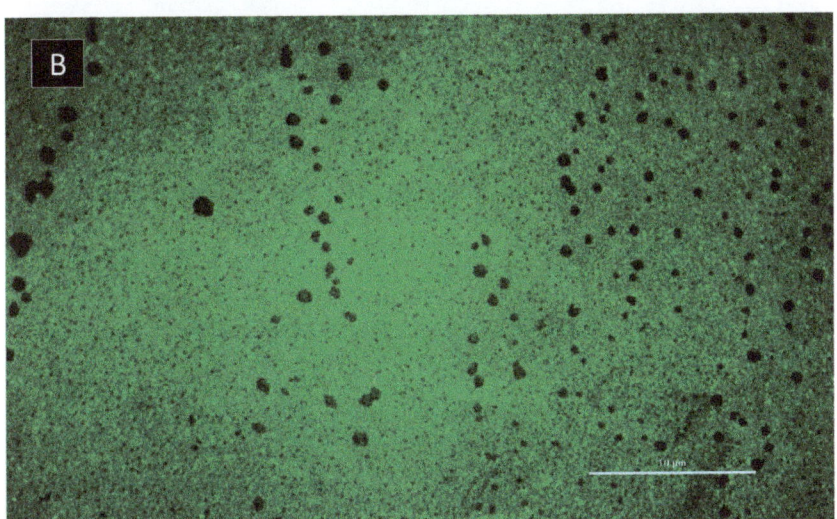

Figure 9. Rhodamine-conA staining of *S. aureus* ATCC 29213 biofilm: (**A**) in the absence of **6** and (**B**) in the presence of **6** after 8 h incubation. Scale bar = 10 µm. Amplification 1000×.

Table 6. Tyrosinase inhibitory activity of **2** and **5–8**.

Compounds	% Inhibition at 200 µM	IC$_{50}$ (µM)
2	11.56 ± 2.05 *	n.d.
5	4.58 ± 0.07 ***	n.d.
6	n.a.	-
7	5.33 ± 0.18 ***	n.d.
8	53.1 ± 1.17 ***	177.03 ± 8.17 **
Kojic acid (positive control)	95.04 ± 0.018 ****	14.00 ± 0.12 ****

Results are given as mean ± SEM of three independent experiments performed in triplicate; n.a.: not active; n.d.: not determined; $p < 0.05$ (*); $p < 0.01$ (**); $p < 0.001$ (***); $p < 0.0001$ (****).

3. Experimental Section

3.1. General Experimental Procedures

The melting points were determined on a Stuart Melting Point Apparatus SMP3 (Bibby Sterilin, Stone, Staffordshire, UK) and are uncorrected. Optical rotations were measured on an ADP410 Polarimeter (Bellingham + Stanley Ltd., Tunbridge Wells, Kent, UK). ^{1}H and ^{13}C NMR spectra were recorded at ambient temperature on a Bruker AMC instrument (Bruker Biosciences Corporation, Billerica, MA, USA) operating at 300 or 500 and 75 or 125 MHz, respectively. High-resolution mass spectra were measured with a Waters Xevo QToF mass spectrometer (Waters Corporations, Milford, MA, USA) coupled to a Waters Aquity UPLC system. A Merck (Darmstadt, Germany) silica gel GF$_{254}$ was used for preparative TLC, and Merck Si gel 60 (0.2–0.5 mm), Li Chroprep silica gel and Sephadex LH 20 were used for column chromatography.

3.2. Fungal Material

The fungus was isolated from a marine sponge *Mycale* sp., which was collected by scuba diving at a depth of 10–15 m from the coral reef at Samae San Island (12°34'36.64" N 100°56'59.69" E), Chonburi province, Thailand, in September 2016. The sponge was washed with sterilized seawater three times, and then dried on a sterile filter paper under sterile aseptic condition. The sponge was cut into small pieces (5 × 5 mm), and four pieces were placed on Petri dish plates containing 15 mL potato dextrose agar (PDA) medium mixed with 300 mg/L of streptomycin sulfate and incubated at room temperature for 7 days. The hyphal tips emerging from sponge pieces were individually transferred onto PDA slant.

The fungal strain KUFA 1047 was identified as *Neosartorya spinosa*, based on morphological characteristics. This identification was confirmed by molecular techniques using internal transcribed spacer (ITS) primers. DNA was extracted from young mycelia following a modified Murray and Thompson method [24]. The universal primer pairs ITS1 and ITS4 were used for ITS gene amplification [25]. PCR reactions were conducted on a thermal cycler and DNA sequencing analyses were performed using the dideoxyribonucleotide chain termination method [26] by Macrogen Inc. (Seoul, South Korea). The DNA sequences were edited using FinchTV software and submitted into the BLAST program for alignment and compared with that of fungal species in the NCBI database (http://www.ncbi.nlm.nih.gov/, accessed on 15 January 2017). Its gene sequences were deposited in GenBank with an accession number MT814287. The pure cultures were maintained at Kasetsart University Fungal Collection, Department of Plant Pathology, Faculty of Agriculture, Kasetsart University, Bangkok, Thailand.

3.3. Extraction and Isolation

The mycelium plugs of *Neosartorya spinosa* KUFA 1047 were transferred into 500 mL Erlenmeyer flasks containing 200 mL of potato dextrose broth (PDB) and incubated on a rotary shaker at 120 rpm for 7 days at room temperature for preparing a mycelial suspension. Fifty 1 L Erlenmeyer flasks, each containing 300 g sterile cooked rice and then inoculated with 20 mL of mycelial suspension in each flask and incubated at room temperature for 30 days. Then, 500 mL of EtOAc were added to each flask and macerated for 7 days and then filtered with Whatman filter paper N°.1 (GE Healthcare UK Limited, Buckinghamshire, UK). The organic solutions were combined and then evaporated under reduced pressure to give 227.8 g of crude EtOAc extracts of *N. spinosa* KUFA 1047. The crude EtOAc extract of *N. spinosa* KUFA 1047 was dissolved in 500 mL of EtOAc and then washed with a 5% NaHCO$_3$ solution (4 × 250 mL). The resulting organic phase was washed with deionized water (3 × 500 mL) and dried with anhydrous Na$_2$SO$_4$, filtered, and evaporated under reduced pressure, to obtain 31.2 g of the crude EtOAc extract, which was applied on a column chromatography of silica gel 60 (350 g) and eluted with mixtures of petrol-CHCl$_3$ and CHCl$_3$-Me$_2$CO, wherein 250 mL fractions (frs) were collected as follows: frs 1–192 (petrol-CHCl$_3$, 3:7), 193–282 (petrol–CHCl$_3$, 1:9), 283–432 (CHCl$_3$–Me$_2$CO, 9:1), and 433–598 (CHCl$_3$–Me$_2$CO, 7:3). Frs 109–155 were combined (980 mg) and applied over a column chromatography of Sephadex LH-20 (15 g) and eluted with MeOH, wherein 35 sub-fractions (sfrs) of 1 mL were collected. Sfrs 9–22 were combined (861.5 mg) and applied over a column chromatography of Sephadex LH-20 (15 g) and eluted with CHCl$_3$, wherein 22 ssfrs of 1 mL were collected. Ssfrs 8–13 were combined (483 mg) and applied over a column chromatography of Sephadex LH-20 (5 g) and eluted with MeOH, wherein 14 frs of 0.25 mL were collected. Frs 5–9 were combined (237.4 mg) and applied over a column chromatography of Sephadex LH-20 (5 g) and eluted with MeOH, wherein 12 sfrs of 0.25 mL were collected. Sfrs 9–12 were combined and to give 36.9 mg of yellow viscous mass of **8**. Frs 156–200 were combined (180.0 mg) and applied over a column chromatography of Sephadex LH-20 (5 g), and eluted with MeOH, wherein 17 sfrs of 1 mL were collected. Sfrs 8–17 were combined (42.8 mg) and applied over a column chromatography of Sephadex LH-20 (5 g), and eluted with MeOH, wherein 19 ssfrs of 0.5 mL were collected. Ssfrs 14–19 were combined and to give 5.4 mg of a mixture of **3** and **4**. Sfrs 5–7 (75.5 mg) from the first Sephadex LH-20 column were combined with ssfrs 3-13 (36.9) of the second Sephadex LH-20 column (112.4 mg) and applied over a column chromatography of Sephadex LH-20 (5 g), and eluted with CHCl$_3$, wherein 22 frs of 1 mL were collected. Frs 8–22 were combined (83.6 mg) and purified by TLC (silica gel 60 G$_{254}$, CHCl$_3$: Me$_2$CO, 9:1) to give 8.8 mg of **7**. Frs 288–291 were combined (226.4 mg) and precipitated in CHCl$_3$ to give 10.3 mg **2**. The mother liquor (209.8 mg) was applied over a column chromatography of Sephadex LH-20 (5 g) and eluted with MeOH, wherein 29 sfrs of 0.25 mL were collected. Sfrs 8–15 were combined (128.4 mg) and applied over a column chromatography of Sephadex LH-20 (5 g) and eluted with CHCl$_3$, wherein 23 ssfrs of 1 mL were collected. Ssfrs 19–23 were combined (43.2 mg) and purified by TLC (silica gel 60 G$_{254}$, petrol: CHCl$_3$: Me$_2$CO, 2: 85:13) to give 14.3 mg of **6**. Frs 293–298 were combined (798.7 mg) and precipitated in CHCl$_3$ to give additional 9.4 mg of **2**. Frs 339–379 were combined (506.6 mg) and purified by TLC (silica gel 60 G$_{254}$, CHCl$_3$: Me$_2$CO, 85:15). One of the bands from the TLC plates (128.4 mg) was applied over a column chromatography of Sephadex LH-20 (5 g) and eluted with MeOH, wherein 19 sfrs of 0.25 mL were collected. Sfrs 4–19 were combined (108.1 mg) and precipitated in CHCl$_3$ to give 39.3 mg of **5**. Frs 299–338 (1.29 g), the mother liquor of frs 293–298 (775.9 mg), and the rest of the TLC bands of frs 339–379 (65.1 mg) were combined (2.13 mg) and applied over a column chromatography of Li Chroprep® silica gel (35 g) and eluted with mixtures of petrol–CHCl$_3$ and CHCl$_3$–Me$_2$CO, wherein 112 sfrs of 100 mL were collected as follow: 1–26 (petrol–CHCl$_3$, 3:7), 27–75 (petrol–CHCl$_3$, 1:9), 76–99 (CHCl$_3$–Me$_2$CO, 9:1), and 100–112 (CHCl$_3$–Me$_2$CO, 7:3). Sfrs 7–8 were combined (41.5 mg) and applied over a column chromatography of Li Chroprep® silica gel (8 g) and eluted with mixtures of petrol–CHCl$_3$ and CHCl$_3$–Me$_2$CO, wherein 33 ssfrs of 25 mL were collected as follow: ssfrs 1–4 (petrol–CHCl$_3$, 1:1), 5–17 (petrol–CHCl$_3$, 3:7), 18–25 (petrol–CHCl$_3$, 1:9), 26–30 (CHCl$_3$–Me$_2$CO, 9:1), and 31–33 (CHCl$_3$–Me$_2$CO, 7:3). Ssfrs 9–11 were combined (7.6 mg) and precipitated in CHCl$_3$ to give 6.6 mg of **1**.

3.3.1. Acetylpenipurdin A (**4**)

For ^{1}H and ^{13}C NMR spectroscopic data (CDCl$_3$, 300 and 75 MHz), see Table 1. (+)-HRESIMS *m/z* 371.1124 (M + H)$^+$ (calcd for C$_{20}$H$_{19}$O$_7$, 329.1131).

3.3.2. Neospinosic Acid (**6**)

Yellow amorphous solid. [α]$_D^{20}$ -166.7 (*c* = 0.042, MeOH). IR (KBr) υ_{max} 3447 (OH), 2956, 2930, 2869, 1683 (CHO), 1653, 1616, 1596, 1472, 1323, and 12792 cm^{-1}. For ^{1}H and ^{13}C spectroscopic data (DMSO-*d6*, 300 and 75 MHz), see Table 2; (+)-HRESIMS *m/z* 417.1915 (M + H)$^+$ (calcd for C$_{23}$H$_{29}$O$_7$, 417.1913); 439.1735 (M + Na)$^+$ (calcd for C$_{23}$H$_{28}$O$_7$Na, 439.1733).

3.3.3. Spinolactone (7)

Yellow viscous oil. $[\alpha]_D^{20}$ -311.5 (c = 0.06, MeOH). IR (KBr) ν_{max} 3423 (OH), 2955, 2927, 2868, 1746, 1596, 1521, 1488, 1470, 1225, and 1202 cm^{-1}. For ^{1}H and ^{13}C spectroscopic data (DMSO-d_6, 500 and 125 MHz), see Table 3; (+)-HRESIMS m/z 373.1652 (M+H)$^+$ (calcd for $C_{21}H_{25}O_6$, 373.1651).

3.4. Electronic Circular Dichroism (ECD)

The experimental UV and ECD spectra of **5** and **7** (*ca.* 1 mg/mL in methanol and acetonitrile) were obtained in a Jasco J-815 CD spectropolarimeter (Jasco Europe S.R.L., Cremella, Italy) with a 0.1 mm cuvette and 12 accumulations. The simulated ECD spectrum was obtained by first determining all the relevant conformers of the (*S*)-**5** computational model. Its conformational space was developed by rotating by 90, 120, or 180 degrees all the single, non-cyclic, bonds, depending on the MM2 torsion energy minima. The large number of conformational degrees of freedom of **5** resulted in a huge number of conformers, which were MM2 minimized with PerkinElmer's Chem3D Ultra 20.1.0.110 (PerkinElmer Inc., Waltham, MA, USA) and ChemScript (PerkinElmer Inc., Waltham, MA, USA) and filtered to eliminate like conformations with VeraChem's Vconf 2.0 (VeraChem LLC, Germantown, MA, USA), resulting in 351 different conformers. Since the MM2 energies of all of these conformers fell within an interval of 3 kcal/mol, many with very similar values, all the 351 conformers were minimized using the semi-empirical method PM6/methanol using Gaussian 16W (Gaussian Inc., Wallingford, NY, USA) and then filtered again. Out of these, 351 PM6 conformers, 20 were found within a 2 kcal/mol interval (about 85% of the population) and were subjected to a final minimization round using the quantum mechanical DFT method B3LYP/6-31G/methanol method (Gaussian 16W), which was also used to calculate its first 70 ECD transitions (TDDFT). The line spectrum for each one of the 20 conformations was built by applying a Gaussian line broadening of 0.3 eV to each computed transition with a constant UV shift of −4 nm. The final ECD spectrum was obtained by the Boltzmann-weighted sum of the 20 line spectra [27].

The simulated ECD spectrum was obtained by first determining all the relevant conformers of the (*S*)-**7** computational model. Its conformational space was developed by rotating by 45 degrees all the single, non-cyclic, bonds for each of the two possible bends about the 7-cycle oxygens. The resulting conformers (over 1000) were MM2 minimized (with PerkinElmer's Chem3D Ultra) and filtered to eliminate like conformations (with VeraChem's Vconf 2.0). The lowest 104 conformers, representing about 99% of MM2 total conformer energy, were further minimized using the PM6/acetonitrile semi-empirical method (Gaussian Inc.'s Gaussian 16W) and filtered. The lowest 96% PM6 energy conformers (21 models) were subjected to a final minimization round using the quantum mechanical DFT method B3LYP/6-31G/acetonitrile method (Gaussian 16W), which was also used to calculate its first 70 ECD transitions (TDDFT). The line spectrum for each one of the 21 conformations was built by applying a Gaussian line broadening of 0.2 eV to each computed transition with a constant UV shift of −5 nm. The final ECD spectrum was obtained by the Boltzmann-weighted sum of the 21 line spectra [27].

3.5. Antibacterial Activity Bioassays

3.5.1. Bacterial Strains and Growth Conditions

Four reference strains obtained from the American Type Culture Collection were included in this study: two Gram-positive (*Staphylococcus aureus* ATCC 29213 and *Enterococcus faecalis* ATCC 29212), two Gram-negative (*Escherichia coli* ATCC 25922 and *Pseudomonas aeruginosa* ATCC 27853), and one clinical isolate (*E. coli* SA/2, an extended-spectrum β-lactamase producer-ESBL) and two environmental isolates: *S. aureus* 74/24 [28], a methicillin-resistant isolate (MRSA), and *E. faecalis* B3/101 [29] a vancomycin-resistant (VRE) isolate. All bacterial strains were cultured in MH agar (MH-BioKar Diagnostics, Allone, France) and incubated overnight at 37 °C before each assay, in order to obtain fresh cultures. Stock solutions of the compounds were prepared in dimethyl sulfoxide (DMSO—

Alfa Aesar, Kandel, Germany), kept at −20 °C, and freshly diluted in the appropriate culture media before each assay. All stock solutions were prepared at final concentration of 10 mg/mL and, in all experiments, in-test concentrations of DMSO were kept below 1%, as recommended by the Clinical and Laboratory Standards Institute [30].

3.5.2. Antimicrobial Susceptibility Testing

The Kirby–Bauer method was used to screen the antimicrobial activity of the compounds according to CLSI recommendations [31]. Briefly, sterile blank paper disks with 6 mm diameter (Liofilchem, Roseto degli Abruzzi, TE, Italy) were impregnated with 15 µg of each compound and placed on MH plates previously inoculated with a bacterial inoculum equal to 0.5 McFarland turbidity. Blank paper disks impregnated with DMSO were used as negative control. MH inoculated plates were incubated for 18–20 h at 37 °C and afterwards the diameter of the inhibition zones was measured in mm.

Minimal inhibitory concentrations (MIC) were determined by the broth microdilution method, as recommended by the CLSI [32]. Two-fold serial dilutions of the compounds were prepared in cation-adjusted Mueller–Hinton broth (CAMHB- Sigma-Aldrich, St. Louis, MO, USA). The tested concentrations ranged from 1 to 64 µg/mL, in order to keep in-test concentrations of DMSO below 1%, avoiding bacterial growth inhibition. Colony-forming unit counts of the inoculum were conducted to ensure that the final inoculum size closely approximated the intended number (5×10^5 CFU/mL). The 96-well U-shaped untreated polystyrene plates were incubated for 16–20 h at 37 °C and the MIC was determined as the lowest concentration of compound that prevented visible growth. During the essays, ceftazidime hidrate (CAZ, Sigma-Aldrich, St. Louis, MO, USA) and kanamycin monosulfate (KAN, Duchefa Biochemie, Haarlem, The Netherlands) were used as positive control of *S. aureus* ATCC 29213 and *E. faecalis* ATCC 29212, respectively. The minimal bactericidal concentration (MBC) was determined by spreading 10 µL of the content of the wells with no visible growth on MH plates. The MBC was determined as the lowest concentration of compound at which no colonies grew after overnight incubation at 37 °C [33]. At least three independent assays were conducted for reference and multidrug-resistant strains.

3.5.3. Antibiotic Synergy Testing

To evaluate the combined effect of the compounds tested with clinically relevant antibacterial drugs, the Kirby–Bauer method was used, as previously described [34]. A set of antibiotic disks (Oxoid, Basingstoke, UK), to which the isolates were resistant, was selected: cefotaxime (CTX, 30 µg) for *E. coli* SA/2, vancomycin (VAN, 30 µg) for *E. faecalis* B3/101, and oxacillin (OXA, 1 µg) for *S. aureus* 66/1. Antibiotic disks impregnated with 15 µg of each compound were placed on seeded MH plates. The controls used included antibiotic disks alone, blank paper disks impregnated with 15 µg of each compound alone, and blank disks impregnated with DMSO. Plates with CTX were incubated for 18–20 h and plates with VAN and OXA were incubated for 24 h at 37 °C [30]. Potential synergy was considered when the inhibition halo of an antibiotic disk impregnated with compound was greater than the inhibition halo of the antibiotic or compound-impregnated blank disk alone.

The combined effect of the compounds and clinically relevant antimicrobial drugs was also evaluated by determining the antibiotic MIC in the presence of each compound. Briefly, when it was not possible to determine an MIC value for the test compound, the MIC of CTX (Duchefa Biochemie, Haarlem, The Netherlands), VAN (Oxoid, Basingstoke, England), and OXA (Sigma-Aldrich, St. Louis, MO, USA) for the respective multidrug-resistant strain was determined in the presence of the highest concentration of each compound tested in previous assays (64 µg/mL). The antibiotic tested was serially diluted, whereas the concentration of each compound was kept fixed. Antibiotic MICs were determined as described above. Potential synergy was considered when the antibiotic MIC was lower in the presence of compound [35]. Fractional inhibitory concentrations (FIC) were calculated as follows: FIC of compound = MIC of compound combined with antibiotic/MIC compound alone, and FIC antibiotic = MIC of antibiotic combined with compound/MIC of antibiotic alone. The FIC index (FICI) was calculated as the sum of each FIC and interpreted as follows: FICI $\leq$ 0.5, "synergy"; 0.5 < FICI $\leq$ 4, "no interaction"; 4 < FICI, "antagonism" [36].

3.5.4. Biofilm Formation Inhibition Assay

The antibiofilm activity of compounds was evaluated through quantification of total biomass, using the crystal violet method, as previously described [34,37]. Briefly, the highest concentration of compound tested in the MIC assay was added to bacterial suspensions of 1×10^6 CFU/mL prepared in unsupplemented Tryptone Soy broth (TSB, Biokar Diagnostics, Allone, Beauvais, France) or TSB supplemented with 1% (p/v) glucose (D-(+)-glucose anhydrous for molecular biology, PanReac AppliChem, Barcelona, Spain) for Gram-positive strains. When it was possible to determine a MIC, concentrations ranging from $2 \times$ MIC to $\frac{1}{4}$ MIC were tested, while keeping in-test concentrations of DMSO below 1%. When it was not possible to determine a MIC, the concentration tested was 64 µg/mL. Controls with appropriate concentration of DMSO, as well as a negative control (TSB or TSB+1% glucose alone), were included. Sterile 96-well flat-bottomed untreated polystyrene microtiter plates were used. After a 24 h incubation at 37 °C, the biofilms were heat-fixed for 1 h at 60 °C and stained with 0.5% (v/v) crystal violet (Química Clínica Aplicada, Amposta, Spain) for 5 min. The stain was resolubilized with 33% (v/v) acetic acid (acetic acid 100%, AppliChem, Darmstadt, Germany) and the biofilm biomass was quantified by measuring the absorbance of each sample at 570 nm in a microplate reader (Thermo Scientific Multiskan® FC, Thermo Fisher Scientific, Waltham, MA, USA). The background absorbance (TSB or TSB+1% glucose without inoculum) was subtracted from the absorbance of each sample and the data are presented as percentage of control. Three independent assays were performed for reference strains, with triplicates for each experimental condition.

3.5.5. Biofilm Viability Assay

Considering the antibiofilm potential of **6**, the metabolic activity of *S. aureus* ATCC 29213 biofilm in presence of **6** at a concentration of 64 µg/mL was assessed using MTT (3-(4,5-dimethylthiazol-2-yl)-2,5-diphenyltetrazolium bromide) assay, as described previously [38,39]. Static biofilm was grown by inoculating 1×10^6 CFU/mL bacteria in sterile 96-well flat-bottomed untreated polystyrene microtiter plates containing TSB supplemented with 1% (w/v) glucose with a positive and a negative controls. After 8 h and 24 h of incubation at 37 °C, non-adherent cells were removed and 100 µL of MTT (5 mg/mL) (Thiazolyl Blue tetrazolium bromide 98%, Alfa Aesar, Kandel, Germany) was added to each well for 2 h at 37 °C. Thereafter, a solubilization solution (16% (w/v) of sodium dodecyl sulfate (SDS for molecular biology, PanReac AppliChem, Barcelona, Spain) and 50% DMSO (v/v) were added to dissolve the formazan product into a colored solution. After overnight dissolution at room temperature, biofilm viability was estimated by measuring absorbance of each sample at 570 nm in a microplate reader (Thermo Scientific Multiskan® FC, Thermo Fisher Scientific, Waltham, MA, USA). Biofilm viability was expressed as percentage of control and at least two different experiments were performed in triplicate.

3.5.6. Biofilm Matrix Visualization

To visualize the extracellular polymeric substances (EPS) matrix of the biofilms, rhodamine-labeled concanavalin A (rhodamine-conA) (Vector Laboratories, Burlingame, CA, USA), which specifically binds to D-(+)-glucose and D-(+)-mannose residues on exopolysaccharide (EPS), was used, as previously described [40]. Interaction between **6** at a concentration of 64 µg/mL and the biofilm of *S. aureus* ATCC 29213 was selected for rhodamine-conA staining, as a consequence of its antibiofilm potential. Briefly, bacterial suspensions of 1×10^6 CFU/mL prepared in TSB supplemented with 1% (w/v) glucose was added to a sterile well chamber (Ibidi, Gräfelfing, Germany). After 8 h of incubation, non-adherent cells were removed from each well and washed with 200 µL of PBS. Then, 100 µL of a rhodamine-conA (10 mg/mL) solution was added to the biofilm for 30 min in the dark at room temperature. Thereafter, the biofilm was washed with 200 µL of PBS and microscopic visualization, using an excitation of 514 nm and an emission wavelength of 600 ± 50 nm.

3.6. Acetylcholinesterase Inhibitory Activity Assay

AChE inhibitory assay was performed according to the Ellman's method [22]. Briefly, 20 µL of 0.22 U/mL AChE in tris buffer (50 mM, pH 8.0) from *Electrophorus electricus* (EC 3.1.1.7, Sigma-Aldrich, St. Louis, MO, USA) was added to the wells containing 10 µL of tested compounds (80 µM in DMSO), 100 µL of 3 mM of 5,5′-dithio-bis-(2-nitrobenzoic acid) (DTNB, Sigma-Aldrich, St. Louis, MO, USA) (in 50 mM tris buffer, pH 8.0), 20 µL of 15 mM acetylthiocholine iodide (Sigma-Aldrich, St. Louis, MO, USA) (in 50 mM tris buffer, pH 8.0), and 100 µL of 50 mM tris buffer (pH 8.0). Absorbance of the colored-end product was measured at 412 nm for 5 min, with 30 s intervals (BioTek Synergy™ HT Microplate Reader, Winooski, VT, USA). Controls containing 10 µL of DMSO instead of the tested compounds and reaction blanks containing 20 µL of buffer (0.1% (w/v) bovine serum albumin in 50 mM Tris-HCl) instead of the enzyme and 10 µL of DMSO instead of the tested compounds were made. In this assay, sample blanks containing 20 µL of buffer (0.1% (w/v) bovine serum albumin in 50 mM Tris-HCl) instead of AChE were also performed. The percentage of enzymatic inhibition was calculated as:

$$\text{Percentage inhibition} = 100 - [(S - So)/(C - Co)] \times 100$$

where C is the absorbance of the control, Co is the absorbance of reaction blank, S is the absorbance in the presence of the tested compounds, and So is the absorbance of sample blanks. All experiments were done in triplicate and galantamine (Sigma-Aldrich, St. Louis, MO, USA), tested at concentrations of 80, 10, 5, and 3.6 µM in DMSO, was used as a positive control as well as for validating the method. The inhibitory activities of the tested compounds toward AChE were expressed as percentage of inhibition as indicated previously. The IC_{50} value of galantamine was obtained by interpolation from a linear regression analysis.

3.7. Tyrosinase Inhibitory Activity Assay

Tyrosinase inhibitory assay was performed according to the method previously described [23]. Briefly, 20 µL of the mushroom tyrosinase (EC 1.14.18.1, Sigma-Aldrich, St. Louis, MO, USA, 480 U/mL) in 20 mM phosphate buffer was added to the wells containing 20 µL of the tested compounds (200 µM in DMSO), and 140 µL of 20 mM phosphate buffer (pH 6.8). After incubation at 25 °C for 10 min, 20 µL of 0.85 mM L-DOPA (Sigma-Aldrich, St. Louis, MO, USA) in phosphate buffer (pH 6.8) was added and the absorbance of the colored-end product was measured at 25 °C, 11 times for 10 min., with 1 min. intervals at 475 nm (BioTek Synergy™ HT Microplate Reader, Winooski, VT USA). Controls containing 20 µL of DMSO instead of the tested compounds, and reaction blanks containing 20 µL of 20 mM phosphate buffer (pH 6.8) instead of tyrosinase, and 20 µL of DMSO instead of the tested compounds were performed. Moreover, sample blanks containing 20 µL of 20 mM phosphate buffer (pH 6.8) instead of tyrosinase were made. The percentage inhibition of tyrosinase activity was calculated as:

$$\text{Percentage inhibition} = 100 \times [1 - (S - So)/(C - Co)]$$

where S is the absorbance in presence of the tested compounds, So is the absorbance of sample blanks, C is the absorbance of the control, and Co is the absorbance of reaction blank. All experiments are done in triplicate and kojic acid (Sigma-Aldrich, Saint Louis, MO, USA) at concentrations of 200, 100, 25, 12.5, 8 and 5 µM was used as a positive control. The inhibitory activities of the compounds towards tyrosinase were expressed as per-centage of inhibition as indicated previously. The IC50 value of kojic acid was obtained by interpolation from a linear regression analysis.

3.8. Statistical Analysis

Data were reported as means ± standard error of the mean (SEM) of at least three independent experiments. Statistical analysis of the results was performed with GraphPad Prism (GraphPad Software, San Diego, CA, USA). Unpaired *t*-test was carried out to test for any significant differences between the means. Differences at the 5% confidence level were considered significant.

4. Conclusions

The EtOAc extract from a solid culture of a marine-derived fungus *Neosartorya spinosa* KUFA1047, isolated from a marine sponge *Mycale* sp. collected in the Gulf of Thailand, furnished five previously reported secondary metabolites *viz*. (*R*)-6-hydroxymellein (**1**), penipurdin A (**2**), acetylquestinol (**3**), tenellic acid C (**5**) and vermixocin A (**8**), in addition to three previously unreported compounds, including acetylpenipurdin A (**4**), neospinosic acid (**6**), and spinolactone (**7**). All the isolated compounds, except **1**, were assayed for in vitro anticholinesterase and anti-tyrosinase activities. Although none of the test compounds exhibited anticholinesterase activity, **2**, **5**, and **7** exhibited weak anti-tyrosinase activity, while **8** showed moderate inhibitory activity against a mushroom tyrosinase. Compounds **2** and **5–8** were also assayed for their antibacterial activity against several reference bacterial species and multidrug-resistant isolates; however, only **7** exhibited antibacterial activity against *Enterococcus faecalis* B3/101 with a MIC value of 64 µg/mL. Since the MBC was more than one-fold higher than the MIC, **7** was suggested to exert a bacteriostatic effect. Interestingly, although **5** and **6** did not exhibit antibacterial activity, they were able to significantly inhibit biofilm formation in three of the four reference strains used in this study. While both **5** and **6** inhibited biofilm formation in *Escherichia coli* ATCC 25922 and *Staphylococcus aureus* ATCC 29213, only **5** inhibited biofilm formation in *E. faecalis* ATCC 29212. Interestingly, **6** exerts more extensive effect, displaying the strongest inhibitory activity in *S. aureus* ATCC 29213. In summary, secondary metabolites isolated from this marine-derived fungus are more preponderant in antibacterial and antibiofilm activities than anticholinesterase activity.

Supplementary Materials: The following are available online at https://www.mdpi.com/article/10.3390/md19080457/s1: Figures S1–S5, S7–S11, S13–S17, S20–S24, S26–S30, S32–S36, and S38–S42: 1D and 2D NMR spectra of compounds **1–8**. Figures S6, S12, S18, S19, S25, S31, S37, and 43: HRMS data for compounds **1–8**. Table S1: ^{1}H and ^{13}C NMR (DMSO-d_6, 300 and 75 MHz) and HMBC assignment for **1**; Table S2. ^{1}H and ^{13}C NMR (DMSO-d_6, 300 and 75 MHz) and HMBC assignment for **2**; Table S3. ^{1}H and ^{13}C NMR (DMSO-d_6, 500 and 125 MHz) and HMBC assignment for **3**; Table S4. ^{1}H and ^{13}C NMR (300 and 75 MHz, DMSO-d_6) and HMBC assignment of **5**; Table S5. ^{1}H and ^{13}C NMR (300 and 75 MHz, CDCl$_3$) and HMBC assignment of **8**.

Author Contributions: A.K. and M.E.S. conceived and designed the experiment and elaborated the manuscript; J.D.M.d.S. performed isolation, purification, and part of structure elucidation of the compounds; T.D. collected, isolated, identified, and cultured the fungus; J.A.P. performed calculations and measurement of ECD spectra and interpretation of the results; H.C. designed and interpreted the result of anticholinesterase and anti-tyrosinase assays; I.C.R. and P.M.C. performed antibacterial and antibiofilm assays; S.M. provided HRMS; A.M.S.S. provided NMR spectra. All authors have read and agreed to the published version of the manuscript.

Funding: This work was funded by the structured program of R&D&I ATLANTIDA—Platform for the monitoring of the North Atlantic Ocean and tools for the sustainable exploitation of the marine resources (reference NORTE-01-0145-FEDER-000040), supported by the North Portugal Regional Operational Programme (NORTE2020), through the European Regional Development Fund (ERDF).

Institutional Review Board Statement: Not applicable.

Informed Consent Statement: Not applicable.

Acknowledgments: We thank Sara Cravo for technical assistance for anticholinesterase and antityrosinase assays. The authors acknowledge the support of the Biochemical and Biophysical Technologies i3S Scientific Platform with the assistance of Frederico Silva and Maria de Fátima Fonseca for the access of Jasco J-815 CD spectropolarimeter.

Conflicts of Interest: The authors declare no conflict of interest.

References

1. Brakhage, A.A. Regulation of fungal secondary metabolism. *Nat. Ver. Microbiol.* **2013**, *11*, 21–32. [CrossRef]
2. Beekman, A.M.; Barrow, R.A. Fungal Metabolites as Pharmaceuticals. *Aust. J. Chem.* **2014**, *67*, 827–843. [CrossRef]
3. Bugni, T.S.; Ireland, C.M. Marine-derived fungi: A chemically and biologically diverse group of microorganisms. *Nat. Prod. Rep.* **2004**, *21*, 143–163. [CrossRef] [PubMed]
4. Prompanya, C.; Fernandes, C.; Cravo, S.; Pinto, M.M.M.; Dethoup, T.; Silva, A.M.S.; Kijjoa, A. A new cyclic hexapeptide and a new isocoumarin derivative from the marine sponge-associated fungus *Aspergillus similanensis* KUFA 0013. *Mar. Drugs.* **2015**, *13*, 1432–1450. [CrossRef]
5. May Zin, W.W.; Prompanya, C.; Buttachon, S.; Kijjoa, A. Bioactive secondary metabolites from a Thai collection of soil and marine-derived fungi of the genera *Neosartorya* and *Aspergillus*. *Curr. Drug Deliv.* **2016**, *13*, 378–388. [CrossRef]
6. Kumla, D.; Aung, T.S.; Buttachon, S.; Dethoup, T.; Gales, L.; Pereira, J.A.; Inácio, Â.; Costa, P.M.; Lee, M.; Sekeroglu, N.; et al. A New Dihydrochromone Dimer and Other Secondary Metabolites from Cultures of the Marine Sponge-Associated Fungi *Neosartorya fennelliae* KUFA 0811 and *Neosartorya tsunodae* KUFC 9213. *Mar. Drugs* **2017**, *15*, 375. [CrossRef] [PubMed]
7. Lucinda, J.; Bessa, L.J.; Buttachon, S.; Dethoup, T.; Martins, R.; Vasconcelos, V.; Kijjoa, A.; Costa, P.M. Neofiscalin A and fiscalin C are potential novel indole alkaloid alternatives for the treatment of multidrug resistant Gram-positive bacterial infections. *FEMS Microbiol. Lett.* **2016**, *363*, fnw150. [CrossRef]
8. Rajachan, O.-T.; Kanokmedhakul, K.; Sanmanoch, W.; Boonlue, S.; Hannongbua, S.; Saparpakorn, P.; Kanokmedhakul, S. Chevalone C analogues and globoscinic acid derivatives from the fungus *Neosartorya spinosa* KKU-1NK1. *Phytochemistry* **2016**, *132*, 68–75. [CrossRef] [PubMed]
9. May Zin, W.W.; Buttachon, S.; Buaruang, J.; Gale, L.; Pereira, J.A.; Pinto, M.M.M.; Silva, A.M.S.; Kijjoa, A. A new meroditerpene and a new tryptoquivaline analog from the algicolous fungus *Neosartorya takakii* KUFC 7898. *Mar. Drugs* **2015**, *13*, 3776–3790. [CrossRef] [PubMed]
10. Islam, M.S.; Ishigami, K.; Watanabe, H. Synthesis of (−)-mellein, (+)-ramulosin, and related natural products. *Tetrahedron* **2007**, *63*, 1074–1079. [CrossRef]
11. Xue, J.; Fu, Y.; Wu, P.; Xu, L.; Huang, R.; Wei, X.; Li, H. Two new anthraquinones from the soil fungus *Penicillium purpurigenum* SC0070. *J. Antibiot.* **2015**, *68*, 598–599. [CrossRef]
12. May Zin, W.W.; Buttachon, S.; Dethoup, T.; Pereira, J.A.; Gales, L.; Inácio, Â.; Paulo, M.; Costa, P.M.; Lee, M.; Sekeroglu, N.; et al. Antibacterial and antibiofilm activities of the metabolites isolated from the culture of the mangrove-derived endophytic fungus *Eurotium chevalieri* KUFA0006. *Phytochemistry* **2017**, *141*, 86–97. [CrossRef]
13. Oh, H.; Kwon, T.O.; Gloer, J.B.; Marvanová, L.; Shearer, S.A. Tenellic Acids A-D: New Bioactive Diphenyl Ether Derivatives from the Aquatic Fungus *Dendrospora tenella*. *J. Nat. Prod.* **1999**, *62*, 580–583. [CrossRef] [PubMed]
14. Proksa, B.; Uhrín, D.; Adamcová, J.; Fuska, J. Vermixocins A and B, two novel metabolites from *Penicillium vermiculatum*. *J. Antibiot.* **1992**, *45*, 1268–1272. [CrossRef]
15. Suzuki, K.; Nozawa, K.; Udagawa, S.; Nakajima, S.; Kawai, K. Penicillide and dehydroisopenicillide from *Talaromyces derxii*. *Phytochemistry* **1991**, *30*, 2096–2098. [CrossRef]
16. Daengrot, C.; Rukachaisirikul, V.; Tadpetch, K.; Phongpaichit, S.; Bowornwiriyapan, K.; Sakayarojc, J.; Shend, X. Penicillanthone and penicillidic acids A-C from the soil-derived fungus *Penicillium aculeatum* PSU-RSPG105. *RSC Adv.* **2016**, *6*, 39700. [CrossRef]
17. Singh, A.J.; Gorka, A.P.; Bokesch, H.R.; Wamiru, A.; O'Keefe, B.R.; Schnermann, M.J.; Gustafson, K.R. Harnessing natural product diversity for fluorophore discovery: Naturally occurring fFluorescent hydroxyanthraquinones from the marine crinoid *Pterometra venusta*. *J. Nat. Prod.* **2018**, *81*, 2750–2755. [CrossRef]
18. Nishida, H.; Tomoda, H.; Cao, J.; Okuda, S.; Omura, S. Purpactins, new inhibitors of acyl-CoA: Cholesterol acyltransferase produced by *Penicillium purpurogenum* II. Structure elucidation of purpactins A, B, C. *J. Antibiot.* **1991**, *44*, 144–151. [CrossRef]
19. Chen, M.; Han, L.; Shao, C.-L.; She, Z.-G.; Wang, C.-Y. Bioactive diphenyl ether derivatives from a gorgonian-derived fungus *Talaromyces* sp. *Chem. Biodivers.* **2015**, *12*, 443–450. [CrossRef]
20. Davey, M.E.; Caiazza, N.C.; O'Toole, G.A. Rhamnolipid surfactant production affects biofilm architecture in *Pseudomonas aeruginosa* PAO1. *J. Bacteriol.* **2003**, *185*, 1027–1036. [CrossRef]
21. Periasamy, S.; Joo, H.-S.; Duong, A.C.; Bach, T.-H.L.; Tan, V.Y.; Chatterjee, S.S.; Cheung, G.Y.C.; Otto, M. How *Staphylococcus aureus* biofilms develop their characteristic structure. *Proc. Natl. Acad. Sci. USA* **2012**, *109*, 1281–1286. [CrossRef]
22. Ellman, G.L.; Courtney, K.D.; Andres, V., Jr.; Featherstone, R.M. A new and rapid colorimetric determination of acetylcholinesterase activity. *Biochem. Pharmacol.* **1961**, *7*, 88–90. [CrossRef]
23. Likhitwitayawuid, K.; Sritularak, B. A new dimeric stilbene with tyrosinase inhibitiory activity from *Artocarpus gomezianus*. *J. Nat. Prod.* **2001**, *64*, 1457–1459. [CrossRef]

24. Murray, M.G.; Thompson, W.F. Rapid isolation of high molecular weight plant DNA. *Nucleic Acids Res.* **1980**, *8*, 4321–4325. [CrossRef]
25. White, T.J.; Bruns, T.; Lee, S.; Taylor, J. Amplification and direct sequencing of fungal ribosomal RNA genes for phylogenetics. In *PCR Protocols: A Guide to Methods and Applications*; Innis, M.A., Gelfand, D.H., Sninsky, J.J., White, T.J., Eds.; Academic Press: New York, NY, USA, 1990; pp. 315–322.
26. Sanger, F.; Nicklen, S.; Coulson, A.R. DNA sequencing with chain-terminating inhibitors. *Proc. Natl. Acad. Sci. USA* **1977**, *72*, 5463–5467. [CrossRef] [PubMed]
27. Stephens, P.J.; Harada, N. ECD Cotton effect approximated by the Gaussian curve and other methods. *Chirality* **2010**, *22*, 229–233. [CrossRef]
28. Simões, R.R.; Aires-de-Sousa, M.; Conceição, T.; Antunes, F.; da Costa, P.M.; de Lencastre, H. High prevalence of EMRSA-15 in Portuguese public buses: A worrisome finding. *PLoS ONE* **2011**, *6*, e17630. [CrossRef] [PubMed]
29. Bessa, L.J.; Barbosa-Vasconcelos, A.; Mendes, Â.; Vaz-Pires, P.; Da Costa, P.M. High prevalence of multidrug-resistant *Escherichia coli* and *Enterococcus* spp. in river water, upstream and downstream of a wastewater treatment plant. *J. Water Health* **2014**, *12*, 426–435. [CrossRef] [PubMed]
30. CLSI. *Performance Standards for Antimicrobial Susceptibility Testing*, 27th ed.; CLSI supplement M100; Clinical and Laboratory Standards Institute: Wayne, PA, USA, 2017.
31. CLSI. *Performance Standards for Antimicrobial Susceptibility Testing*, 11th ed.; CLSI document M02-A11; Clinical and Laboratory Standards Institute: Wayne, PA, USA, 2012.
32. CLSI. *Methods for Dilution Antimicrobial Susceptibility Tests for Bacteria That Grow Aerobically*, 10th ed.; CLSI document M07-A10; Clinical and Laboratory Standards Institute: Wayne, PA, USA, 2015.
33. CLSI. *Methods for Determining Bactericidal Activity of Antimicrobial Agents*; Approved Guideline, CLSI Document M26-A; Clinical and Laboratory Standards Institute: Wayne, PA, USA, 1999.
34. Kumla, D.; Dethoup, T.; Gales, L.; Pereira, J.A.; Freitas-Silva, J.; Costa, P.M.; Silva, A.; Pinto, M.M.; Kijjoa, A. Erubescensoic Acid, a new polyketide and a xanthonopyrone SPF-3059-26 from the culture of the marine sponge-associated fungus *Penicillium erubescens* KUFA 0220 and antibacterial activity evaluation of some of its constituents. *Molecules* **2019**, *24*, 208. [CrossRef]
35. Buttachon, S.; Ramos, A.A.; Inácio, Â.; Dethoup, T.; Gales, L.; Lee, M.; Costa, P.M.; Silva, A.M.S.; Sekeroglu, N.; Rocha, E.; et al. Bis-indolyl benzenoids, hydroxypyrrolidine derivatives and other constituents from cultures of the marine sponge-associated fungus *Aspergillus candidus* KUFA0062. *Mar. Drugs* **2018**, *16*, 119. [CrossRef] [PubMed]
36. Odds, F.C. Synergy, antagonism, and what the chequer board puts between them. *J. Antimicrob. Chemother.* **2003**, *52*, 1. [CrossRef]
37. Stepanović, S.; Vuković, D.; Hola, V.; Di Bonaventura, G.; Djuki'c, S.; Cirković, I.; Ruzicka, F. Quantification of biofilm in microtiter plates: Overview of testing conditions and practical recommendations for assessment of biofilm production by staphylococci. *Apmis* **2007**, *115*, 891–899. [CrossRef] [PubMed]
38. Grela, E.; Kozłowska, J.; Grabowiecka, A. Current methodology of MTT assay in bacteria—A review. *Acta Histochem.* **2018**, *120*, 303–311. [CrossRef] [PubMed]
39. Riss, T.L.; Moravec, R.A.; Niles, A.L.; Duellman, S.; Benink, H.A.; Worzella, T.J.; Minor, L. Cell viability assays. In *The Assay Guidance Manual [Internet]*; Markossian, S., Grossman, A., Brimacombe, K., Arkin, M., Auld, D., Austin, C.P., Baell, J., Chung, T.D.Y., Coussens, N.P., Dahlin, J.L., et al., Eds.; Eli Lilly & Company and the National Center for Advancing Translational Sciences: Bethesda, MD, USA, 2004; 1 May 2013; Last Update: 1 July 2016. Available online: https://www.ncbi.nlm.nih.gov/books/NBK144065/ (accessed on 17 June 2021).
40. Bessa, L.J.; Grande, R.; Di Iorio, D.; Di Giulio, M.; Di Campli, E.; Cellini, L. *Helicobacter pylori* free-living and biofilm modes of growth: Behavior in response to different culture media. *Apmis* **2013**, *121*, 149–160. [CrossRef] [PubMed]

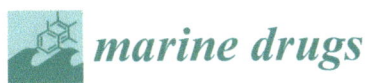

Review

Structures and Biological Activities of Diketopiperazines from Marine Organisms: A Review

Zhiqiang Song, Yage Hou, Qingrong Yang, Xinpeng Li and Shaohua Wu *

State Key Laboratory for Conservation and Utilization of Bio-Resources in Yunnan, Key Laboratory for Southwest Microbial Diversity of the Ministry of Education, School of Life Sciences, Yunnan Institute of Microbiology, Yunnan University, Kunming 650091, China; songzhiqiang@mail.ynu.edu.cn (Z.S.); houyage@126.com (Y.H.); yangqingrong132@163.com (Q.Y.); lixinpeng10086@126.com (X.L.)
* Correspondence: shhwu@ynu.edu.cn

Abstract: Diketopiperazines are potential structures with extensive biological functions, which have attracted much attention of natural product researchers for a long time. These compounds possess a stable six-membered ring, which is an important pharmacophore. The marine organisms have especially been proven to be a wide source for discovering diketopiperazine derivatives. In recent years, more and more interesting bioactive diketopiperazines had been found from various marine habitats. This review article is focused on the new 2,5-diketopiperazines derived from marine organisms (sponges and microorganisms) reported from the secondary half-year of 2014 to the first half of the year of 2021. We will comment their chemical structures, biological activities and sources. The objective is to assess the merit of these compounds for further study in the field of drug discovery.

Keywords: natural products; chemical structures; diketopiperazines; biological activities

Citation: Song, Z.; Hou, Y.; Yang, Q.; Li, X.; Wu, S. Structures and Biological Activities of Diketopiperazines from Marine Organisms: A Review. *Mar. Drugs* **2021**, *19*, 403. https://doi.org/10.3390/md19080403

Academic Editors: RuAngelie Edrada-Ebel, Chang-Yun Wang and Bin-Gui Wang

Received: 6 July 2021
Accepted: 18 July 2021
Published: 21 July 2021

Publisher's Note: MDPI stays neutral with regard to jurisdictional claims in published maps and institutional affiliations.

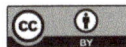

Copyright: © 2021 by the authors. Licensee MDPI, Basel, Switzerland. This article is an open access article distributed under the terms and conditions of the Creative Commons Attribution (CC BY) license (https://creativecommons.org/licenses/by/4.0/).

1. Introduction

The 2,5-diketopiperazines (DKPs), the smallest cyclic dipeptides from the double condensations of two α-amino acids, are abundant in nature and possess a six-membered piperazine rigid backbone [1,2]. The formation of two peptide bonds in DKPs are catalyzed by two major enzymes, the nonribosomal peptide synthetases (NRPSs, >100 kDa) and cyclodipeptide synthases (CDPSs, 30 kDa) [3]. These three-dimensional molecular skeletons carry different substituents, which overcome the planar limitations of most conventional drugs and play an important role in drug discovery [4]. Recently, the interest in DKPs is still high because they have not only antimicrobial, antitumor and antiviral activities [5], but also a relatively rare treatment of ischemic brain injury [6], quorum-sensing signaling [7,8], anti-Alzheimer [9], inhibition of microtubule polymerization [10] and haemosuppressor activity [11].

Bicyclomycin is a classic DKP antibiotic that has been used to treat diarrhea in humans and bacterial diarrhea in calves and pigs and it is also a rho (a member of the RecA-type ATPase) inhibitor [12–14]. Chaetocin is a specific DKP dimer containing sulfurs as the first inhibitor of a lysine-specific histone methyltransferase SU(VAR)3-9, which could reduce the H3 isoform trimethylated at the Lys9 (H3K9me3) level and this compound has also been reported to have potent antimyeloma activity [15–17]. Recently, chaetocin is proved to be able to increase the efficiency of the efficient epigenetic reprogramming via reducing the aberrant level of H3K9me3 to enhance the developmental competence of porcine somatic cell nuclear transfer embryos. It promotes osteogenic differentiation in mesenchymal stem cells [16,18,19]. Plinabulin (formerly named as NPI-2358), a marine-derived DKP, is currently in a phase 3 trial in combination with docetaxel in non-small cell lung cancer (NCT02504489) [20–22]. In addition, some DKPs possess an ability to cross the blood–brain barrier via a passive diffusion process as an ideal candidate for new therapeutic agents for brain diseases [23,24]. As of August 2012, there are approximately 150 global patents related to DKPs and its derivatives, and DKPs are present in nearly 50 bio-complexes in the Research Collaboratory for the Structural Bioinformatics Protein Data Bank [25,26]. DKPs are diamonds in the rough and have huge potential in future therapies.

There have been several reviews reported on DKPs until now. Cao et al. summarized chemical diversity and the biological function of indolediketopiperazines from marine-derived fungi [27]. Gomes et al. summed up marine-derived DKP dimers with their structures and biological activity [28]. From 1972 to the first half of the year of 2014, 214 DKPs from marine sources have been reported [5,29]. However, there is no relevant review for summarizing the comprehensive DKPs from a marine source from 2014 to now. On this basis, we now summarize a total of 241 marine-derived DKPs from the second half of 2014 to the first half of 2021 in this paper. In addition, a total of 55 marine-derived variable DKP derivatives from 2011 to the first half of 2021 are also summarized here.

2. Chemical Structures of Diketopiperazines from Marine Organisms

The 241 DKPs from different sources including sponges, bacteria, actinomycetes and fungi are shown in Table 1.

Table 1. The bioactivities, sources and habitats of DKPs during 2014–2021.

Sources	Compounds	Bioactivities	Species	Habitats	Refs
Sponge	Cyclo-(R-Pro-6-hydroxyl-S-Ile) (1)	- [a]	Callyspongia sp.	South China Sea	[30]
	Geobarrettin A (2)	-	G. barrette	Iceland	[31]
	Geobarrettin B (3)	Anti-inflammatory	G. barrette	Iceland	[32]
	Tedanizaine A (4)	-	Tedania sp.	Guangdong	[32]
	(−)-Cyclo(L-trans-Hyp-L-Ile) (5)	-	A. sinoxea	Larak Island	[33]
Bacteria	Cyclo(Trp-Ser) (6)	Antimicrobial Antiquorum sensing	R. aquimaris QSI02	Yellow Sea	[34]
	Cyclo(Pro-Val) (7)	-	G. antarctica PI12	Antarctica	[35]
	(−)-Cyclo(Pro-Tyr) (8)	-	G. antarctica PI12	Antarctica	[35]
	(−)-Cyclo(Pro-Phe) (9)	-	G. antarctica PI12	Antarctica	[35]
	(+)-Cyclo(Pro-Leu) (10)	-	G. antarctica PI12	Antarctica	[35]
	(3S,6S)-3,6-Diisobutylpiperazine-2,5-dione (11)	Antimicrobial	Bacillus sp. SPB7	S. officinalis	[36]
	Gallaecimonamide A (12)	Antimicrobial	G. mangrovi HK-28	Mangrove sediment	[37]
	Gallaecimonamide A (13)	-	G. mangrovi HK-28	Mangrove sediment	[37]
	Gallaecimonamide A (14)	-	G. mangrovi HK-28	Mangrove sediment	[37]
	cis-Cyclo(Pro-3-chloro-Tyr) (15)	-	B. subtilis BI0980	Kerkyra and Erikoussa	[38]
	trans-Cyclo(Pro-3-chloro-Tyr) (16)	-	B. subtilis BI0980	Kerkyra and Erikoussa	[38]
	cis-Cyclo(3-chloro-Tyr-Ile) (17)	-	B. subtilis BI0980	Kerkyra and Erikoussa	[38]
Actinomycetes	iso-Naseseazine B (18)	Antimicrobial	Streptomyces sp. SMA-1	Yellow Sea	[39]
	Naseseazine A (19)	Antiplasmodial	Streptomyces sp. USC-636	Marine sediment	[40]
	Naseseazine B (20)	Antiplasmodial	Streptomyces sp. USC-636	Marine sediment	[40]
	Naseseazine C (21)	Antiplasmodial	Streptomyces sp. USC-636	Marine sediment	[40]
	(6R,3Z)-3-Benzylidene-6-isobutyl-1-methyl piperazine-2,5-dione (22)	-	Streptomyces sp. strain SCSIO 04496	South China Sea	[41]

Table 1. Cont.

Sources	Compounds	Bioactivities	Species	Habitats	Refs
	Demethylmaremycins (23–28)	-	*Streptomyces* sp. B9173	Pacific coast	[42]
	3-(3-Hydroxy-4-methoxybenzyl)-6-isobutyl-2,5-diketopiperazine (29)	Cytotoxicity	*Streptomyces* sp. MNU FJ-36	*Katsuwonus* sp.	[43]
	3-(1,3-Benzodioxol-5-ylmethyl)-6-isobutyl-2,5-diketopiperazine (30)	Cytotoxicity	*Streptomyces* sp. MNU FJ-36	*Katsuwonus* sp.	[43]
	3-(1,3-Benzodioxol-5-ylmethyl)-6-isopropyl-2,5-diketopiperazine (31)	Cytotoxicity	*Streptomyces* sp. MNU FJ-36	*Katsuwonus* sp.	[43]
	maculosin-*O*-α-L-rhamnopyranoside (32)	Antimicrobial	*Streptomyces* sp. ZZ446	Coastal soil	[44, 45]
	Actinozine A (33)	Antimicrobial Cytotoxicity	*Streptomyces* species Call-36	*Callyspongia* species	[46]
	Streptodiketopiperazine A (34)	Antimicrobial	*Streptomyces* sp. SY1965	Mariana Trench sediment	[47]
	Streptodiketopiperazine A (35)	Antimicrobial	*Streptomyces* sp. SY1965	Mariana Trench sediment	[47]
	Cyclo-(4-*trans*-6-dihydroxy-proline-D-leucine) (36)	-	*M. variabilis* C-03	*Palythoa tuberculosa*	[48]
	Nocarazepine A (37)	-	*A. caerulea*	*Anthogorgia caerulea*	[49]
	Photopiperazine A (38)	Cytotoxicity	Strain AJS-327	Sponge fragment	[50]
	Photopiperazine B (39)	Cytotoxicity	Strain AJS-327	Sponge fragment	[50]
	Photopiperazine C (40)	Cytotoxicity	Strain AJS-327	Sponge fragment	[50]
	Photopiperazine D (41)	Cytotoxicity	Strain AJS-327	Sponge fragment	[50]
	Cyclo-(D-8-acetoxyl-Pro-L-Leu) (42)	Pancreatic lipase enzyme inhibition	*Treptomyces* sp. SCSIO 41400	Mangrove derived-soil	[51]
Fungus	Graphiumin A (43)	-	*Graphium* sp. OPMF00224	Sediment	[52]
	Graphiumin B (44)	-	*Graphium* sp. OPMF00224	Sediment	[52]
	Graphiumin C (45)	Virulence factors inhibitor	*Graphium* sp. OPMF00224	Sediment	[52]
	Graphiumin D (46)	Virulence factors inhibitor	*Graphium* sp. OPMF00224	Sediment	[52]
	Graphiumin E (47)	Virulence factors inhibitor	*Graphium* sp. OPMF00224	Sediment	[52]
	Graphiumin F (48)	-	*Graphium* sp. OPMF00224	Sediment	[52]
	Graphiumin G (49)	Virulence factors inhibitor	*Graphium* sp. OPMF00224	Sediment	[52]
	Graphiumin H (50)	Virulence factors inhibitor	*Graphium* sp. OPMF00224	Sediment	[52]
	Graphiumin I (51)	Virulence factors inhibitor	*Graphium* sp. OPMF00224	Sediment	[53]
	Graphiumin J (52)	Virulence factors inhibitor	*Graphium* sp. OPMF00224	Sediment	[53]
	Cladosporin A (53)	Cytotoxicity	*Cladosporium* sp.	Sediment	[54]
	Cladosporin B (54)	Cytotoxicity	*Cladosporium* sp.	Sediment	[54]

Table 1. Cont.

Sources	Compounds	Bioactivities	Species	Habitats	Refs
	12,13-Dihydroxy-fumitremorgin C (**55**)	-	*A. alternate* HK-25	Sediment	[55]
	Gliotoxin (**56**)	-	*A. alternate* HK-25	Sediment	[55]
	Demethoxyfumitremorgin C (**57**)	-	*A. alternate* HK-25	Sediment	[55]
	Bisdethiobis(methylthio)gliotoxin (**58**)	-	*A. alternate* HK-25	Sediment	[55]
	Fumitremorgin C (**59**)	-	*A. alternate* HK-25	Sediment	[55]
	Haenamindole (**60**)	Antiviral	*Penicillium* sp. KCB12F005	Sediment	[56]
	Dichotocejpin A (**61**)	Cytotoxicity α-glucosidase inhibitor	*D. cejpii* FS110	Sediment	[57, 58]
	Dichotocejpin B (**62**)	-	*D. cejpii* FS110	Sediment	[57, 58]
	Dichotocejpin C (**63**)	-	*D. cejpii* FS110	Sediment	[57, 58]
	Cristazine (**64**)	Antioxidant Cytotoxicity	*C. cristatum*	Sediment	[59, 60]
	Eutypellazine A (**65**)	Antiviral	*Eutypella* sp. MCCC 3A00281	Sediment	[61]
	Eutypellazine B (**66**)	Antiviral	*Eutypella* sp. MCCC 3A00281	Sediment	[61]
	Eutypellazine C (**67**)	Antiviral	*Eutypella* sp. MCCC 3A00281	Sediment	[61]
	Eutypellazine D (**68**)	Antiviral	*Eutypella* sp. MCCC 3A00281	Sediment	[61]
	Eutypellazine E (**69**)	Antiviral	*Eutypella* sp. MCCC 3A00281	Sediment	[61]
	Eutypellazine F (**70**)	Antiviral	*Eutypella* sp. MCCC 3A00281	Sediment	[61]
	Eutypellazine G (**71**)	Antiviral	*Eutypella* sp. MCCC 3A00281	Sediment	[61]
	Eutypellazine H (**72**)	Antiviral	*Eutypella* sp. MCCC 3A00281	Sediment	[61]
	Eutypellazine I (**73**)	Antiviral	*Eutypella* sp. MCCC 3A00281	Sediment	[61]
	Eutypellazine J (**74**)	Antiviral	*Eutypella* sp. MCCC 3A00281	Sediment	[61]
	Eutypellazine K (**75**)	Antiviral	*Eutypella* sp. MCCC 3A00281	Sediment	[61]
	Eutypellazine L (**76**)	Antiviral	*Eutypella* sp. MCCC 3A00281	Sediment	[61]
	Eutypellazine M (**77**)	-	*Eutypella* sp. MCCC 3A00281	Sediment	[61]
	Eutypellazine N (**78**)	-	*Eutypella* sp. MCCC 3A00281	Sediment	[62]
	Eutypellazine O (**79**)	-	*Eutypella* sp. MCCC 3A00281	Sediment	[62]
	Eutypellazine P (**80**)	-	*Eutypella* sp. MCCC 3A00281	Sediment	[62]
	Eutypellazine Q (**81**)	-	*Eutypella* sp. MCCC 3A00281	Sediment	[62]
	Eutypellazine R (**82**)	-	*Eutypella* sp. MCCC 3A00281	Sediment	[62]
	Eutypellazine S (**83**)	-	*Eutypella* sp. MCCC 3A00281	Sediment	[62]
	Fusaperazine F (**84**)	Cytotoxicity	*P. crustosum* HDN153086	Sediment	[63]

Table 1. Cont.

Sources	Compounds	Bioactivities	Species	Habitats	Refs
	Roquefortine J (**85**)	Cytotoxicity	*P. granulatum* MCCC 3A00475	Sediment	[64, 65]
	(+)-7,8-Epoxy-brevianamide Q (**86**)	-	*A. versicolor* MF180151	Sediment	[66]
	(−)-7,8-Epoxy-brevianamide Q (**87**)	-	*A. versicolor* MF180151	Sediment	[66]
	(+)-8-Hydroxy-brevianamide R (**88**)	-	*A. versicolor* MF180151	Sediment	[66]
	(−)-8-Hydroxy-brevianamide R (**89**)	-	*A. versicolor* MF180151	Sediment	[66]
	(+)-8-Epihydroxy-brevianamide R (**90**)	-	*A. versicolor* MF180151	Sediment	[66]
	(−)-8-Epihydroxy-brevianamide R (**91**)	-	*A. versicolor* MF180151	Sediment	[66]
	Raistrickindole A (**92**)	Antiviral	*P. raistrickii* IMB17-034	Sediment	[67]
	5′-Hydroxy-6′-ene-epicoccin G (**93**)	-	*E. nigrum* SD-388	Sediment	[68]
	7-Methoxy-7′-hydroxyepicoccin G (**94**)	-	*E. nigrum* SD-388	Sediment	[68]
	8′-Acetoxyepicoccin D (**95**)	-	*E. nigrum* SD-388	Sediment	[68]
	7′-Demethoxyrostratin C (**96**)	Cytotoxicity	*E. nigrum* SD-388	Sediment	[68]
	(+)-5-hydroxydiphenylalazine A (**97**)	-	*E. nigrum* SD-388	Sediment	[68]
	(−)-5-hydroxydiphenylalazine A (**98**)	-	*E. nigrum* SD-388	Sediment	[68]
	(+) Eurotinoid A (**99**)	Antioxidant	*Eurotium* sp. SCSIO F452	Sediment	[69]
	(−) Eurotinoid A (**100**)	Antioxidant	*Eurotium* sp. SCSIO F452	Sediment	[69]
	(+) Eurotinoid B (**101**)	Antioxidant	*Eurotium* sp. SCSIO F452	Sediment	[69]
	(−) Eurotinoid B (**102**)	Antioxidant	*Eurotium* sp. SCSIO F452	Sediment	[69]
	(+) Eurotinoid C (**103**)	Antioxidant	*Eurotium* sp. SCSIO F452	Sediment	[69]
	(−) Eurotinoid C (**104**)	Antioxidant	*Eurotium* sp. SCSIO F452	Sediment	[69]
	Versicamide A (**105**)	-	*A. versicolor* HDN08-60	Sediment	[70]
	Versicamide B (**106**)	-	*A. versicolor* HDN08-60	Sediment	[70]
	Versicamide C (**107**)	-	*A. versicolor* HDN08-60	Sediment	[70]
	Versicamide D (**108**)	-	*A. versicolor* HDN08-60	Sediment	[70]
	Versicamide E (**109**)	-	*A. versicolor* HDN08-60	Sediment	[70]
	Versicamide F (**110**)	-	*A. versicolor* HDN08-60	Sediment	[70]
	Versicamide G (**111**)	-	*A. versicolor* HDN08-60	Sediment	[70]
	Versicamide H (**112**)	Cytotoxicity	*A. versicolor* HDN08-60	Sediment	[70]
	Rubrumline A (**113**)	-	*E. rubrum*	Sediment	[71]
	Rubrumline B (**114**)	-	*E. rubrum*	Sediment	[71]
	Rubrumline C (**115**)	-	*E. rubrum*	Sediment	[71]
	Rubrumline D (**116**)	Antiviral	*E. rubrum*	Sediment	[71]
	Rubrumline E (**117**)	-	*E. rubrum*	Sediment	[71]
	Rubrumline F (**118**)	-	*E. rubrum*	Sediment	[71]
	Rubrumline G (**119**)	-	*E. rubrum*	Sediment	[71]
	Rubrumline H (**120**)	-	*E. rubrum*	Sediment	[71]

Table 1. *Cont.*

Sources	Compounds	Bioactivities	Species	Habitats	Refs
	Rubrumline I (**121**)	-	*E. rubrum*	Sediment	[71]
	Rubrumline J (**122**)	-	*E. rubrum*	Sediment	[71]
	Rubrumline K (**123**)	-	*E. rubrum*	Sediment	[71]
	Rubrumline L (**124**)	-	*E. rubrum*	Sediment	[71]
	Rubrumline M (**125**)	-	*E. rubrum*	Sediment	[71]
	Rubrumline N (**126**)	-	*E. rubrum*	Sediment	[71]
	Rubrumline O (**127**)	-	*E. rubrum*	Sediment	[71]
	12β-Hydroxy-13α-ethoxyverruculogen TR-2 (**128**)	-	*Penicillium* sp. DT-F29	Sediment	[72]
	12β-Hydroxy-13α-butoxyethoxyverruculogen TR-2 (**129**)	-	*Penicillium* sp. DT-F29	Sediment	[72]
	Hydrocycloprostatin A (**130**)	-	*Penicillium* sp. DT-F29	Sediment	[72]
	Hydrocycloprostatin B (**131**)	-	*Penicillium* sp. DT-F29	Sediment	[72]
	25-Hydroxyfumitremorgin B (**132**)	-	*Penicillium* sp. DT-F29	Sediment	[72]
	12β-Hydroxy-13α-butoxyethoxyfumitremorgin B (**133**)	-	*Penicillium* sp. DT-F29	Sediment	[72]
	12β-Hydroxy-13α-methoxyverruculogen (**134**)	BRD4 protein inhibition	*Penicillium* sp. DT-F29	Sediment	[72]
	26α-Hydroxyfumitremorgin A (**135**)	-	*Penicillium* sp. DT-F29	Sediment	[72]
	25-Hydroxyfumitremorgin A (**136**)	-	*Penicillium* sp. DT-F29	Sediment	[72]
	Diprostatin A (**137**)	BRD4 protein inhibition	*Penicillium* sp. DT-F29	Sediment	[72]
	(+) variecolortin A (**138**)	Antioxidant	*Eurotium* sp. SCSIO F452	Sediment	[73]
	(−) variecolortin A (**139**)	-	*Eurotium* sp. SCSIO F452	Sediment	[73]
	(+) variecolortin B (**140**)	Cytotoxicity	*Eurotium* sp. SCSIO F452	Sediment	[73]
	(−) variecolortin B (**141**)	-	*Eurotium* sp. SCSIO F452	Sediment	[73]
	(+) variecolortin C (**142**)	Cytotoxicity	*Eurotium* sp. SCSIO F452	Sediment	[73]
	(−) variecolortin C (**143**)	-	*Eurotium* sp. SCSIO F452	Sediment	[73]
	Eurotiumin A (**144**)	Antioxidant	*Eurotium* sp. SCSIO F452	Sediment	[74]
	Eurotiumin B (**145**)	Antioxidant	*Eurotium* sp. SCSIO F452	Sediment	[74]
	Eurotiumin C (**146**)	Antioxidant	*Eurotium* sp. SCSIO F452	Sediment	[74]
	6-Acetylmonodethiogliotoxin (**147**)	NF-κB inhibitor	*D. cejpii*	*Callyspongia* cf. *C. flammea*	[75]
	6-Acetylbisdethiobis(methylthio)gliotoxin (**148**)	NF-κB inhibitor	*D. cejpii*	*Callyspongia* cf. *C. flammea*	[75]
	5a,6-Anhydrobisdethiobis(methyl-thio)gliotoxin (**149**)	NF-κB inhibitor	*D. cejpii*	*Callyspongia* cf. *C. flammea*	[75]
	Peniciadametizine A (**150**)	Antimicrobial	*P. adametzioides* AS-53	Unidentified sponge	[76]

Table 1. Cont.

Sources	Compounds	Bioactivities	Species	Habitats	Refs
	peniciadametizine B (151)	Antimicrobial	*P. adametzioides* AS-53	Unidentified sponge	[76]
	Cyclo-(2-hydroxy-Pro-Gly) (152)	-	*Simplicillium* sp. YZ-11	*H. perleve*	[77]
	Fellutanine A (153)	-	*N. glabra* KUFA 0702	*Mycale* sp.	[78]
	Asperflocin (154)	Cytotoxicity	*A. versicolor* 16F-11	*P. fusca*	[79]
	Unnamed diketopiperazine dimer (155)	Anti-inflammatory	*A. violaceofuscus*	*Reniochalina* sp.	[80]
	Waspergillamide B (156)	-	*A. ochraceus*	*A. oroides*	[81]
	Penicillivinacine (157)	Cytotoxicity	*P. vinaceum*	*H. erectus*	[82]
	Adametizine A (158)	Antimicrobial Brine shrimp lethality	*P. adametzioides* AS-53	unidentified sponge	[83]
	Adametizine B (159)	Antimicrobial Brine shrimp lethality	*P. adametzioides* AS-53	unidentified sponge	[83]
	SF5280-415 (160)	Enzyme inhibition	*Aspergillus* sp. SF-5280	unidentified sponge	[84]
	Penicimutide (161)	Cytotoxicity	*P. purpurogenum* G59	Bohai Bay	[85]
	Penicimutanin C (162)	Cytotoxicity	*P. purpurogenum* G59	Bohai Bay	[86]
	Waikikiamide A (163)	Cytotoxicity	*Aspergillus* sp. FM242	Waikiki beach	[87]
	Waikikiamide B (164)	-	*Aspergillus* sp. FM242	Waikiki beach	[87]
	Waikikiamide C (165)	Cytotoxicity	*Aspergillus* sp. FM242	Waikiki beach	[87]
	5S-Hydroxynorvaline-S-Ile (166)	-	*Penicillium* sp. GD6	*B. gymnorrhiza*	[88]
	3S-Hydroxylcyclo(S-Pro-S-Phe) (167)	-	*Penicillium* sp. GD6	*B. gymnorrhiza*	[88]
	Cyclo(S-Phe-S-Gln) (168)	-	*Penicillium* sp. GD6	*B. gymnorrhiza*	[88]
	(−)-Asperginulin A (169)	-	*Aspergillus* sp. SK-28	*K. candel*	[89]
	(+)-Asperginulin A (170)	Antifouling	*Aspergillus* sp. SK-28	*K. candel*	[89]
	Saroclazine A (171)	Cytotoxicity	*S. kiliense* HDN11-84	*T. populnea*	[90]
	Saroclazine B (172)	-	*S. kiliense* HDN11-84	*T. populnea*	[90]
	Saroclazine C (173)	-	*S. kiliense* HDN11-84	*T. populnea*	[90]
	Brocazine A (174)	Cytotoxicity	*P. brocae* MA-231	*A. marina*	[91]
	Brocazine B (175)	Cytotoxicity	*P. brocae* MA-231	*A. marina*	[91]
	Brocazine C (176)	Cytotoxicity	*P. brocae* MA-231	*A. marina*	[91]
	Brocazine D (177)	Cytotoxicity	*P. brocae* MA-231	*A. marina*	[91]
	Brocazine E (178)	-	*P. brocae* MA-231	*A. marina*	[91]
	Brocazine F (179)	-	*P. brocae* MA-231	*A. marina*	[91]
	Penicibrocazine A (180)	-	*P. brocae* MA-231	*A. marina*	[92]
	Penicibrocazine B (181)	-	*P. brocae* MA-231	*A. marina*	[92]
	Penicibrocazine C (182)	Antimicrobial	*P. brocae* MA-231	*A. marina*	[92]
	Penicibrocazine D (183)	-	*P. brocae* MA-231	*A. marina*	[92]
	Penicibrocazine E (184)	Antimicrobial	*P. brocae* MA-231	*A. marina*	[92]
	Spirobrocazine A (185)	Antimicrobial	*P. brocae* MA-231	*A. marina*	[93]
	Spirobrocazine B (186)	-	*P. brocae* MA-231	*A. marina*	[93]
	Spirobrocazine C (187)	Antimicrobial	*P. brocae* MA-231	*A. marina*	[93]
	Brocazine G (188)	Antimicrobial Cytotoxicity	*P. brocae* MA-231	*A. marina*	[93]
	Pseudellone A (189)	-	*P. ellipsoidea* F42−3	*L. crassum*	[94]
	Pseudellone B (190)	-	*P. ellipsoidea* F42−3	*L. crassum*	[94]

Table 1. Cont.

Sources	Compounds	Bioactivities	Species	Habitats	Refs
	Pseuboydone C (**191**)	Cytotoxicity	*P. boydii* F19-1	*L. crassum*	[95]
	Pseuboydone D (**192**)	-	*P. boydii* F19-1	*L. crassum*	[95]
	Dichocerazine A (**193**)	-	*D. cejpii* F31-1	*L. crassum*	[96]
	Dichocerazine B (**194**)	-	*D. cejpii* F31-1	*L. crassum*	[96]
	11-Methylneoechinulin E (**195**)	Cytotoxicity	*Aspergillus* sp. EGF 15-0-3	South China Sea	[97]
	Variecolorin M (**196**)	Cytotoxicity	*Aspergillus* sp. EGF 15-0-3	South China Sea	[97]
	(+)-Variecolorin G (**197**)	Cytotoxicity	*Aspergillus* sp. EGF 15-0-3	South China Sea	[97]
	(+)-Neoechinulin A (**198**)	Cytotoxicity	*Aspergillus* sp. EGF 15-0-3	South China Sea	[97]
	16α-Hydroxy-17β-methoxy-deoxydihydroisoaustamide (**199**)	-	*P. dimorphosporum* KMM 4689	South China Sea	[98]
	16β-Hydroxy-17α-methoxy-deoxydihydroisoaustamide (**200**)	-	*P. dimorphosporum* KMM 4689	South China Sea	[98]
	16β,17α-dihydroxy-deoxydihydroisoaustamide (**201**)	-	*P. dimorphosporum* KMM 4689	South China Sea	[98]
	16α-hydroxy-17α-methoxy-deoxydihydroisoaustamide (**202**)	Enhance cell viability	*P. dimorphosporum* KMM 4689	South China Sea	[98]
	16α,17α-dihydroxy-deoxydihydroisoaustamide (**203**)	Enhance cell viability	*P. dimorphosporum* KMM 4689	South China Sea	[98]
	16,17-dihydroxy-deoxydihydroisoaustamide (**204**)	Enhance cell viability	*P. dimorphosporum* KMM 4689	South China Sea	[98]
	3β-Hydroxy-deoxyisoaustamide (**205**)	-	*P. dimorphosporum* KMM 4689	South China Sea	[98]
	Pseudellone D (**206**)	-	*P. ellipsoidea* F42-3	*L. crissum*	[99]
	Dehydroxymethylbis(dethio)bis(methylthio)gliotoxin (**207**)	-	*T. virens* Y13-3	*G. vermiculophylla*	[100]
	(3*S*,6*R*)-6-(Para-hydroxybenzyl)-1,4-dimethyl-3,6-bis(methylthio)piperazine-2,5-dione (**208**)	-	*T. virens* Y13-3	*G. vermiculophylla*	[100]
	Methylcordysinin A (**209**)	-	*T. asperellum* cf44-2	*Sargassum* sp.	[101]
	Citriperazine A (**210**)	-	*Penicillium* sp. KMM 4672	*Padina* sp.	[102]
	Citriperazine B (**211**)	-	*Penicillium* sp. KMM 4672	*Padina* sp.	[102]
	Citriperazine C (**212**)	-	*Penicillium* sp. KMM 4672	*Padina* sp.	[102]
	Citriperazine D (**213**)	-	*Penicillium* sp. KMM 4672	*Padina* sp.	[102]
	(+) Acrozines A (**214**)	Antiacetylcholinesterase	*A. luteoalbus* TK-43	*C. fragile*	[103]
	(−) Acrozines A (**215**)	Antiacetylcholinesterase	*A. luteoalbus* TK-43	*C. fragile*	[103]
	(+) Acrozines B (**216**)	Antimicrobial	*A. luteoalbus* TK-43	*C. fragile*	[103]
	(−) Acrozines B (**217**)	-	*A. luteoalbus* TK-43	*C. fragile*	[103]
	(+) Acrozines C (**218**)	-	*A. luteoalbus* TK-43	*C. fragile*	[103]
	(−) Acrozines C (**219**)	-	*A. luteoalbus* TK-43	*C. fragile*	[103]
	Cyclo(L-5-MeO-Pro-L-5-MeO-Pro) (**220**)	Antimicrobial	*T. asperellum* A-YMD-9-2	*G. verrucose*	[104]
	Pretrichodermamide D (**221**)	-	*Penicillium* sp. KMM 4672	*Padina* sp.	[105]
	Pretrichodermamide E (**222**)	-	*Penicillium* sp. KMM 4672	*Padina* sp.	[105]

Table 1. Cont.

Sources	Compounds	Bioactivities	Species	Habitats	Refs
	Pretrichodermamide F (223)	-	*Penicillium* sp. KMM 4672	*Padina* sp.	[105]
	N-(4′-hydroxyprenyl)-cyclo(alanyltryptophyl) (224)	-	*E. cristatum* EN-220	*S. thunbergia*	[106]
	Isovariecolorin I (225)	Brine shrimp lethal	*E. cristatum* EN-220	*S. thunbergia*	[106]
	30-Hydroxyechinulin (226)	-	*E. cristatum* EN-220	*S. thunbergia*	[106]
	29-Hydroxyechinulin (227)	-	*E. cristatum* EN-220	*S. thunbergia*	[106]
	(+)-Brevianamide X (228)	-	*A. versicolor* OUCMDZ-2738	*E. prolifera*	[107]
	(−)-Brevianamide X (229)	-	*A. versicolor* OUCMDZ-2738	*E. prolifera*	[107]
	Isoechinulin D (230)	-	*E. rubrum* MPUC136	/ [b]	[108]
	Spirotryprostatin G (231)	Cytotoxicity	*P. brasilianum* HBU-136	Bohai Sea	[109]
	Cyclotryprostatin F (232)	Cytotoxicity	*P. brasilianum* HBU-136	Bohai Sea	[109]
	Cyclotryprostatin G (233)	Cytotoxicity	*P. brasilianum* HBU-136	Bohai Sea	[109]
	Penilline C (234)	-	*P. chrysogenum* SCSIO 07007	Western Atlantic	[110]
	Emestrin L (235)	-	*A. terreus* RA2905	*A. pulmonica*	[111]
	Emestrin M (236)	Antimicrobial	*A. terreus* RA2905	*A. pulmonica*	[111]
	Aspamide A (237)	-	*A. versicolor* DY180635	*C. haematocheir*	[112]
	Aspamide B (238)	-	*A. versicolor* DY180635	*C. haematocheir*	[112]
	Aspamide C (239)	-	*A. versicolor* DY180635	*C. haematocheir*	[112]
	Aspamide D (240)	-	*A. versicolor* DY180635	*C. haematocheir*	[112]
	Penicillatide B (241)	Cytotoxicity Antimicrobial	*Penicillium* sp.	*Didemnum* sp.	[113]

[a] The bioactivity was not mentioned; [b] the habitat was not mentioned.

2.1. Sponge

Cyclo-(R-Pro-6-hydroxyl-S-Ile) (**1**) was a new DKP isolated from the sponge *Callyspongia* sp., which was collected from the South China Sea. Compound **1** showed no antibacterial activity against the tested *Bacillus subtilis*, *Staphylococcus aureus* and *Escherichia coli* [30]. Geobarrettins A (**2**) and B (**3**), two new DKPs, were obtained from the sub-Arctic sponge *Geodia barrette*, which was collected at the west of Iceland (-388 m). Before coculturing with allogeneic CD4$^+$ T cells, the maturing human dendritic cells (DCs) were processed by compound **3** with a dose of 10 μg/mL and then reduced the IFN-γ of T cell secretion. Compound **3** had no effect on the DCs secretion of IL-10 but induced the IL-12p40. This above data demonstrated that compound **3** possessed an overall anti-inflammatory activity and may be used to treat the Th1 type inflammation [31]. A novel sulfur-containing DKP, tedanizaine A (**4**), was collected from the marine sponge *Tedania* sp. at a depth of 10 m in Zhanjiang, Guangdong province. Compound **4** bearing a thiazolidine unit was separated by integrating molecular networking and became the second example of thiodiketopiperazine. However, the evaluation of cytotoxicity activities did not reveal the inhibitory activity of compound **4** on the growth of the tested A549 (lung carcinoma) and RAW 246.7 (macrophage) cell lines [32]. (−)-Cyclo(L-trans-Hyp-L-Ile) (**5**) was a new DKP isolated from the marine sponge *Axinella sinoxea*, collected from a reef habitat around Larak Island, Persian Gulf. Compound **5** had no influence on methicillin-resistant *Staphylococcus* *aureus* (MRSA) in the dose of 100 μg/mL [33]. All 5 DKPs from sponge described above are presented in Figure 1.

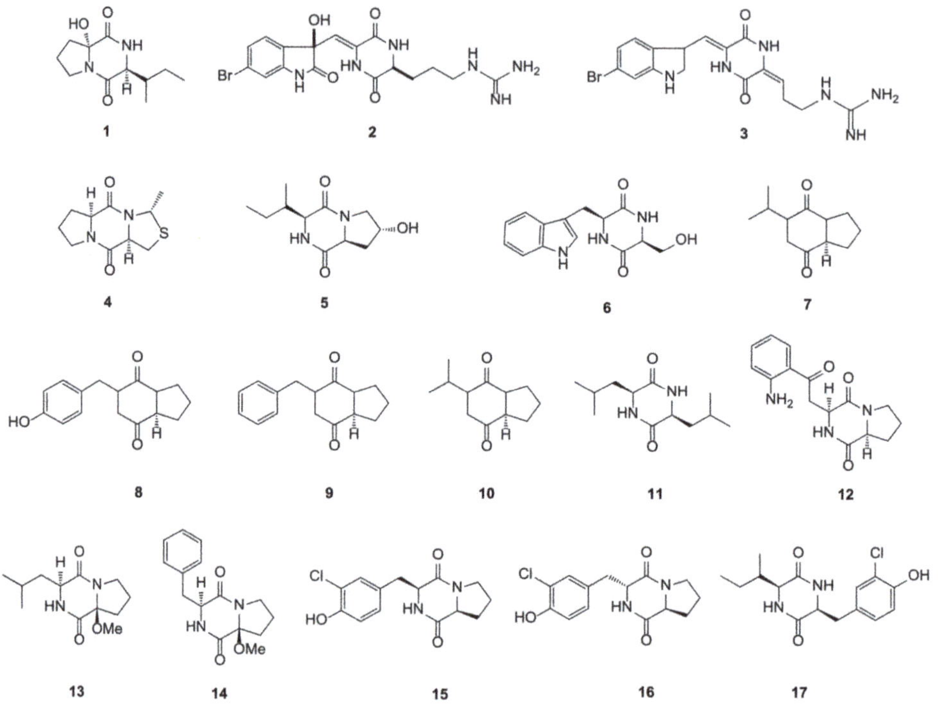

Figure 1. DKP structures from sponge (**1–5**) and bacteria (**6–17**).

2.2. Bacteria

Cyclo (Trp-Ser) (**6**) was a novel DKP from *Rheinheimera aquimaris* QSI02, in the Yellow Sea of Qingdao, which was active against *E. coli*, *Chromobacterium violaceum* CV026 and *Pseudomonas aeruginosa* PA01 with the minimum inhibitory concentration (MIC) values of 6.4, 3.2 and 6.4 mg/mL, respectively. Compound **6** possessed antiquorum sensing activity, which could decrease the QS-regulated violacein and pyocyanin production by 67% and 65% in *C. violaceum* CV026 and *P. aeruginosa*. Based on the molecular docking results, compared with the natural signaling molecule, compound **6** was easier to combine with the CviR receptor, but opposite in the LasR receptor. These consequences indicated that compound **6** may become a potential inhibitor to control the quorum sensing (QS) system [34]. Four novel DKPs were isolated from psychrophilic yeast *Glaciozyma antarctica* PI12, which was collected from a marine environment in Antarctica, and they were named as cyclo(Pro-Val) (**7**), (−)-cyclo(Pro-Tyr) (**8**), (−)-cyclo(Pro-Phe) (**9**) and (+)-cyclo(Pro-Leu) (**10**). However, all these compounds reported in the present study were not subjected to further bioactivity studies [35]. (3*S*,6*S*)-3,6-diisobutylpiperazine-2,5-dione (**11**) was firstly displayed from a sponge-associated bacterium *Bacillus* sp. SPB7, which was isolated from the sponge *Spongia officinalis*. Compound **11** exhibited antimicrobial activity against *E. coli* and *S. aureus* subsp. *aureus* with the MIC values of 16 and 22 μg/mL, respectively [36]. Gallaecimonamides A–C (**12–14**) were three new DKPs collected from the marine bacterium *Gallaecimonas mangrovi* HK-28, which was isolated from the mangrove sediment from Haikou, Hainan Province, China. Compound **12** showed significant selectively antimicrobial activity against *V. harveyi* with the MIC value of 50 μM [37]. Three novel chlorine-containing DKPs namely *cis*-cyclo(Pro-3-chloro-Tyr) (**15**), *trans*-cyclo(Pro-3-chloro-Tyr) (**16**) and *cis*-cyclo(3-chloro-

Tyr-Ile) (**17**) were isolated from *Bacillus subtilis* BI0980 collected from a depth of 18 m marine sediment between the islands of Kerkyra and Erikoussa. Compounds **15** and **16** showed no inhibitory activity for the tested fungi (*Candida albicans* and *Aspergillus niger*) [38]. All 12 DKPs from bacteria described above are presented in Figure 1.

2.3. Actinomycetes

A novel DKP, iso-naseseazine B (**18**), was isolated from the medium of *Streptomyces* sp. SMA-1 from the marine sediment of the Yellow Sea, China. Compound **18** could oppose the fluconazole-resistant *C. albicans* and the diameter of the inhibition zone was 9 mm [39]. The other *Streptomyces* sp. USC-636 strain was collected from marine sediment in Sunshine Coast, QLD, Australia. Naseseazine C (**21**) was extracted from the culture of this strain, which exhibited a novel C-6′/C-3 linkage between the two DKP subunits and possessed the activity of antiplasmodial with an IC_{50} value of 3.52 µM. However, the analog naseseazines A (**19**) and B (**20**) inhibited the malaria parasite at a dose of 20 µM. The special linkage between C-6′ and C-3 may be critical to increase bioactivity [40]. (6R,3Z)-3-benzylidene-6-isobutyl-1-methyl piperazine-2,5-dione (**22**), a new DKP, was produced by the *Streptomyces* sp. strain SCSIO 04496, which was collected from a deep-sea sediment sample of the South China Sea [41]. ΔmarF, the methyltransferase gene of maremycins, knockout in strain *Streptomyces* sp. B9173 (collected from the pacific coast of Chile) obtained the mutant LS26. Six new demethylmaremycins (**23–28**) were isolated from the mutant LS26, however, the specific name of these compounds could not be found [42]. *Streptomyces* sp. MNU FJ-36 was collected from the *Katsuwonus* sp. intestinal fabric. Three novel compounds, 3-(3-hydroxy-4-methoxybenzyl)-6-isobutyl-2,5-diketopiperazine (**29**), 3-(1,3-benzodioxol-5-ylmethyl)-6-isobutyl-2,5-diketopiperazine (**30**) and 3-(1,3-benzodioxol-5-ylmethyl)-6-isopropyl-2,5-diketopiperazine (**31**), were isolated from the *Streptomyces* sp. MNU FJ-36. All of these compounds **29–31** could inhibit the growth of the A549 cell lines with IC_{50} values of 89.4, 35.4 and 28.4 mg/mL, respectively. Compounds **30** and **31** also exhibited a weak cytotoxicity against the HCT-116 (human colon carcinoma) cell lines with IC_{50} values of 75.4 and 45.4 mg/mL, respectively [43]. A novel DKP glycosidem, maculosin-*O*-α-L-rhamnopyranoside (**32**), was discovered from the *Streptomyces* sp. ZZ446, which was collected in coastal soil from Zhoushan Islands, Zhejiang Province. Compound **32** possessed antimicrobial activity against MRSA, *E. coli* and *C. albicans* with MIC values of 37, 28 and 26 µg/mL, respectively [44,45]. Actinozine A (**33**) was a new DKP, which was isolated from the *Streptomyces* species Call-36 from the Red Sea sponge *Callyspongia* species. Compound **33** exhibited a moderate antimicrobial activity against *S. aureus* and *C. albicans* with inhibition zones of 23 and 19 mm at 100 µg/disc, respectively, and showed a weak activity for the HCT-116 (IC_{50} = 146 µM) and MCF-7 (breast cancer, IC_{50} = 88.8 µM) cell lines [46]. *Streptomyces* sp. SY1965 was collected from the Mariana Trench sediment-associated at a depth of 11,000 m and two new DKPs, streptodiketopiperazines A (**34**) and B (**35**) were isolated from the strain. The crude extraction of this strain from the Gauze's liquid medium with sea salt could suppress the human glioma U87MG and U251 cells with an inhibition rate of over 100%. Both compounds **34** and **35** exhibited antifungal activity against *C. albicans* with a MIC value of 42 µg/mL [47].

A novel DKP, cyclo-(4-*trans*-6-dihydroxy-proline-D-leucine) (**36**), was discovered from the *Microbulbifer variabilis* C-03, which isolated from the *Palythoa tuberculosa* in the intertidal zone of Wanlitong [48]. One novel DKP namely nocarazepine A (**37**) was isolated from the *Nocardiopsis alba* collected from the gorgonian *Anthogorgia caerulea*, which was sampled from the coast of Xieyang Island, Guangxi Province [49]. Strain AJS-327 was a rare actinomycete (maybe a new linkage within *Streptomycetaceae*) and collected from the sponge fragment on the beach from La Jolla, CA. It was proved to be a likely novel species because it exhibited an extremely poor 16S rRNA sequence similarity to other members of the actinomycete family *Streptomycetaceae*. Four new DKPs, photopiperazines A–D (**38–41**), were isolated from this strain. The olefin geometrical isomers of these four compounds could be interconverted under light conditions, on account of the photopiperazines being sensitive to light. In terms of activity, the mixture of four compounds included compounds **38** (33.5%), **39** (39.7%), **40** (8.4%) and **41** (18.4%). This mixture exhibited a remarkable activity to the cancer cell of U87 (glioblastoma brain cancer), SHOV3 (ovarian cancer), MDA-MB-231(breast cancer) and HCT116 (human colon carcinoma) with IC_{50} values of 1.2×10^{-4}, 2.2×10^{-4}, 1.6 and 1.6 µg/mL, respectively [50]. Cyclo-(D-8-acetoxyl-Pro-L-Leu) (**42**) was a novel DKP isolated from *Treptomyces* sp. SCSIO 41400, which was obtained from a mangrove derived-soil from the Fuli Mangrove Bay Wetland Park, Haikou, Hainan Province of China. Compound **42** could anchor in the binding site of the pancreatic lipase (PL) enzyme and then prevent the substrate from entering and inhibit the PL enzyme activity with an IC_{50} value of 27.3 µg/mL [51]. All 25 DKPs from the actinomycetes described above are presented in Figure 2.

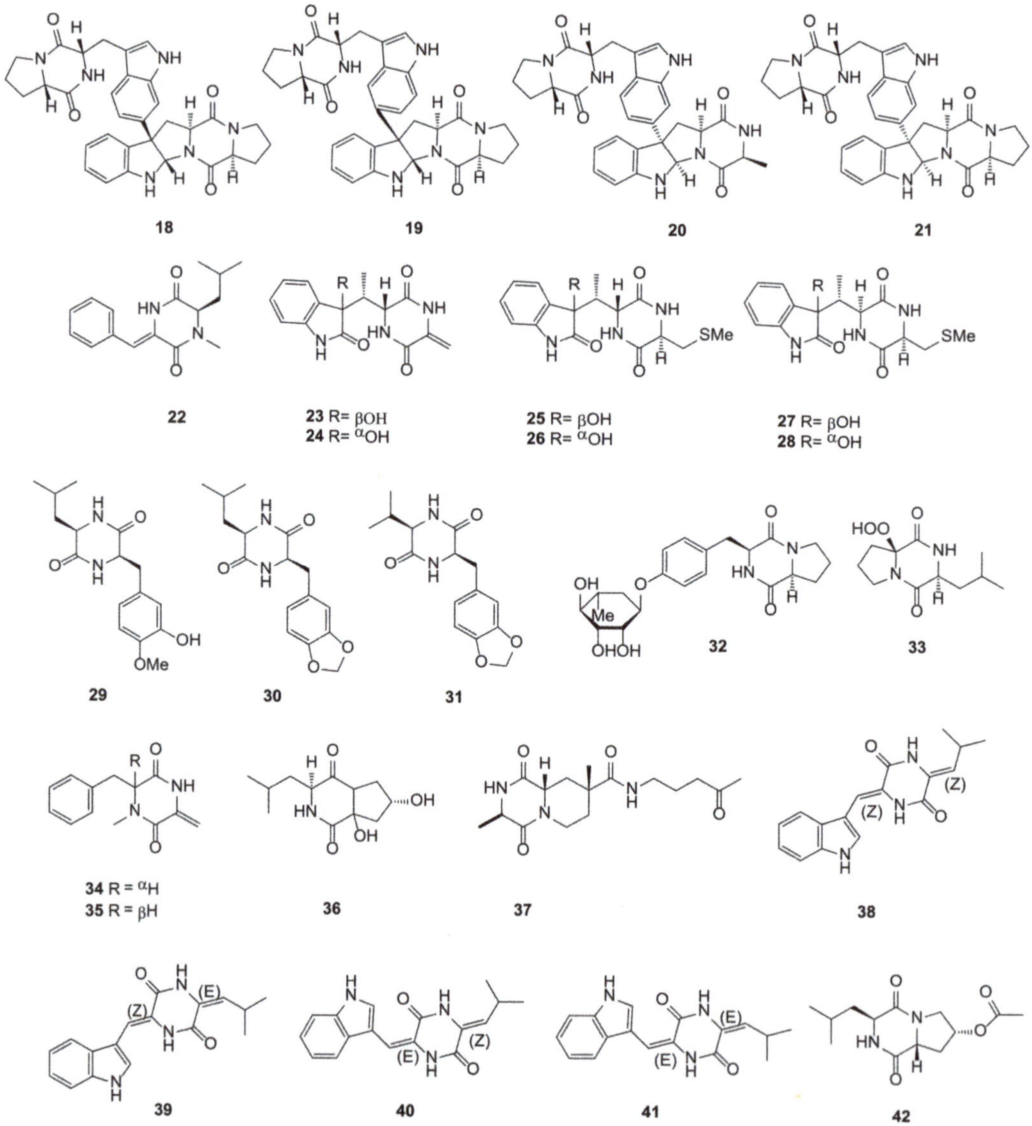

Figure 2. DKP structures from actinomycetes (**18**–**42**).

2.4. Fungi

2.4.1. Fungi from Sediment Origin

Graphiumins A–J (**43–52**), ten new sulfur-containing DKPs, were isolated from the fungus *Graphium* sp. OPMF00224 collected from a depth of 17 m marine sediment on Ishigaki Island, Okinawa, Japan. Compounds **45–47** and **49–52** exhibited no inhibition for MRSA; however, they could inhibit the production of the yellow pigment (virulence factors of MRSA) with a white zone of 10, 14, 10, 12, 11, 24 and 23 mm (50 µg/8 mm) [52,53]. Gu et al. firstly utilized the high-speed countercurrent chromatography (HSCCC) to separate and purify the marine fungus secondary metabolites and then two new sulfur-containing DKPs named cladosporins A (**53**) and B (**54**) were discovered from the marine fungus *Cladosporium* sp. collected from marine sediment in Yangshashan Bay, Ningbo, Zhejiang Province, China. Compounds **53** and **54** showed cytotoxicity activities against HepG2 (hepatocellular carcinoma) cell lines with the IC_{50} values of 21 and 48 µg/mL, respectively. The marine fungus *Alternaria alternate* HK-25 was isolated from mangrove sediment (Sanya, Hainan, China). By using HSCCC, five DKPs named 12,13-dihydroxy-fumitremorgin C (**55**), gliotoxin (**56**), demethoxyfumitremorgin C (**57**), bisdethiobis(methylthio)gliotoxin (**58**) and fumitremorgin C (**59**) were isolated from *A. alternate* HK-25 and first discovered from fungi. Purities of these compounds were all above 94% [54,55].

Haenamindole (**60**) was discovered from the fungus *Penicillium* sp. KCB12F005 isolated from a marine sediment on the coast of Haenam, Korea. Compound **60** exhibited weak inhibitory activity against hepatitis C virus with the IC_{50} value of 76.3 µM [56,57]. Dichotocejpins A–C (**61–63**), three novel DKPs, were isolated from the fungus *Dichotomomyces cejpii* FS110 collected from a depth of 3941 m sediment in the South China Sea. Compound **61** exhibited weak cytotoxicity against SF-268 (human glioma), MCF-7 and HepG2 tumor cell lines with IC_{50} values of 35.7, 29.5 and 28.9 µM, respectively, and showed remarkably more α-glucosidase inhibition activity than acarbose (oral antidiabetic agent, IC_{50} = 463 µM) with the IC_{50} value of 138 µM [58]. Cristazine (**64**) was discovered from the fungus *Chaetomium cristatum*, which was isolated from a marine mudflat on Suncheon Bay, Korea. Compound **64** exhibited antioxidant activity against 2,2-diphenyl-1-picrylhydrazyl (DPPH) with the IC_{50} value of 19 µM, which was similar to ascorbic acid (positive control, IC_{50} = 20 µM). It also possessed potent cytotoxicity activities against Hela (cervical carcinoma) and A431 (epidermoid carcinoma) cell lines with the IC_{50} value of 0.5 µM. Compound **64** could trigger the death of the apoptotic cell via the Type I death receptor pathway and inhibit the cell cycle progression by arresting the G_1/S phase and upregulating the inhibitory proteins of cyclin-dependent kinases. By these two ways, compound **64** could inhibit the growth of A431 cells [59,60].

Nineteen novel DKPs namely eutypellazines A–S (**65–83**) were isolated from fungus *Eutypella* sp. MCCC 3A00281, which was collected from a depth of 5610 m of marine sediment from the South Atlantic Ocean. Compounds **65–76** could inhibit the replication of human immunodeficiency virus type 1 (HIV-1) with the IC_{50} values ranging 3.2–18.2 µM. A sulfide bridge existing in compounds **65–67** and **71–72** (IC_{50} = 10.7–18.2 µM) might be the reason for exhibiting lower inhibitory activities than compounds **68–69** and **73–76** (IC_{50} = 3.2–8.7 µM). Compound **74** exhibited the ability to reactivate the latent HIV-1 transcription, which was rarely discovered from nature products. These compounds may become new anti-HIV candidates via modifying the original new scaffolds [61,62]. Fusaperazine F (**84**) was isolated from the fungus *Penicillium crustosum* HDN153086 collected from the Prydz Bay sediment of the Antarctic and showed cytotoxicity activity against K562 cell lines (human chronic myelogenous leukemia cells, IC_{50} = 12.7 µM) [63]. Roquefortine J (**85**) was another new DKP discovered from the fungus *Penicillium granulatum* MCCC 3A00475 isolated from a -2284 m deep-sea sediment from the Prydz Bay of Antarctica and exhibited moderate cytotoxicity activity against HepG2 cell lines with an IC_{50} value of 19.5 µM [64,65]. Three pairs of new DKPs namely (±)-7,8-epoxy-brevianamide Q (**86–87**), (±)-8-hydroxy-brevianamide R (**88–89**) and (±)-8-epihydroxy-brevianamide R (**90–91**) were isolated from the fungus *Aspergillus versicolor* MF180151, which was collected from a sediment in Bohai Sea, China. However, these compounds showed no antimicrobial activities [66].

Raistrickindole A (**92**), a novel DKP containing indole tetraheterocyclic ring system, was discovered from the fungus *Penicillium raistrickii* IMB17-034 obtained from a mangrove swamp sediment in Sanya, Hainan Province, China. Compound **92** exhibited the inhibitory activity against hepatitis C virus (HCV) with the EC_{50} value of 5.7 µM [67]. 5′-hydroxy-6′-ene-epicoccin G (**93**), 7-methoxy-7′-hydroxyepicoccin G (**94**), 8′-acetoxyepicoccin D (**95**), 7′-demethoxyrostratin C (**96**) and (±)-5-hydroxydiphenylalazines A (**97–98**) were five new DKPs and isolated from the fungus *Epicoccum nigrum* SD-388, which was collected from a depth of 4500 m of sediment in the West Pacific. Compound **96** possessed the excellent cytotoxicity activity against Huh7.5 (liver tumor) cell lines with an IC_{50} value of 9.52 µM, however, it also inhibited the growth of human normal liver LO2 cell lines. The disulfide bridge in the main structure may be crucial for its activity [68]. (±) Eurotinoids A (**99–100**), (±) eurotinoids B (**101–102**) and (±) eurotinoids C (**103–104**), three pairs of novel DKPs spirocyclic alkaloid enantiomers, were isolated from the fungus *Eurotium* sp. SCSIO F452 obtained from the sediment sample in South China Sea. These compounds showed excellent antioxidant activities against DPPH with the IC_{50} values between 5.8 and 24.9 µM [69].

Seven novel DKPs, versicamides A−G (**105−111**), were isolated from the fungus *Aspergillus versicolor* HDN08-60 collected from the marine sediment in the South China Sea. Versicamide H (**112**) was obtained from the methylation reaction of **111**. Only compound **112** showed modest cytotoxicity activities against the HL-60, HCT-116, Hela and K562 cell lines with IC_{50} values of 8.7, 17.7, 19.4 and 22.4 µM, respectively, and compound **112** exhibited selective PTK inhibitory activity with the highest inhibitory rate of 60% at a concentration of 10 µM. Compound **112** had stronger activities than compounds **105–111**, which might be attributed to an unprecedented skeleton featuring a 2,5-dihydro-1H-azepino-[4,3-b]quinoline system [70]. Fifteen novel DKPs namely rubrumlines A–O (**113–127**) were isolated from the fungus *Eurotium rubrum*, which was collected from a depth of 2067 m marine sediment in the South Atlantic Ocean. Compound **116** possessed antivirus activity against the influenza A/WSN/33 virus with the inhibitory rate of 52.64% [71]. Ten new DKPs, 12β-hydroxy-13α-ethoxyverruculogen TR-2 (**128**), 12β-hydroxy-13α-butoxyethoxyverruculogen TR-2 (**129**), hydrocycloprostatin A (**130**), hydrocycloprostatin B (**131**), 25-hydroxyfumitremorgin B (**132**), 12β-hydroxy-13α-butoxyethoxyfumitremorgin B (**133**), 12β-hydroxy-13α-methoxyverruculogen (**134**), 26α-hydroxyfumitremorgin A (**135**), 25-hydroxyfumitremorgin A (**136**) and diprostatin A (**137**) were isolated from the coculture of the fungus *Penicillium* sp. DT-F29 with the bacteria *Bacillus* sp. B31, which were collected from the marine sediments of Dongtou County and Changzhi Island, respectively. In a dose of 20 µM, compounds **133** and **137** showed remarkable BRD4 protein inhibitory activities [72].

Three novel pairs of spirocyclic DKPs namely (±) variecolortins A−C (**138−143**) were obtained from the fungus *Eurotium* sp. SCSIO F452, which was isolated from marine sediment in the South China Sea. Compound **138** had a 2-oxa-7-azabicyclo[3.2.1]octane core, which was an unprecedented highly functionalized seco-anthronopyranoid carbon skeleton. In addition, compounds **139** and **140** had a rare 6/6/6/6 tetracyclic cyclohexene−anthrone carbon scaffold. Compound **138** showed remarkable antioxidant activity against DPPH with an IC_{50} value of 58.4 µM. Compound **140** and **142** exhibited modest cytotoxicity activities against SF-268 (IC_{50} = 12.5 and 15.0 µM) and HepG2 (IC_{50} = 30.1 and 37.3 µM) cell lines. The preliminary molecular docking study revealed that the potential antioxidative target of compounds **138** and **139** might be peroxiredoxin and the potential cytotoxic target of compounds **140** and **142** might be farnesyltransferase [73]. Eurotiumins A–C (**144–146**), three new DKP alkaloids, were also isolated from the fungus *Eurotium* sp. SCSIO F452. Compounds **144–146** showed antioxidant activities against DPPH with IC_{50} values of 37, 69 and 13 µM, respectively. Based on these results, the absolute configurations of the C-2 and C-3 of compounds **144** and **145** might have an influence on antioxidant activities [74]. All 104 DKPs from sediment-derived fungi described above are presented in Figures 3–5.

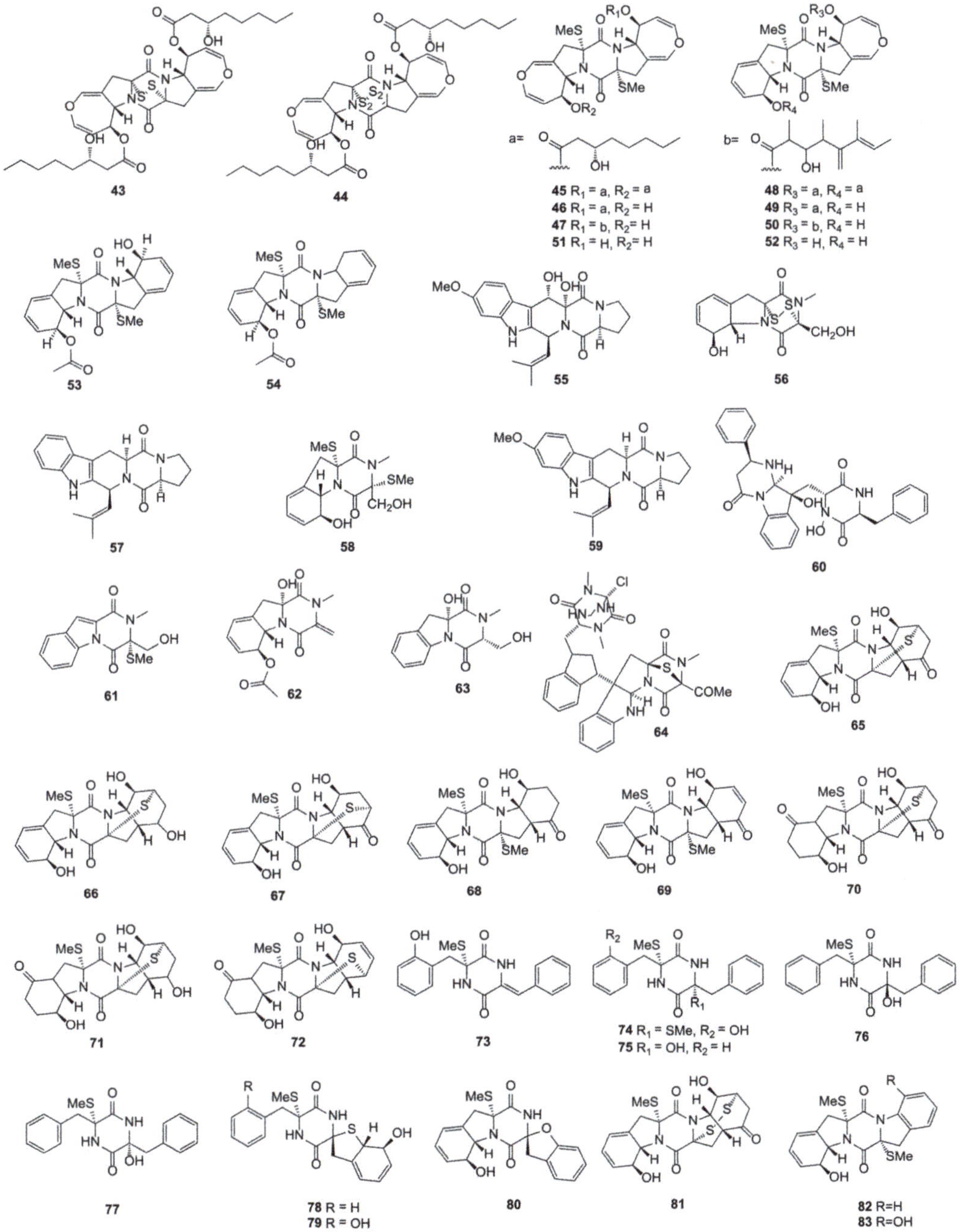

Figure 3. DKP structures from sediment-derived fungi (**43**–**83**).

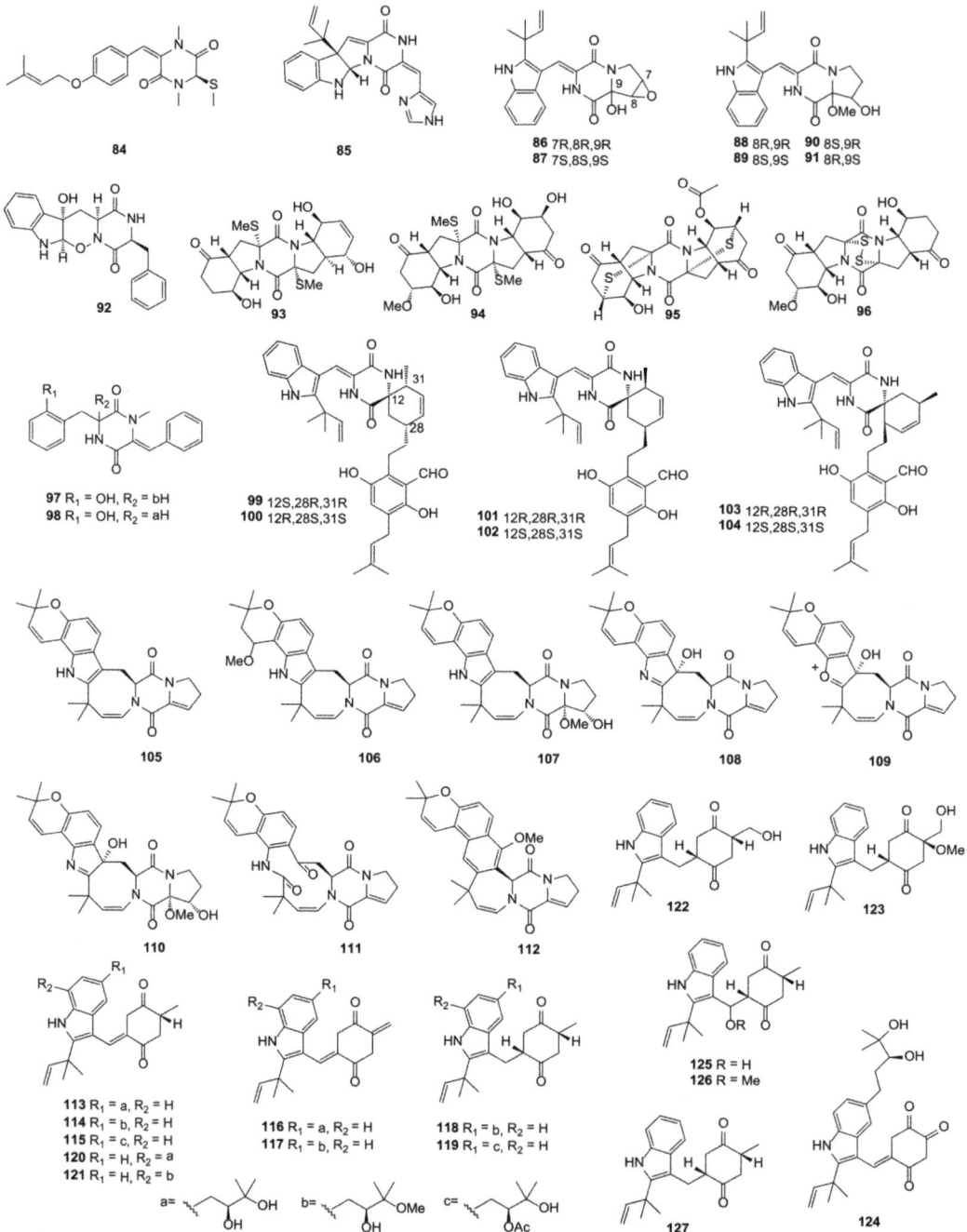

Figure 4. DKP structures from sediment-derived fungi (**84**–**127**).

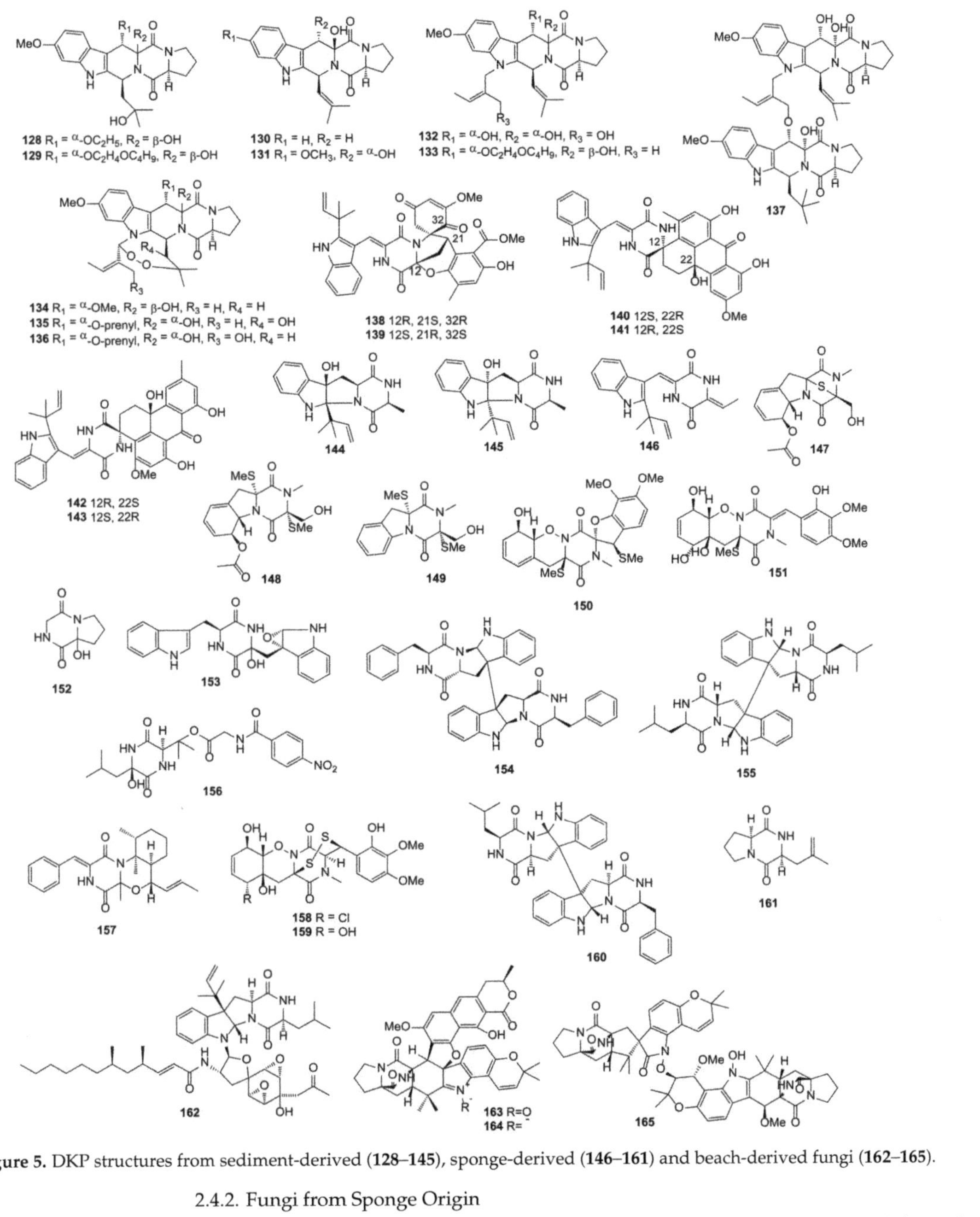

Figure 5. DKP structures from sediment-derived (**128–145**), sponge-derived (**146–161**) and beach-derived fungi (**162–165**).

2.4.2. Fungi from Sponge Origin

A novel DKP namely 6-acetylmonodethiogliotoxin (**147**) was obtained from the fungus *Dichotomomyces cejpii*, which was collected from the marine sponge *Callyspongia* cf. *C. flammea* at Bare Island, Sydney, Australia. Two DKPs previously only known as semisynthetic compounds, 6-acetylbisdethiobis(methylthio)gliotoxin (**148**) and 5a,6-anhydrobisdethiobis(methylthio)gliotoxin (**149**), were found in nature for the first time. In human chronic myeloid leukemia cells, compounds **147** and **148** showed downregulated

TNFα-induced NF-κB activity with the IC$_{50}$ values of 38.5 and 65.7 μM, respectively [75]. Peniciadametizine A (**150**) and B (**151**) were isolated from the fungus *Penicillium adametzioides* AS-53 collected from an unidentified sponge in Hainan Island of China. Compound **150** had a unique spiro[furan-2,7'-pyrazino[1,2-b][1,2]oxazine] skeleton, which was found from a natural source for the first time and compound **151** was the highly oxygenated analogue of **150**. In a dose of 100 μg/mL, compounds **150** and **151** could kill *Artemia salina* with the lethal ratio of 45.5 and 62.4%, respectively. These two compounds also showed antifungal activity against *Alternaria brassicae* with MIC values of 4.0 and 32.0 μg/mL, respectively [76]. Cyclo-(2-hydroxy-Pro-Gly) (**152**), a novel minor DKP, was obtained from the fungus *Simplicillium* sp. YZ-11, which was collected from an intertidal sponge *Hymeniacidon perleve* from Dalian, Liaoning Province, China [77]. *Neosartorya glabra* KUFA 0702 was isolated from the sponge *Mycale* sp. collected from 15 to 20 m coral reef at Samaesarn Island and a new DKP, fellutanine A (**153**), was obtained. Compound **153** showed no antibacterial (MIC > 256 μg/mL) or antifungal (MIC > 512 μg/mL) activity against the tested microbe including *E. coli* ATCC 25922, *Staphylococcus aureus* ATCC 25923, *A. fumigatus* ATCC 46645, *Trichophyton rubrum* ATCC FF5 and *C. albicans* ATCC 10231 [78]. Asperflocin (**154**), a novel asymmetric DKP dimer, was isolated from the fungus *Aspergillus versicolor* 16F-11, which was obtained from the sponge *Phakellia fusca* from Yongxing Island in the South China Sea. Compound **154** could inhibit the A375 (human melanoma) cell lines growth with the IC$_{50}$ value of 10.29 ± 2.37 μM [79].

One novel DKP dimer (**155**) possessing the same planar structure and different stereochemistry with an unnamed and ambiguous compound was isolated from the fungus *Aspergillus violaceofuscus*, which was collected from sponge *Reniochalina* sp. from Xisha Islands in the South China Sea. In a dose of 10 μM, compound **155** exhibited anti-inflammatory activity via decreasing LPS-induced expression of IL-10 in THP-1 cells with inhibitory rates of 78.1% [80]. Waspergillamide B (**156**), a new DKP containing an unusual *p*-nitrobenzoic acid structure, was obtained from the fungus *Aspergillus ochraceus* collected from the sponge *Agelas oroides* from the Mediterranean. Compound **156** had no cytotoxic activity against A2780 (human ovarian carcinoma) cell lines [81]. One new DKP alkaloid namely penicillivinacine (**157**) was obtained from the fungus *Penicillium vinaceum* that was isolated from the marine sponge *Hyrtios erectus* from Yanbu. Compound **157** exhibited significant cytotoxicity activity against MDA-MB-231 cell lines with an IC$_{50}$ value of 18.4 μM [82]. Adametizines A (**158**) and B (**159**), two novel sulfur-containing DKPs, were separated from the fungus *Penicillium adametzioides* AS-53, which was isolated from an unidentified marine sponge collected from Hainan Island of China. Compound **158** could inhibit the growth of brine shrimp (*A. salina*) with the LD$_{50}$ (lethal dose 50%) value of 4.8 μM. In addition, compound **158** showed antimicrobial activities against *Staphylococcus aureus*, *Aeromonas hydrophilia* and *V. parahaemolyticus* with an MIC value of 8 μg/mL and compound **159** showed antimicrobial activities against *S. aureus* with an MIC value of 64 μg/mL. These results revealed that the Cl substitution at C-7 remarkably increased the brine shrimp lethality and antimicrobial activity [83]. SF5280-415 (**160**) was a novel DKP dimer and isolated from the fungus *Aspergillus* sp. SF-5280, which was obtained from an unidentified sponge at Cheju Island, Korea. Compound **160** showed enzyme inhibitory activity against the PTP1B enzyme with an IC$_{50}$ value of 14.2 μM [84]. All 14 DKPs from sponge-derived fungi described above are presented in Figure 5.

2.4.3. Fungi from Beach Origin

A novel DKP namely penicimutide (**161**) was obtained from a neomycin-resistant mutant fungus *Penicillium purpurogenum* G59, which was isolated from a soil sample from the tideland of Bohai Bay. In a dose of 100 μg/mL, compound **161** exhibited excellent cytotoxicity activity against HeLa cell lines with an inhibition rate of 39.4% [85]. Penicimutanin C (**162**), a new DKP contained alkaloidal, was isolated from the neomycin-resistant mutant strain 3-f-31 fungus *P. purpurogenum* G59. Compound **162** exhibited cytotoxic activities against HeLa, BGC-823 (gastric adenocarcinoma), MCF-7, K562 and HL-60 (acute promyelocytic leukemia) cell lines with IC$_{50}$ values of 11.9, 5.0, 8.6, 8.7 and 6.0 µM, respectively. In a dose of 100 µg/mL, compound **162** showed cytotoxicity activities against these five cell lines with inhibition rates of 88.1%, 83.9%, 80.5%, 87.7% and 87.3%, respectively [86].

Waikikiamides A−C (**163**−**165**) were obtained from the fungus *Aspergillus* sp. FM242 collected from a sample at Waikiki beach in Oahu, Honolulu, Hawaii. Compounds **163** and **164** contained a new skeleton with a hendecacyclic ring system and compound **165** was composed of two notoamide analogs with an N-O-C bridge to feature the unique heterodimer. Compounds **163** possessed antiproliferative activities against HT1080 (fibrosarcoma), PC3 (prostatic tumor), Jurkat (immortalized T lymphocyte) and A2780S cell lines with IC$_{50}$ values of 0.519, 1.855, 0.62 and 0.78 µM, respectively. Compound **165** exhibited antiproliferative activities against these four cell lines with IC$_{50}$ values of 1.135, 1.805, 1.79 and 1.127 µM, respectively. Compound **164** showed no activities to these four cell lines. The reason for the difference in activity was that compounds **163** and **165** possessed an N–O bond but compound **164** did not [87]. All 5 DKPs from fungi of beach origin described above are presented in Figure 5.

2.4.4. Fungi from Mangrove Origin

A new DKP namely 5S-hydroxynorvaline-S-Ile (**166**), together with two firstly discovered in nature namely 3S-hydroxylcyclo(S-Pro-S-Phe) (**167**) and cyclo(S-Phe-S-Gln) (**168**), were obtained from mangrove endophytic fungus *Penicillium* sp. GD6, which was isolated from the stem bark of *Bruguiera gymnorrhiza* collected from Zhanjiang, China. These compounds showed no activity against the tested MRSA [88]. (−)-asperginulin A (**169**) and (+)-asperginulin A (**170**), two dimers DKPs that contained enantiomeric indole, were isolated from the mangrove endophytic fungus *Aspergillus* sp. SK-28, which was obtained from *Kandelia candel* from the Shankou Mangrove Nature Reserve in Guangxi Province, China. Compound **170** could inhibit the growth of the barnacle *Balanus reticulatus* with antifouling activity and low toxicity [89]. Three novel DKPs, saroclazines A−C (**171**−**173**), were isolated from the fungus *Sarocladium kiliense* HDN11-84, which was obtained from a root soil sample of mangrove *Thespesia populnea* from Guangxi Province, China. Compound **171** exhibited cytotoxicity activity against Hela cell lines with the IC$_{50}$ value of 4.2 µM [90].

Fifteen novel DKPs, brocazines A−F (**174**−**179**), penicibrocazines A−E (**180**−**184**), spirobrocazines A−C (**185**−**187**) and brocazine G (**188**) were obtained from the fungus *Penicillium brocae* MA-231, which was isolated from the marine mangrove plant *Avicennia marina* in Hainan Island. Compounds **174**–**177** showed potent cytotoxic activities against Du145 (human prostate carcinoma), Hela, HepG2, MCF-7, NCI-H460 (human non-small cell lung cancer), SGC-7901 (human gastric carcinoma), SW1990 (human pancreatic adenocarcinoma) and U251 cell lines with the IC$_{50}$ values in the range of 0.89–12.4 µM [91]. Compounds **182** and **184** exhibited antimicrobial activities against *S. aureus* and *Gaeumannomyces graminis* with the MIC values ranging from 0.25 to 32.0 µg/mL, respectively, and compound **183** also showed antimicrobial activities against *S. aureus* and *Micrococcus luteus* with the MIC values of 0.25 µg/mL [92]. In addition, compounds **185** and **187** showed modest antimicrobial activities against *E. coli* and *Vibrio harveyi* with the MIC values in the range of 32–64 µg/mL. Compound **188** exhibited significant cytotoxic activities against A2780 and A2780 CisR cell lines with the IC$_{50}$ values of 664 and 661 nM, respectively, and had potent antimicrobial activity against *S. aureus* with an MIC value of 0.25 µg/mL [91,93]. These results showed that compounds possessing two double bonds at C-6 and C-6' or one double bond at C-6/6' conjugating with a keto group at C-5/5' might exhibit higher cytotoxic or antimicrobial activity. All 23 DKPs from mangrove-derived fungi described above are presented in Figure 6.

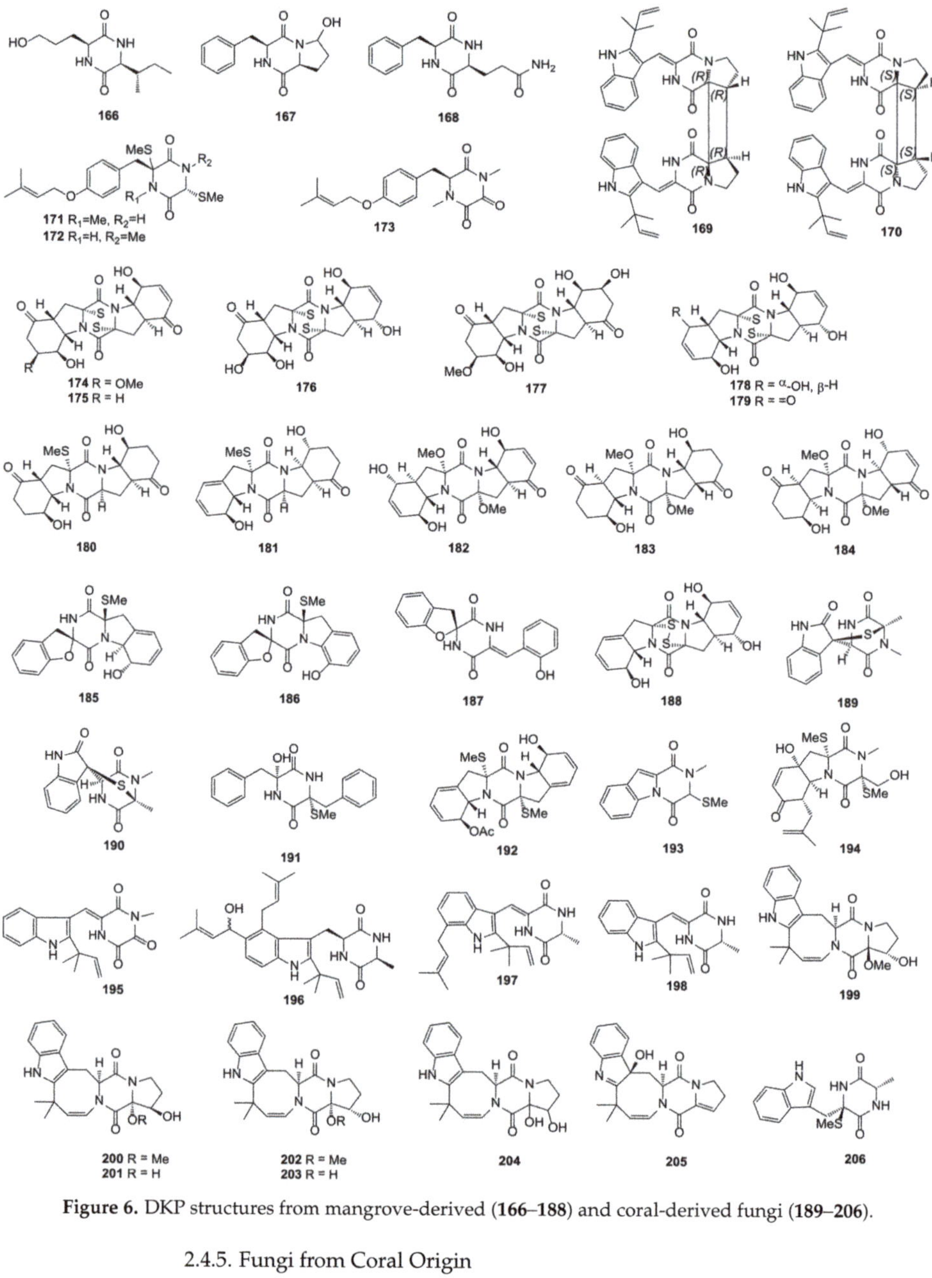

Figure 6. DKP structures from mangrove-derived (**166–188**) and coral-derived fungi (**189–206**).

2.4.5. Fungi from Coral Origin

Pseudellones A (**189**) and B (**190**), two new DKPs containing an irregular bridge, were separated from the fungus *Pseudallescheria ellipsoidea* F42−3 derived from the soft coral *Lobophytum crassum* in Hainan Sanya National Coral Reef Reserve, China [94]. Pseuboydones C (**191**) and D (**192**) were isolated from the fungus *Pseudallescheria boydii* F19-1 collected from the soft coral *L. crassum*. Compound **191** exhibited remarkable cytotoxic activity against Sf9 cell lines with an IC_{50} value of 0.7 µM [95]. Fungus *Dichotomomyces cejpii* F31-1 was collected from the soft coral *L. crassum* and two novel DKPs namely dichocerazines A (**193**) and B (**194**) were then obtained from the GPY medium (added L-tryptophan and L-phenylalanine) of the fungus. These two compounds showed no activity for the tested HCT116, RD (human rhabdomyosarcoma), ACHN (human renal carcinoma) and A2780T cell lines [96]. Three new DKPs alkaloids namely 11-methylneoechinulin E (**195**), variecolorin M (**196**) and (+)-variecolorin G (**197**) and a DKP first discovered in nature namely (+)-neoechinulin A (**198**) were obtained from the fungus *Aspergillus* sp. EGF 15-0-3, which was isolated from a soft coral in the South China Sea. Compounds **195–198** showed cytotoxic activity against NCI-H1975 gefitinib resistance cell lines at the concentration of 50 μM [97].

16α-hydroxy-17β-methoxy-deoxydihydroisoaustamide (**199**), 16β-hydroxy-17α-methoxy-deoxydihydroisoaustamide (**200**), 16β,17α-dihydroxy-deoxydihydroisoaustamide (**201**), 16α-hydroxy-17α-methoxy-deoxydihydroisoaustamide (**202**), 16α,17α-dihydroxy-deoxydihydroisoaustamide (**203**), 16,17-dihydroxy-deoxydihydroisoaustamide (**204**) and 3β-hydroxy-deoxyisoaustamide (**205**), seven new DKPs containing a prenylated indole ring, were obtained from the fungus *Penicillium dimorphosporum* KMM 4689, which was separated from an unidentified soft coral in the South China Sea. When the murine neuroblastoma Neuro-2a cells were treated with the mixture of 500 μM paraquat (PQ) and 1 μM each of compounds **202**, **203** and **204**, the cell viability was increased by 38.6%, 30.3% and 36.5%, respectively, compared with the treatment of PQ alone. The hydroxy groups at C-16 and C-17 played a key role in neuroprotective activity by the analysis of structure–activity relationships [98]. Pseudellone D (**206**), a novel DKP alkaloid possessing a rare monomethylthio group, was isolated from the fungus *Pseudallescheria ellipsoidea* F42-3 sourced from the soft coral *Lobophytum crissum* [99]. All 18 DKPs from coral-derived fungi described above are presented in Figure 6.

2.4.6. Fungi from Alga Origin

Dehydroxymethylbis(dethio)bis(methylthio)gliotoxin (**207**) and (3S,6R)-6-(para-hydroxybenzyl)-1,4-dimethyl-3,6-bis(methylthio)piperazine-2,5-dione (**208**), two novel sulphurated DKPs, were obtained from the fungus *Trichoderma virens* Y13-3 derived from the marine red alga *Gracilaria vermiculophylla* in Yangma Island [100]. Methylcordysinin A (**209**) was separated from *Trichoderma asperellum* cf44-2, which was collected from brown alga *Sargassum* sp. in Zhoushan Islands [101]. Four new DKP alkaloids named citriperazines A-D (**210–213**) were separated from *Penicillium* sp. KMM 4672 obtained from the Vietnamese marine brown algae *Padina* sp. [102]. Compounds **207–213** showed no inhibitory activities for the tested bacteria or cancer cell lines. The endophytic fungus *Acrostalagmus luteoalbus* TK-43 was isolated from the green algal *Codium fragile* collected in Sinop, Turkey, and six novel N-methoxy-containing indole DKPs, namely (±) acrozines A–C (**214–219**), were obtained from the strain. Compound **216** exhibited moderate antimicrobial activity against the plant pathogen *Fusarium solani* (MIC = 32 μg/mL). Compounds **214** and **215** possessed antiacetylcholinesterase activities with the IC_{50} values of 2.3 and 13.8 μM, respectively. This result indicated that the bioactivity was concerned with the absolute configurations of these compounds [103].

One new DKP namely cyclo(L-5-MeO-Pro-L-5-MeO-Pro) (**220**) was isolated from the fungus *Trichoderma asperellum* A-YMD-9-2, which was obtained from marine macroalga *Gracilaria verrucose* collected from Yangma Island. Compound **220** exhibited inhibitory activities against *Chattonella marina*, *Heterosigma akashiwo*, *Karlodinium veneficum* and *Prorocentrum donghaiense* with the EC_{50} values of 47.3, 276, 327 and 351 μM, respectively [104]. Three novel sulfur-containing DKPs namely pretrichodermamides D–F (**221–223**) were separated from the fungus *Penicillium* sp. KMM 4672, which was obtained from the Vietnamese brown alga *Padina* sp. These compounds did not show potent activities for the human prostate cancer 22Rv1 cells [105]. Four new DKP alkaloids namely N-(4′-hydroxyprenyl)-cyclo(alanyltryptophyl) (**224**), isovariecolorin I (**225**), 30-hydroxyechinulin (**226**) and 29-hydroxyechinulin (**227**) were obtained from the fungus *Eurotium cristatum* EN-220, which was collected from marine alga *Sargassum thunbergia* on the coast of Qingdao, China. Compound **225** showed brine shrimp (*A. salina*) lethal activity with the LD$_{50}$ value of 19.4 μg/mL and had moderate antioxidative activities with an IC$_{50}$ value of 20.6 μg/mL [106]. (±)-Brevianamides X (**228** and **229**) were obtained from the fungus *Aspergillus versicolor* OUCMDZ-2738 isolated from alga *Enteromorpha prolifera*, which was collected from Shilaoren beach, Qingdao, China, and showed no antimicrobial activities [107]. All 23 DKPs from alga-derived fungi described above are presented in Figure 7.

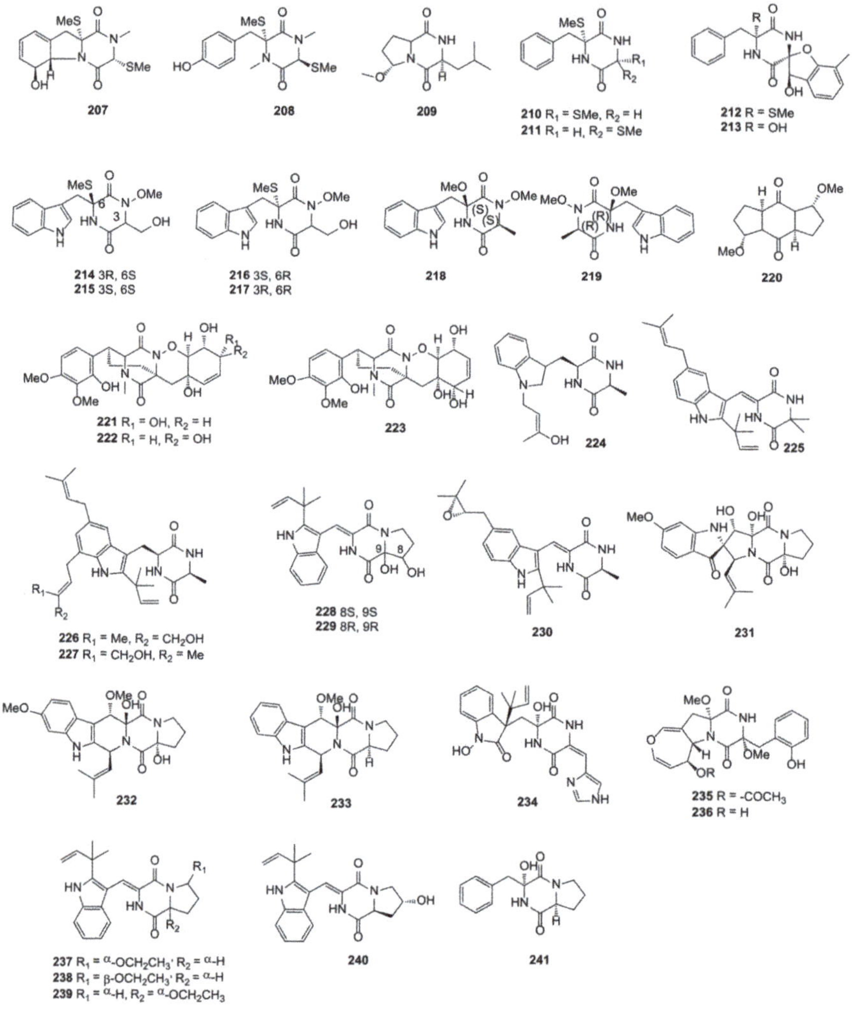

Figure 7. DKP structures from alga-derived (**207–229**) and other sourced fungi (**230–241**).

2.4.7. Fungi from Other Origin

One novel DKP namely isoechinulin D (**230**) was isolated from the marine fungus *Eurotium rubrum* MPUC136, which was collected from the seaweed in Chosei-mura, Chosei-gun, Chiba Prefecture, Japan, and showed weak inhibitory activity against melanin synthesis with an IC$_{50}$ value of 60 μM [108]. Spirotryprostatin G (**231**), cyclotryprostatins F (**232**) and G (**233**), three new DKPs alkaloids, were isolated from the fungus *Penicillium brasilianum* HBU-136 separated from the Bohai Sea. Compound **231** showed excellent cytotoxic activity against HL-60 cell lines with an IC$_{50}$ value of 6.0 μM and compounds **232** and **233** exhibited remarkable cytotoxic activity against MCF-7 cell lines with IC_{50} values of 7.6 and 10.8 μM, respectively [109]. A new DKP alkaloid namely penilline C (**234**) was obtained from the fungus *Penicillium chrysogenum* SCSIO 07007, which was isolated from a deep-sea hydrothermal vent environment sample of Western Atlantic [110]. Emestrins L (**235**) and M (**236**), two novel DKPs, were separated from the fungus *Aspergillus terreus* RA2905, which was obtained from the sea hare *Aplysia pulmonica* from the Weizhou coral reefs in the South China Sea. Compound **236** showed antifungal activity against *P. aeruginosa* ATCC 27853 with the MIC value of 64 μg/mL [111].

Aspamides A–D (**237–240**), four novel DKPs alkaloids, were separated from the endophyte fungus *Aspergillus versicolor* DY180635, which was isolated from the sea crab *Chiromantes haematocheir* from the intertidal zone of Zhoushan, Zhejiang, China. For the virtual screening on the 3CL hydrolase (Mpro) of SARS-CoV-2 (potential drug target to fight COVID-19), the docking scores of compounds **237** and **238** were −5.389 and −4.772, respectively, and the score of positive control ritonavir was −7.039. In the future, these two compounds may be helpful in fighting COVID-19 [112]. One novel DKP namely penicillatide B (**241**) was isolated from the fungus *Penicillium* sp., which was collected from the Red Sea tunicate *Didemnum* sp. Compound **241** showed moderate cytotoxic activity against the HCT-116 cell lines with an IC_{50} value of 23.0 μM and exhibited modest antimicrobial activities against *S. aureus* and *V. anguillarum* with inhibition zones of 19 and 20 mm, respectively [113]. All 12 DKPs from fungi sourced from other origins described above are presented in Figure 7.

3. Chemical Structures of Diketopiperazine Derivatives from Marine Organisms

Diketopiperazine derivatives are further modified on the basis of the six-membered piperazine rigid backbone. The following 54 DKP derivatives were described in this paper, of which 53 lacked a carbonyl group and 1 lacked two carbonyl groups in the skeleton (Table 2).

Table 2. The bioactivities, strains and habitats of diketopiperazine derivatives during 2011–2021.

Sources	Compounds	Bioactivities	Species	Habitats	Refs
Actinomycetes	Isomethoxyneihumicin (**242** and **243**)	Cytotoxicity	*N. alba* KM6-1	Marine sediment	[114]
	Nocazine F (**244**)	Cytotoxicity	*Nocardiopsis* sp. YIM M13066	Deep-sea sediment	[115]
	Nocazine G (**245**)	Cytotoxicity Antimicrobial	*Nocardiopsis* sp. YIM M13066	Deep-sea sediment	[115]
	Streptopyrazinone A (**246**)	Antimicrobial	*Streptomyces* sp. ZZ446	Coastal soil	[44]
	Streptopyrazinone B (**247**)	Antimicrobial	*Streptomyces* sp. ZZ446	Coastal soil	[44]
	Streptopyrazinone C (**248**)	Antimicrobial	*Streptomyces* sp. ZZ446	Coastal soil	[44]
	Streptopyrazinone D (**249**)	Antimicrobial	*Streptomyces* sp. ZZ446	Coastal soil	[44]
	Streptopyrazinone (**250**)	Cytotoxicity	*Streptomyces* sp. B223	Marine sediment	[116]
	Nocazine A (**251**)	-	*N. dassonvillei* HR10-5	Estuary of Yellow River	[117]
	Nocazine B (**252**)	-	*N. dassonvillei* HR10-5	Estuary of Yellow River	[117]
Fungus	Varioloid A (**253**)	Antimicrobial	*P. variotii* EN-291	*G. turuturu*	[118]
	Varioloid B (**254**)	Antimicrobial	*P. variotii* EN-291	*G. turuturu*	[118]
	Oxepinamide H (**255**)	Transcriptional activation	*A. puniceus* SCSIO z021	Deep-sea sediment	[119]
	Oxepinamide I (**256**)	Transcriptional activation	*A. puniceus* SCSIO z021	Deep-sea sediment	[119]
	Oxepinamide J (**257**)	Transcriptional activation	*A. puniceus* SCSIO z021	Deep-sea sediment	[119]
	Oxepinamide K (**258**)	-	*A. puniceus* SCSIO z021	Deep-sea sediment	[119]
	Puniceloid A (**259**)	Transcriptional activation	*A. puniceus* SCSIO z021	Deep-sea sediment	[119]

Table 2. Cont.

Sources	Compounds	Bioactivities	Species	Habitats	Refs
	Puniceloid B (260)	Transcriptional activation	A. puniceus SCSIO z021	Deep-sea sediment	[119]
	Puniceloid C (261)	Transcriptional activation	A. puniceus SCSIO z021	Deep-sea sediment	[119]
	Puniceloid D (262)	Transcriptional activation Enzyme inhibition	A. puniceus SCSIO z021	Deep-sea sediment	[119]
	Protuboxepin C (263)	Cytotoxicity	Aspergillus sp. SCSIO XWS02F40	Callyspongia sp.	[120,121]
	Protuboxepin D (264)	Cytotoxicity	Aspergillus sp. SCSIO XWS02F40	Callyspongia sp.	[120,121]
	Pyranamide A (265)	-	A. versicolor SCSIO 41016	Sponge	[122]
	Pyranamide A (266)	-	A. versicolor SCSIO 41016	Sponge	[122]
	Pyranamide A (267)	-	A. versicolor SCSIO 41016	Sponge	[122]
	Pyranamide A (268)	-	A. versicolor SCSIO 41016	Sponge	[122]
	Secopyranamide C (269)	-	A. versicolor SCSIO 41016	Sponge	[122]
	Protuboxepin F (270)	Cytotoxicity	A. versicolor SCSIO 41016	Sponge	[122]
	Protuboxepin G (271)	-	A. versicolor SCSIO 41016	Sponge	[122]
	Protuboxepin H (272)	-	A. versicolor SCSIO 41016	Sponge	[122]
	Protuboxepin I (273)	-	A. versicolor SCSIO 41016	Sponge	[122]
	Protuboxepin J (274)	-	A. versicolor SCSIO 41016	Sponge	[122]
	Chrysopiperazine A (275)	-	P. chrysogenum	D. gemmacea	[123]
	Chrysopiperazine B (276)	-	P. chrysogenum	D. gemmacea	[123]
	Chrysopiperazine C (277)	-	P. chrysogenum	D. gemmacea	[123]
	Quinadoline D (278)	-	Penicillium sp. L129	L. sinense	[124]
	Aspamide F (279)	-	A. versicolor DY180635	C. haematocheir	[110]
	Aspamide G (280)	-	A. versicolor DY180635	C. haematocheir	[110]
	Polonimide A (281)	Enzyme inhibition	P. polonicum	Bohai Sea	[125]
	Polonimide B (282)	Enzyme inhibition	P. polonicum	Bohai Sea	[125]
	Polonimide C (283)	Enzyme inhibition	P. polonicum	Bohai Sea	[125]
	Protuboxepin K (284)	Enzyme inhibition	Aspergillus sp. BFM-0085	Marine sediment	[126]
	Varioxepine B (285)	Cytotoxicity	A. terreus	S. subviride	[127]
	3-Hydroxyprotuboxepin K (286)	Enzyme inhibition	A. creber EN-602	R. confervoides	[128]
	3,15-Hehydroprotuboxepin K (287)	Antimicrobial	A. creber EN-602	R. confervoides	[128]
	Versiamide A (288)	Antimicrobial	A. creber EN-602	R. confervoides	[128]
	Protuboxepin A (289)	Cytotoxicity	Aspergillus sp. SF-5044	Sediment	[129,130]
	Protuboxepin B (290)	-	Aspergillus sp. SF-5044	Sediment	[129,130]
	Carnequinazoline A (291)	-	A. carneus KMM 4638	L. sachalinensis	[131]
	Carnequinazoline B (292)	-	A. carneus KMM 4638	L. sachalinensis	[131]
	Carnequinazoline C (293)	-	A. carneus KMM 4638	L. sachalinensis	[131]
	Fumiquinazoline K (294)	-	A. fumigatus KMM 4631	Sinularia sp.	[132]
	3-[6-(2-Methylpropyl)-2-oxo-1H-pyrazin-3-yl]propanamide (295)	-	A. versicolor OUCMDZ-2738	E. prolifera	[107]

[a] The bioactivity was not mentioned.

3.1. Actinomycetes

A mixture of two new tautomers DKP derivatives named isomethoxyneihumicin (**242** and **243**) were obtained from the actinomycete *Nocardiopsis alba* KM6-1, which was collected from marine sediment in Chichijima, Ogasawara, Japan. The mixture showed excellent cytotoxic activity against Jurkat cell lines with the IC_{50} value of 6.98 µM and in a dose of 15 µM, compounds **242** and **243** made the cell cycle of Jurkat cell lines staying in the G2/M phase with the inhibition ratio of 66% in 12 h. These consequences indicated that the mixed compounds inhibited the growth of Jurkat cell lines via arresting the cell cycle at the G2/M phase [114]. Two novel DKP derivatives namely nocazines A (**244**) and B (**245**) were isolated from *Nocardiopsis dassonvillei* HR10-5, which was obtained from marine sediment in the estuary of Yellow River, Dongying, China. However, compounds **244** and **245** did not exhibit cytotoxic or antimicrobial activities for the tested cancer cell lines and microorganisms [115].

Nocazines F (**246**) and G (**247**), two novel DKP derivatives, were isolated from the *Nocardiopsis* sp. YIM M13066, which was collected from the deep-sea sediment. Compound **246** showed remarkable cytotoxic activities against the human cancer cell lines H1299 (non-small cell lung cancer), Hela, HL7702, MCF-7, PC3 and U251 with IC_{50} values of 3.87, 4.77, 7.10, 3.86 and 8.17 µM, respectively. Compound **247** also showed excellent cytotoxic activities against the human cancer cell lines H1299, Hela, HL7702 (human derived liver), MCF-7, PC3 and U251 with the IC_{50} values of 2.60, 3.97, 8.73, 6.67 and 16.7 µM, respectively, and exhibited modest antimicrobial activity against *B. subtilis* ATCC 6051 with the MIC value of 25.8 µM [116]. Streptopyrazinones A–D (**248–251**) were four new DKP derivatives and isolated from *Streptomyces* sp. ZZ446, which was collected from a coastal soil sample from Zhoushan Islands. Compounds **248–251** exhibited moderate antimicrobial activities against *C. albicans* and MRSA with the MIC values of 35–45 and 58–65 µg/mL, respectively [44]. One novel tricyclic DKP derivative namely strepyrazinone (**252**) was obtained from *Streptomyces* sp. B223, which was isolated from the marine sediment of Laizhou Bay. Compound **252** displayed remarkable cytotoxic activity against the HCT-116 cell lines with the IC_{50} value of 0.34 µM [117]. All 11 DKP derivatives from actinomycetes described above are presented in Figure 8.

3.2. Fungi

Varioloids A (**253**) and B (**254**) were two novel oxepine-containing DKP derivatives and obtained from the endophytic fungus *Paecilomyces variotii* EN-291, which was collected from red alga *Grateloupia turuturu* on the coast of Qingdao. Compounds **253** and **254** showed significant antimicrobial activities against *F. graminearum* with the MIC values of 8 and 4 µg/mL, respectively. In addition, compounds **253** and **254** also inhibited the growth of *A. hydrophila*, *E. coli*, *M. luteus*, *S. aureus*, *V. anguillarum*, *V. harveyi* and *V. parahaemolyticus* with the MIC values in the range of 16–64 µg/mL [118]. Four novel oxepine-containing DKP derivatives namely oxepinamides H−K (**255–258**) and four novel 4-quinazolinone DKP derivatives namely puniceloids A−D (**259–262**) were isolated from the fungus *Aspergillus puniceus* SCSIO z021, which was collected from deep-sea sediment in Okinawa Trough. Compounds **255–257** and **259–262** exhibited remarkable transcriptional activation of liver X receptor α with the EC_{50} values of 1.7–16 µM. This result suggested that the transcriptional activation activity of these compounds would be decreased when the benzene ring was converted into an oxepin unit. In addition, compound **262** possessed enzyme inhibitory activities against seven enzymes including TCPTP, SHP1, MEG2, SHP2, PTP1B, IDO1 and LDHA with the IC_{50} values in the range of 14–87 µM [119].

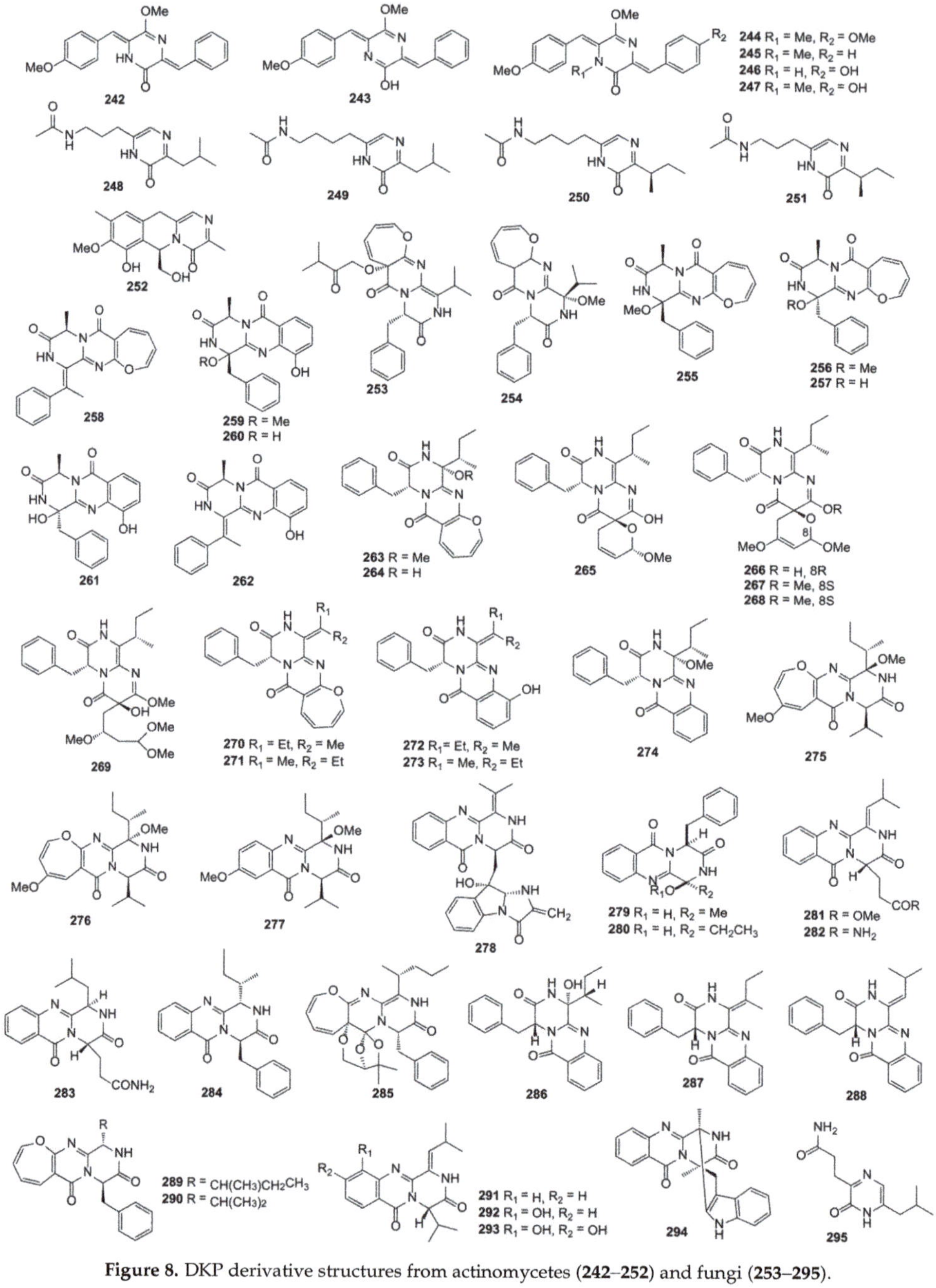

Figure 8. DKP derivative structures from actinomycetes (**242–252**) and fungi (**253–295**).

Protuboxepins C (**263**) and D (**264**), two novel oxepin-containing DKP derivatives, were obtained from the fungus *Aspergillus* sp. SCSIO XWS02F40, which was isolated from the sponge *Callyspongia* sp. from the sea area near Xuwen County, Guangdong Province, China. Compounds **263** and **264** showed moderate cytotoxic activities against Hela cell lines with the IC$_{50}$ values of 61 and 114 µM, respectively [120,121]. Pyranamides A–D (**265–**

268), secopyranamide C (**269**) and protuboxepins F−J (**270–274**), ten novel DKP derivatives, were isolated from the marine sponge-derived fungus *Aspergillus versicolor* SCSIO 41016, which was also separated from *Callyspongia* sp. Compound **270** showed modest cytotoxic activities against the ACHN, OS-RC-2 and 786-O cell lines (three renal carcinoma cell lines) with the IC$_{50}$ values of 27, 34.9 and 47.1 µM, respectively [122]. Chrysopiperazines A–C (**275–277**) were three new DKP derivatives and obtained from the fungus *Penicillium chrysogenum*, which was collected from gorgonian *Dichotella gemmacea* in South China Sea. The oxepine-containing DKPs were found from the genus *Penicillium* for the first time [123]. One novel DKP derivative namely quinadoline D (**278**) was isolated from the fungus *Penicillium* sp. L129, which was collected from the rhizosphere-soil of *Limonium sinense* (Girald) Kuntze from Yangkou Beach, Qingdao, China [124]. Two novel DKP derivatives namely aspamides F (**279**) and G (**280**) were isolated from the endophyte fungus *A. versicolor* DY180635. For the virtual screening on the 3CL hydrolase of SARS-CoV-2, the docking scores of compounds **279** and **280** were −5.146 and −4.962, respectively [112].

Polonimides A–C (**281–283**), three novel quinazoline-containing DKP derivatives, were isolated from the fungus *Penicillium polonicum* obtained from the Bohai Sea. Compounds **281–283** showed potent chitinase inhibitory activity against GH18 chitinase *Of*Chi-h with the inhibition rates of 91.9%, 79.1% and 86.1%, respectively [125]. Protuboxepin K (**284**) was obtained from the fungus *Aspergillus* sp. BFM-0085, which was collected from a marine sediment sample of Tokyo Bay. In mutant bone morphogenetic protein (BMP) receptor-carrying C2C12 (R206H) cells, compound **284** exhibited the BMP-induced alkaline phosphatase inhibitory activity with the IC$_{50}$ value of 4.7 µM [126]. One novel oxepine-containing DPK derivative namely varioxepine B (**285**) was isolated from the fungus *Aspergillus terreus*, which was collected from soft coral *Sarcophyton subviride* on Xisha Island. Compound **285** showed excellent inhibitory activity against Con A-induced murine splenocytes with the inhibition rates of 20%, 28%, 23% and 80% at the concentration of 64, 128, 256 and 512 nM, respectively, and had no effect on cell viability at the concentration of 100 µM. Meanwhile, compound **285** also remarkably decreased the cytokine (interferon-γ, interleukin-2 and tumor necrosis factor-α) production by activating murine splenocytes. Furthermore, compound **285** showed significant inhibitory activity against anti-CD3/anti-CD28 mAb-induced murine splenocytes, human T cell proliferation and Th1/Th2 cytokine production [127].

Three novel DKP derivatives namely 3-hydroxyprotuboxepin K (**286**), 3,15-dehydroprotuboxepin K (**287**) and versiamide A (**288**) were isolated from the fungus *Aspergillus creber* EN-602 derived from marine red alga *Rhodomela confervoides* on the coast of Qingdao, China. Compound **286** showed enzyme inhibitory activity against the angiotensin converting enzyme with the IC$_{50}$ value of 22.4 µM. In addition, compound **287** exhibited antimicrobial activities against *Edwardsiella tarda*, *E. coli*, *M. luteus*, *P. aeruginosa* and *V. harveyi* with the MIC values in the range of 8–64 µg/mL and compound **288** exhibited antimicrobial activities against *A. hydrophila*, *E. coli*, *M. luteus* and *P. aeruginosa* with the MIC values between 16 and 64 µg/mL [128]. Protuboxepins A (**289**) and B (**290**) were two novel oxepin-containing DKP derivatives and were isolated from the fungus *Aspergillus* sp. SF-5044, which was collected from the intertidal sediment from Dadaepo Beach, Busan, Korea. Compound **289** exhibited weak cytotoxic activities against HL-60, MDA-MB-231, Hep3B (human liver carcinoma), 3Y1 and K562 cell lines with the IC$_{50}$ values of 75, 130, 150, 180 and 250 µM, respectively. Compound **289** possessed a disrupting microtubule dynamics ability and induced apoptosis in cancer because it could bind to α,β-tubulin and stabilize tubulin polymerization and then leading to chromosome misalignment and metaphase arrest in cancer [129,130].

Carnequinazolines A–C (**291–293**), three novel DKP derivatives, were separated from the fungus *Aspergillus carneus* KMM 4638 collected from the marine brown alga *Laminaria sachalinensis*, which was isolated from Kunachir Island. Compounds **291** and **292** had no cytotoxicity and antimicrobial activities [131]. One novel alkaloid DKP derivative namely fumiquinazoline K (**294**) was obtained from the fungus *Aspergillus fumigatus* KMM

4631, which was separated from soft coral *Sinularia* sp. in Kuril islands, and showed no enzyme inhibition and cytotoxic activities [132]. 3-[6-(2-Methylpropyl)-2-oxo-1H-pyrazin-3-yl]propanamide (**295**) was obtained from the fungus *Aspergillus versicolor* OUCMDZ-2738, and exhibited no antimicrobial and α-glucosidase inhibitory activity [107]. All 43 DKP derivatives from fungi described above are presented in Figure 8.

4. Characteristics of Bioactive Diketopiperazines and Their Derivatives from Marine Organisms

In this review, 241 DKPs and 54 DKP derivatives isolated from marine organisms were summarized, among which fungi and actinomycetes were the most abundant sources. These marine organisms come from a wide range of sources and the red dots (Figure 9) and yellow dots (Figure 10) represent the collection points for marine biological samples, which produced DKPs and DKP derivatives, respectively. DKPs and DKP derivatives of fungi sources were 199 (82.6%) and 43 (79.6%), respectively, and those of actinomycetes sources were 25 (10.4%) and 11 (20.4%), respectively (Figure 11a,b). In addition, DKPs of sponge and bacteria sources were 5 (2.1%) and 12 (5%), respectively (Figure 11a).

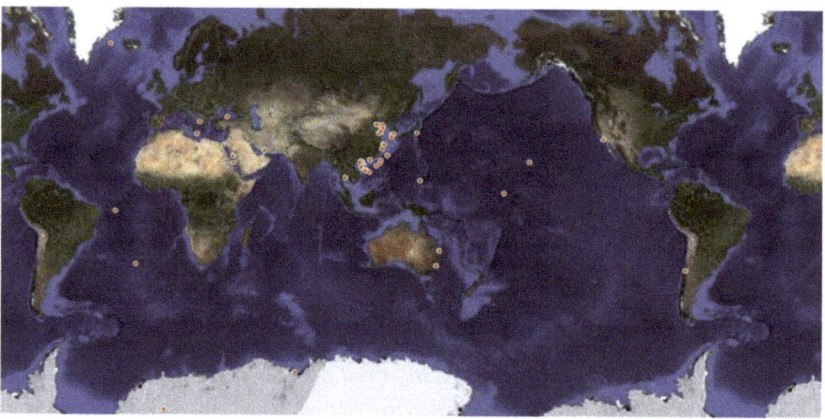

Figure 9. Collection points for marine biological samples producing DKPs (red dots).

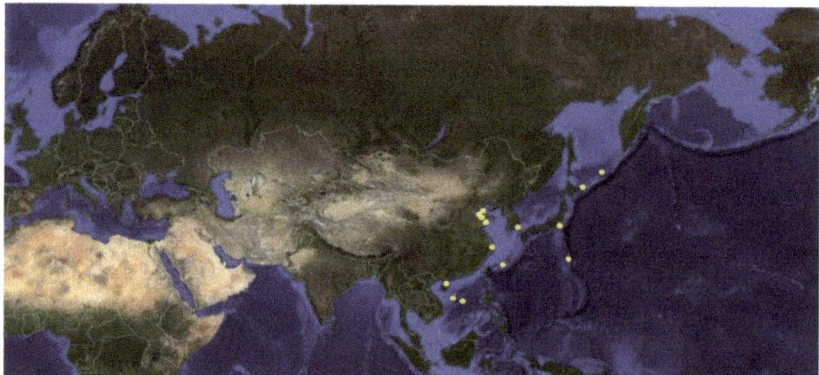

Figure 10. Collection points for marine biological samples producing DKP derivatives (yellow dots).

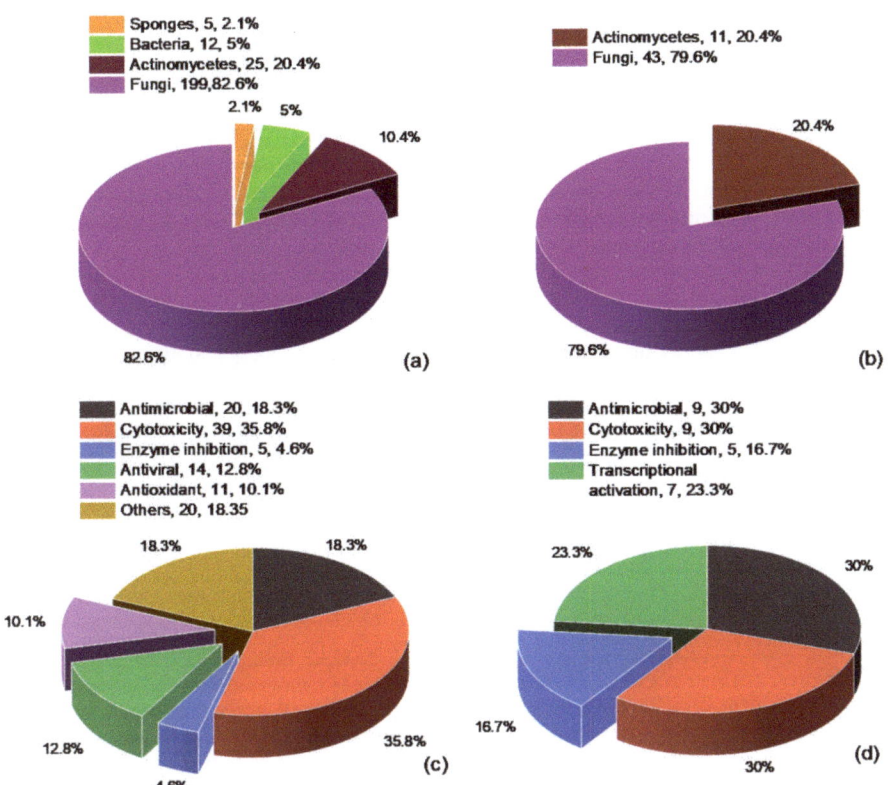

Figure 11. The proportion of DKPs from sponges, bacteria, actinomycetes and fungi (**a**); the proportion of DKP derivatives from actinomycetes and fungi (**b**); the proportion of antimicrobial, cytotoxicity, enzyme inhibition, antiviral, antioxidant and other activities of DKPs (**c**); the proportion of antimicrobial, cytotoxicity, enzyme inhibition and transcriptional activation activities of DKP derivatives (**d**).

These DKPs had antimicrobial (20, 18.3%), cytotoxic (39, 35.8%), enzyme inhibition (5, 4.6%), antiviral (14, 12.8%), antioxidant (11, 10.1%) and other activities (20, 18.3%) (Figure 11c). Furthermore, these DKP derivatives also had antimicrobial (9, 30%), cytotoxicity (9, 30%), enzyme inhibition (5, 16.7%) activities and a possessed transcriptional activation (7, 23.3%) effect (Figure 11d). Subtle differences in chemical structures are closely related to the bioactivity. For example, compound **96** possessing a unique disulfide bridge in the six-membered piperazine skeleton showed much more significant cytotoxic activity than compounds **93–95**, **97** and **98**. Compounds **163** and **165** exhibited remarkable antiproliferative activities but compound **164** was inactive, which indicated that the N–O bond played an important role for their bioactivity. In addition, the absolute configurations might be closely associated with the activity intensity. For instance, the antioxidant activity of compounds **144** (IC$_{50}$ = 37 μM) and **145** (IC$_{50}$ = 69 μM) were relevant to the absolute configurations of C-2 and C-3. Different substituents in the same chemical skeleton may lead to different activities. For example, compound **158** bearing a Cl atom at C-7 exhibited stronger antimicrobial and brine shrimp inhibition activity than compound **159**.

5. Conclusions

In recent years, the number of papers and patents related to DKPs is on the rise continuously and many novel DKPs had been isolated from marine sources. More and more researchers are turning their attention to the six-membered ring rigid structure with great potential for biological activity. It is a heterocyclic scaffold with restricted conformation, which can control stereochemistry at up to four positions. These features provide its potential to break the planarity of traditional drugs. Natural DKPs have more interesting structural complexity and biological characteristics and possibly can be further chemically synthesized or modified to increase their activity, promoting the natural product and synthetic chemistry to complement each other. In addition, DKPs can be used as the quorum sensing signal molecule of *Shewanella baltica* (a kind of unique microorganism produced during transporting the large yellow croaker at 4 °C) and inhibiting the production of DKPs can slow down the spoilage of the large yellow croaker [7]. Furthermore, thaxtomin A has good herbicidal activity and achieves an herbicidal purpose by inhibiting cellulose synthesis [133]. With the tremendous advancement of technology, the known compound can be initially eliminated through the Global Natural Products Social (GNPS) molecular networking project [134]. It would be helpful for targeting directly to discover new natural DKPs and further enrich the library of DKPs.

To sum up, DKPs are potential bioactive chemical substances that are valuable for further exploration from natural sources, especially from marine environments. The conversion of promising bioactive DKPs into clinical drugs for the treatment of diseases needs much more time and energy for researchers. DKPs are regarded as unprocessed diamonds, attracting scientists to take efforts to study their pharmacological properties and therapeutic effects.

Author Contributions: Z.S. wrote the paper, Y.H., Q.Y. and X.L. checked the paper, S.W. verified the content. All authors have read and agreed to the published version of the manuscript.

Funding: This research was funded by the National Natural Science Foundation of China (grant number 81860634), Applied Basic Research Key Project of Yunnan Province (grant number 202001BB050029), Major Science and Technology Projects of Yunnan Province (Digitalization, development and application of biotic resource, grant number 202002AA100007), Project of Innovative Research Team of Yunnan Province (grant number 202005AE160005), and Science Research Foundation of Yunnan Province Education Department (grant number 2021Y041).

Institutional Review Board Statement: Not applicable.

Informed Consent Statement: Not applicable.

Data Availability Statement: All data in this article is openly available without any restrictions.

Conflicts of Interest: The authors declare no conflict of interest.

References

1. Zhao, K.L.; Xing, R.R.; Yan, X.H. Cyclic dipeptides: Biological activities and self-assembled materials. *Pept. Sci.* **2021**, *113*, 13. [CrossRef]
2. Zhao, P.C.; Xue, Y.; Li, J.H.; Li, X.; Zu, X.Y.; Zhao, Z.Q.; Quan, C.S.; Gao, W.N.; Feng, S.X. Non-lipopeptide fungi-derived peptide antibiotics developed since 2000. *Biotechnol. Lett.* **2019**, *41*, 651–673. [CrossRef] [PubMed]
3. Borgman, P.; Lopez, R.D.; Lane, A.L. The expanding spectrum of diketopiperazine natural product biosynthetic pathways containing cyclodipeptide synthases. *Org. Biomol. Chem.* **2019**, *17*, 2305–2314. [CrossRef] [PubMed]
4. Borthwick, A.D. 2,5-Diketopiperazines: Synthesis, reactions, medicinal chemistry, and bioactive natural products. *Chem. Rev.* **2012**, *112*, 3641–3716. [CrossRef] [PubMed]
5. Huang, R.; Zhou, X.; Xu, T.; Yang, X.; Liu, Y. Diketopiperazines from marine organisms. *Chem. Biodivers.* **2010**, *7*, 2809–2829. [CrossRef] [PubMed]
6. Guan, J. Insulin-like growth factor-1 and its derivatives: Potential pharmaceutical application for ischemic brain injury. *Recent Pat. CNS Drug Discov.* **2008**, *3*, 112–127. [CrossRef] [PubMed]
7. Zhu, J.L.; Zhang, Y.W.; Deng, J.M.; Jiang, H.Y.; Zhuang, L.M.; Ye, W.; Ma, J.Y.; Jiang, J.Y.; Feng, L.F. Diketopiperazines synthesis gene in *Shewanella baltica* and roles of diketopiperazines and resveratrol in quorum sensing. *J. Agric. Food Chem.* **2019**, *67*, 12013–12025. [CrossRef] [PubMed]
8. Feng, L.; Bi, W.; Chen, S.; Zhu, J.; Liu, X. Regulatory function of sigma factors RpoS/RpoN in adaptation and spoilage potential of *Shewanella baltica*. *Food Microbiol.* **2021**, *97*, 103755. [CrossRef]
9. Turkez, H.; Cacciatore, I.; Arslan, M.E.; Fornasari, E.; Marinelli, L.; Di Stefano, A.; Mardinoglu, A. Histidyl-proline diketopiperazine isomers as multipotent anti-alzheimer drug candidates. *Biomolecules* **2020**, *10*, 737. [CrossRef] [PubMed]

10. Ding, Z.P.; Li, F.F.; Zhong, C.J.; Li, F.; Liu, Y.Q.; Wang, S.X.; Zhao, J.C.; Li, W.B. Structure-based design and synthesis of novel furan-diketopiperazine-type derivatives as potent microtubule inhibitors for treating cancer. *Bioorg. Med. Chem.* **2020**, *28*, 16. [CrossRef]
11. Deigin, V.; Ksenofontova, O.; Yatskin, O.; Goryacheva, A.; Ignatova, A.; Feofanov, A.; Ivanov, V. Novel platform for the preparation of synthetic orally active peptidomimetics with hemoregulating activity. II. Hemosuppressor activity of 2,5-diketopiperazine-based cyclopeptides. *Int. Immunopharmacol.* **2020**, *81*, 106185. [CrossRef] [PubMed]
12. Kamiya, T.; Maeno, S.; Hashimoto, M.; Mine, Y. Bicyclomycin, a new antibiotic. II. Structural elucidation and acyl derivatives. *J. Antibiot.* **1972**, *25*, 576–581. [CrossRef]
13. Kohn, H.; Widger, W. The molecular basis for the mode of action of bicyclomycin. *Curr. Drug Targets Infect. Disord.* **2005**, *5*, 273–295. [CrossRef] [PubMed]
14. De Carvalho, M.P.; Abraham, W.R. Antimicrobial and biofilm inhibiting diketopiperazines. *Curr. Med. Chem.* **2012**, *19*, 3564–3577. [CrossRef]
15. Hauser, D.; Weber, H.P.; Sigg, H.P. Isolation and configuration of chaetocin. *Helv. Chim. Acta.* **1970**, *53*, 1061–1073. [CrossRef]
16. Greiner, D.; Bonaldi, T.; Eskeland, R.; Roemer, E.; Imhof, A. Identification of a specific inhibitor of the histone methyltransferase SU(VAR)3-9. *Nat. Chem. Biol.* **2005**, *1*, 143–145. [CrossRef]
17. Isham, C.R.; Tibodeau, J.D.; Jin, W.; Xu, R.F.; Timm, M.M.; Bible, K.C. Chaetocin: A promising new antimyeloma agent with in vitro and in vivo activity mediated via imposition of oxidative stress. *Blood* **2008**, *109*, 2579–2588. [CrossRef]
18. Jeong, P.S.; Sim, B.W.; Park, S.H.; Kim, M.J.; Kang, H.G.; Nanjidsuren, T.; Lee, S.; Song, B.S.; Koo, D.B.; Kim, S.U. Chaetocin improves pig cloning efficiency by enhancing epigenetic reprogramming and autophagic activity. *Int. J. Mol. Sci.* **2020**, *21*, 4836. [CrossRef]
19. Liang, Y.D.; Liu, X.; Zhou, R.P.; Song, D.W.; Jiang, Y.Z.; Xue, W.W. Chaetocin promotes osteogenic differentiation via modulating Wnt/Beta-Catenin signaling in mesenchymal stem cells. *Stem. Cells. Int.* **2021**, *2021*, 6. [CrossRef]
20. Nicholson, B.; Lloyd, G.K.; Miller, B.R.; Palladino, M.A.; Kiso, Y.; Hayashi, Y.; Neuteboom, S.T.C. NPI-2358 is a tubulin-depolymerizing agent: In-vitro evidence for activity as a tumor vascular-disrupting agent. *Anti-Cancer Drugs* **2006**, *17*, 25–31. [CrossRef]
21. Heist, R.; Aren, O.; Millward, M.; Mainwaring, P.; Mita, A.; Mita, M.; Bazhenova, L.; Blum, R.; Polikoff, J.; Gadgeel, S.; et al. Phase 1/2 study of the vascular disrupting agent (VDA) plinabulin (NPI-2358) combined with docetaxel in patients with non-small cell lung cancer (NSCLC). *Mol. Cancer Ther.* **2009**, *8*, 3. [CrossRef]
22. Natoli, M.; Herzig, P.; Bejestani, E.P.; Buchi, M.; Ritschard, R.; Lloyd, G.K.; Mohanlal, R.; Tonra, J.R.; Huang, L.; Heinzelmann, V.; et al. Plinabulin, a distinct microtubule-targeting chemotherapy, promotes M1-Like macrophage polarization and nti-tumor immunity. *Front. Oncol.* **2021**, *11*, 14. [CrossRef] [PubMed]
23. Cornacchia, C.; Cacciatore, I.; Baldassarre, L.; Mollica, A.; Feliciani, F.; Pinnen, F. 2,5-Diketopiperazines as neuroprotective agents. *Mini-Rev. Med. Chem.* **2012**, *12*, 2–12. [CrossRef] [PubMed]
24. Virgone-Carlotta, A.; Dufour, E.; Bacot, S.; Ahmadi, M.; Cornou, M.; Moni, L.; Garcia, J.; Chierici, S.; Garin, D.; Marti-Batlle, D.; et al. New diketopiperazines as vectors for peptide protection and brain delivery: Synthesis and biological evaluation. *J. Label. Compd. Radiopharm.* **2016**, *59*, 517–530. [CrossRef]
25. Wang, Y.; Wang, P.; Ma, H.G.; Zhu, W.M. Developments around the bioactive diketopiperazines: A patent review. *Expert Opin. Ther. Pat.* **2013**, *23*, 1415–1433. [CrossRef] [PubMed]
26. Apostolopoulos, V.; Bojarska, J.; Chai, T.T.; Elnagdy, S.; Kaczmarek, K.; Matsoukas, J.; New, R.; Parang, K.; Lopez, O.P.; Parhiz, H.; et al. A global review on short peptides: Frontiers and perspectives. *Molecules* **2021**, *26*, 430. [CrossRef]
27. Cao, J.; Wang, B.-G. Chemical diversity and biological function of indolediketopiperazines from marine-derived fungi. *Mar. Life Sci. Technol.* **2020**, *2*, 31–40. [CrossRef]
28. Gomes, N.G.M.; Pereira, R.B.; Andrade, P.B.; Valentao, P. Double the chemistry, double the fun: Structural diversity and biological activity of marine-derived diketopiperazine dimers. *Mar. Drugs* **2019**, *17*, 551. [CrossRef] [PubMed]
29. Huang, R.M.; Yi, X.X.; Zhou, Y.Y.; Su, X.D.; Peng, Y.; Gao, C.H. An update on 2,5-diketopiperazines from marine organisms. *Mar. Drugs* **2014**, *12*, 6213–6235. [CrossRef]
30. Yang, B.; Huang, J.X.; Lin, X.P.; Zhang, Y.Y.; Tao, H.M.; Liu, Y.H. A new diketopiperazine from the marine sponge callyspongia species. *Molecules* **2010**, *15*, 871–877. [CrossRef]
31. Di, X.X.; Rouger, C.; Hardardottir, I.; Freysdottir, J.; Molinski, T.F.; Tasdemir, D.; Omarsdottir, S. 6-Bromoindole derivatives from the icelandic marine sponge geodia barretti: Isolation and anti-inflammatory activity. *Mar. Drugs* **2018**, *16*, 437. [CrossRef] [PubMed]
32. Zhang, H.; Lai, W.; Guan, Z.B.; Liao, X.J.; Zhao, B.X.; Xu, S.H. A new thiodiketopiperzaine from the marine sponge *Tedania* sp. *Nat. Prod. Res.* **2019**, *34*, 1113–1117. [CrossRef] [PubMed]
33. Kouchaksaraee, R.M.; Farimani, M.M.; Li, F.J.; Nazemi, M.; Tasdemir, D. Integrating molecular networking and (1)H NMR spectroscopy for isolation of bioactive metabolites from the Persian Gulf Sponge *Axinella sinoxea*. *Mar. Drugs* **2020**, *18*, 366. [CrossRef] [PubMed]
34. Sun, S.W.; Dai, X.Y.; Sun, J.; Bu, X.G.; Weng, C.H.; Li, H.; Zhu, H. A diketopiperazine factor from *Rheinheimera aquimaris* QSI02 exhibits anti-quorum sensing activity. *Sci. Rep.* **2016**, *6*, 39637. [CrossRef]

35. Andi, R.R.; Muntaz, A.B.; Nurul, N.A.R.; Abdul, M.A.M.; Azira, M.; Rozida, M.K. Diketopiperazine produced by psychrophilic yeast *Glaciozyma antarctica* PI12. *Malays. J. Anal. Sci.* **2017**, *21*. [CrossRef]
36. Bhattacharya, D.; Lai, T.K.; Saha, A.; Selvin, J.; Mukherjee, J. Structural elucidation and antimicrobial activity of a diketopiperazine isolated from a Bacillus sp. associated with the marine sponge *Spongia officinalis*. *Nat. Prod. Res.* **2019**, *10*, 1–9. [CrossRef]
37. Ding, L.J.; Xu, P.; Zhang, W.Y.; Yuan, Y.; He, X.P.; Su, D.Q.; Shi, Y.T.; Naman, C.B.; Yan, X.J.; Wu, B.; et al. Three new diketopiperazines from the previously uncultivable marine bacterium *Gallaecimonas mangrovi* HK-28 cultivated by iChip. *Chem. Biodivers.* **2020**, *17*, 6. [CrossRef] [PubMed]
38. Harizani, M.; Katsini, E.; Georgantea, P.; Roussis, V.; Ioannou, E. New chlorinated 2,5-diketopiperazines from marine-derived bacteria isolated from sediments of the eastern Mediterranean Sea. *Molecules* **2020**, *25*, 509. [CrossRef] [PubMed]
39. Xiong, Z.Q.; Liu, Q.X.; Pan, Z.L.; Zhao, N.; Feng, Z.X.; Wang, Y. Diversity and bioprospecting of culturable actinomycetes from marine sediment of the Yellow Sea, China. *Arch. Microbiol.* **2014**, *197*, 299–309. [CrossRef]
40. Buedenbender, L.; Grkovic, T.; Duffy, S.; Kurtboke, D.I.; Avery, V.M.; Carroll, A.R. Naseseazine C, a new anti-plasmodial dimeric diketopiperazine from a marine sediment derived *Streptomyces* sp. *Tetrahedron. Lett.* **2016**, *57*, 5893–5895. [CrossRef]
41. Luo, M.H.; Tang, G.L.; Ju, J.H.; Lu, L.C.; Huang, H.B. A new diketopiperazine derivative from a deep sea-derived *Streptomyces* sp. SCSIO 04496. *Nat. Prod. Res.* **2016**, *30*, 138–143. [CrossRef] [PubMed]
42. Lan, Y.X.; Zou, Y.; Huang, T.T.; Wang, X.Z.; Brock, N.L.; Deng, Z.X.; Lin, S.J. Indole methylation protects diketopiperazine configuration in the maremycin biosynthetic pathway. *Sci. China Chem.* **2016**, *59*, 1224–1228. [CrossRef]
43. Ou, Y.X.; Huang, J.F.; Li, X.M.; Kang, Q.J.; Pan, Y.T. Three new 2,5-diketopiperazines from the fish intestinal *Streptomyces* sp. MNU FJ-36. *Nat. Prod. Res.* **2016**, *30*, 1771–1775. [CrossRef]
44. Chen, M.X.; Chai, W.Y.; Zhu, R.Y.; Song, T.F.; Zhang, Z.Z.; Lian, X.Y. Streptopyrazinones A–D, rare metabolites from marine-derived *Streptomyces* sp ZZ446. *Tetrahedron* **2018**, *74*, 2100–2106. [CrossRef]
45. Chen, S.L.; Zhang, D.; Chen, M.X.; Zhang, Z.Z.; Lian, X.Y. A rare diketopiperazine glycoside from marine-sourced *Streptomyces* sp. ZZ446. *Nat. Prod. Res.* **2018**, *34*, 1046–1050. [CrossRef] [PubMed]
46. Shaala, L.A.; Youssef, D.T.A.; Badr, J.M.; Harakeh, S.M.; Genta-Jouve, G. Bioactive diketopiperazines and nucleoside derivatives from a sponge-derived *Streptomyces* species. *Mar. Drugs* **2019**, *17*, 584. [CrossRef] [PubMed]
47. Yi, W.W.; Qin, L.; Lian, X.Y.; Zhang, Z.Z. New antifungal metabolites from the Mariana Trench sediment-associated actinomycete *Streptomyces* sp. SY1965. *Mar. Drugs* **2020**, *18*, 385. [CrossRef]
48. Lin, C.K.; Wang, Y.T.; Hung, E.M.; Yang, Y.L.; Lee, J.C.; Sheu, J.H.; Liaw, C.C. Butyrolactones and diketopiperazines from marine microbes: Inhibition effects on dengue virus Type 2 replication. *Planta Med.* **2017**, *83*, 158–163. [CrossRef] [PubMed]
49. Zhou, H.Y.; Yang, X.M.; Li, F.; Yi, X.X.; Yu, L.; Gao, C.H.; Huang, R.M. A new diketopiperazine of *Nocardiopsis* alba isolated from *Anthogorgia caerulea*. *Chem. Nat. Compd.* **2017**, *53*, 338–340. [CrossRef]
50. Kim, M.C.; Cullum, R.; Machado, H.; Smith, A.J.; Yang, I.; Rodvold, J.J.; Fenical, W. Photopiperazines A–D, photosensitive interconverting diketopiperazines with significant and selective activity against U87 glioblastoma cells, from a rare, marine-derived actinomycete of the family *Streptomycetaceae*. *J. Nat. Prod.* **2019**, *82*, 2262–2267. [CrossRef] [PubMed]
51. Song, M.M.; Xie, Y.H.; Chen, W.H.; Hu, Y.W.; Zhao, K.; Liu, Y.H.; Huang, X.L.; Liu, Q.C.; Wang, J.F. Diketopiperazine and enterotoxin analogues from the mangrove derived-soil *Streptomyces* sp. SCSIO 41400 and their biological evaluation. *Nat. Prod. Res.* **2020**, 1–8. [CrossRef]
52. Fukuda, T.; Shinkai, M.; Sasaki, E.; Nagai, K.; Kurihara, Y.; Kanamoto, A.; Tomoda, H. Graphiumins, new thiodiketopiperazines from the marine-derived fungus *Graphium* sp. OPMF00224. *J. Antibiot.* **2015**, *68*, 620–627. [CrossRef] [PubMed]
53. Fukuda, T.; Nagai, K.; Kurihara, Y.; Kanamoto, A.; Tomoda, H. Graphiumins I and J, new thiodiketopiperazines from the marine-derived fungus *Graphium* sp. OPMF00224. *J. Antibiot.* **2015**, *21*, 255–260. [CrossRef] [PubMed]
54. Gu, B.B.; Zhang, Y.Y.; Ding, L.J.; He, S.; Wu, B.; Dong, J.D.; Zhu, P.; Chen, J.J.; Zhang, J.R.; Yan, X.J. Preparative separation of sulfur-containing diketopiperazines from marine fungus *Cladosporium* sp. using high-speed counter-current chromatography in stepwise elution mode. *Mar. Drugs* **2015**, *13*, 354–365. [CrossRef] [PubMed]
55. He, X.P.; Ding, L.J.; Yi, M.Q.; Xu, J.Z.; Zhou, X.Z.; Zhang, W.Y.; He, S. Separation of five diketopiperazines from the marine fungus *Alternaria alternate* HK-25 by high-speed counter-current chromatography. *J. Sep. Sci.* **2019**, *42*, 2510–2516. [CrossRef] [PubMed]
56. Kim, J.W.; Ko, S.K.; Son, S.; Shin, K.S.; Ryoo, I.J.; Hong, Y.S.; Oh, H.; Hwang, B.Y.; Hirota, H.; Takahashi, S.; et al. Haenamindole, an unusual diketopiperazine derivative from a marine-derived *Penicillium* sp. KCB12F005. *Bioorg. Med. Chem. Lett.* **2015**, *25*, 5398–5401. [CrossRef]
57. Hawas, U.W.; El-Kassem, L.T.A. Anticancer and antiviral diketopiperazine produced by the Red Sea endophytic fungus *Penicillium chrysogenum*. *Lett. Org. Chem.* **2019**, *16*, 409–414. [CrossRef]
58. Fan, Z.; Sun, Z.H.; Liu, Z.; Chen, Y.C.; Liu, H.X.; Li, H.H.; Zhang, W.M. Dichotocejpins A–C: New diketopiperazines from a deep-sea-derived fungus *Dichotomomyces cejpii* FS110. *Mar. Drugs* **2016**, *14*, 164. [CrossRef] [PubMed]
59. Yun, K.; Khong, T.T.; Leutou, A.S.; Kim, G.D.; Hong, J.; Lee, C.H.; Son, B.W. Cristazine, a new cytotoxic dioxopiperazinealkaloid from themudflat-sediment-derived fungus *Chaetomium cristatum*. *Chem. Pharm. Bull.* **2016**, *64*, 59–62. [CrossRef]
60. Jo, M.J.; Patil, M.P.; Jung, H.I.; Seo, Y.B.; Lim, H.K.; Son, B.W.; Kim, G.D. Cristazine, a novel dioxopiperazine alkaloid, induces apoptosis via the death receptor pathway in A431 cells. *Drug. Dev. Res.* **2019**, *80*, 504–512. [CrossRef]
61. Niu, S.W.; Liu, D.; Shao, Z.Z.; Proksch, P.; Lin, W.H. Eutypellazines N–S, new thiodiketopiperazines from a deep sea sediment derived fungus *Eutypella* sp. with anti-VRE activities. *Tetrahedron Lett.* **2017**, *58*, 3695–3699. [CrossRef]

62. Niu, S.W.; Liu, D.; Shao, Z.Z.; Proksch, P.; Lin, W.H. Eutypellazines A–M, thiodiketopiperazine-type alkaloids from deep sea derived fungus *Eutypella* sp. MCCC 3A00281. *RSC. Adv.* **2017**, *7*, 33580–33590. [CrossRef]
63. Liu, C.C.; Zhang, Z.Z.; Feng, Y.Y.; Gu, Q.Q.; Li, D.H.; Zhu, T.J. Secondary metabolites from Antarctic marine-derived fungus *Penicillium crustosum* HDN153086. *Nat. Prod. Res.* **2018**, *33*, 414–419. [CrossRef]
64. Niu, S.W.; Wang, N.; Xie, C.L.; Fan, Z.W.; Luo, Z.H.; Chen, H.F.; Yang, X.W. Roquefortine J, a novel roquefortine alkaloid, from the deep-sea-derived fungus *Penicillium granulatum* MCCC 3A00475. *J. Antibiot.* **2018**, *71*, 658–661. [CrossRef] [PubMed]
65. Niu, S.W.; Fan, Z.W.; Xie, C.L.; Liu, Q.M.; Luo, Z.H.; Liu, G.M.; Yang, X.W. Spirograterpene A, a tetracyclic spiro-diterpene with a fused 5/5/5/5 ring system from the deep-sea-derived fungus *Penicillium granulatum* MCCC 3A00475. *J. Nat. Prod.* **2017**, *80*, 2174–2177. [CrossRef]
66. Hu, J.S.; Li, Z.; Gao, J.Y.; He, H.T.; Dai, H.Q.; Xia, X.K.; Liu, C.H.; Zhang, L.X.; Song, F.H. New diketopiperazines from a marine-derived fungus strain *Aspergillus versicolor* MF180151. *Mar. Drugs* **2019**, *17*, 262. [CrossRef]
67. Li, J.; Hu, Y.Y.; Hao, X.M.; Tan, J.L.; Li, F.; Qiao, X.R.; Chen, S.Z.; Xiao, C.L.; Chen, M.H.; Peng, Z.G.; et al. Raistrickindole A, an anti-HCV oxazinoindole alkaloid from *Penicillium raistrickii* IMB17-034. *J. Nat. Prod.* **2019**, *82*, 1391–1395. [CrossRef]
68. Chi, L.P.; Li, X.M.; Li, L.; Li, X.; Wang, B.G. Cytotoxic thiodiketopiperazine derivatives from the deep sea-derived fungus *Epicoccum nigrum* SD-388. *Mar. Drugs* **2020**, *18*, 160. [CrossRef] [PubMed]
69. Zhong, W.M.; Wang, J.F.; Wei, X.Y.; Fu, T.D.; Chen, Y.C.; Zeng, Q.; Huang, Z.H.; Huang, X.N.; Zhang, W.M.; Zhang, S.; et al. Three pairs of new spirocyclic alkaloid enantiomers from the marine-derived fungus *Eurotium* sp. SCSIO F452. *Front. Chem.* **2019**, *7*, 350. [CrossRef] [PubMed]
70. Peng, J.X.; Gao, H.Q.; Li, J.; Ai, J.; Geng, M.Y.; Zhang, G.J.; Zhu, T.J.; Gu, Q.Q.; Li, D.H. Prenylated indole diketopiperazines from the marine-derived fungus *Aspergillus versicolor*. *J. Org. Chem.* **2014**, *79*, 7895–7904. [CrossRef] [PubMed]
71. Chen, X.Q.; Si, L.L.; Liu, D.; Proksch, P.; Zhang, L.H.; Zhou, D.M.; Lin, W.H. Neoechinulin B and its analogues as potential entry inhibitors of influenza viruses, targeting viral hemagglutinin. *Eur. J. Med. Chem.* **2015**, *93*, 182–195. [CrossRef]
72. Yu, L.Y.; Ding, W.J.; Wang, Q.Q.; Ma, Z.J.; Xu, X.W.; Zhao, X.F.; Chen, Z. Induction of cryptic bioactive 2,5-diketopiperazines in fungus *Penicillium* sp. DT-F29 by microbial co-culture. *Tetrahedron* **2017**, *73*, 907–914. [CrossRef]
73. Zhong, W.M.; Wang, J.F.; Shi, X.F.; Wei, X.Y.; Chen, Y.C.; Zeng, Q.; Xiang, Y.; Chen, X.Y.; Tian, X.P.; Xiao, Z.H.; et al. Eurotiumins A–E, five new alkaloids from the marine-derived fungus *Eurotium* sp. SCSIO F452. *Mar. Drugs* **2018**, *16*, 136. [CrossRef] [PubMed]
74. Zhong, W.M.; Wang, J.F.; Wei, X.Y.; Chen, Y.C.; Fu, T.D.; Xiang, Y.; Huang, X.N.; Tian, X.P.; Xiao, Z.H.; Zhang, W.M.; et al. Variecolortins A–C, three pairs of spirocyclic diketopiperazine enantiomers from the marine-derived fungus *Eurotium* sp. SCSIO F452. *Org. Lett.* **2018**, *20*, 4593–4596. [CrossRef] [PubMed]
75. Harms, H.; Orlikova, B.; Ji, S.; Nesaei-Mosaferan, D.; Konig, G.M.; Diederich, M. Epipolythiodiketopiperazines from the marine derived fungus *Dichotomomyces cejpii* with NF-kappa B inhibitory potential. *Mar. Drugs* **2015**, *13*, 4949–4966. [CrossRef]
76. Liu, Y.; Mandi, A.; Li, X.M.; Meng, L.H.; Kurtan, T.; Wang, B.G. Peniciadametizine A, a dithiodiketopiperazine with a unique spiro furan-2,7′-pyrazino 1,2-b 1,2 oxazine skeleton, and a related analogue, peniciadametizine B, from the marine sponge-derived fungus *Penicillium adametzioides*. *Mar. Drugs* **2015**, *13*, 3640–3652. [CrossRef]
77. Yan, B.F.; Fang, S.T.; Li, W.Z.; Liu, S.J.; Wang, J.H.; Xia, C.H. A new minor diketopiperazine from the sponge-derived fungus *Simplicillium* sp. YZ-11. *Nat. Prod. Res.* **2015**, *29*, 2013–2017. [CrossRef] [PubMed]
78. Zin, W.W.M.; Buttachon, S.; Dethoup, T.; Fernandes, C.; Cravo, S.; Pinto, M.M.M.; Gales, L.; Pereira, J.A.; Silva, A.M.S.; Sekeroglu, N.; et al. New cyclotetrapeptides and a new diketopiperzine derivative from the marine sponge-associated fungus *Neosartorya glabra* KUFA 0702. *Mar. Drugs* **2016**, *14*, 136. [CrossRef]
79. Gu, B.B.; Gui, Y.H.; Liu, L.; Su, Z.Y.; Jiao, W.H.; Li, L.; Sun, F.; Wang, S.P.; Yang, F.; Lin, H.W. A new asymmetric diketopiperazine dimer from the sponge-associated fungus *Aspergillus versicolor* 16F-11. *Magn. Reson. Chem.* **2019**, *57*, 49–54. [CrossRef]
80. Liu, J.T.; Gu, B.B.; Yang, L.J.; Yang, F.; Lin, H.W. New Anti-inflammatory cyclopeptides from a sponge-derived fungus *Aspergillus violaceofuscus*. *Front. Chem.* **2018**, *6*, 226. [CrossRef] [PubMed]
81. Frank, M.; Ozkaya, F.C.; Muller, W.E.G.; Hamacher, A.; Kassack, M.U.; Lin, W.H.; Liu, Z.; Proksch, P. Cryptic secondary metabolites from the sponge-associated fungus *Aspergillus ochraceus*. *Mar. Drugs* **2019**, *17*, 99. [CrossRef]
82. Asiri, I.A.M.; Badr, J.M.; Youssef, D.T.A. Penicillivinacine, antimigratory diketopiperazine alkaloid from the marine-derived fungus *Penicillium vinaceum*. *Phytochem. Lett.* **2015**, *13*, 53–58. [CrossRef]
83. Liu, Y.; Li, X.M.; Meng, L.H.; Jiang, W.L.; Xu, G.M.; Huang, C.G.; Wang, B.G. Bisthiodiketopiperazines and acorane sesquiterpenes produced by the marine-derived fungus *Penicillium adametzioides* AS-53 on different culture media. *J. Nat. Prod.* **2015**, *78*, 1294–1299. [CrossRef]
84. Cho, K.H.; Sohn, J.H.; Oh, H. Isolation and structure determination of a new diketopiperazine dimer from marine-derived fungus *Aspergillus* sp. SF-5280. *Nat. Prod. Res.* **2017**, *32*, 214–221. [CrossRef] [PubMed]
85. Wang, N.; Cui, C.B.; Li, C.W. A new cyclic dipeptide penicimutide: The activated production of cyclic dipeptides by introduction of neomycin-resistance in the marine-derived fungus *Penicillium purpurogenum* G59. *Arch. Pharm. Res.* **2016**, *39*, 762–770. [CrossRef]
86. Wang, N.; Dong, Y.; Yang, Y.; Xu, R.; Li, C.W.; Cui, C.B. Penicimutanin C, a new alkaloidal compound, isolated from a neomycin-resistant mutant 3-f-31 of *Penicillium purpurogenum* G59. *Chem. Biodivers.* **2020**, *17*, 8. [CrossRef] [PubMed]

87. Wang, F.Q.; Sarotti, A.M.; Jiang, G.D.; Huguet-Tapia, J.C.; Zheng, S.L.; Wu, X.H.; Li, C.S.; Ding, Y.S.; Cao, S.G. Waikikiamides A–C: Complex diketopiperazine dimer and diketopiperazine-polyketide hybrids from a hawaiian marine fungal strain *Aspergillus* sp. FM242. *Org. Lett.* **2020**, *22*, 4408–4412. [CrossRef]
88. Jiang, C.S.; Zhou, Z.F.; Yang, X.H.; Lan, L.F.; Gu, Y.C.; Ye, B.P.; Guo, Y.W. Antibacterial sorbicillin and diketopiperazines from the endogenous fungus *Penicillium* sp. GD6 associated Chinese mangrove *Bruguiera gymnorrhiza*. *Chin. J. Nat. Med.* **2018**, *16*, 358–365. [CrossRef]
89. Cai, R.L.; Jiang, H.M.; Xiao, Z.; Cao, W.H.; Yang, T.; Liu, Z.M.; Lin, S.E.; Long, Y.H.; She, Z.G. (−)- and (+)-Asperginulin A, a pair of indole diketopiperazine alkaloid dimers with a 6/5/4/5/6 pentacyclic skeleton from the mangrove endophytic fungus *Aspergillus* sp. SK-28. *Org. Lett.* **2019**, *21*, 9633–9636. [CrossRef] [PubMed]
90. Li, F.; Guo, W.Q.; Wu, L.; Zhu, T.J.; Gu, Q.Q.; Li, D.H.; Che, Q. Saroclazines A–C, thio-diketopiperazines from mangrove-derived fungi *Sarocladium kiliense* HDN11-84. *Arch. Pharm. Res.* **2017**, *41*, 30–34. [CrossRef] [PubMed]
91. Meng, L.H.; Li, X.M.; Lv, C.T.; Huang, C.G.; Wang, B.G. Brocazines A–F, cytotoxic bisthiodiketopiperazine derivatives from *Penicillium brocae* MA-231, an endophytic fungus derived from the marine mangrove plant *Avicennia marina*. *J. Nat. Prod.* **2014**, *77*, 1921–1927. [CrossRef]
92. Meng, L.H.; Zhang, P.; Li, X.M.; Wang, B.G. Penicibrocazines A–E, five new sulfide diketopiperazines from the marine-derived endophytic fungus *Penicillium brocae*. *Mar. Drugs* **2015**, *13*, 276–287. [CrossRef]
93. Meng, L.H.; Wang, C.Y.; Mandi, A.; Li, X.M.; Hu, X.Y.; Kassack, M.U.; Kurtan, T.; Wang, B.G. Three diketopiperazine alkaloids with spirocyclic skeletons and one bisthiodiketopiperazine derivative from the mangrove-derived endophytic fungus *Penicillium brocae* MA-231. *Org. Lett.* **2016**, *18*, 5304–5307. [CrossRef] [PubMed]
94. Liu, W.; Li, H.J.; Xu, M.Y.; Ju, Y.C.; Wang, L.Y.; Xu, J.; Yang, D.P.; Lan, W.J. Pseudellones A–C, three alkaloids from the marine-derived fungus *Pseudallescheria ellipsoidea* F42-3. *Org. Lett.* **2015**, *17*, 5156–5159. [CrossRef] [PubMed]
95. Lan, W.J.; Wang, K.T.; Xu, M.Y.; Zhang, J.J.; Lam, C.K.; Zhong, G.H.; Xu, J.; Yang, D.P.; Li, H.J.; Wang, L.Y. Secondary metabolites with chemical diversity from the marine-derived fungus *Pseudallescheria boydii* F19-1 and their cytotoxic activity. *RSC Adv.* **2016**, *6*, 76206–76213. [CrossRef]
96. Chen, Y.X.; Xu, M.Y.; Li, H.J.; Zeng, K.J.; Ma, W.Z.; Tian, G.B.; Xu, J.; Yang, D.P.; Lan, W.J. Diverse secondary metabolites from the marine-derived fungus *Dichotomomyces cejpii* F31-1. *Mar. Drugs* **2017**, *15*, 339. [CrossRef]
97. Wei, X.; Feng, C.; Wang, S.Y.; Zhang, D.M.; Li, X.H.; Zhang, C.X. New indole diketopiperazine alkaloids from soft coral-associated epiphytic fungus *Aspergillus* sp. EGF 15-0-3. *Chem. Biodivers.* **2020**, *17*, 11. [CrossRef]
98. Zhuravleva, O.I.; Antonov, A.S.; Trang, V.T.D.; Pivkin, M.V.; Khudyakova, Y.V.; Denisenko, V.A.; Popov, R.S.; Kim, N.Y.; Yurchenko, E.A.; Gerasimenko, A.V.; et al. New deoxyisoaustamide derivatives from the coral-derived fungus *Penicillium dimorphosporum* KMM 4689. *Mar. Drugs* **2021**, *19*, 32. [CrossRef]
99. Wang, K.T.; Xu, M.Y.; Liu, W.; Li, H.J.; Xu, J.; Yang, D.P.; Lan, W.J.; Wang, L.Y. Two additional new compounds from the marine-derived fungus *Pseudallescheria ellipsoidea* F42-3. *Molecules* **2016**, *21*, 442. [CrossRef]
100. Shi, Z.Z.; Miao, F.P.; Fang, S.T.; Yin, X.L.; Ji, N.Y. Sulfurated diketopiperazines from an algicolous isolate of *Trichoderma virens*. *Phytochem. Lett.* **2018**, *27*, 101–104. [CrossRef]
101. Song, Y.P.; Miao, F.P.; Fang, S.T.; Yin, X.L.; Ji, N.Y. Halogenated and nonhalogenated metabolites from the marine-alga-endophytic fungus *Trichoderma asperellum* cf44-2. *Mar. Drugs* **2018**, *16*, 266. [CrossRef]
102. Yurchenko, A.N.; Berdyshev, D.V.; Smetanina, O.F.; Ivanets, E.V.; Zhuravleva, O.I.; Rasin, A.B.; Khudyakova, Y.V.; Popov, R.S.; Dyshlovoy, S.A.; von Amsberg, G.; et al. Citriperazines A–D produced by a marine algae-derived fungus *Penicillium* sp. KMM 4672. *Nat. Prod. Res.* **2019**, *34*, 1118–1123. [CrossRef] [PubMed]
103. Cao, J.; Li, X.M.; Meng, L.H.; Konuklugil, B.; Li, X.; Li, H.L.; Wang, B.G. Isolation and characterization of three pairs of indolediketopiperazine enantiomers containing infrequent N-methoxy substitution from the marine algal-derived endophytic fungus *Acrostalagmus luteoalbus* TK-43. *Bioorg. Chem.* **2019**, *90*, 103030. [CrossRef] [PubMed]
104. Song, Y.; Miao, F.; Yin, X.; Ji, N. Three nitrogen-containing metabolites from an algicolous isolate of *Trichoderma asperellum*. *Mar. Life Sci. Technol.* **2020**, *2*, 155–160. [CrossRef]
105. Yurchenko, A.N.; Smetanina, O.F.; Ivanets, E.V.; Kalinovsky, A.I.; Khudyakova, Y.V.; Kirichuk, N.N.; Popov, R.S.; Bokemeyer, C.; von Amsberg, G.; Chingizova, E.A.; et al. Pretrichodermamides D–F from a marine algicolous fungus *Penicillium* sp. KMM 4672. *Mar. Drugs* **2016**, *14*, 122. [CrossRef] [PubMed]
106. Du, F.Y.; Li, X.; Li, X.M.; Zhu, L.W.; Wang, B.G. Indolediketopiperazine alkaloids from *Eurotium cristatum* EN-220, an endophytic fungus isolated from the marine alga *Sargassum thunbergii*. *Mar. Drugs* **2017**, *15*, 24. [CrossRef]
107. Liu, W.; Wang, L.P.; Wang, B.; Xu, Y.C.; Zhu, G.L.; Lan, M.M.; Zhu, W.M.; Sun, K.L. Diketopiperazine and diphenylether derivatives from marine algae-derived *Aspergillus versicolor* OUCMDZ-2738 by epigenetic activation. *Mar. Drugs* **2018**, *17*, 6. [CrossRef]
108. Kamauchi, H.; Kinoshita, K.; Sugita, T.; Koyama, K. Conditional changes enhanced production of bioactive metabolites of marine derived fungus *Eurotium rubrum*. *Bioorg. Med. Chem. Lett.* **2016**, *26*, 4911–4914. [CrossRef]
109. Zhang, Y.H.; Geng, C.; Zhang, X.W.; Zhu, H.J.; Shao, C.L.; Cao, F.; Wang, C.Y. Discovery of bioactive indole-diketopiperazines from the marine-derived fungus *Penicillium brasilianum* aided by genomic information. *Mar. Drugs* **2019**, *17*, 514. [CrossRef]

110. Han, W.R.; Cai, J.; Zhong, W.M.; Xu, G.M.; Wang, F.Z.; Tian, X.P.; Zhou, X.J.; Liu, Q.C.; Liu, Y.H.; Wang, J.F. Protein tyrosine phosphatase 1B (PTP1B) inhibitors from the deep-sea fungus *Penicillium chrysogenum* SCSIO 07007. *Bioorg. Chem.* **2020**, *96*, 103646. [CrossRef]
111. Wu, J.S.; Shi, X.H.; Yao, G.S.; Shao, C.L.; Fu, X.M.; Zhang, X.L.; Guan, H.S.; Wang, C.Y. New thiodiketopiperazine and 3,4-dihydroisocoumarin derivatives from the marine-derived fungus *Aspergillus terreus*. *Mar. Drugs* **2020**, *18*, 132. [CrossRef]
112. Ding, Y.; Zhu, X.J.; Hao, L.L.; Zhao, M.Y.; Hua, Q.; An, F.L. Bioactive indolyl diketopiperazines from the marine derived endophytic *Aspergillus versicolor* DY180635. *Mar. Drugs* **2020**, *18*, 338. [CrossRef]
113. Youssef, D.T.A.; Alahdal, A.M. Cytotoxic and antimicrobial compounds from the marine-derived fungus, *Penicillium* Species. *Molecules* **2018**, *23*, 394. [CrossRef] [PubMed]
114. Fukuda, T.; Takahashi, M.; Nagai, K.; Harunari, E.; Imada, C.; Tomoda, H. Isomethoxyneihumicin, a new cytotoxic agent produced by marine *Nocardiopsis* alba KM6-1. *J. Antibiot.* **2017**, *70*, 590–594. [CrossRef] [PubMed]
115. Fu, P.; Liu, P.P.; Qu, H.J.; Wang, Y.; Chen, D.F.; Wang, H.; Li, J.; Zhu, W.M. Alpha-pyrones and diketopiperazine derivatives from the marine-derived actinomycete *Nocardiopsis dassonvillei* HR10-5. *J. Nat. Prod.* **2011**, *74*, 2219–2223. [CrossRef] [PubMed]
116. Sun, M.W.; Chen, X.T.; Li, W.J.; Lu, C.H.; Shen, Y.M. New diketopiperazine derivatives with cytotoxicity from *Nocardiopsis* sp YIM M13066. *J. Antibiot.* **2017**, *70*, 795–797. [CrossRef]
117. Zhang, L.; Feng, L.L.; Wang, G.F.; Yang, Q.L.; Fu, X.Z.; Li, Z.; Liu, M.; Kou, L.J.; Xu, B.; Xie, Z.P.; et al. Strepyrazinone, a tricyclic diketopiperazine derivative with cytotoxicity from a marine-derived actinobacterium. *J. Asian Nat. Prod. Res.* **2020**, 1–7. [CrossRef] [PubMed]
118. Zhang, P.; Li, X.M.; Wang, J.N.; Wang, B.G. Oxepine-containing diketopiperazine alkaloids from the algal-derived endophytic fungus *Paecilomyces variotii* EN-291. *Helv.Chim. Acta.* **2015**, *98*, 800–804. [CrossRef]
119. Liang, X.; Zhang, X.L.; Lu, X.H.; Zheng, Z.H.; Ma, X.; Qi, S.H. Diketopiperazine-type alkaloids from a deep-sea-derived *Aspergillus puniceus* fungus and their effects on liver X receptor alpha. *J. Nat. Prod.* **2019**, *82*, 1558–1564. [CrossRef]
120. Tian, Y.Q.; Lin, S.N.; Zhou, H.; Lin, S.T.; Wang, S.Y.; Liu, Y.H. Protuboxepin C and protuboxepin D from the sponge-derived fungus *Aspergillus* sp. SCSIO XWS02F40. *Nat. Prod. Res.* **2018**, *32*, 2510–2515. [CrossRef] [PubMed]
121. Tian, Y.Q.; Lin, X.P.; Wang, Z.; Zhou, X.F.; Qin, X.C.; Kaliyaperumal, K.; Zhang, T.Y.; Tu, Z.C.; Liu, Y.H. Asteltoxins with antiviral activities from the marine sponge-derived fungus *Aspergillus* sp. SCSIO XWS02F40. *Molecules* **2015**, *21*, 34. [CrossRef] [PubMed]
122. Luo, X.W.; Chen, C.M.; Tao, H.M.; Lin, X.P.; Yang, B.; Zhou, X.F.; Liu, Y.H. Structurally diverse diketopiperazine alkaloids from the marine-derived fungus *Aspergillus versicolor* SCSIO 41016. *Org. Chem. Front.* **2019**, *6*, 736–740. [CrossRef]
123. Xu, W.F.; Mao, N.; Xue, X.J.; Qi, Y.X.; Wei, M.Y.; Wang, C.Y.; Shao, C.L. Structures and absolute configurations of diketopiperazine alkaloids chrysopiperazines A–C from the gorgonian-derived *Penicillium chrysogenum* fungus. *Mar. Drugs* **2019**, *17*, 250. [CrossRef] [PubMed]
124. Zhang, H.M.; Ju, C.X.; Li, G.; Sun, Y.; Peng, Y.; Li, Y.X.; Peng, X.P.; Lou, H.X. Dimeric 1,4-benzoquinone derivatives with cytotoxic activities from the marine-derived fungus *Penicillium* sp. L129. *Mar. Drugs* **2019**, *17*, 383. [CrossRef] [PubMed]
125. Guo, X.C.; Zhang, Y.H.; Gao, W.B.; Pan, L.; Zhu, H.J.; Cao, F. Absolute configurations and chitinase inhibitions of quinazoline-containing diketopiperazines from the marine-derived fungus *Penicillium polonicum*. *Mar. Drugs* **2020**, *18*, 479. [CrossRef]
126. Ohte, S.; Shiokawa, T.; Koyama, N.; Katagiri, T.; Imada, C.; Tomoda, H. A new diketopiperazine-like inhibitor of bone morphogenetic protein-induced osteoblastic differentiation produced by marine-derived *Aspergillus* sp. BFM-0085. *J. Antibiot.* **2020**, *73*, 554–558. [CrossRef] [PubMed]
127. Qi, C.X.; Tan, X.S.; Shi, Z.Y.; Feng, H.; Sun, L.J.; Hu, Z.X.; Chen, G.; Zhang, Y.H. Discovery of an oxepine-containing diketopiperazine derivative active against Concanavalin A-Induced Hepatitis. *J. Nat. Prod.* **2020**, *83*, 2672–2678. [CrossRef] [PubMed]
128. Li, H.-L.; Yang, S.-Q.; Li, X.-M.; Li, X.; Wang, B.-G. Structurally diverse alkaloids produced by *Aspergillus creber* EN-602, an endophytic fungus obtained from the marine red alga Rhodomela confervoides. *Bioorg. Chem.* **2021**, *110*, 104822. [CrossRef] [PubMed]
129. Lee, S.U.; Asami, Y.; Lee, D.; Jang, J.-H.; Ahn, J.S.; Oh, H. Protuboxepins A and B and Protubonines A and B from the Marine-Derived Fungus *Aspergillus* sp. SF-5044. *J. Nat. Prod.* **2011**, *74*, 1284–1287. [CrossRef]
130. Asami, Y.; Jang, J.H.; Soung, N.K.; He, L.; Moon, D.O.; Kim, J.W.; Oh, H.; Muroi, M.; Osada, H.; Kim, B.Y.; et al. Protuboxepin A, a marine fungal metabolite, inducing metaphase arrest and chromosomal misalignment in tumor cells. *Bioorg. Med. Chem.* **2012**, *20*, 3799–3806. [CrossRef]
131. Zhuravleva, O.I.; Afiyatullov, S.S.; Denisenko, V.A.; Ermakova, S.P.; Slinkina, N.N.; Dmitrenok, P.S.; Kim, N.Y. Secondary metabolites from a marine-derived fungus *Aspergillus carneus* blochwitz. *Phytochemistry* **2012**, *80*, 123–131. [CrossRef] [PubMed]
132. Afiyatullov, S.S.; Zhuravleva, O.I.; Antonov, A.S.; Kalinovsky, A.I.; Pivkin, M.V.; Menchinskaya, E.S.; Aminin, D.L. New metabolites from the marine-derived fungus *Aspergillus fumigatus*. *Nat. Prod. Commun.* **2012**, *7*, 497–500. [CrossRef] [PubMed]
133. Wang, L.Q.; Wang, M.Y.; Fu, Y.D.; Huang, P.J.; Kong, D.K.; Niu, G.Q. Engineered biosynthesis of thaxtomin phytotoxins. *Crit. Rev. Biotechnol.* **2020**, *40*, 1163–1171. [CrossRef] [PubMed]
134. Wang, M.X.; Carver, J.J.; Phelan, V.V.; Sanchez, L.M.; Garg, N.; Peng, Y.; Nguyen, D.D.; Watrous, J.; Kapono, C.A.; Luzzatto-Knaan, T.; et al. Sharing and community curation of mass spectrometry data with global natural products social molecular networking. *Nat. Biotechnol.* **2016**, *34*, 828–837. [CrossRef] [PubMed]

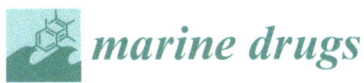

Article

Four New Chromones from the Endophytic Fungus *Phomopsis asparagi* DHS-48 Isolated from the Chinese Mangrove Plant *Rhizophora mangle*

Chengwen Wei [1], Chunxiao Sun [2], Zhao Feng [1], Xuexia Zhang [1] and Jing Xu [1,2,*]

[1] School of Chemical Engineering and Technology, Hainan University, Haikou 570228, China; weichengwen@hainanu.edu.cn (C.W.); fz329077397@163.com (Z.F.); zhangxuexia@hainanu.edu.cn (X.Z.)
[2] School of Medicine and Pharmacy, Ocean University of China, Qingdao 266003, China; scx@stu.ouc.edu.cn
* Correspondence: happyjing3@hainanu.edu.cn; Tel.: +86-898-6627-9226

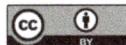

Citation: Wei, C.; Sun, C.; Feng, Z.; Zhang, X.; Xu, J. Four New Chromones from the Endophytic Fungus *Phomopsis asparagi* DHS-48 Isolated from the Chinese Mangrove Plant *Rhizophora mangle*. *Mar. Drugs* 2021, 19, 348. https://doi.org/10.3390/md19060348

Academic Editors: RuAngelie Edrada-Ebel, Chang-Yun Wang and Bin-Gui Wang

Received: 5 June 2021
Accepted: 16 June 2021
Published: 19 June 2021

Publisher's Note: MDPI stays neutral with regard to jurisdictional claims in published maps and institutional affiliations.

Copyright: © 2021 by the authors. Licensee MDPI, Basel, Switzerland. This article is an open access article distributed under the terms and conditions of the Creative Commons Attribution (CC BY) license (https://creativecommons.org/licenses/by/4.0/).

Abstract: Four new chromones, phomochromenones D–G (**1–4**), along with four known analogues, diaporchromone A (**5**), diaporchromanone C (**6**), diaporchromanone D (**7**), and phomochromenone C (**8**), were isolated from the culture of *Phomopsis asparagi* DHS-48 from Chinese mangrove *Rhizophora mangle*. Their structures were elucidated on the basis of comprehensive spectroscopic analysis. The absolute configurations of **1** and **4** were assigned on the basis of experimental and calculated electronic circular dichroism (ECD) data, and those of enantiomers **2** and **3** were determined by a modified Mosher's method and basic hydrolysis. To the best of our knowledge, phomochromenones D–F (**1–4**) possessing a 3-substituted-chroman-4-one skeleton are rarely found in natural sources. Diaporchromone A (**5**) showed moderate to weak immunosuppressive activity against T and/or B lymphocyte cells with IC_{50} of 34 μM and 117 μM.

Keywords: mangrove endophytic fungi; *Phomopsis* sp.; chromenones; immunosuppressive activity

1. Introduction

Marine-derived fungi are morphologically and physiologically adapted to harsh environmental stresses, such as high salinity, high temperature, extreme tides, oxygen pressure, high humidity, and light and air limitations, which have increasingly attracted the attention of both pharmaceutical and natural product chemists in recent decades [1,2]. Fungi colonized in mangrove forests, which comprise the second largest ecological group of marine fungi, have especially adapted their metabolic mechanisms to the unique properties of the marine environment via the generation of a large variety of structurally unprecedented and biologically interesting metabolites of pharmaceutical importance [3–5]. One fungal genus which is especially productive with regard to the accumulation of a diverse array of mostly bioactive compounds is *Phomopsis*. Chemical investigation of this fungal genus has resulted in the discovery of over 70 potentially bioactive secondary metabolites, such as subintestinal vessel plexus (SIV) accelerator phomopsis-H76 A [6], cytotoxic phomopchalasins B and C [7], mycoepoxydiene [8], dicerandrols [9], antibiotic phomoxanthone A [10], phomodiol [11], phompsichalasin [12], antimicrotubule phomosidin [13], and anti-inflammatory phomol [14]. As part of our ongoing investigation on bioactive metabolites from mangrove endophytic fungi [15–19], *Phomopsis asparagi* DHS-48 was isolated from a fresh root of the mangrove plant *Rhizophora mangle*. Four new chromones (**1–4**), and five known compounds, including diaporchromone A (**5**) [20], diaporchromanone C (**6**) [20], diaporchromanone D (**7**) [20], and phomochromenone C (**8**) [21] (Figure 1) were isolated from the EtOAc extract of *P. asparagi* after fermentation on a solid rice medium containing sea salt. Herein, we report the isolation, structural elucidation, and exploration on the biological activities of compounds **1–8**.

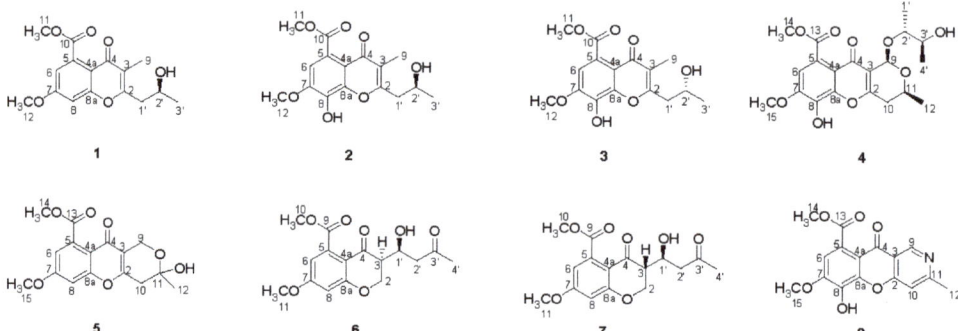

Figure 1. The chemical structures of compounds 1–8.

2. Results and Discussion

Phomochromenone D (**1**), a white amorphous powder, has the molecular formula $C_{16}H_{19}O_6$, established by HR-ESIMS (m/z 307.1139, calcd. for $[M+H]^+$ 307.1182), implying eight degrees of unsaturation. The UV absorption maxima at 219, 245, 295 nm indicated that **1** could be a chromone derivative. The 1D NMR data of **1** (Table 1) indicated that six of the eight units of unsaturation came from four carbon–carbon double bonds and two carbonyls. Therefore, the other two units of unsaturation come from two rings. The ^{1}H NMR spectrum of **1** showed the presence of two meta-coupled aromatic protons at δ_H 6.92 (d, J = 2.4 Hz, H-6) and δ_H 7.10 (d, J = 2.4 Hz, H-8), one methine at δ_H 4.25 (m, H-2′), one methylene at δ_H 2.92 (dd, J = 14.0, 8.0 Hz, H_a-1′) and 2.60 (dd, J = 14.0, 5.1 Hz, H_b-1′), and two methyl at δ_H 2.02 (s, H_3-9) and 1.29 (d, J = 6.3 Hz, H_3-3′), and two methoxy at δ_H 3.917 (s, H_3-11) and δ_H 3.924 (s, H_3-12),. The ^{13}C NMR and DEPT spectra showed 16 carbon resonances corresponding to two sp^2 methine (δ_C 114.52 and 102.3), ten sp^2 quaternary (δ_C 165.1, 164.8, 159.5, 135.9, 119.1, 114.49, one carbonyl at δ_C 171.4, one conjugated carbonyl at δ_C 178.4), one oxygenated methine (δ_C 67.1), two methoxy (δ_C 57.0, 53.5), one methylene (δ_C 42.6), and two methyl (δ_C 23.7, 10.3) carbons. The HMBC correlation (Figure 2) from H-6 to C-5, C-7, and C-10, and from H-8 to C-7, C-4a and C-8a indicated the presence of the chromone moiety. Moreover, HMBC correlations from H_3-9 to C-2, C-3 and C-4; and from H_2-1′ to C-2 and C-3, suggested that a 2-hydroxypropyl group was attached to C-2 of the chromone core. The absolute configuration of C-2′ of **1** was determined by the comparison of its experimental and time-dependent density functional theory (TDDFT)-calculated electronic circular dichroism spectrum. The experimental ECD spectrum (CH_3OH) for 2′S-**1** matched well with the calculated spectrum (Figure 3), which confirmed the unambiguous assignment of the absolute configuration of **1** as S, and the trivial name, phomochromenone D, was assigned.

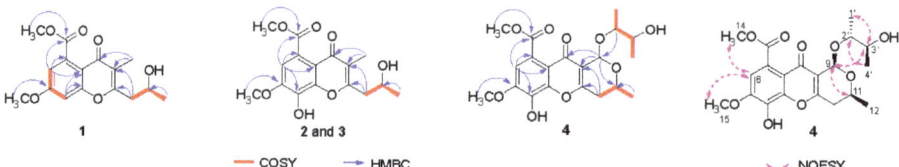

Figure 2. Selected 2D NMR of compounds **1–4**.

Table 1. ^{1}H (400 MHz) and ^{13}C (125 MHz) NMR spectroscopic data for **1–4** in CD$_3$OD.

Position	1		2/3		4	
	δ_C, Type	δ_H (J in Hz)	δ_C, Type	δ_H (J in Hz)	δ_C, Type	δ_H (J in Hz)
2	164.8, C		164.8, C		166.7, C	
3	119.1, C		118.2, C		116.8, C	
4	178.4, C		178.9, C		176.8, C	
4a	135.9, C		115.4, C		116.5, C	
5	114.5, C		123.2, C		123.0, C	
6	114.6, CH	6.92, d, 2.4	110.0, CH	7.07, s	110.3, CH	7.09, s
7	165.1, C		151.4, C		152.6, C	
8	102.3, CH	7.10, d, 2.4	138.2, C		140.3, C	
8a	159.5, C		147.1, C		147.2, C	
9	10.3, CH$_3$	2.02, s	10.2, CH$_3$	2.02, s	96.9, CH	5.73, s
10	171.4, C		172.4, C		35.2, CH$_2$	H$_a$ 2.77, dd, 17.9, 3.7 H$_b$ 2.68, dd, 17.9, 10.7
11	53.5, CH$_3$	3.92, s	53.5, CH$_3$	3.89, s	63.9, CH	4.40, m
12	57.0, CH$_3$	3.92, s	57.2, CH$_3$	3.96, s	20.8, CH$_3$	1.37, d, 6.2
13					172.1, C	
14					53.3, CH$_3$	3.87, s
15					57.2, CH$_3$	3.96, s
1′	42.6, CH$_2$	H$_a$ 2.92, dd, 14.0, 8.0 H$_b$ 2.83, dd, 14.0, 5.1	42.4, CH$_2$	H$_a$ 2.95, dd, 14.1, 7.9 H$_b$ 2.83, dd, 14.1, 5.1	18.8, CH$_3$	1.19, d, 6.0
2′	67.1, CH	4.25, m	67.1, CH	4.29, m	83.4, CH	3.60, m
3′	23.7, CH$_3$	1.29, d, 6.3	23.6, CH$_3$	1.29, d, 6.3	73.4, CH	3.54, m
4′					18.3, CH$_3$	1.13, d, 6.0

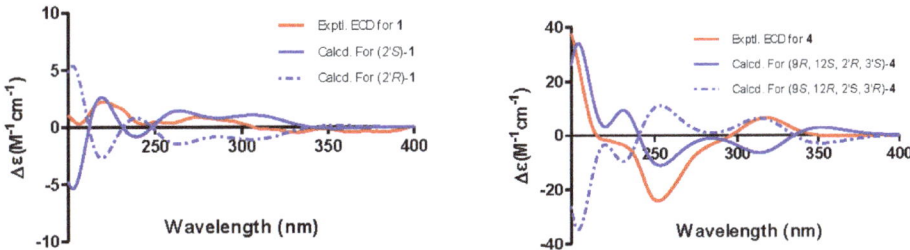

Figure 3. Experimental and calculated ECD spectra of **1** and **4**.

Phomochromenones E (**2**) and F (**3**) were isolated as a mixture of two enantiomers and shared the same NMR data, ^{1}H-^{1}H COSY and HMBC spectra. Based on the HR-ESIMS ion detected at *m/z* 321.0989 (calcd. for [M−H]$^−$, 321.0974), the mixture (**2/3**) had the same molecular formula of C$_{16}$H$_{18}$O$_7$ (i.e., differing from that of **1** by an additional hydroxyl group). The ^{1}H and ^{13}C NMR spectrum clearly indicated that this hydroxyl group was attached at C-6. Supporting evidence for this assignment was obtained from the downfield chemical shifts of C-8 (δ_C 138.2, s) and the absence of the proton signal of H-6 in **2/3** (δ_H 7.10, d, *J* = 2.4 Hz for H-8 and δ_C 102.3, d for C-8 in **1**, respectively). Moreover, the presence of a hydroxyl group at C-8 was corroborated by the observed HMBC correlation from H-6 (δ_H 7.10, d, *J* = 2.4 Hz) to C-8, C-7 (δ_C 151.4), C-5 (δ_C 123.2), C-4a (δ_C 115.4), and C-10 (δ_C 172.4). However, the antipode rotation and ECD were detected, which suggested the mixture was not an optically pure compound. Since the chiral phase HPLC (CHIRALPAK IC) did not afford the separation of these two enantiomers, a modified Mosher's experiment was performed to obtain its MPA esters. The products of Mosher's reactions were subsequently analyzed by UPLC-ESI-MS through a RP-C$_{18}$ chromatography column to afford two pairs of diastereomeric esters (*R*-MPA-**2**/*R*-MPA-**3** and *S*-MPA-**2**/*S*-MPA-**3**) (Figure 4). The spectral non-equivalences in ^{1}H NMR chemical shifts between (*R*)- and (*S*)-MPA esters ($\Delta\delta = \delta_R - \delta_S$) indicated a 2′-*S* configuration for (+)-**2** (positive for H-9 and negative for H-3′) and a 2′-*R* configuration for (−)-**3** (negative for H-9 and positive for H-3′) (Figure 4). The (*R*)- and (*S*)-MPA esters of **2**/**3** was further separated by semi-prep. RP-C$_{18}$ HPLC (40% CH$_3$CN/H$_2$O, 0.2% HCOOH) to afford *R*-MTPA-**2**/*S*-MTPA-**3** (t_R 18.8 min) and *R*-MPA-**3**/*S*-MPA-**2** (t_R 19.2 min). Compounds **2** and **3** were successfully obtained by chromatography after alkaline hydrolysis of *R*-MPA-**2**/*S*-MPA-**2** and *R*-MPA-**3**/*S*-MPA-**3**, respectively. Therefore, enantiomers **2** and **3** were successfully isolated and assigned the names phomochromenone E and phomochromenone F, respectively.

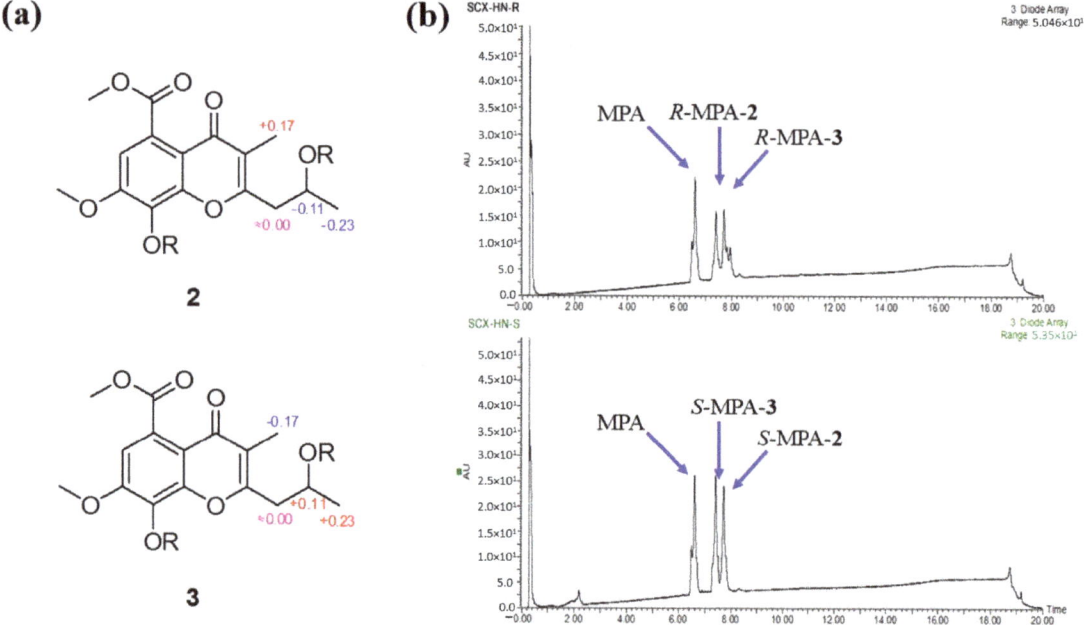

Figure 4. (**a**) $\Delta\delta$ ($=\delta_R - \delta_S$) values for (*R*)- and (*S*)- MPA esters of **2** and **3**. (**b**) UPLC analysis profile of (*R*)- and (*S*)- MPA esters of **2** and **3** over a 20 min gradient as follows: T = 0.0, 5% B; T = 15.0, 95% B; T = 17.0, 100% B, T = 18.0, 100% B, and T = 18.1, 5% B, and T = 20.0, 5% B (A, MQ+0.2% HCOOH; B, MeOH+0.2% HCOOH).

Phomochromenone G (**4**) was obtained as a white amorphous powder and had a molecular formula of C$_{20}$H$_{24}$O$_9$, as determined by its HR-ESIMS (*m/z* 431.1314, calcd. for [M+Na]$^+$ 431.1318), indicating nine degrees of unsaturation. The ^{1}H NMR spectrum showed resonances for one singlet aromatic proton at δ_H 7.09 (s, H-6); four methine protons at δ_H 5.73(s, H-9), δ_H 4.40 (m, H-11), δ_H 3.60 (m, H-1′), and δ_H 3.54 (m, H-2′); one methylene at δ_H 2.77 (dd, *J* = 17.9, 3.7 Hz, H$_a$-10) and 2.68 (dd, *J* = 17.9, 10.7 Hz, H$_b$-10); three methyl at δ_H 1.37 (d, *J* = 6.2 Hz, H$_3$-12), δ_H 1.13 (d, *J* = 6.0 Hz, H$_3$-3′), and δ_H 1.19 (d, *J* = 6.0 Hz, H$_3$-4′); two methoxy groups at δ_H 3.96(s, H$_3$-15) and δ_H 3.87(s, H$_3$-14). The ^{13}C NMR and DEPT spectra showed 20 carbon signals, including a keto group, an ester carbonyl group, eight olefinic carbon signals (including four oxygenated carbons), three oxy-methines, one methylene, two methoxy group, and three methyl group. Comparison of the NMR data of **4** with those of phomochromenone B [21], previously isolated from endophytic fungus *Phomopsis* sp. HNY29-2B derived from mangrove plant *Acanthus ilicifolius* Linn, revealed that both compounds differed with regard to the nature of the side chain at C-1, where the hydroxyl group of the latter was replaced by the 3-hydroxybutan-2-yloxyl group of **3**. This was confirmed through ^{1}H-^{1}H COSY correlations of H$_3$-4′/ H-1′/ H-2′/ H$_3$-3′ and HMBC correlations (Figure 2) from H-9 to C-11(δ_C 63.9), C-4(δ_C 176.8), C-2(δ_C 166.7), and C-1′(δ_C 67.1). The relative configuration of **4** was based on the NOESY correlations as indicated in Figure 2. The NOESY correlations of H-9 to H-11, H$_3$-1′ and H-3′; H-11 to H$_3$-1′; and H$_3$-4′ to H-2′ indicated that H-9, H-11, H$_3$-1′, and H$_3$-4′ were on the opposite side of the H$_3$-12, H-2′, and H$_3$-4′. The absolute configuration of **4** were also determined by comparing experimental and calculated electronic circular dichroism (ECD) spectra for the truncated model (9R, 12S, 2′R, 3′S)-**4** and the truncated model (9S, 12R, 2′S, 3′R)-**4** using time-dependent density functional theory (TDDFT). The theoretical spectrum of **4** showed an excellent fit with the experimental plot recorded in MeOH (Figure 3), which supported the absolute configuration to be 9R, 12S, 2′R, 3′S. Thus, the structure of **4** was determined and named phomochromenone F.

Our primary application of immunosuppressive activity screening indicated that a crude extract of *P. asparagi* DHS-48 showed strong inhibitory of splenic lymphocyte growth with IC$_{50}$ of 6 μg/mL. An immunosuppressive assay showed that compound **5** exhibited moderate to weak inhibitory activity against ConA-induced T and LPS-induced B murine splenic lymphocytes *in vitro* with IC$_{50}$ values of 34 and 117 μM, respectively (Table 2, Figure 5), whereas the other investigated compounds showed no obvious inhibitory effect. The cytotoxicity of **5** was tested in splenocyte cultures for 72 h using the tetrazolium salt-based CCK-8 assay. The results showed that it inhibited splenic lymphocyte growth with relatively lower toxicity (IC$_{50}$ 47μM), at which the survival of normal splenic cells was slightly influenced in comparison with that of CsA (IC$_{50}$ 11 μM). The results showed that compound **5** with a 1,3,4,10-tetrahydropyrano[4,3-b]chromene nucleus displayed significant immunosuppressive activity compared to compounds (1–3, 6, 7) with a chromone nucleus and compound **8** with a 10H-chromeno[3,2-c]pyridine nucleus. The additional 11-OH group in **5** is essential for its stimulated splenic lymphocyte inhibitory compared to compound **4**.

Table 2. Immunosuppressive activities of isolated compounds 1–8.

Compound	Cytotoxicity [a] IC$_{50}$ (μM) [b]	ConA-Induced T-Cell Proliferation IC$_{50}$ (μM) [b]	LPS-Induced B-Cell Proliferation IC$_{50}$ (μM) [b]
5	47	34	117
1–4, 6–8	-	-	-
CsA [c]	11	4	25

[a] Cell viability on murine splenocytes was tested by using CCK-8 method. [b] Data are presented as mean ± SD (n = 3) in μM. [c] Positive control.

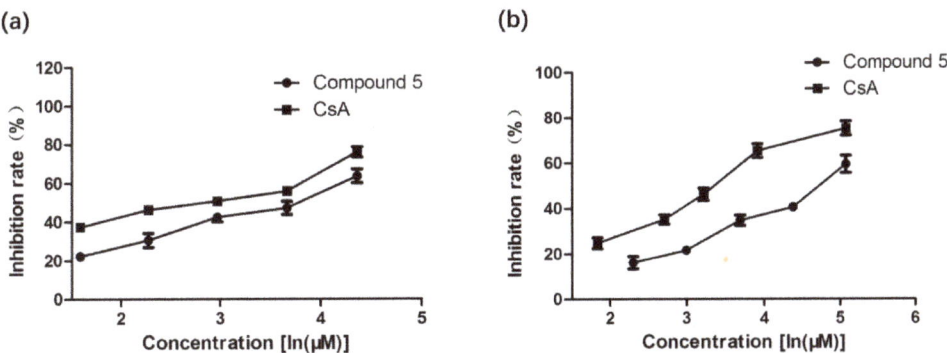

Figure 5. Effect of **5** on mouse splenocytes viability and proliferation. (**a**) Effect of **5** on the viability of T lymphocyte cells. (**b**) Effect of **5** on the viability of B lymphocyte cells. All values are expressed as mean ± SD. n = 3.

3. Materials and Methods

3.1. General Procedures

Specific rotations were obtained on a WYA-2S digital Abbe refractometer (Shanghai Physico-optical Instrument Factory, Shanghai, China). UV spectra were determined using a Shimadzu UV-2401 PC spectrophotometer (Shimadzu Corporation, Tokyo, Japan), while CD spectra were measured on a JASCO J-715 spectra polarimeter (Japan Spectroscopic, Tokyo, Japan). ^{1}H, ^{13}C and 2D NMR spectra were recorded on a Bruker AV 400 NMR spectrometer using TMS as an internal standard. High-resolution ESI-MS were performed on an LTQ Orbitrap XL instrument (Thermo Fisher Scientific, Bremen, Germany) using peak matching. TLC and column chromatography (CC) were carried out over silica gel (200–400 mesh, Qingdao Marine Chemical Inc., Qingdao, China), or a Sephadex-LH-20 (18−110 μm, Merck, Darmstadt, Germany), respectively. UPLC analysis (Waters Corporation, Milford, MA, USA) was recorded using a Waters system equipped in ESI mode on an Acquity UPLC H-Class connected to an SQ Detector 2 mass spectrometer using a BEH RP C_{18} column (2.1 × 50 mm, 1.7 μm, 0.5 mL/min). Semi-preparative HPLC was performed using a Waters equipped with a 2998 PDA detector (Waters Corporation, Milford, MA, USA) and a RP C_{18} column (YMC-Pack ODS-A, 10 × 250 mm, 5 μm, 3 mL/min).

3.2. Fungal Material

Endophytic fungus *Phomopsis asparagi* was isolated with PDA medium from the fresh root of the mangrove plant *Rhizophora mangle*, collected in October 2015 in Dong Zhai Gang-Mangrove Garden on Hainan Island, China. The fungus (strain no.DHS-8) was identified using a molecular biological protocol by DNA amplification and sequencing of the ITS region (GenBank Accession no.MT126606) [22]. A voucher strain was deposited at one of the authors' laboratories (J.X.).

3.3. Extraction Isolation

The fungus was fermented onto auto autoclaved rice solid-substrate medium (thirty 1000 mL Erlenmeyer flasks, each containing 100 g of rice and 100 mL of 0.3% of saline water) and incubated for 28 days at 28 °C. In total, 140 flasks of culture were extracted three times with EtOAc and the filtrate was evaporated under reduced pressure to yield crude extract (65 g). The crude extract was partitioned with petroleum ether (PE), dichloromethane, ethyl acetate (EA), and n-butyl alcohol (BA). The dichloromethane fraction and ethyl acetate fraction were combined (30 g), then chromatographed on silica gel column chromatography using gradient elution with a CH_2Cl_2-MeOH mixture of increasing polarity (100:0–0:100, v/v) to afford 8 fractions (Fr. 1–Fr. 8). Fr. 2 was subjected to open silica gel CC using gradient elution with CH_2Cl_2-EtOAc (4:1–1:1, v/v) to yield fractions Fr. 2.1–2.6. Fr. 2.4 and Fr. 2.5 were purified by semi-preparative reversed-phase HPLC using MeOH-H_2O (60:40, v/v) to afford **8** (5.0 mg) and **5** (4.8 mg), respectively. Fr. 3.4 was separated by silica gel CC using CH_2Cl_2-EtOAc (2:1, v/v) and was subsequently subjected to Sephadex LH-20 CC using MeOH as an eluent to give Fr. 3.4.5, followed by gradient elution MeOH-H_2O (70:30–0:100, v/v) with semi-preparative reversed-phase HPLC to obtain **1** (1.2 mg) and a mixture of diaporchromanone C (**6**) and D (**7**) (5.1 mg). Purification of Fr. 4 was isolated using CC over silica gel CC using CH_2Cl_2-EtOAc (1:1, v/v) to afford Fr. 4.1–Fr. 4.6. Fr. 4.5 was purified using RP-18 with a MeOH−H_2O (70:30, v/v) and then separated by semi-preparative reversed-phase HPLC with MeOH-H_2O (50:50, v/v) to yield **2/3** (5.1 mg). Fr. 6.2, collected from Fr. 6, was subjected to silica gel CC with gradient elution of CH_2Cl_2-EtOAc (100:6–100:8, v/v) to give Fr. 6.2.1–Fr. 6.2.3. Fr. 6.2.2 was further separated by semi-preparative HPLC (MeOH-H_2O, 55:45, v/v) to obtain **4** (3.0 mg).

3.4. Compound Characterization Data

Phomochromenone D (**1**): white amorphous powder (MeOH); $[\alpha]^{20}_D - 13$ (c 0.001, MeOH); UV (MeOH) λ_{max} 219, 245, 295 nm; ^{1}H and ^{13}C NMR data, see Tables 1 and 2, respectively; HR-ESI-MS m/z 307.1179 [M+H]$^+$ (calcd. for $C_{16}H_{19}O_6$, 307.1182).

Phomochromenone E (**2**): yellow gum (MeOH); $[\alpha]^{20}_D$ +17 (c 0.001, MeOH); UV (MeOH) λ_{max} 220, 245, 294 nm; ^{1}H NMR data, see Table 1; HR-ESI-MS m/z 321.0989 [M−H]$^−$ (calcd. for $C_{16}H_{17}O_7$, 321.0974).

Phomochromenone F (**3**): yellow gum (MeOH); $[\alpha]^{20}_D$ − 19 (c 0.0008, MeOH); UV (MeOH) λ_{max} 220, 245, 294 nm; ^{1}H NMR data, see Table 1; HR-ESI-MS m/z 321.0989 [M−H]$^−$ (calcd. for $C_{16}H_{17}O_7$, 321.0974).

Preparation of MPA Esters of **2/3** by Mosher's Method. The mixture of compounds **2** and **3** (1.5 mg) was treated with (*R*)- or (*S*)-MPA (1.0 mg) with DCC (1.0 mg) and DMAP (0.3 mg) in anhydrous CH_2Cl_2 (0.5 mL). After being stirred at room temperature for 4 h at 0 °C, the solvent from the reaction mixture was removed in vacuo to furnish a residue, which was then subjected to semi-preparative RP-HPLC eluting with CH_3CN-H_2O (40:60, 0.2% HCOOH) to obtain *R*-MTPA-**2**/*S*-MTPA-**3** (t_R 18.8 min) and *R*-MPA-**3**/*S*-MPA-**2** (t_R 19.2 min).

(*R*)-MPA ester of **2**: yellow gum (MeOH); ^{1}H NMR(400 MHz, CD$_3$OD) δ_H 7.63–7.41 (m, 5H), 7.25–7.18 (m, 5H), 7.22 (s, 1H), 5.26 (s, 1H), 4.98 (m, 1H), 4.68 (s, 1H), 3.94 (s, 3H), 3.92 (s, 3H), 3.55 (s, 3H), 3.20 (s, 3H), 2.77 (m, 1H), 2.62 (m, 1H), 1.92 (s, 3H), 1.09 (d, *J* = 6.2, 3H); HR-ESI-MS m/z 619.2164 [M + H]$^+$ (calcd. for $C_{34}H_{35}O_{11}$, 619.2179).

(*S*)-MPA ester of **2**: yellow gum (MeOH); 7.72–7.40 (m, 5H), 7.16 (s, 1H), 7.05–6.82 (m, 5H), 5.30 (s, 1H), 4.64 (s, 1H), 4.28 (m, 1H), 3.96 (s, 3H), 3.85 (s, 3H), 3.55 (s, 3H), 3.27 (s, 3H), 2.88 (m, 1H), 2.61 (m, 1H), 1.75 (s, 3H), 1.32 (d, *J* = 6.1, 3H); HR-ESI-MS m/z 619.2172 [M+H]$^+$ (calcd. for $C_{34}H_{35}O_{11}$, 619.2179).

(*R*)-MPA ester of **3**: yellow gum (MeOH); ^{1}H NMR(400 MHz, CD$_3$OD) δ_H 7.65–7.42 (m, 5H), 7.16 (s, 1H), 7.05–6.82 (m, 5H), 5.30 (s, 1H), 4.64 (s, 1H), 4.28 (m, 1H), 3.96 (s, 3H), 3.85 (s, 3H), 3.55 (s, 3H), 3.27 (s, 3H), 2.88 (m, 1H), 2.62 (m, 1H), 1.75 (s, 3H), 1.32 (d, *J* = 6.2, 3H); HR-ESI-MS m/z 619.2184 [M+H]$^+$ (calcd. for $C_{34}H_{35}O_{11}$, 619.2179).

(*S*)-MPA ester of **3**: yellow gum (MeOH); ^{1}H NMR(400 MHz, CD$_3$OD) δ_H 7.63–7.41 (m, 5H), 7.25–7.19 (m, 5H), 7.22 (s, 1H), 5.26 (s, 1H), 4.98 (m, 1H), 4.68 (s, 1H), 3.94 (s, 3H), 3.92 (s, 3H), 3.55 (s, 3H), 3.20 (s, 3H), 2.77 (m, 1H), 2.60 (m, 1H), 1.92 (s, 3H), 1.09 (d, *J* = 6.2, 3H); HR-ESI-MS m/z 619.2157 [M+H]$^+$ (calcd. for $C_{34}H_{35}O_{11}$, 619.2179).

Preparation of phomochromenones E(**2**) and F(**3**). (*R*)- and (*S*)-MPA ester of **2** were combined (1.2 mg) and dissolved in 10% NaOH (1.0 mL) and stirred for 1 h at room temperature (rt). The reaction mixture was extracted with EtOAc repeatedly and the organic layer was evaporated in vacuo to give optically pure (+)-**2** (0.7 mg). Similarly, (−)-**3** (0.8 mg) was prepared from the alkaline hydrolysis of (*R*)- and (*S*)-MPA ester of **3** (totally 1.0 mg) in the same manner.

Phomochromenone G (**4**): white amorphous powder (MeOH); $[\alpha]^{20}_D$ − 15 (c 0.001, MeOH); UV (MeOH) λ_{max} 205, 241, 303 nm; ^{1}H and ^{13}C NMR data, see Tables 1 and 2, respectively; HR-ESI-MS m/z 431.1314 [M+Na]$^+$ (calcd. for $C_{20}H_{24}O_9Na$, 431.1318).

Diaporchromone A (**5**): yellow gum (CHCl$_3$); $[\alpha]^{20}_D$ − 40 (c 0.001, MeOH); UV (MeOH) λ_{max} 219, 294 nm; ^{1}H NMR(400 MHz, CDCl$_3$) δ_H 6.89(1H, d, *J* = 2.3Hz, H-6), 6.87(1H, d, *J* = 2.3 Hz, H-8), 4.72(2H, m, H-9), 3.98(3H, s, H-14), 3.90(3H, s, H-15), 2.86(1H, dd, *J* = 17.4 Hz, *J* = 2.8 Hz, 10-Ha), 2.76(1H, dd, *J* = 17.4 Hz, *J* = 9.8 Hz, 10-Hb), 1.63(3H, s, H-12); ^{13}C-NMR (100 MHz, CDCl$_3$) δ_C 173.7 (C-4), 169.8 (C-13), 163.2 (C-7), 158.4 (C-2), 158.0 (C-8a), 134.7 (C-5), 115.6 (C-3), 114.4 (C-4a), 113.0 (C-6), 101.7 (C-8), 95.4 (C-11), 57.5 (C-9), 56.2 (C-15), 53.2 (C-14), 37.1 (C-10), 29.4 (C-12). ESI-MS m/z 321.09 [M+H]$^+$.

Diaporchromanone C (**6**): yellow gum (CHCl$_3$); UV (MeOH) λ_{max} 215, 239, 275, 315 nm; ^{1}H NMR(400MHz, CDCl$_3$) δ_H 6.54(1H, d, *J* = 2.4 Hz, H = 6), 6.46(1H, d, *J* = 2.4 Hz, H = 8), 4.71(1H, dd, *J* = 11.6 Hz, *J* = 6.3 Hz, 2-Ha), 4.57(1H, dd, *J* = 11.6 Hz, *J* = 3.9 Hz, 2-Hb), 4.38 (1H, ddd, *J* = 8.5 Hz, *J* = 8.5 Hz, *J* = 2.9 Hz, H-1′), 3.94(3H, s, H-10), 3.84(3H, s, H-11), 2.66(1H, ddd, *J* = 8.5 Hz, *J* = 6.3 Hz, *J* = 3.9 Hz, H-3), 2.88(1H, dd, *J* = 18.1 Hz, *J* = 2.9 Hz, 2′-Ha), 2.71(1H, dd, *J* = 18.1 Hz, *J* = 8.5 Hz, 2′-Hb), 2.18(3H, s, H-4′); ^{13}C NMR (125MHz, CDCl$_3$) δ_C 210.0 (C-3′), 190.2 (C-4), 169.7 (C-9), 165.5 (C-8a), 164.0 (C-7), 136.3 (C-5), 111.7 (C-4a), 109.8 (C-6), 102.0 (C-8), 68.2 (C-2), 64.0 (C-1′), 56.1 (C-11), 53.1 (C-10), 50.6 (C-3), 47.7 (C-2′), 30.9 (C-4′). ESI-MS m/z 323.09 [M+H]$^+$.

Diaporchromanone D (**7**): yellow gum (CHCl$_3$); UV (MeOH) λ_{max} 215, 239, 275, 315 nm; ^{1}H NMR(400MHz, CDCl$_3$) δ_H 6.56(1H, d, J = 2.4 Hz, H = 6), 6.46(1H, d, J = 2.4 Hz, H = 8), 4.60(1H, dd, J = 11.5 Hz, J = 5.1 Hz, 2-Ha), 4.51(1H, ddd, J = 8.7 Hz, J = 5.1 Hz, J = 3.6 Hz, H-1′), 4.47 (1H, dd, J = 11.5 Hz, J = 9.6 Hz, 2-Hb), 3.93(3H, s, H-10), 3.85(3H, s, H-11), 2.96(1H, ddd, J = 9.6 Hz, J = 5.1 Hz, J = 5.1 Hz, H-3), 2.80(1H, dd, J = 17.3 Hz, J = 8.7 Hz, 2′-Ha), 2.74(1H, dd, J = 17.3 Hz, J = 3.6 Hz, 2′-Hb), 2.18(3H, s, H-4′); ^{13}C NMR (125MHz, CDCl$_3$) δ_C 208.8 (C-3′), 190.9 (C-4), 169.7 (C-9), 165.6 (C-8a), 164.1 (C-7), 136.3 (C-5), 112.3 (C-4a), 109.8 (C-6), 102.2 (C-8), 68.6 (C-2), 66.4 (C-1′), 56.1 (C-11), 53.1 (C-10), 49.6 (C-3), 46.8 (C-2′), 31.0 (C-4′). ESI-MS m/z 323.09 [M+H]$^+$.

Phomochromenone C (**8**): yellow gum (MeOH); UV (MeOH) λ_{max} 206, 236, 308 nm; ^{1}H NMR (400 MHz, CD$_3$OD) δ_H 9.34(1H, s, H-1), 7.30(1H, s, H-4), 6.98(1H, s, H-8), 4.06(3H, s, H-14), 4.02(3H, s, H-13), 2.70(3H, s, H-3); ^{13}C-NMR (125MHz, CD3OD) δ_C 176.3 (C-10), 171.7(C-12), 165.4 (C-3), 162.9 (C-4a), 153.9 (C-7), 150.1 (C-1), 146.6 (C-5a), 139.1 (C-6), 124.6 (C-9), 116.7 (C-10a), 115.4 (C-9a), 112.7 (C-4), 109.6 (C-8), 57.3 (C-14), 53.4 (C-13), 24.4 (C-11). ESI-MS m/z 316.12 [M+H]$^+$.

3.5. Computational Analyses

Conformational analysis of the enantiomers of compounds **1** and **4** established by NOESY analyses were carried out using optimization and spectrum calculation. Conformational searches were carried out by means of the MM+ method in Hyper Chem 8.0 software (Hyperchem Release 8.0, Hypercube, Inc., Gainesville, FL, USA). The lowest energy conformers within 2 kcal/mol were subjected to further DFT calculations. The geometries of the conformers were optimized at the B3LYP/6-31+G(d,p) level in the gas phase using the Gaussian 09 program (Gaussian Inc., Wallingford, CT, USA). The theoretical calculation of ECD was conducted with IEFPCM solvent model for CH$_3$OH using TDDFT at the B3LYP/6-31+G(d,p) level for all conformers of compounds (see Supplementary Materials). Boltzmann-weighted ECD spectra was obtained using SpecDis1.70.1 software (University of Würzburg, Würzburg, Germany).

3.6. Preparation of Spleen Lymphocytes

Female BALB/c mice (6–8 weeks old, 20 ± 2 g) were purchased from the Department of Laboratory Animal Science (Hainan Medicinal University, China). The mice were sacrificed by cervical dislocation, and their spleens were collected in complete RPMI 1640 medium, which was minced with surgical scissors in a germ-free condition. The suspension was then filtered through a sterile sieve mesh to obtain the single cell suspension. After centrifugation (1000 rpm at 4 °C for 5 min), the resulting cells were treated with erythrocytes lysis buffer, followed by washing twice with cold phosphate-buffered saline (PBS). Then, the cells were adjusted to the concentration of 5×10^6 cells/mL and resuspended in RPMI 1640 medium supplemented with 10% heat-inactivated fetal bovine serum (FBS).

3.7. Cell Viability Assay

Cell viability of compounds **1–8** were measured using the tetrazolium salt-based CCK-8 assay according to a previously described protocol with some modifications [23]. Spleen lymphocytes were seeded into 96-well plates at a density of 2×10^6 cells/mL onto 96-well plates containing 100 μL of RPMI1640 complete medium (triplicate wells). Then, the cells were treated with 100 μL of various concentrations (3 μg/mL, 6 μg/mL, 12 μg/mL, 25 μg/mL, 50 μg/mL) of isolated compounds or cyclosporine (CsA) at 37 °C with a 5% CO$_2$ incubator for 44 h. At the end of the culture, the cell culture plate was removed and observed under an inverted microscope followed by 20 μL of CCK-8 reagent (5 mg/mL). The cells were further incubated for 4 h at 37 °C with 5% CO$_2$. The optical density was measured at 450 nm on a microplate reader.

3.8. Immunosuppressive Assay

Compounds **1–8** were evaluated for immunosuppressive activity against the proliferation of concanavalin A (ConA)-induced T and lipopolysaccharide (LPS)-induced B murine splenic lymphocyte in vitro using a CCK-8 method according to previously reported methods [24]. Cyclosporine A was used as a positive control.

Supplementary Materials: The following are available online at https://www.mdpi.com/article/10.3390/md19060348/s1. Figures S1–S36: Copies of HR-ESI-MS, 1D- and 2D-NMR spectra of **1–4**. Tables S1–S4: Gibbs free energies^a and equilibrium populations^b of low-energy conformers of **1** and **4**; Cartesian coordinates for the low-energy reoptimized MMFF conformers of **1** and **4** at B3LYP/6-31G(d,p) level of theory in gas.

Author Contributions: J.X. conceived and designed the experiments; C.W. and Z.F. isolated the metabolites; C.S. elucidated structures; X.Z. performed the bioactivity assays; J.X. and C.W. wrote the paper. All authors have read and agreed to the published version of the manuscript.

Funding: This work was supported by the Finance Science and Technology Project of Hainan Province (ZDKJ202018), the National Natural Science Foundation of China (No. 81973229/81660584), High-level Talents Programs of Hainan Province (2019RC006), and Key Project of the Education Department of Hainan Province (Hnky2019ZD-6).

Institutional Review Board Statement: All experiments conducted on animal material were approved by the Ethics Committee of the Hainan University (HNUAUCC-2021-00082, Feb. 19th, 2021), and all methods used were compliant with the regulations of the Ethics Committee.

Informed Consent Statement: Not applicable.

Data Availability Statement: Data is contained within the article or Supplementary Materials.

Conflicts of Interest: The authors declare no conflict of interest.

References

1. Xu, J.; Yi, M.; Ding, L.; He, S. A Review of Anti-Inflammatory Compounds from *Marine Fungi*, 2000–2018. *Mar. Drugs.* **2019**, *17*, 636–660. [CrossRef]
2. Bugni, T.S.; Ireland, C.M. Marine-derived fungi: A chemically and biologically diverse group of microorganisms. *Nat. Prod. Rep.* **2004**, *21*, 143–163. [CrossRef]
3. Xu, J. Bioactive natural products derived from mangrove-associated microbes. *RSC Adv.* **2015**, *5*, 841–892. [CrossRef]
4. Xu, J. Biomolecules Produced by Mangrove-Associated Microbes. *Curr. Med. Chem.* **2011**, *18*, 5224–5266. [CrossRef]
5. Zhou, J.; Xu, J. *Mangrove Ecosystem Ecology and Function*. InTechOpen Book Chapter: Chemistry and Biodiversity of Rhizophora-Derived Endophytic Fungi; InTechOpen: London, UK, 2018; Volume 8, pp. 165–184. ISBN 978-1-78984-277-7.
6. Yang, J.X.; Fang, X.; Huang, C.; Jing, L.; She, Z.; Zhong, P.; Lin, Y. Metabolites from the mangrove endophytic fungus *Phomopsis* sp. *Eur. J. Org. Chem.* **2010**, *41*, 3692–3695. [CrossRef]
7. Yan, B.C.; Wang, W.G.; Hu, D.B.; Sun, X.K.; Ling, M.; Li, X.N.; Du, X.; Luo, S.H.; Liu, Y.; Li, Y. Phomopchalasins a and b, two cytochalasans with polycyclic-fused skeletons from the endophytic fungus *phomopsis* sp shj2. *Org. Lett.* **2016**, *18*, 1108–1111. [CrossRef] [PubMed]
8. Prachya, S.; Wiyakrutta, S.; Sriubolmas, N.; Ngamrojanavanich, N.; Mahidol, C.; Ruchirawat, S.; Kittakoop, P. Cytotoxic mycoepoxydiene derivatives from an endophytic fungus *phomopsis* sp. isolated from hydnocarpus anthelminthicus. *Planta Med.* **2007**, *73*, 1418–1420. [CrossRef]
9. Wagenaar, M.M.; Clardy, J. Dicerandrols, new antibiotic and cytotoxic dimers produced by the fungus *phomopsis* l ongicolla isolated from an endangered mint. *J. Nat. Prod.* **2001**, *64*, 1006–1009. [CrossRef]
10. Elsässer, B.; Krohn, K.; Flörke, U.; Root, N.; Aust, H.J.; Draeger, S.; Schulz, B.; Antus, S.; Kurtán, T. New oblongolides isolated from the endophytic fungus *phomopsis* sp. from melilotus dentata from the shores of the baltic sea. *Eur. J. Org. Chem.* **2005**, 4563–4570. [CrossRef]
11. Horn, W.S.; Schwartz, R.E.; Simmonds, M.S.J.; Blaney, W.M. Isolation and characterization of phomodiol, a new antifungal from *phomopsis*. *Tetrahedron Lett.* **1994**, *35*, 6037–6040. [CrossRef]
12. Horn, W.S.; Simmonds, M.S.J.; Schwartz, R.E.; Blaney, W.M. Phomopsichalasin, a Novel Antimicrobial Agent from an Endophytic *Phomopsis* sp. *Tetrahedron Lett.* **1995**, *51*, 3969–3978. [CrossRef]
13. Kobayashi, H.; Meguro, S.; Yoshimoto, T.; Namikoshi, M. Absolute structure, biosynthesis, and anti-microtubule activity of phomopsidin, isolated from a marine-derived fungus *Phomopsis* sp. *Tetrahedron.* **2003**, *59*, 455–459. [CrossRef]
14. Weber, D.; Sterner, O.; Anke, T.; Gorzalczancy, S.; Martino, V.; Acevedo, C. Phomol, a new antiinflammatory metabolite from an endophyte of the medicinal plant erythrina crista-galli. *J. Antibiot.* **2004**, *57*, 559–563. [CrossRef] [PubMed]

15. Xu, Z.Y.; Xiong, B.X.; Xu, J. Chemical investigation of secondary metabolites produced by mangrove endophytic fungus phyllosticta capitalensis. *Nat. Prod. Res.* **2019**, *35*, 1561–1565. [CrossRef]
16. Zhou, J.; Li, G.; Deng, Q.; Zheng, D.Y.; Yang, X.B.; Xu, J. Cytotoxic constituents from the mangrove endophytic *Pestalotiopsis* sp. induce G(0)/G(1) cell cycle arrest and apoptosis in human cancer cells. *Nat. Prod. Res.* **2018**, *32*, 2968–2972. [CrossRef]
17. Xu, Z.Y.; Wu, X.; Li, G.; Feng, Z.; Xu, J. Pestalotiopisorin B, a new isocoumarin derivative from the mangrove endophytic fungus *Pestalotiopsis* sp. HHL101. *Nat. Prod. Res.* **2020**, *34*, 1002–1007. [CrossRef] [PubMed]
18. Hemberger, Y.; Xu, J.; Wray, V.; Proksch, P.; Wu, J.; Bringmann, G. Pestalotiopens A and B: Stereochemically Challenging Flexible Sesquiterpene-Cyclopaldic Acid Hybrids from *Pestalotiopsis* sp. *Chem. Eur. J.* **2013**, *19*, 15556–15564. [CrossRef]
19. Deng, Q.; Li, G.; Sun, M.Y.; Yang, X.; Xu, J. A new antimicrobial sesquiterpene isolated from endophytic fungus *Cytospora* sp. from the Chinese mangrove plant *Ceriops tagal*. *Nat. Prod. Res.* **2020**, *34*, 1404–1408. [CrossRef]
20. Cui, H.; Ding, M.; Huang, D.; Zhang, Z.; Liu, H.; Huang, H.; She, Z. Chroman-4-one and pyrano[4,3-b]chromenone derivatives from the mangrove endophytic fungus *diaporthe phaseolorum* sks019. *Rsc Advances.* **2017**, *7*, 20128–20134. [CrossRef]
21. Ding, B.; Wang, Z.Y.; Xia, G.P.; Huang, X.S.; Fang, C. Three new chromone derivatives produced by *phomopsis* sp. hny29-2b from *acanthus ilicifolius linn*. *Chin. J. Chem.* **2017**, 1889–1893. [CrossRef]
22. Zhou, J.; Diao, X.; Wang, T.; Chen, G.; Lin, Q.; Yang, X.; Xu, J. Phylogenetic diversity and antioxidant activities of culturable fungal endophytes associated with the mangrove species *Rhizophora stylosa* and *R. mucronata* in the South China Sea. *PLoS ONE* **2018**, *13*, e0197359. [CrossRef]
23. Cen, J.R.; Shi, M.S.; Yang, Y.F.; Fu, Y.X.; Zhou, H.L.; Wang, M.; Su, Z.; Wei, Q.; Mccormick, D.L. Isogarcinol is a new immunosuppressant. *PLoS ONE* **2013**, *8*, e66503. [CrossRef]
24. Xu, Z.Y.; Zhang, X.X.; Ma, J.K.; Yang, Y.; Zhou, J.; Xu, J. Secondary metabolites produced by mangrove endophytic fungus *Aspergillus fumigatus* HQD24 with immunosuppressive activity. *Biochem. Syst. Ecol.* **2020**, *93*, 104166. [CrossRef]

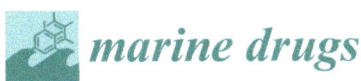

Review

Marine Polysaccharides as a Versatile Biomass for the Construction of Nano Drug Delivery Systems

Ying Sun [1], Xiaoli Ma [2] and Hao Hu [1,*]

[1] Institute of Biomedical Materials and Engineering, College of Materials Science and Engineering, Qingdao University, Qingdao 266071, China; sunying150996@163.com
[2] Qingdao Institute of Measurement Technology, Qingdao 266000, China; maxiaoli1989@yeah.net
* Correspondence: huhao@qdu.edu.cn

Abstract: Marine biomass is a treasure trove of materials. Marine polysaccharides have the characteristics of biocompatibility, biodegradability, non-toxicity, low cost, and abundance. An enormous variety of polysaccharides can be extracted from marine organisms such as algae, crustaceans, and microorganisms. The most studied marine polysaccharides include chitin, chitosan, alginates, hyaluronic acid, fucoidan, carrageenan, agarose, and Ulva. Marine polysaccharides have a wide range of applications in the field of biomedical materials, such as drug delivery, tissue engineering, wound dressings, and sensors. The drug delivery system (DDS) can comprehensively control the distribution of drugs in the organism in space, time, and dosage, thereby increasing the utilization efficiency of drugs, reducing costs, and reducing toxic side effects. The nano-drug delivery system (NDDS), due to its small size, can function at the subcellular level in vivo. The marine polysaccharide-based DDS combines the advantages of polysaccharide materials and nanotechnology, and is suitable as a carrier for different pharmaceutical preparations. This review summarizes the advantages and drawbacks of using marine polysaccharides to construct the NDDS and describes the preparation methods and modification strategies of marine polysaccharide-based nanocarriers.

Keywords: marine polysaccharide; drug delivery system; nanocarrier; cancer therapy

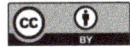

1. Introduction

Because the human body has a complex physiological environment and defense capabilities, whether it is administered by oral, intramuscular, or intravenous injection, the utilization of drugs has been severely weakened [1]. The hydrophilicity and hydrophobicity of drug molecules determine the absorption, distribution, metabolism, and excretion of drugs in the body [2]. The hydrophobic structure in some drug molecules, such as benzene rings, can increase the hydrophobicity of the drug. The development of nano-drug delivery systems (NDDSs) brings hope to overcome the above obstacles. The drug molecules can be encapsulated in the interior or adsorbed on the surface by physical action or can be connected to the framework or matrix of the nanocarrier by chemical bonding [3,4]. At present, nanocarriers have been widely used to deliver drugs [5], peptides [6], and nucleic acids [7]. Nanocarriers can (1) help drugs avoid rapid clearance during circulation and prolong their time in the blood [8], (2) be enriched at the lesion site through enhanced permeability and retention effect (EPR effect) or active targeting, which improves the utilization of drugs and reduces toxic and side effects [9], and (3) realize the controlled release of drugs through internal (e.g., pH) or external (e.g., radiation) stimulation signals [10]. Some DDSs have realized the transformation from laboratory to clinical [11].

The materials for constructing nanocarriers need to have good biocompatibility and biodegradability. A large number of organic and inorganic materials have been studied to construct carriers [12,13]. As a kind of natural polymer, polysaccharides are non-toxic, biodegradable, and rich in reserves, and have shown great application prospects in the fields of biology, medicine and pharmaceuticals [14–16]. Polysaccharides have various resources from terrestrial and marine animals, plants, and microorganisms. Marine polysaccharides bear important physiological functions in marine organisms and are an important type of biomass. Compared with polysaccharides extracted from the land, polysaccharides extracted from marine organisms (shells, crabs, shrimps, sharks, squids, seaweed, etc.) have absolute advantages in terms of biodiversity and simple preparation process. Marine polysaccharides and their derivatives are excellent substrates for the construction of DDSs.

Some marine polysaccharides have biological activities, such as anti-tumor, antiviral, anti-cardiovascular disease, and immune regulatory effects [17,18]. For example, hyaluronic acid (HA) can be specifically targeted to the CD44 receptor that is overexpressed on many tumor cells [19]. Chitosan (CS) has effective antibacterial ability [20]. Besides, there are a large number of active functional groups on the backbone of marine polysaccharides, such as hydroxyl, amino, and carboxylic acid groups. Marine polysaccharides can be chemically modified through these active sites to expand their application fields [21]. Drug molecules can be conjugated to the backbone of polysaccharide molecules through cleavable chemical bonds [22]. The charged drug molecules can form nanoparticles with charged polysaccharides through electrostatic interaction [23,24]. Drug molecules can be encapsulated in the internal cavities of micelles formed by polysaccharide-based amphiphilic polymers through hydrophobic interaction [25]. The construction of the marine polysaccharide-based DDS can make DDSs possess the various advantages of nanoscale systems while also possessing the properties of polysaccharides.

This review summarizes the advantages and disadvantages of marine polysaccharides and introduces the preparation and modification methods of marine polysaccharide-based DDSs in detail. We look forward to the future applications of marine polysaccharides, and hope that this review will inspire the research and development of marine polysaccharide products.

2. Characteristics of Marine Polysaccharides

2.1. Structure and Classification

Polysaccharides are a class of carbohydrates with complex and large molecular structures. Polysaccharides are formed by the dehydration of multiple monosaccharide molecules. The structural units of polysaccharides are connected by glycoside bonds. Common glycoside bonds include α-1,4-, β-1,4- and α-1,6-glycosidic bonds. The structural unit can be connected into a straight chain or a branched chain. The straight chain is generally connected by α-1,4-glycosidic bonds (such as starch) or β-1,4-glycosidic bonds (such as cellulose); the connection point in the branched chain is often α-1,6-glycosidic bonds [26,27]. The polysaccharides composed of single monosaccharide are defined as homopolysaccharides, such as starch, cellulose, and glycogen [26]. The polysaccharides composed of diverse monosaccharides are called heteropolysaccharides such as HA, chondroitin, and alginate (Alg) [28–30]. Marine polysaccharides can be divided into marine animal polysaccharides, marine plant polysaccharides, and marine microbial polysaccharides, according to their sources. There are many kinds of active polysaccharides isolated from marine animals, such as chitin in crustaceans, chondroitin sulfate in cartilaginous fish bones, sulfated polysaccharides in sea cucumbers and starfish, and glycosamines in mollusks, scallops, clams, and abalones. The seaweeds (such as brown algae, red algae, and green algae) are the main source of marine plant polysaccharides. Brown algae are rich in algin and fucoidan; red algae mainly contain carrageenan and agar polysaccharides; the Ulva polysaccharide is the main ingredient in green algae. Marine microbial polysaccharides are polysaccharides produced by marine bacteria, microalgae, or fungi. The chemical structure, source, and feature of typical marine polysaccharides are summarized in Table 1.

2.2. Advantages of Marine Polysaccharide-Based DDSs

Biocompatibility, biodegradability, low immunogenicity, and high natural availability are recognized advantages of marine polysaccharides [31,32]. The presence of multifunctional groups (such as hydroxyl, carboxyl, and amine) on the molecular backbone makes it easy to be modified by chemical, biochemical, or enzymatic modification (Figure 1). Common construction methods include: (i) esterification of hydroxyl groups with acylating agents; etherification of hydroxyl groups with alkylation agents; oxidation of primary alcohols to carboxyl groups; oxidation of vicinal secondary hydroxyl groups to aldehydes; (ii) ester bonds consist of hydroxyl groups linked to carboxyl groups; amide bonds consist of carboxyl groups linked to amino groups; hydrazone bond formed by the reaction of -COOH and -NHNH$_2$; (iii) interaction between amino groups and hydroxyl or carboxyl groups. Drug molecules can be grafted onto polysaccharides through the reaction with the active groups on the polysaccharides. Carboxymethyl groups can be introduced into the polysaccharide backbone through the esterification reaction of polysaccharides and carboxylic acid derivatives. Carboxymethylation can increase the solubility and electronegativity of polysaccharides. In addition, some types of marine polysaccharides have unique physicochemical properties and pharmacological effects due to their unique structure. For instance, CS is the only alkaline polysaccharide in nature. The amino groups in its molecular chain can combine with protons to generate cations in weak acid solutions, thus having a broad-spectrum antibacterial activity [33,34]. Some marine polysaccharides retain several recognition functions, permitting specific receptor recognition or adhesion, as well as providing neutral coatings with low surface energy and avoiding non-specific protein adsorption. HA can recognize the CD44 receptor on the cell surface [35]. The carrier with the negative surface can prevent the adhesion of proteins in the blood and prolong the circulation time of the carrier. Marine polysaccharides such as HA and Alg exhibit negative charge under physiological conditions, and in some cases, can be used as a substitute for poly(ethylene glycol) (PEG) segments. The mentioned advantages make marine polysaccharides an ideal candidate material for the design and preparation of DDSs.

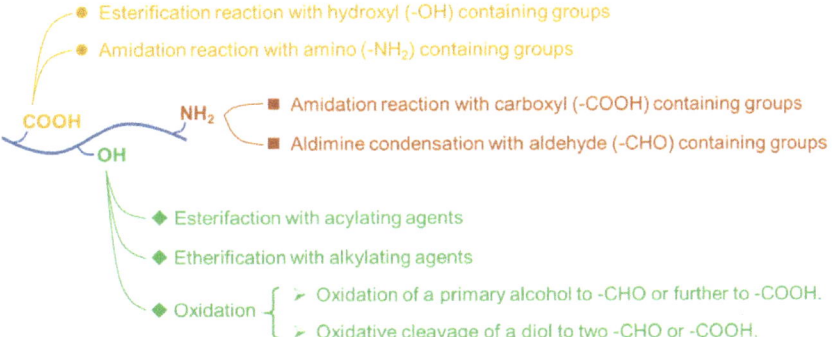

Figure 1. Overview of polysaccharide derivatization.

2.3. Drawbacks of Using Polysaccharide in Drug Delivery

Although many marine polysaccharide-based products, such as wound dressings and dermal filler, have been used clinically, most of these products are used in vitro or in specific locations in the body [36,37]. As for the carrier, it is usually required to have a clear structure and clear metabolism in the body [38,39]. Marine polysaccharide-based materials are at a disadvantage in this regard. Because the source of marine polysaccharides is destined to have its molecular weight and structure susceptible to the season and place of production [40]. Even though high-quality and stable products can be obtained through industrial refinement, it is usually accompanied by a substantial increase in cost. In addition, due to the uncertainty of selecting model drugs in most studies, it is necessary to fully study the interaction between drug molecules, polysaccharides, and the human body, including absorption, distribution, metabolism, and excretion.

Some marine polysaccharides have poor solubility in common solvents, which limits the chemical modification of polysaccharides. For example, CS can only be dissolved in some dilute inorganic or organic acids. Only by reducing the molecular weight or making hydrophilic modification can the water solubility of CS be increased [41]. Alg is soluble in an aqueous solution, but after multiple steps of modification, its solubility in an aqueous solution is usually greatly reduced. Considering these drawbacks, the design of DDSs based on marine polysaccharides should be considered holistically.

In fact, some of the drawbacks mentioned above are not only the existence of marine polysaccharide-based DDSs, but carriers of other materials also face these problems. Therefore, starting from the bottom, optimizing the design, flexible modification, the all-around carrier may be obtained. Figure 2 summarizes the advantages and disadvantages of marine polysaccharides in the construction of DDSs.

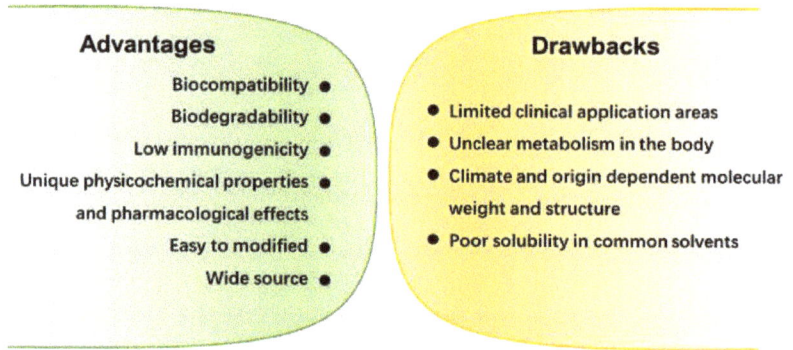

Figure 2. Advantages and disadvantages of marine polysaccharides in the construction of DDSs.

3. Preparation and Modification of the Marine Polysaccharide-Based DDS

3.1. Preparation of Marine Polysaccharide-Based Nanoparticles (NPs)

The preparation of marine polysaccharide-based NPs can be categorized as self-assembly and covalent crosslinking. Self-assembled NPs are formed under the action of non-covalent bonds. The driving force mainly includes polyelectrolyte complexation, hydrophobic interaction, and ionic interactions [21,42]. There are many ways to achieve covalent crosslinking, such as chemical crosslinking and radiation crosslinking [43,44]. Depending on the synthesis method, the obtained NPs can be nanogels, micelles, or vesicles [45–47].

3.1.1. Polyelectrolyte Complexation (PEC)

Marine polysaccharides containing ionizable groups can be classified as natural polyelectrolytes. The polyelectrolyte complexation is formed by electrostatic interaction between oppositely charged components. Naturally charged polysaccharides can easily form PEC with oppositely charged polyelectrolytes. The only cationic polysaccharide, CS, can form PEC with negative polysaccharides, peptides, and polyacrylic acid family [48]. Furthermore, CS can also form complexes with nucleic acids, serving as a matrix for gene carriers [49]. However, it should be noted that due to the poor water solubility of CS, more studies have been conducted on CS derivatives, such as glycol chitosan [50,51]. Malhotra et al. used sodium hydride to catalyze the etherification reaction between chlorinated chitosan and methyl-PEG, and PEG-grafted chitosan was successfully synthesized [50]. Under physiological conditions, some groups become negatively charged after ionization, such as the carboxylate in HA and Alg, and the sulfonate in chondroitin sulfate, thus that polysaccharide molecules can interact with positively charged polymers [52,53]. Figure 3a shows a schematic diagram of the formation of NPs by electrostatic interaction between CS and semi-flexible polyethylene glycol [54]. The molecular weight and flexibility of each component will affect the particle size. Similarly, the NPs formed by the complexation of CS and nucleic acid are also affected by factors such as the ratio of nitrogen to phosphorus and pH (Figure 3b) [55]. At a low N/P ratio, cationic compounds are not enough to compress nucleic acids into nanoparticles, and loose complexes with low transfection and low toxicity efficiency can be formed through weak electrostatic interaction. As the N/P ratio increases, when the cationic compounds reach a sufficient amount, compact complexes with ideal transfection efficiency but quite a cytotoxicity can be formed [7]. Both the nucleic acid and the cell membrane are negatively charged, thus the charge of the carrier not only affects the loading of the nucleic acid but also affects the affinity of the nanocarrier and the cell membrane. These positively charged nanocarriers are easily attached to the cell membrane surface and then taken up by the cell. The main advantage of this method for preparing marine polysaccharide-based NPs is a simple operation. NPs can be formed in situ by simply mixing two polyelectrolytes with opposite charges in a solution. However, the stability of the complex requires attention. The formation and stability of the PEC depend on the structure, molecular weight, surface charge density, and mixing ratio of the polyelectrolyte. External conditions such as pH, temperature, ionic strength, and solvent properties also affect the preparation process of NPs.

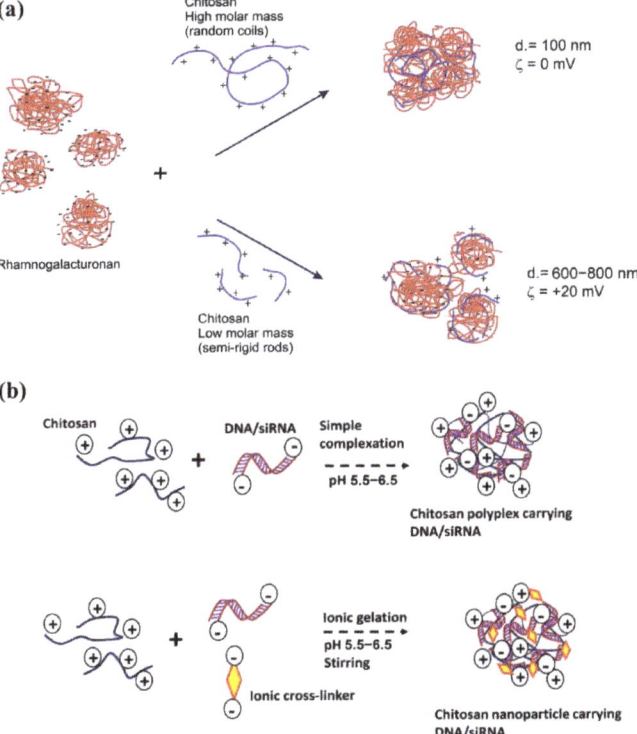

Figure 3. (**a**) Schematic representation of the effect of CS molar mass on the particle size of PEC formed with semi-flexible polynion, adapted from [54]. (**b**) Common preparation methods of chitosan nanocarrier for DNA/siRNA delivery. Adapted from [55].

3.1.2. Hydrophobic Interaction

Micelle is a thermodynamically stable nanosystem self-assembled of amphiphilic polymers in an aqueous solution. The hydrophobic cavity of the micelle can be loaded with poorly water-soluble drugs to realize the solubilization of the drug; the hydrophilic shell of the micelle can protect the drug from non-specific uptake by the reticuloendothelial system and prolong the retention of the drug in the blood circulation. When hydrophilic polysaccharides are grafted with hydrophobic fragments, amphiphilic copolymers based on polysaccharides are obtained [56,57]. Commonly used hydrophobic fragments include cholesterol, steroid acids, deoxycholic acid, and hydrophobic polymers [58]. The hydroxyl, amino, and carboxyl groups on the polysaccharide backbone are common sites for connecting hydrophobic fragments. When in an aqueous solution, to achieve the minimum free energy, the hydrophobic segment can spontaneously form micelles or self-aggregates through the interaction between the intermolecular and intramolecular hydrophobic parts [58]. For instance, Zhong et al. used HA (M_W ~ 9.5 kDa) as the hydrophilic segment to prepare endosomal pH-activatable paclitaxel prodrug micelles for active targeting and effective treatment of CD44-overexpressing human breast cancer xenografts in nude mice (Figure 4) [59]. The in vivo pharmacokinetics and biodistribution studies showed that the HA-shelled acid-activatable paclitaxel prodrug micelles (HA-dOG-PTX-PM) had a prolonged circulation time in the nude mice and a remarkably high accumulation in the MCF-7 tumor (6.19%ID/g at 12 h post-injection). The size and thermodynamic stability of micelles depend on the ratio of hydrophilic and hydrophobic parts.

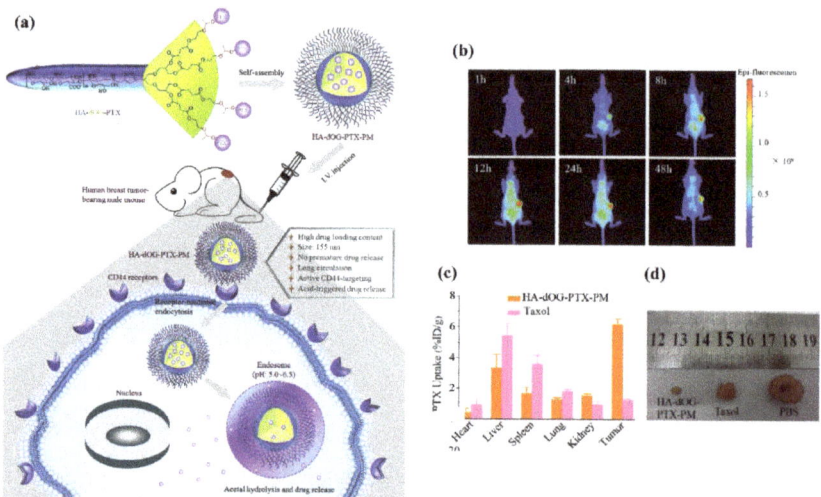

Figure 4. (**a**) Endosomal pH-activatable HA-bdendritic oligoglycerol (HA-dOG-PTX-PM) for active CD44-targeted paclitaxel (PTX) delivery in vivo; (**b**) in vivo fluorescence images of MCF-7 human breast tumor-bearing nude mice at different time points following injection of DIR-loaded HA-dOG-PTX-PM; (**c**) quantification of PTX accumulated in tumor and different organs using HPLC measurements. PTX uptake is expressed as injected dose per gram of tissue (%ID/g). Data are presented as mean ± SD (*n* = 3); (**d**) photographs of typical tumor blocks collected from different treatment groups of mice on day 29. Adapted from [59].

3.1.3. Ionic Interaction

The ionic interaction is also a kind of electrostatic interaction. The polyelectrolyte polysaccharide interacts with oppositely charged ions to crosslink [60]. Ionic interaction strategy is the most useful method to crosslink Alg. Alg is a polysaccharide containing beta-D-mannuronate (M) and alpha-L-guluronate (G) building blocks. In the presence of divalent cations, such as Cu^{2+} or Ca^{2+}, the G blocks of adjacent Alg chains could be cooperatively chelated [61]. For example, Zhang et al. prepared a gene carrier (denoted as Ca^{2+}/(Alg/PEI/DNA) NPs) with calcium ions crosslinked sodium alginate as a protective layer [62]. As shown in Figure 5, sodium alginate, which was further crosslinked by Ca^{2+}, was chosen as the shielding material to improve the stability of PEI/DNA complexes. Compared to PEI/DNA complexes and Alg/PEI/DNA complexes, $Ca^{2+}/(Alg/PEI/DNA)$ NPs exhibited enhanced stability, which was confirmed by the in vitro and in vivo. Furthermore, the pharmacokinetic study indicated that $Ca^{2+}/(Alg/PEI/DNA)$ NPs exhibited longer circulation time in blood, which would be beneficial to the EPR effect of NPs and could realize improved NPs accumulation at the tumor site. Factors that may affect the formation of NPs through ionic crosslinking include the molecular weight and type of polysaccharide, the ionic strength and pH of the solvent, and the ratio of ionic crosslinker to the polysaccharide [63,64]. NPs crosslinked by divalent chelation alone may not provide sufficient swelling capacity or mechanical properties because divalent ions will leak from the NPs into the surrounding medium.

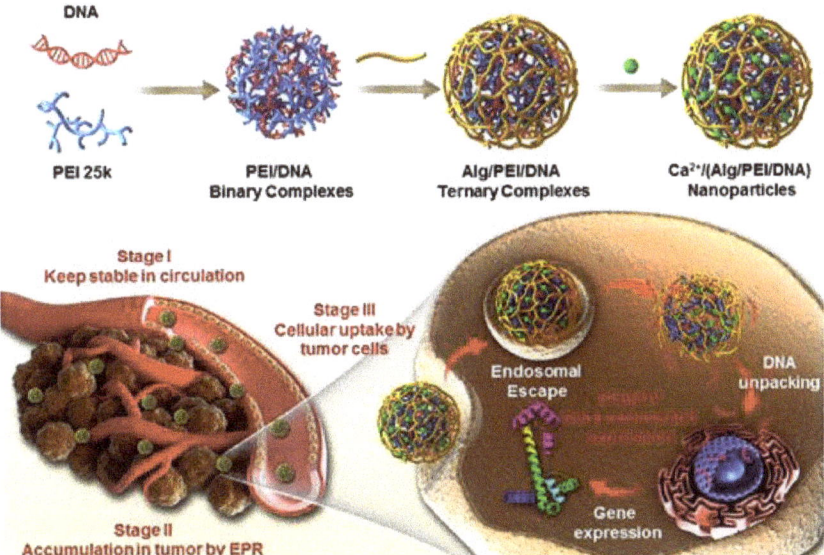

Figure 5. Preparation of $Ca^{2+}/(Alg/PEI/DNA)$ NPs and the schematic illustration of the in vivo transportation process of $Ca^{2+}/(Alg/PEI/DNA)$ NPs. Adapted from [62].

3.1.4. Covalent Crosslinking

The NPs after covalent crosslinking are more compact and stable. The crosslinked polysaccharide-based NPs can be used as a DDS to avoid premature dissociation and drug leakage. Usually, the reactive functional groups (such as hydroxyl, amino, and carboxylic acid groups) on the polysaccharide molecular backbone are used as crosslinking sites. The complementary group can be on the chain of another component, or an additional small molecule crosslinker can be used. Covalent crosslinking strategies mainly include Schiff-base reaction, radical polymerization, click chemistries, and photoreaction [65,66]. The vicinal glycols in some marine polysaccharides can be specifically oxidized cleavage by periodate to form aldehyde groups that could subsequently react with amine groups. The Schiff-base reaction is the most commonly used method for preparing CS-based NPs [67,68]. Molecules with more than two active groups may be used as crosslinking agents. The two aldehyde groups of glutaraldehyde can efficiently react with the amino groups on the macromolecular chain to achieve crosslinking. Schiff-base (imine) linkages would be hydrolyzed under acidic conditions, which is related to the degradation of the DDS and the controlled release of drugs. It should be noted that aldehyde groups are toxic to cells and can cause severe inflammation in the body. If crosslinking agents containing aldehyde groups are introduced during the preparation process, especially small molecule crosslinking agents (e.g., glutaraldehyde), the residual crosslinking agents should be completely removed, and the biocompatibility of the DDS needs to be strictly evaluated. Dialysis and washing against distilled water are common methods to remove residual crosslinking agents. Marine polysaccharides containing carboxyl groups (such as HA and Alg) can be crosslinked by the condensation reaction of -COOH/-OH or -COOH/-NH$_2$. Ester bonds or amide bonds are formed as linkages to connect different molecular chains [28]. The polysaccharide can also be modified in advance to introduce other chemically reactive groups. Alg is usually crosslinked through ionic interaction, but the carboxyl group on its backbone can also be modified [69]. More and more new types of crosslinking agents or methods have been reported to solve the conflict between crosslinking efficiency and toxicity, such as silane coupling agents, amine-reactive disuccinimidyl tartrate, and horseradish peroxidase-catalyzed crosslinking [70–72].

Crosslinking methods, including physical crosslinking and chemical crosslinking methods, are the most effective methods for preparing marine polysaccharide NPs. There are other methods for preparing polysaccharide particles, such as the precipitation/coagulation method, solvent evaporation method, and spray drying method [73–75]. However, the particle size obtained by these methods is relatively large and uneven. The DDS prepared by these methods is suitable for mucosal absorption administration on the skin, eyes, cavities, etc., but is not suitable for intravenous administration.

3.2. Modification of Polysaccharide-Based NPs

A qualified DDS needs to have good dispersion stability, biocompatibility, stealth during the circulation in the body, and targeting of the lesion [76,77]. Although polysaccharide-based NPs have some inherent properties, such as good biocompatibility, to be a perfect carrier, they need to be modified to be endowed with new functions and meet the requirements of biomedical applications. Therefore, surface modification is another important step in the preparation of the polysaccharide-based DDS.

Similar to the description in the covalent crosslinking section, the modification of polysaccharide-based NPs is also based on the reactive groups in the molecule. However, compared to covalent crosslinking, the methodology used in the modification process is more flexible. Taking the functional groups on the backbone as a starting point, the polysaccharide couples to other molecules through the reaction between the functional groups [78,79]. The main methods of polysaccharide modification are the formation of esters or ethers using saccharides hydroxyl groups as nucleophiles, the chemical oxidation of primary alcohols to aldehydes or carboxylic acids, the enzymatic oxidation of primary alcohols to uronic acid, the formation of amide bonds between the saccharides carboxyl group and heteroatomic nucleophiles, as well as the nucleophilic reactions or Schiff-base reaction of the amines [21,80]. Physical adsorption is also one of the methods for surface modification, but it is usually used for the modification of charged polysaccharide (e.g., CS, HA, Alg) [81]. The modification process may be achieved through one or more steps.

3.2.1. Modification of Functional Molecules on Marine Polysaccharide-Based NPs

The purpose of the functional modification is to change the in vivo process of NPs after intravenous injection, thus that they can have long circulation or targeting functions, thereby enhancing drug efficacy and reducing adverse reactions. For marine polysaccharide-based NPs, giving DDSs the ability to target lesions actively is the main research content. Coupling or adsorbing appropriate ligands (including antibodies, haptens, lectins, folic acid, etc.) on the surface of NPs, DDSs can be directed to specific cells using the strong affinity of the ligands to specific receptors on the cell surface [82]. For example, the surface of CS-based NPs can be efficiently targeted to tumors after being conjugated with folic acid [83]. In addition, there are also reports that graft drug molecules on the polysaccharide backbone to achieve drug delivery. As illustrated in Figure 6a, Jafari et al. reported a fucoidan (M_W ~70 kDa)-based DDS for minimizing the side effects of doxorubicin (Dox) with the help of active targeting toward P-selectin [84]. P-selectin, which plays an important role in metastasis by enhancing the adhesion of cancer cells to endothelium and activated platelets in distant organs, is overexpressed on many cancer types. The fucoidan-doxorubicin conjugate (FU-Dox NPs) showed a well-controlled size distribution and sustained release. The active targeting capability of FU-Dox NPs toward P-selectin resulted in enhanced cellular uptake and cytotoxicity against the MDA-MB-231 cell line with high P-selectin expression compared to the MDA-MB-468 cell line with low P-selectin expression Figure 6b. To achieve a controlled release of the pendant, cleavable bonds will be introduced into the DDS. For example, disulfide bonds or imine bonds were introduced between the functional molecules and the polysaccharide backbone to realize the response release of the tumor microenvironment [85–87].

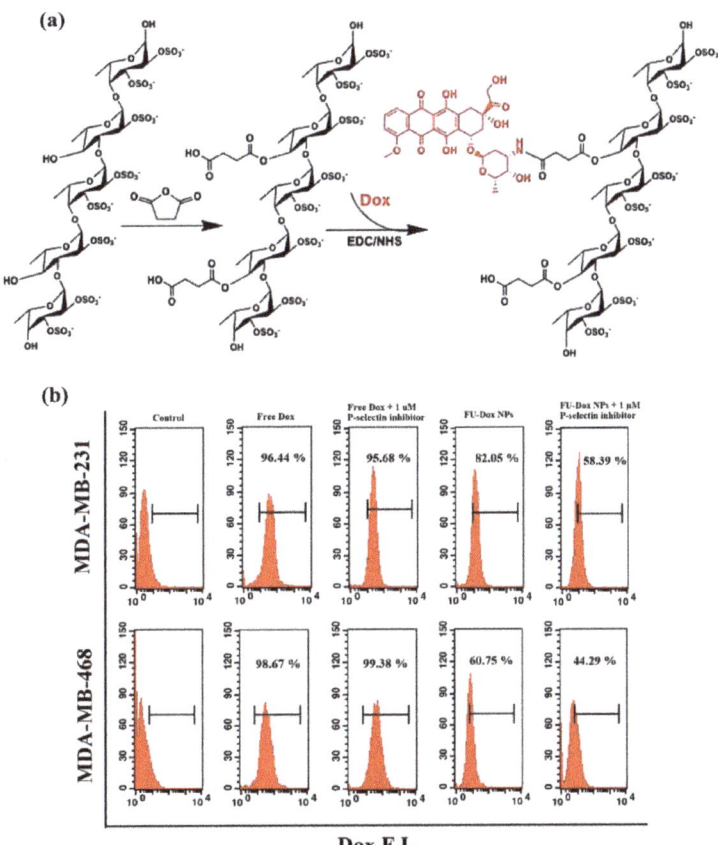

Figure 6. (**a**) Synthesis route of fucoidan-doxorubicin conjugate (FU-Dox NPs) developed by direct conjugation of Dox to the fucoidan backbone; (**b**) flow cytometry analysis of the cellular uptake of FU-Dox NPs after pretreatment with 1 µM P-selectin inhibitor, KF 38789, for MDA-MB-231 and MDA-MB-468 cell lines. Adapted from [84].

Table 1. The chemical structure, source, and feature of typical marine polysaccharides.

Polysaccharides	Structure	Source	Feature	Reference
Chitosan (CS)		Extracted from shrimp and crab	CS is a deacetylated chitin derivative, consisting of β-1,4-linked glucosamine (2-amino-2-deoxy-β-D-glucose) and minor amounts of N-acetyl glucosamine.	[20,41]
Hyaluronic Acid (HA)		Extracted from fish eye and mussel	HA is a linear negatively charged polysaccharide constituted repeating monosaccharide unit of N-acetyl-D-glucosamine and D-glucuronic acid, which is linked together via alternating β-1,3 and β-1,4 glycosidic bonds.	[28]
Alginate (Alg)		Extracted from brown algae	Alg is a well-known linear anion polyelectrolyte polysaccharide consisting of β-D-Mannuronic acid (M units) and α-L-Guluronic acid (G units).	[29,53]
Chondroitin sulfate		Extracted from fish cartilage	Chondroitin sulfate composed of an alternating disaccharide units of N-acetylgalactosamine and glucuronic acid, which joined together through β-(1→3) glycosidic bonds.	[30,37]
Fucoidan		Extracted from brown algae	Fucoidan derived from kelp is formed by the sulfated fucose linked by α-(1→3) glycosidic bonds, while the fucoidan derived from fucus and ascophyllum is linked by α-(1→3) and α-(1→4) glycosidic bonds.	[68,84]
Ulva		Extracted from green algae	Ulva is dominated by repeating disaccharide units, where uronic acid, either D-glucuronic acid or L-iduronic acid, or D-xylose is linked to L-rhamnose-3-sulfate through 1, 4-glycosidic bonds.	[37]
Carrageenan (λ) Carrageenan (ι) Carrageenan (κ)		Extracted from red algae	Carrageenan is mainly formed by alternately connecting disaccharide units composed of α-(1→4)-D-galactopyranose or β-(1→3)-D-galactopyranose of substitution of sulfate groups.	[37]

3.2.2. Grafting Polymer Chains onto Marine Polysaccharides

Grafting polymer chains on the macromolecular backbone can effectively change the properties of marine polysaccharides. The introduction of polymer chains can be divided into two strategies: "graft from" and "graft to" [88,89]. The "graft from" strategy mainly takes the active group on the polysaccharide backbone as the initiation site and introduces functional side chains through atom transfer radical polymerization (ATRP) and reversible addition-fragmentation chain transfer polymerization (RAFT), including cationic components for nucleic acid delivery, PEGylated, and zwitterionic moieties for shielding effects, and functional species for bioimaging applications as well as bioresponsive drug release applications [15]. Ping et al. used ATRP to functionalize CS in a well-controlled manner [90]. As shown in Figure 7a, a series of new degradable cationic polymers (termed as PDCS) composed of biocompatible CS (M_w ~ 150 kDa; degree of deacetylation: 83%) backbones and poly((2-dimethyl amino)ethyl methacrylate) (P(DMAEMA)) side chains of different length were designed as highly efficient gene vectors via ATRP. In comparison with high-molecular-weight P(DMAEMA) and 'gold-standard' PEI (25 kDa), the PDCS vectors showed considerable buffering capacity in the pH range of 7.4 to 5. They were capable of mediating much more efficient gene transfection at low N/P ratios (Figure 7b). At their own optimal N/P ratios for transfection, the PDCS/pDNA complexes showed much lower cytotoxicity (Figure 7c). The "graft to" strategy is usually based on more reactive reactions such as click chemistry reactions [47]. The properties of DDSs can be controlled by regulation of the length of the polymer segment [15].

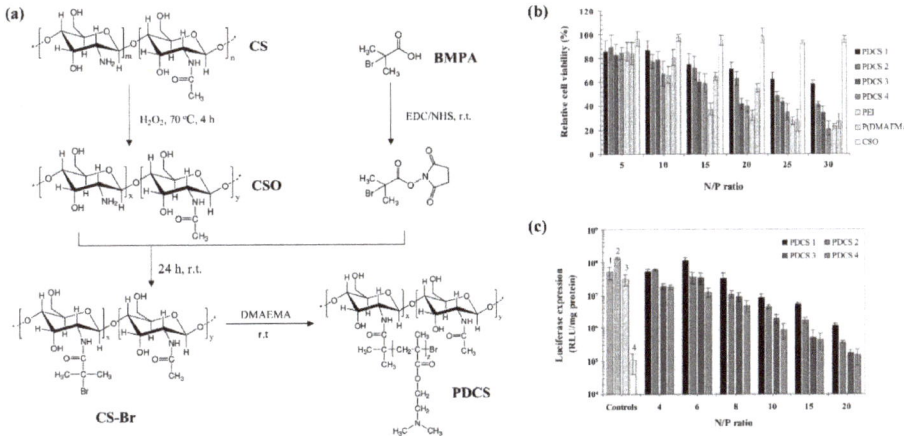

Figure 7. (a) Route of the synthesis of P(DMAEMA) functionalized CS (PDCS); (b) Cell viability of PDCS/pDNA polyplexes at different N/P ratios in COS7, where polyethylenimine (PEI) (25 kDa), P(DMAEMA) and chitosan oligomers (CSO) polyplexes were used as controls. (mean ± SD, n = 4); (c) in vitro gene transfection efficiency of PDCS/pDNA polyplexes in comparison with those mediated by PEI (25 kDa) (control 1) at N/P ratio of 10, ExGen 500 (control 2) at N/P ratio of 6, P(DMAEMA) (control 3) at N/P ratio of 10, and CSO (control 4) at N/P ratio of 20 in COS7 cell line in the presence of serum. (mean ± SD, n = 3). Adapted from [90].

4. Conclusions and Perspectives

Marine polysaccharides are gifts from nature. The development and utilization of marine polysaccharides are one of the ways to realize the high value of marine resources. The inherent natural properties of marine polysaccharides, such as biodegradability and biocompatibility, make marine polysaccharide-based nanocarriers a high potential platform for developing DDS. The marine polysaccharide-based DDS integrates the advantages of nanotechnology and is suitable as a carrier for different pharmaceutical preparations. From the bench to industrialization is not a simple process. It is necessary to further optimize the extraction and purification process of marine polysaccharides and integrate upstream and downstream resources. With the development and mutual penetration of related disciplines such as chemistry, biology, physics, and pharmacy, the application fields of marine polysaccharide products have gradually expanded, for example, in the fields of tissue engineering, scaffold materials, and wound accessories. There are already a large number of products based on marine polysaccharides, such as clinical wound dressings (e.g., Hemcon Gauze, Regenecare HA) and health products (e.g., Move Free joint health supplements). However, the marine polysaccharide-based DDS still has a long way to go to clinical application. As technical issues such as preparation, quality standards, and route of administration are resolved, marine polysaccharide-based products will have great development prospects.

Author Contributions: All authors designed the concept of the manuscript. Y.S. collected information and wrote the manuscript. X.M. collected information and contributed to visualization. H.H. contributed to reviewing and editing of the manuscript. All authors have read and agreed to the published version of the manuscript.

Funding: This research was funded by the National Natural Science Foundation of China (51703105) and the China Postdoctoral Science Foundation (2018M630752).

Institutional Review Board Statement: Not applicable.

Informed Consent Statement: Not applicable.

Data Availability Statement: Data sharing not applicable.

Conflicts of Interest: There are no conflict to declare.

Abbreviations

DDS	Drug delivery system
NDDS	Nano drug delivery system
HA	Hyaluronic acid
CS	Chitosan
CSO	Chitosan oligomers
Alg	Alginate
NPs	Nanoparticles
PEC	Polyelectrolyte complexation
PTX	Paclitaxel
EPR	Enhanced permeability and retention
Dox	Doxorubicin
ATRP	Atom transfer radical polymerization
RAFT	Reversible addition-fragmentation chain transfer polymerization
P(DMAEMA)	Poly((2-dimethyl amino)ethyl methacrylate)
PEI	Polyethylenimine

References

1. Sun, Q.H.; Zhou, Z.X.; Qiu, N.S.; Shen, Y.Q. Rational design of cancer nanomedicine: Nanoproperty integration and synchronization. *Adv. Mater.* **2017**, *29*, 1606628. [CrossRef] [PubMed]
2. Cong, H.L.; Zhou, L.P.; Meng, Q.Y.; Zhang, Y.X.; Yu, B.; Shen, Y.Q.; Hu, H. Preparation and evaluation of PAMAM dendrimer-based polymer gels physically cross-linked by hydrogen bonding. *Biomater. Sci.* **2019**, *7*, 3918–3925. [CrossRef]
3. Park, K. Controlled drug delivery systems: Past forward and future back. *J. Control. Release* **2014**, *190*, 3–8. [CrossRef] [PubMed]
4. Sun, Y.Z.; Jing, X.D.; Ma, X.L.; Feng, Y.L.; Hu, H. Versatile types of polysaccharide-based drug delivery systems: From strategic design to cancer therapy. *Int. J. Biol. Macromol.* **2020**, *21*, 9159.
5. Meng, Q.Y.; Cong, H.L.; Hu, H.; Xu, F.J. Rational design and latest advances of codelivery systems for cancer therapy. *Mater. Today Bio.* **2020**, *7*, 100056. [CrossRef] [PubMed]
6. Kovalainen, M.; Monkare, J.; Riikonen, J.; Pesonen, U.; Vlasova, M.; Salonen, J.; Lehto, V.P.; Jarvinen, K.; Herzig, K.H. Novel delivery systems for improving the clinical use of peptides. *Pharmacol. Rev.* **2015**, *67*, 541–561. [CrossRef] [PubMed]
7. Hu, H.; Yuan, W.; Liu, F.S.; Cheng, G.; Xu, F.J.; Ma, J. Redox-responsive polycation-functionalized cotton cellulose nanocrystals for effective cancer treatment. *ACS Appl. Mater. Interfaces* **2015**, *7*, 8942–8951. [CrossRef] [PubMed]
8. Sun, Y.; Hu, H.; Jing, X.; Meng, Q.Y.; Yu, B.; Cong, H.L.; Shen, Y.Q. Co-delivery of chemotherapeutic drugs and cell cycle regulatory agents using nanocarriers for cancer therapy. *Sci. China Mater* **2021**, 1–12. [CrossRef]
9. Kumari, P.; Ghosh, B.; Biswas, S. Nanocarriers for cancer-targeted drug delivery. *J. Drug Target.* **2016**, *24*, 179–191. [CrossRef]
10. Sun, Y.; Ma, X.; Hu, H. Application of Nano-Drug Delivery System Based on Cascade Technology in Cancer Treatment. *Int. J. Mol. Sci.* **2021**, *22*, 5698. [CrossRef]
11. Bulbake, U.; Doppalapudi, S.; Kommineni, N.; Khan, W. Liposomal formulations in clinical use: An updated review. *Pharmaceutics* **2017**, *9*, 12. [CrossRef]

12. Liu, Y.L.; Chen, D.; Shang, P.; Yin, D.C. A review of magnet systems for targeted drug delivery. *J. Control. Release* **2019**, *302*, 90–104. [CrossRef]
13. Wang, Y.; Zhao, Q.F.; Han, N.; Bai, L.; Li, J.; Liu, J.; Che, E.X.; Hu, L.; Zhang, Q.; Jiang, T.Y.; et al. Mesoporous silica nanoparticles in drug delivery and biomedical applications. *Nanomedicine* **2015**, *11*, 313–327. [CrossRef] [PubMed]
14. Meng, Q.Y.; Sun, Y.; Cong, H.L.; Hu, H.; Xu, F.J. An overview of chitosan and its application in infectious diseases. *Drug Deliv. Transl. Res.* **2021**, 1–12. [CrossRef]
15. Hu, Y.; Li, Y.; Xu, F.J. Versatile functionalization of polysaccharides via polymer grafts: From design to biomedical applications. *Acc. Chem. Res.* **2017**, *50*, 281–292. [CrossRef] [PubMed]
16. Guo, X.; Wang, Y.; Qin, Y.M.; Shen, P.L.; Peng, Q. Structures, properties and application of alginic acid: A review. *Int. J. Biol. Macromol.* **2020**, *162*, 618–628. [CrossRef] [PubMed]
17. Manivasagan, P.; Oh, J. Marine polysaccharide-based nanomaterials as a novel source of nanobiotechnological applications. *Int. J. Biol. Macromol.* **2016**, *82*, 315–327. [CrossRef]
18. Cardoso, M.J.; Costa, R.R.; Mano, J.F. Marine origin polysaccharides in drug delivery systems. *Mar. Drugs* **2016**, *14*, 34. [CrossRef]
19. Oh, E.J.; Park, K.; Kim, K.S.; Kim, J.; Yang, J.A.; Kong, J.H.; Lee, M.Y.; Hoffman, A.S.; Hahn, S.K. Target specific and long-acting delivery of protein, peptide, and nucleotide therapeutics using hyaluronic acid derivatives. *J. Control. Release* **2010**, *141*, 2–12. [CrossRef] [PubMed]
20. Moeini, A.; Pedram, P.; Makvandi, P.; Malinconico, M.; d'Ayala, G.G. Wound healing and antimicrobial effect of active secondary metabolites in chitosan-based wound dressings: A review. *Carbohydr. Polym.* **2020**, *233*, 115839. [CrossRef] [PubMed]
21. Debele, T.A.; Mekuria, S.L.; Tsai, H.C. Polysaccharide based nanogels in the drug delivery system: Application as the carrier of pharmaceutical agents. *Mater. Sci. Eng. C* **2016**, *68*, 964–981. [CrossRef] [PubMed]
22. Meng, Q.Y.; Hu, H.; Zhou, L.P.; Zhang, Y.X.; Yu, B.; Shen, Y.Q.; Cong, H.L. Logical design and application of prodrug platforms. *Polym. Chem.* **2019**, *10*, 306–324. [CrossRef]
23. Nitta, S.K.; Numata, K. Biopolymer-Based Nanoparticles for Drug/Gene Delivery and Tissue Engineering. *Int. J. Mol. Sci.* **2013**, *14*, 1629–1654. [CrossRef] [PubMed]
24. Huh, M.S.; Lee, E.J.; Koo, H.; Yhee, J.Y.; Oh, K.S.; Son, S.; Lee, S.; Kim, S.H.; Kwon, L.C.; Kim, K. Polysaccharide-based Nanoparticles for Gene Delivery. *Top. Curr. Chem.* **2017**, *375*, 31. [CrossRef]
25. Liu, Y.; Sun, J.; Zhang, P.; He, Z. Amphiphilic polysaccharide-hydrophobicized graft polymeric micelles for drug delivery nanosystems. *Curr. Med. Chem.* **2011**, *18*, 2638–2648. [CrossRef]
26. Habibi, Y.; Lucia, L.A.; Rojas, O.J. Cellulose nanocrystals: Chemistry, self-assembly, and applications. *Chem. Rev.* **2010**, *110*, 3479–3500. [CrossRef]
27. Perez, S.; Bertoft, E. The molecular structures of starch components and their contribution to the architecture of starch granules: A comprehensive review. *Starch/Staerke* **2010**, *62*, 389–420. [CrossRef]
28. Collins, M.N.; Birkinshaw, C. Hyaluronic acid based scaffolds for tissue engineering-A review. *Carbohydr. Polym.* **2013**, *92*, 1262–1279. [CrossRef]
29. Lee, K.Y.; Mooney, D.J. Alginate: Properties and biomedical applications. *Prog. Polym. Sci.* **2012**, *37*, 106–126. [CrossRef]
30. Muzzarelli, R.A.A.; Greco, F.; Busilacchi, A.; Sollazzo, V.; Gigante, A. Chitosan, hyaluronan and chondroitin sulfate in tissue engineering for cartilage regeneration: A review. *Carbohydr. Polym.* **2012**, *89*, 723–739. [CrossRef]
31. Yu, Y.; Shen, M.Y.; Song, Q.Q.; Xie, J.H. Biological activities and pharmaceutical applications of polysaccharide from natural resources: A review. *Carbohydr. Polym.* **2018**, *183*, 91–101. [CrossRef] [PubMed]
32. Hu, H.; Xu, F.J. Rational design and latest advances of polysaccharide-based hydrogels for wound healing. *Biomater. Sci.* **2020**, *8*, 2084–2101. [CrossRef] [PubMed]
33. Rabea, E.I.; Badawy, M.E.T.; Stevens, C.V.; Smagghe, G.; Steurbaut, W. Chitosan as antimicrobial agent: Applications and mode of action. *Biomacromolecules* **2003**, *4*, 1457–1465. [CrossRef] [PubMed]
34. Dash, M.; Chiellini, F.; Ottenbrite, R.M.; Chiellini, E. Chitosan-A versatile semi-synthetic polymer in biomedical applications. *Prog. Polym. Sci.* **2011**, *36*, 981–1014. [CrossRef]
35. Lesley, J.; Hyman, R.; English, N.; Catterall, J.B.; Turner, G.A. CD44 in inflammation and metastasis. *Glycoconj. J.* **1997**, *14*, 611–622. [CrossRef]
36. Gupta, A.; Kowalczuk, M.; Heaselgrave, W.; Britland, S.T.; Martin, C.; Radecka, I. The production and application of hydrogels for wound management: A review. *Eur. Polym. J.* **2019**, *111*, 134–151. [CrossRef]
37. Jing, X.; Sun, Y.D.; Ma, X.; Hu, H. Marine polysaccharides: Green and recyclable resources as wound dressings. *Mater. Chem. Front.* **2021**. [CrossRef]
38. Elsabahy, M.; Wooley, K.L. Design of polymeric nanoparticles for biomedical delivery applications. *Chem. Soc. Rev.* **2012**, *41*, 2545–2561. [CrossRef]
39. Haag, R.; Kratz, F. Polymer therapeutics: Concepts and applications. *Angew. Chem. Int. Ed.* **2006**, *45*, 1198–1215. [CrossRef]
40. Garcia-Gonzalez, C.A.; Alnaief, M.; Smirnova, I. Polysaccharide-based aerogels-promising biodegradable carriers for drug delivery systems. *Carbohydr. Polym.* **2011**, *86*, 1425–1438. [CrossRef]
41. Pillai, C.K.S.; Paul, W.; Sharma, C.P. Chitin and chitosan polymers: Chemistry, solubility and fiber formation. *Prog. Polym. Sci.* **2009**, *34*, 641–678. [CrossRef]

42. Liu, M.; Li, H.; Wang, X.; Jing, L.; Jiang, P.; Li, Y. Experimental study of the vascular normalization window for tumors treated with apatinib and the efficacy of sequential chemotherapy with apatinib in lung cancer-bearing mice and patients. *Cancer Med.* **2020**, *9*, 2660–2673. [CrossRef]
43. Li, M.Q.; Tang, Z.H.; Zhang, D.W.; Sun, H.; Liu, H.Y.; Zhang, Y.; Zhang, Y.Y.; Chen, X.S. Doxorubicin-loaded polysaccharide nanoparticles suppress the growth of murine colorectal carcinoma and inhibit the metastasis of murine mammary carcinoma in rodent models. *Biomaterials* **2015**, *51*, 161–172. [CrossRef]
44. Zhao, L.; Mitomo, H. Hydrogels of dihydroxypropyl chitosan crosslinked with irradiation at paste-like condition. *Carbohydr. Polym.* **2009**, *76*, 314–319. [CrossRef]
45. Soni, K.S.; Desale, S.S.; Bronich, T.K. Nanogels: An overview of properties, biomedical applications and obstacles to clinical translation. *J. Control. Release* **2016**, *240*, 109–126. [CrossRef]
46. Zhang, N.; Wardwell, P.R.; Bader, R.A. Polysaccharide-based micelles for drug delivery. *Pharmaceutics* **2013**, *5*, 329–352. [CrossRef]
47. Schatz, C.; Louguet, S.; Le Meins, J.F.; Lecommandoux, S. Polysaccharide-block-polypeptide copolymer vesicles: Towards synthetic viral capsids. *Angew. Chem. Int. Ed.* **2009**, *48*, 2572–2575. [CrossRef] [PubMed]
48. Hamman, J.H. Chitosan based polyelectrolyte complexes as potential carrier materials in drug delivery systems. *Mar. Drugs* **2010**, *8*, 1305–1322. [CrossRef] [PubMed]
49. Mao, S.R.; Sun, W.; Kissel, T. Chitosan-based formulations for delivery of DNA and siRNA. *Adv. Drug Deliv. Rev.* **2010**, *62*, 12–27. [CrossRef]
50. Malhotra, M.; Lane, C.; Tomaro-Duchesneau, C.; Shyamali, S.; Prakash, S. A novel method for synthesizing PEGylated chitosan nanoparticles: Strategy, preparation, and in vitro analysis. *Int. J. Nanomed.* **2011**, *6*, 485–494.
51. Chen, S.; Deng, J.; Zhang, L.M. Cationic nanoparticles self-assembled from amphiphilic chitosan derivatives containing poly(amidoamine) dendrons and deoxycholic acid as a vector for co-delivery of doxorubicin and gene. *Carbohydr. Polym.* **2021**, *258*, 117706. [CrossRef] [PubMed]
52. Yin, X.; Xie, H.G.; Li, R.X.; Yan, S.G.; Yin, H. Regulating association strength between quaternary ammonium chitosan and sodium alginate via hydration. *Carbohydr. Polym.* **2021**, *255*, 117390. [CrossRef]
53. Mirtic, J.; Ilas, J.; Kristl, J. Influence of different classes of crosslinkers on alginate polyelectrolyte nanoparticle formation, thermodynamics and characteristics. *Carbohydr. Polym.* **2018**, *181*, 93–102. [CrossRef] [PubMed]
54. Magalhaes, G.A.; Neto, E.M.; Sombra, V.G.; Richter, A.R.; Abreu, C.; Feitosa, J.P.A.; Paula, H.C.B.; Goycoole, F.M.; de Paula, R.C.M. Chitosan/Sterculia striata polysaccharides nanocomplex as a potential chloroquine drug release device. *Int. J. Biol. Macromol.* **2016**, *88*, 244–253. [CrossRef] [PubMed]
55. Babu, A.; Ramesh, R. Multifaceted applications of chitosan in cancer drug delivery and therapy. *Mar. Drugs* **2017**, *15*, 96. [CrossRef]
56. Wu, J.L.; Tian, G.X.; Yu, W.J.; Jia, G.T.; Sun, T.Y.; Gao, Z.Q. pH-Responsive hyaluronic acid-based mixed micelles for the hepatoma-targeting delivery of doxorubicin. *Int. J. Mol. Sci.* **2016**, *17*, 364. [CrossRef] [PubMed]
57. Shen, Y.; Li, Q.; Tu, J.S.; Zhu, J.B. Synthesis and characterization of low molecular weight hyaluronic acid-based cationic micelles for efficient siRNA delivery. *Carbohydr. Polym.* **2009**, *77*, 95–104. [CrossRef]
58. Mizrahy, S.; Peer, D. Polysaccharides as building blocks for nanotherapeutics. *Chem. Soc. Rev.* **2012**, *41*, 2623–2640. [CrossRef] [PubMed]
59. Zhong, Y.N.; Goltsche, K.; Cheng, L.; Xie, F.; Meng, F.H.; Deng, C.; Zhong, Z.Y.; Haag, R. Hyaluronic acid-shelled acid-activatable paclitaxel prodrug micelles effectively target and treat CD44-overexpressing human breast tumor xenografts in vivo. *Biomaterials* **2016**, *84*, 250–261. [CrossRef]
60. Zhang, Y.; Cai, L.L.; Li, D.; Lao, Y.H.; Liu, D.Z.; Li, M.Q.; Ding, J.X.; Chen, X.S. Tumor microenvironment-responsive hyaluronate-calcium carbonate hybrid nanoparticle enables effective chemotherapy for primary and advanced osteosarcomas. *Nano Res.* **2018**, *11*, 4806–4822. [CrossRef]
61. Akay, S.; Heils, R.; Trieu, H.K.; Smirnova, I.; Yesil-Celiktas, O. An injectable alginate-based hydrogel for microfluidic applications. *Carbohydr. Polym.* **2017**, *161*, 228–234. [CrossRef]
62. Zhang, Y.; Lin, L.; Liu, L.; Liu, F.; Maruyama, A.; Tian, H.Y.; Chen, X.S. Ionic-crosslinked polysaccharide/PEI/DNA nanoparticles for stabilized gene delivery. *Carbohydr. Polym.* **2018**, *201*, 246–256. [CrossRef] [PubMed]
63. Gan, Q.; Wang, T.; Cochrane, C.; McCarron, P. Modulation of surface charge, particle size and morphological properties of chitosan-TPP nanoparticles intended for gene delivery. *Colloids Surf. B* **2005**, *44*, 65–73. [CrossRef]
64. Ma, Z.S.; Yeoh, H.H.; Lim, L.Y. Formulation pH modulates the interaction of insulin with chitosan nanoparticles. *J. Pharm. Sci.* **2002**, *91*, 1396–1404. [CrossRef] [PubMed]
65. Zhang, X.; Malhotra, S.; Molina, M.; Haag, R. Micro- and nanogels with labile crosslinks-from synthesis to biomedical applications. *Chem. Soc. Rev.* **2015**, *44*, 1948–1973. [CrossRef] [PubMed]
66. Liu, Z.H.; Jiao, Y.P.; Wang, Y.F.; Zhou, C.R.; Zhang, Z.Y. Polysaccharides-based nanoparticles as drug delivery systems. *Adv. Drug Deliv. Rev.* **2008**, *60*, 1650–1662. [CrossRef]
67. Zhao, W.F.; Huang, X.L.; Wang, Y.L.; Sun, S.D.; Zhao, C.S. A recyclable and regenerable magnetic chitosan absorbent for dye uptake. *Carbohydr. Polym.* **2016**, *150*, 201–208. [CrossRef] [PubMed]

68. da Silva, L.; Todaro, V.; do Carmo, F.A.; Frattani, F.S.; de Sousa, V.P.; Rodrigues, C.R.; Sathler, P.C.; Cabral, L.M. A promising oral fucoidan-based antithrombotic nanosystem: Development, activity and safety. *Nanotechnology* **2018**, *29*, 165102. [CrossRef] [PubMed]
69. Lee, C.; Shin, J.; Lee, J.S.; Byun, E.; Ryu, J.H.; Um, S.H.; Kim, D.I.; Lee, H.; Cho, S.W. Bioinspired, Calcium-free alginate hydrogels with tunable physical and mechanical properties and improved biocompatibility. *Biomacromolecules* **2013**, *14*, 2004–2013. [CrossRef]
70. Nguyen, M.H.; Tran, T.T.; Hadinoto, K. Controlling the burst release of amorphous drug-polysaccharide nanoparticle complex via crosslinking of the polysaccharide chains. *Eur. J. Pharm. Biopharm.* **2016**, *104*, 156–163. [CrossRef]
71. Mocanu, G.; Mihai, D.; Legros, M.; Picton, L.; LeCerf, D. New polysaccharide-based microparticles crosslinked with siloxane: Interactions with biologically active substances. *J. Bioact. Compat. Polym.* **2008**, *23*, 82–94. [CrossRef]
72. Khanmohammadi, M.; Sakai, S.; Taya, M. Characterization of encapsulated cells within hyaluronic acid and alginate microcapsules produced via horseradish peroxidase-catalyzed crosslinking. *J. Biomater. Sci. Polym. Ed.* **2019**, *30*, 295–307. [CrossRef]
73. Calvo, P.; RemunanLopez, C.; VilaJato, J.L.; Alonso, M.J. Novel hydrophilic chitosan-polyethylene oxide nanoparticles as protein carriers. *J. Appl. Polym. Sci.* **1997**, *63*, 125–132. [CrossRef]
74. Park, S.; Hwang, S.; Lee, J. pH-responsive hydrogels from moldable composite microparticles prepared by coaxial electro-spray drying. *Chem. Eng. J.* **2011**, *169*, 348–357. [CrossRef]
75. Imam, M.E.; Bernkop-Schnurch, A. Controlled drug delivery systems based on thiolated chitosan microspheres. *Drug Dev. Ind. Pharm.* **2005**, *31*, 557–565. [CrossRef]
76. Zahin, N.; Anwar, R.; Tewari, D.; Kabir, M.T.; Sajid, A.; Mathew, B.; Uddin, M.S.; Aleya, L.; Abdel-Daim, M.M. Nanoparticles and its biomedical applications in health and diseases: Special focus on drug delivery. *Environ. Sci. Pollut. Res.* **2020**, *27*, 19151–19168. [CrossRef] [PubMed]
77. Molavi, F.; Barzegar-Jalali, M.; Hamishehkar, H. Polyester based polymeric nano and microparticles for pharmaceutical purposes: A review on formulation approaches. *J. Control. Release* **2020**, *320*, 265–282. [CrossRef] [PubMed]
78. Li, D.; Peng, X.R.; Chen, L.; Ding, J.X.; Chen, X.S. One-step synthesis of targeted acid-labile polysaccharide prodrug for efficiently intracellular drug delivery. *ACS Biomater. Sci. Eng.* **2018**, *4*, 539–546. [CrossRef] [PubMed]
79. Pilipenko, I.M.; Korzhikov-Vlakh, V.A.; Zakharova, N.V.; Urtti, A.; Tennikova, T.B. Thermo- and pH-sensitive glycosaminoglycans derivatives obtained by controlled grafting of poly(N-isopropylacrylamide). *Carbohydr. Polym.* **2020**, *248*, 116764. [CrossRef] [PubMed]
80. Li, S.; Xiong, Q.; Lai, X.; Li, X.; Wan, M.; Zhang, J.; Yan, Y.; Cao, M.; Lu, L.; Guan, J.; et al. Molecular modification of polysaccharides and resulting bioactivities. *Compr. Rev. Food Sci. Food Saf.* **2015**, *15*, 237–250. [CrossRef] [PubMed]
81. Correa, S.; Boehnke, N.; Barberio, A.E.; Deiss-Yehiely, E.; Shi, A.; Oberlton, B.; Smith, S.G.; Zervantonakis, I.; Dreaden, E.C.; Hammond, P.T. Tuning nanoparticle interactions with ovarian cancer through layer-by-layer modification of surface chemistry. *Acs Nano* **2020**, *14*, 2224–2237. [CrossRef] [PubMed]
82. Muhamad, N.; Plengsuriyakarn, T.; Na-Bangchang, K. Application of active targeting nanoparticle delivery system for chemotherapeutic drugs and traditional/herbal medicines in cancer therapy: A systematic review. *Int. J. Nanomed.* **2018**, *13*, 3921–3935. [CrossRef] [PubMed]
83. Fathi, M.; Zangabad, P.S.; Aghanejad, A.; Barar, J.; Erfan-Niya, H.; Omidi, Y. Folate-conjugated thermosensitive O-maleoyl modified chitosan micellar nanoparticles for targeted delivery of erlotinib. *Carbohydr. Polym.* **2017**, *172*, 130–141. [CrossRef] [PubMed]
84. Jafari, M.; Sriram, V.; Xu, Z.Y.; Harris, G.M.; Lee, J.Y. Fucoidan-doxorubicin nanoparticles targeting p-selectin for effective breast cancer therapy. *Carbohydr. Polym.* **2020**, *249*, 116837. [CrossRef] [PubMed]
85. Cao, J.; Zheng, H.R.; Hu, R.; Liao, J.H.; Fei, Z.M.; Wei, X.; Xiong, X.; Zhang, F.L.; Zheng, H.; Li, D. pH-Responsive nanoparticles based on covalently grafted conjugates of carboxymethyl chitosan and daunorubicin for the delivery of anti-cancer drugs. *J. Biomed. Nanotechnol.* **2017**, *13*, 1647–1659. [CrossRef]
86. Curcio, M.; Diaz-Gomez, L.; Cirillo, G.; Nicoletta, F.P.; Leggio, A.; Iemma, F. Dual-targeted hyaluronic acid/albumin micelle-like nanoparticles for the vectorization of doxorubicin. *Pharmaceutics* **2021**, *13*, 304. [CrossRef]
87. Lee, S.J.; Jeong, Y.I. Hybrid nanoparticles based on chlorin e6-conjugated hyaluronic acid/poly(L-histidine) copolymer for theranostic application to tumors. *J. Mater. Chem. B* **2018**, *6*, 2851–2859. [CrossRef] [PubMed]
88. Tizzotti, M.; Charlot, A.; Fleury, E.; Stenzel, M.; Bernard, J. Modification of polysaccharides through controlled/living radical polymerization grafting-towards the generation of high performance hybrids. *Macromol. Rapid Commun.* **2010**, *31*, 1751–1772. [CrossRef]
89. Singh, V.; Kumar, P.; Sanghi, R. Use of microwave irradiation in the grafting modification of the polysaccharides-A review. *Prog. Polym. Sci.* **2012**, *37*, 340–364. [CrossRef]
90. Ping, Y.; Liu, C.D.; Tang, G.P.; Li, J.S.; Li, J.; Yang, W.T.; Xu, F.J. Functionalization of chitosan via atom transfer radical polymerization for gene delivery. *Adv. Funct. Mater.* **2010**, *20*, 3106–3116. [CrossRef]

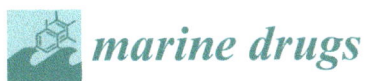

Article

Antiproliferative Illudalane Sesquiterpenes from the Marine Sediment Ascomycete *Aspergillus oryzae*

Raha Orfali [1,*], Shagufta Perveen [1,*], Muhammad Farooq Khan [2], Atallah F. Ahmed [1,3], Mohammad A. Wadaan [2], Areej Mohammad Al-Taweel [1], Ali S. Alqahtani [1,4], Fahd A. Nasr [4], Sobia Tabassum [5], Paolo Luciano [6], Giuseppina Chianese [6], Jyh-Horng Sheu [7,8] and Orazio Taglialatela-Scafati [6,*]

1 Department of Pharmacognosy, College of Pharmacy, King Saud University, P.O. Box 2457, Riyadh 11451, Saudi Arabia; afahmed@ksu.edu.sa (A.F.A.); amaltaweel@ksu.edu.sa (A.M.A.-T.); alalqahtani@ksu.edu.sa (A.S.A.)
2 Bio-Products Research Chair, Department of Zoology, College of Science, King Saud University, P.O. Box 2455, Riyadh 11451, Saudi Arabia; fmuhammad@ksu.edu.sa (M.F.K.); wadaan@ksu.edu.sa (M.A.W.)
3 Department of Pharmacognosy, Faculty of Pharmacy, Mansoura University, Mansoura 35516, Egypt
4 Medicinal, Aromatic and Poisonous Plants Research Center, College of Pharmacy, King Saud University, P.O. Box 2455, Riyadh 11451, Saudi Arabia; fnasr@ksu.edu.sa
5 Interdisciplinary Research Centre in Biomedical Materials (IRCBM), Lahore Campus, COMSATS University Islamabad, Islamabad 44000, Pakistan; sobiatabassum@cuilahore.edu.pk
6 Department of Pharmacy, School of Medicine and Surgery, University of Naples Federico II, Via Montesano 49, 80131 Naples, Italy; pluciano@unina.it (P.L.); g.chianese@unina.it (G.C.)
7 Department of Marine Biotechnology and Resources, National Sun Yat-sen University, Kaohsiung 80424, Taiwan; sheu@mail.nsysu.edu.tw
8 Department of Medical Research, China Medical University Hospital, China Medical University, Taichung 40447, Taiwan
* Correspondence: rorfali@ksu.edu.sa (R.O.); shakhan@ksu.edu.sa (S.P.); scatagli@unina.it (O.T.-S.)

Abstract: The new asperorlactone (**1**), along with the known illudalane sesquiterpene echinolactone D (**2**), two known pyrones, 4-(hydroxymethyl)-5-hydroxy-2*H*-pyran-2-one (**3**) and its acetate **4**, and 4-hydroxybenzaldehyde (**5**), were isolated from a culture of *Aspergillus oryzae*, collected from Red Sea marine sediments. The structure of asperorlactone (**1**) was elucidated by HR-ESIMS, 1D, and 2D NMR, and a comparison between experimental and DFT calculated electronic circular dichroism (ECD) spectra. This is the first report of illudalane sesquiterpenoids from *Aspergillus* fungi and, more in general, from ascomycetes. Asperorlactone (**1**) exhibited antiproliferative activity against human lung, liver, and breast carcinoma cell lines, with IC_{50} values < 100 µM. All the isolated compounds were also evaluated for their toxicity using the zebrafish embryo model.

Keywords: *Aspergillus oryzae*; marine fungus; illudalane sesquiterpenes; antiproliferative activity; zebrafish toxicity

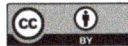

1. Introduction

The marine environment is an unsurpassed casket of chemodiversity and a prolific source of biologically active compounds with potential medicinal applications [1]. In the last 50 years, scientists all over the world have dedicated their efforts to uncover the potential of marine metabolites, succeeding in the isolation of thousands of natural products with peculiar architectures and interesting bioactivities [2]. As per April 2021, the marine pharmacology arsenal [3] includes 15 approved drugs (mainly for cancer treatment), seven compounds in phase I, 12 compounds in phase II, and 5 compounds in phase III clinical trials, the latter including plitidepsin, recently proposed for COVID-19 symptomatic treatment [4,5]. Sponges and tunicates are undoubtedly the most intensely studied marine organisms, but it is now clear that marine microbes, isolated from sediments or from symbiotic plants or invertebrates, constitute a rich source for secondary metabolites. In this context, although terrestrial fungi are more explored, in comparison to their marine counterparts, a surprising number of structurally unique compounds have been isolated from fungi living in marine habitats [6]. The peculiar properties of the marine environment with regard to nutrients, temperature, and competition, are likely crucial factors in improving the ability of marine fungi to elaborate compounds with promising bioactivities, especially suited for antibiotic and anticancer applications [7].

The genus *Aspergillus* is one of the most abundant among marine ascomycetes, characterized by high salt tolerance, fast growth rate, and the capacity to adapt to diverse habitats. Marine *Aspergillus* fungi produce a wide range of secondary metabolites belonging to different classes and are endowed with a broad array of biological activities of industrial and pharmaceutical interest [8,9]. As a part of our ongoing research activity aimed at the isolation of bioactive compounds from terrestrial and marine fungi [10–13], *A. oryzae* samples obtained from the sediments of the Red Sea, along the coasts of Saudi Arabia, were chemically investigated. This study resulted in the isolation of two illudalane sesquiterpenes, the new asperorlactone (**1**) and the known echinolactone D (**2**), along with two rare pyrone derivatives (**3–4**) and 4-hydroxybenzaldehyde (**5**). These compounds were evaluated for their antiproliferative activity against three human carcinomas (lung, liver, and breast) cell lines. Chemotherapeutics used in cancer treatment are often characterized by marked toxic effects on normal cells. Less than 2% of compounds emerging from in vitro drug screening could enter clinical trials since the majority of the newly developed leads fail in preclinical testing due to their toxicity in experimental animal models [14]. In vitro drug screening methods are prevalently used in order to characterize the bioactivity and the toxicity of new compounds, while testing their safety in suitable animal models prior to clinical trials would save time and money. Since a high throughput screening approach is not feasible in higher animals, zebrafish constitute a valid option for preclinical testing and have shown quite reproducible results. It is predicted that, following further development of technologies, zebrafish will play a key role in speeding up the emergence of precision medicine [15,16]. On these bases, the isolated compounds **1–5** have been tested for their zebrafish animal toxicity, and results are reported herein.

2. Results and Discussion

2.1. Extraction and Structural Identification

A. oryzae samples were isolated from the Red Sea sediment collected at a depth of—50 m off Jeddah, Saudi Arabia. Fermentation of the fungus on solid rice medium and extraction with EtOAc afforded a brownish residue, which was chromatographed by using silica gel and RP-18 column chromatography, affording one new (**1**) and four known (**2–5**) compounds (Figure 1).

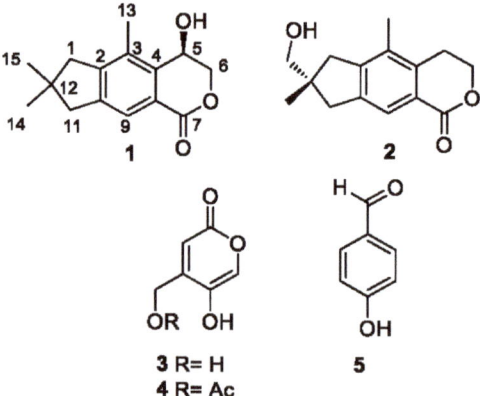

Figure 1. Chemical structures of metabolites isolated from *A. oryzae*.

The known compounds were identified as echinolactone D (**2**) [17], 4-(hydroxymethyl)-5-hydroxy-2*H*-pyran-2-one (**3**) [18], (5-hydroxy-2-oxo-2*H*-pyran-4-yl)methyl acetate (**4**) [16], and 4-hydroxybenzaldehyde (**5**), by a comparison of their spectroscopic data with those reported in the literature. The illudalane echinolactone D (**2**) had been isolated before from mycelia of the fungus *Echinodontium japonicum* [17] and from the wood decomposing fungus *Granulobasidium vellereum* [19], and therefore, this is its first report from a marine source. Compound **3** is a rare isomeric analog of kojic acid for which only three reports were present in the literature, all from *Aspergillus* fungi (marine *A. flavus* [18], terrestrial *A. niger* [20], and freshwater *A. austroafricanus* [21]).

Asperorlactone (**1**) was isolated as a colorless oil with molecular formula $C_{15}H_{18}O_3$, determined by HR-ESIMS. The ^{13}C NMR and DEPT spectra of **1** (Table 1) showed the presence of one lactone carbonyl (δ_C 166.5), one aromatic methine (δ_C 123.1), one oxymethine (δ_C 60.8), one sp^3 (δ_C 39.3) and five sp^2 (δ_C 122.7, 132.2, 136.2, 144.3, 150.1) nonprotonated carbons, three sp^3 methylenes (δ_C 46.5, 47.1, 72.7, the latter O-bearing), and three methyl groups (δ_C 13.1, 27.5 × 2). On the basis of these data, the seven unsaturation equivalents required by the molecular formula of **1** could be accommodated by the presence of a benzene ring and of two additional rings, including a lactone.

The ^1H NMR spectrum of **1** (Table 1) showed only one aromatic methine signal (δ_H 7.75), two methyl singlets (δ_H 1.19 × 2), an arylmethyl at δ_H 2.37 (s, 3H), and two pairs of methylenes around δ_H 2.80–2.83. The single-spin system of **1** included a diastereoptopic hydroxymethylene (δ_H 4.52 and 4.63), and an oxymethine signal (δ_H 4.95). Having associated all these proton signals to those of the directly linked carbons with the 2D NMR HSQC experiment, the illudalane type sesquiterpenes skeleton of compound **1** could be established by following the correlation network of the 2D NMR HMBC spectrum (Figure 2) (see Supplementary Materials).

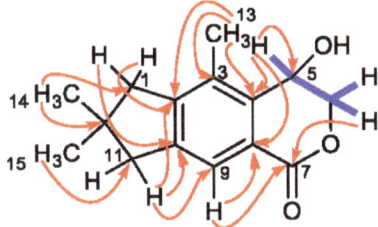

Figure 2. COSY (blue) and key HMBC (red arrows) correlations for compound **1**.

Table 1. ^1H (700 MHz) and ^{13}C (175 MHz) NMR data for asperorlactone (**1**) in CD_3OD.

Positions	δ_H (Mult., *J* in Hz)	δ_C, Type
1a	2.83 (overlapped)	46.5, CH_2
1b	2.81 (d, 17.5)	
2	-	150.1, C
3	-	132.2, C
4	-	136.2, C
5	4.95 (dd, 1.0, 2.1)	60.8, CH
6	4.63 (dd, 1.0, 12.0)	72.7, CH_2
	4.52 (dd, 2.1, 12.0)	
7	-	166.5, C
8	-	122.7, C
9	7.75 (s)	123.1, CH
10	-	144.3, C
11	2.82 (overlapped)	47.1, CH_2
12	-	39.3, C
13	2.37 (s)	13.1, CH_3

Table 1. *Cont.*

Positions	δ_H (Mult., *J* in Hz)	δ_C, Type
14	1.19 (s)	27.5, CH_3
15	1.19 (s)	27.5, CH_3

In particular, correlations of H-9 with C-8 and the lactone C-7, of H-5 with C-4 and C-8, and of H_2-6 with C-7 defined the structure of the hydroxyisochroman-1-one moiety of asperorlactone. The structure of the condensed dimethylated five-membered ring was deduced from the correlation of H_3-14/H_3-15 with C-1, C-11, and C-12 and of H_2-1 and H_2-11 with C-2 and C-10. Finally, the remaining methyl group was attached at C-3, following its correlations with C-2, C-3, and C-4.

Asperorlactone (**1**) is an optically active compound ($[\alpha]_D^{23}$ − 19.8) with a single stereocenter (C-5). We first tried to define the absolute configuration of **1** by employing the modified Mosher's method [22]; however, all the attempts to obtain the formation of the MTPA esters from the corresponding chloride failed. Most likely, the reaction of the bulky MTPA group with the hydroxyl group at C-5 was hindered by the methyl group present on the condensed aromatic ring. Therefore, we decided to rely on computational calculations, reasoning that comparison between experimental and quantum mechanically calculated ECD spectrum could provide an unambiguous indication on the absolute configuration of **1**.

The structure of **1** was subjected to a geometry and energy optimization using DFT with the mPW1PW91/6-311+G (d,p) functional and basis set combination using the Gaussian 09 software. The reasonably populated conformations, their relative energy, and the equilibrium room-temperature Boltzmann populations are reported in Figure 3. The two major conformers **1a** and **1b**, accounting for 99.5% of the total population, differ almost exclusively for the pseudorotation of the five-membered ring.

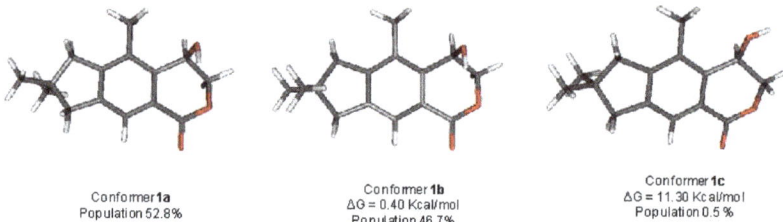

Figure 3. The reasonably populated conformers **1a**–**1c** of **1** and their calculated Boltzmann population.

TDDFT calculations were run using the functional CAM-B3LYP and the basis sets 6-31G (d,p) including at least 30 excited states in all cases, and using IEF-PCM for MeOH. The rotatory strength values were summed after a Boltzmann statistical weighting, and Δε values were calculated by forming sums of Gaussian functions centered at the wavelengths of the respective electronic transitions and multiplied by the corresponding rotatory strengths. Thus, the ECD spectra for *R*-**1** and *S*-**1** were obtained (Figure 4). The extensive similarity of the first with the experimental ECD spectrum allowed us a confident assignment of the absolute configuration of asperorlactone as 5*R*.

The isolation of asperorlactone (**1**), as well as of the related echinolactone D (**2**), is of great relevance because, to our knowledge, this is the first report of illudalane-type sesquiterpenes from an ascomycete (*A. oryzae*), since this class of metabolites has, until now, been found exclusively in basidiomycetes.

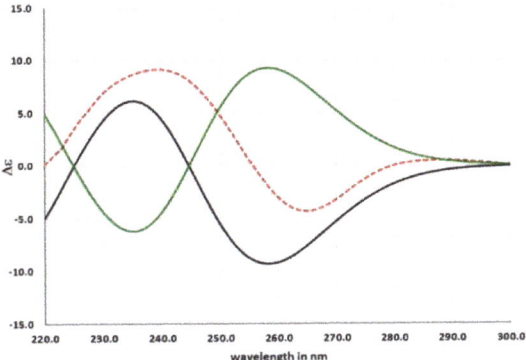

Figure 4. Experimental ECD curve of asperorlactone (red) and calculated ECD curves for *R*-**1** (black) and *S*-**1** (green).

It has been reported that illudalanes derive biosynthetically from a humulene precursor that, upon cyclization, would generate a protoilludane that finally would rearrange to form the illudalane derivative [23]. In the light of this hypothesis, a possible biosynthesis of asperorlactone is reported in Figure 5, where illudol [24] is a key intermediate that could afford **1** by dehydration, oxidation, and four-membered ring opening.

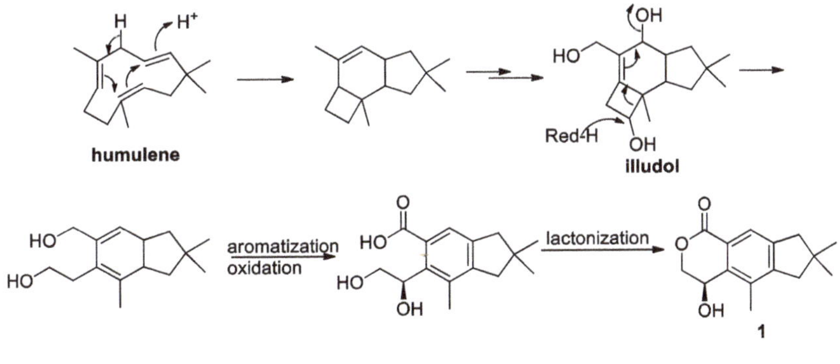

Figure 5. Postulated biosynthesis of asperorlactone (**1**).

2.2. Pharmacological and Toxicological Evaluation of the Isolated Compounds

Illudalane sesquiterpenes, obtained from different sources, have been reported to possess several biological properties, with a special focus on anticancer activities [25,26]. This prompted us to evaluate the antiproliferative activity of compounds **1–5** against three human cancer cell lines, namely, lung carcinoma (A549), liver carcinoma (HepG2), and breast carcinoma (MCF7). The obtained IC_{50} values are presented in Table 2. Compounds **1–5** generally showed moderate antiproliferative activity against all tested cell lines, invariably with higher potency against lung carcinoma, as compared to liver or breast carcinoma. As shown in Table 1, asperorlactone (**1**) and compound **2** were the most potent compounds against three cancer cell lines, with the single exception of the activity of **5** against the MCF-7 cell line. Additionally, interesting is the comparison between compounds **3** and **4**, evidencing that acetylation improves the activity against A549 and HepG2.

Table 2. Antiproliferative activity of compounds **1–5** against three human cancer cell lines.

Compound	IC_{50} (µM) for the Different Carcinoma Cell Lines		
	A549 (Lung)	HepG2 (Liver)	MCF-7 (Breast)
1	72.7 ± 1.1	86.6 ± 3.2	106.5 ± 4.2
2	55.7 ± 2.5	148.4 ± 5.6	128.0 ± 2.8
3	208.5 ± 6.8	220.4 ± 3.6	225.4 ± 5.1
4	89.4 ± 2.3	126.8 ± 6.4	170.7 ± 4.5
5	97.5 ± 2.6	242.6 ± 6.4	158.2 ± 5.5
Doxorubicin	2.1 ± 0.08	2.2 ± 0.15	1.9 ± 0.05

As anticipated, screening in zebrafish embryos provides an excellent environment in which the toxicity of a compound on noncancer cells and systems could be predicted. Thus, the zebrafish embryos model was used to evaluate the animal toxicity of compounds **1–5** (Figure 6). The LC_{50} values (the concentration required to kill 50% of embryos) of all the tested compounds were higher than the 1 mg/mL range, indicating their safety on noncancer cells and selectivity indices >50. The zebrafish embryos that were treated with compounds **2**, **3**, and **5** did not exhibit any observable toxicity, and they developed normally up to 3 days post treatment. On the other hand, compound **4**, for which the initial development and growth of zebrafish embryos was normal, induced the death of 100% of treated embryos after 24 h post treatment. The zebrafish embryos that were treated with more than 200 µM compound **1** (higher than IC_{50}) developed normally; however, the embryos exhibited cardiac toxicity (cardiac edema and cardiac hypertrophy, black arrow in Figure 6) after 2 days post treatment.

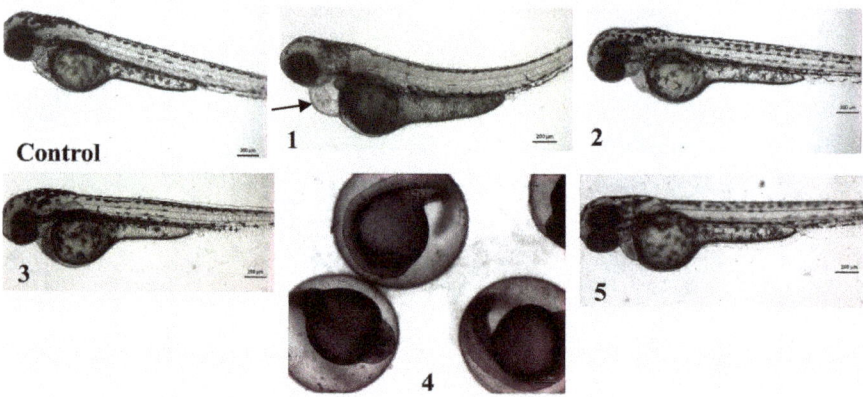

Figure 6. In vivo screening of compounds **1–5** in zebrafish embryos. Representative micrograph of embryos at 3 days poster fertilization, which were treated with compounds **1–5**. The zebrafish embryos treated with compounds **2**, **3**, and **5** developed normally, and there were no obvious differences in morphology and growth between control and treated embryos. The zebrafish embryos treated with >200 µM of **1**, however, had cardiac edema and cardiac hypertrophy (black arrow). The zebrafish embryos treated with compound **4** developed normally but were found dead on day 2. All the images are in same magnification, scale is 200 µm.

3. Materials and Methods

3.1. Fungal Material

Aspergillus oryzae was isolated from the marine sediment collected at −50 m off Jeddah, Red Sea, Saudi Arabia, in October 2018. The fungal identification was conducted by DNA amplification and sequencing of the internal transcribed spacer region (GenBank accession

No. MH608347) followed by a subsequent BLAST search in NCBI according to the protocol described before [27]. The specimen of the fungal strain was deep-frozen and deposited at the authors' lab (R.O., S.P.).

3.2. Fermentation, Extraction, and Isolation

A. oryzae was cultivated in 20 Erlenmeyer flasks on solid rice medium containing (100 g rice, 3.5 g sea salt, and 110 mL of demineralized water). After autoclaving at 121 °C for 20 min and then cooling to room temperature, each flask was inoculated and then incubated at 20 °C under static conditions. After four weeks, 500 mL EtOAc was added to each flask to stop the fermentation and extract. The total extract was collected after the flasks had been shaken at 150 rpm for 8 h on a laboratory shaker. The obtained crude extract after evaporation of the EtOAc (7 g) was then partitioned between n-hexane and MeOH. The polar phase was then subjected to Sephadex LH-20 column (100 × 2.5 cm) using 100% methanol as an eluting solvent. Similar fractions were combined with each other according to TLC readings and further purified by semipreparative HPLC using gradient system MeOH-H$_2$O from 40:60 to 70:30 in 30 min to afford **1** (3.5 mg), **2** (5.0 mg), **3** (7.0 mg), **4** (5.0 mg), and **5** (2.6 mg).

Asperorlactone (**1**). Colorless oil; $[\alpha]_D^{23}$ −19.8 (c 0.6, MeOH); UV λ_{max} (MeOH) nm (log ε): 230 (4.6); ECD λ_{max} (MeOH) nm (Δε): 238 (+ 9.6), 265 (−4.8); ^{1}H NMR (700 MHz, CD$_3$OD), and ^{13}C NMR (175 MHz, CD$_3$OD); see Table 1; ESIMS m/z 269.1150 [M + Na]$^+$ (calc. for C$_{15}$H$_{18}$ O$_3$ Na m/z 269.1154).

3.3. Computational Calculations

A preliminary conformational search on each stereoisomer was performed by Simulated Annealing in the INSIGHT II package. The MeOH solution phases were mimicked through the value of the corresponding dielectric constant. Using the steepest descent followed by quasi-Newton–Raphson method (VA09A) the conformational energy was minimized. Restrained simulations were carried out for 500 ps using the CVFF force field as implemented in Discovery software (Version 4.0 Accelrys, San Diego, USA). The simulation started at 1000 K, and then the temperature was decreased stepwise to 300 K. The final step was again the energy minimization, performed in order to refine the conformers obtained, using the steepest descent and the quasi-Newton–Raphson (VA09A) algorithms successively. Both dynamic and mechanic calculations were carried out by using 1 (kcal/mol)/Å 2 flat well distance restraints. In total, 100 structures were generated. TDDFT calculations were run using the functional CAM-B3LYP and the basis sets 6-31G (d,p) including at least 30 excited states in all cases, and using IEF-PCM for MeOH. The rotatory strength values were summed after a Boltzmann statistical weighting, and Δε values were calculated by forming sums of Gaussian functions centered at the wavelengths of the respective electronic transitions and multiplied by the corresponding rotatory strengths. The ECD spectra that were obtained were UV-corrected and compared with the experimental ones.

3.4. In Vitro Antiproliferative Activity

The antiproliferative activity of compounds was measured using MTT (3-(4, 5-dimethylthiazol-2-yl)-2,5-diphenyltetrazolium bromide) assay. A549 (lung), HepG2 (liver), and MCF-7 (breast) cancer cells were purchased from the American Type Cell Collection (ATCC, Manassas, VA, USA). The cells were seeded at 5×10^4 cells/well (in 100 µL of DMEM) in 96-well microplates. After 24 h incubation at 37 °C, serial dilution (15–250 µM) of each compound was added and incubated for 48 h. Thereafter, 10 µL of the MTT solution (5 mg/mL) was added to each well. After 4 h incubation with the MTT solution, a volume of 100 µL of acidified isopropanol was added to solubilize the formazan product and incubated on a shaker for a further 10 min. Reduced MTT was assayed at 570 nm using a microplate reader (BioTek, Winoosky, VT, USA). Control groups received the same amount of DMSO (0.1%), untreated cells were used as a negative control, whereas cells treated with doxorubicin were used as a positive control. The IC$_{50}$ (concentration that caused more than 50% inhibition of proliferation) was calculated from a dose-dependent curve. The cell viability percent was calculated = mean absorbance of treated sample/mean absorbance of control ×100.

3.5. Zebrafish Toxicity Screening

Wild-type zebrafish strain AB/Tuebingen TAB-14(AB/TuebingenTAB-14) (Catalog ID: ZL1438) were obtained from zebrafish international resource center and grown in an animal facility at the Department of Zoology, King Saud University, Riyadh, Kingdom of Saudi Arabia. The fish were maintained and bred following guidelines of the Institutional Animal Care and Use Committee (ICUAC) and zebrafish book. The fertilized embryos were obtained by natural pairwise breeding of adult fish. The fertilized embryos were sorted, dead embryos were removed, and synchronous stage embryos were used for screening.

A stock solution of 25 mM was made by dissolving the compounds in molecular biology grade DMSO (Sigma Aldrich, St. Louis, MI, USA). Zebrafish embryos were exposed to serial dilution (1, 5, 15, 45, 150, and 300 µM) of each compound. The embryos were remained exposed to the compounds for 3 days, and the embryos medium containing the compounds were changed every day. The response of the embryos toward mortality, and embryonic toxicity (teratogenicity) was monitored once after 12 h and then after every 24 h until the end of the experiment. The experiment was repeated at least three times (triplicate biological repeats) by using a new batch of embryos every time. LC_{50} for zebrafish embryonic toxicity was calculated by using an updated Probit analysis by Finney method [28].

4. Conclusions

Samples of *A. oryzae*, obtained from the Red Sea sediments collected off Jeddah, Saudi Arabia, afforded the first illudalane sesquiterpenoids isolated from an ascomycete, including the new asperorlactone (**1**), characterized by hydroxylation of the lactone ring. Elucidation of the structure and absolute configuration of this compound needed application of ESIMS and NMR spectral analyses and computational calculations of ECD spectra. The isolated compounds showed moderate antiproliferative activity against three human carcinoma cell lines (lung, liver, and breast). The zebrafish embryo model was used to evaluate the animal toxicity of compounds and selected echinolactone D (**2**) and the rare pyrone **3** as targets worthy of further investigation.

Supplementary Materials: The following are available online at https://www.mdpi.com/article/10.3390/md19060333/s1, Figures S1–S5: 1D and 2D NMR spectra of asperorlactone (**1**).

Author Contributions: Conceptualization, R.O., S.P., and O.T.-S.; methodology, M.F.K., F.A.N., S.P., and A.F.A.; software, A.M.A.-T. and P.L.; validation, S.T.; formal analysis, M.F.K., F.A.N., R.O., and G.C.; investigation, M.F.K., F.A.N., P.L., and G.C.; resources A.S.A. and M.A.W.; writing—original draft preparation M.F.K., F.A.N., and O.T.-S.; writing—review and editing A.S.A., M.A.W., and O.T.-S.; funding acquisition M.F.K., M.A.W., and J.-H.S. All authors have read and agreed to the published version of the manuscript.

Funding: This study was funded by the Deanship of Scientific Research, King Saud University, through the Vice Deanship of Scientific Research Chairs.

Institutional Review Board Statement: In this study, only zebrafish embryos were used which aged less than 5 days post fertilization, and hence, as reported in *Reprod. Toxicol.* **2012**, *33*, 128–132, doi:10.1016/j.reprotox.2011.06.121, they are exempted to take the ethical approval from ethical committee for the use and care of laboratory animals.

Informed Consent Statement: Not applicable.

Data Availability Statement: The data presented in this study are available in the article and Supplementary Material.

Conflicts of Interest: The authors declare no conflict of interest.

References

1. Montaser, R.; Luesch, H. Marine natural products: A new wave of drugs? *Future Med. Chem.* **2011**, *3*, 1475–1489. [CrossRef]
2. Carroll, A.R.; Copp, B.R.; Davis, R.A.; Keyzers, R.A.; Prinsep, M.R. Marine natural products. *Nat. Prod. Rep.* **2019**, *36*, 122–173. [CrossRef]
3. Available online: https://www.marinepharmacology.org (accessed on 25 May 2021).
4. White, K.M.; Rosales, R.; Yildiz, S.; Kehrer, T.; Miorin, L.; Moreno, E.; Jangra, S.; Uccellini, M.B.; Rathnasinghe, R.; Coughlan, L.; et al. Plitidepsin has potent preclinical efficacy against SARS-CoV-2 by targeting the host protein eEF1A. *Science* **2021**, *371*, 926–931. [CrossRef] [PubMed]
5. Taglialatela-Scafati, O. New hopes for drugs against COVID-19 come from the sea. *Mar. Drugs* **2021**, *19*, 104. [CrossRef] [PubMed]
6. Bugni, T.S.; Ireland, C.M. Marine-derived fungi: A chemically and biologically diverse group of microorganisms. *Nat. Prod. Rep.* **2004**, *21*, 143–163. [CrossRef] [PubMed]
7. Gomes, N.G.M.; Lefranc, F.; Kijjoa, A.; Kiss, R. Can some marine-derived fungal metabolites become actual anticancer agents? *Mar. Drugs* **2015**, *13*, 3950–3991. [CrossRef]
8. Yoon, J.; Kikuma, T.; Maruyama, J.; Kitamoto, K. Enhanced production of bovine chymosin by autophagy deficiency in the filamentous fungus *Aspergillus oryzae*. *PLoS ONE* **2013**, *8*, e62512. [CrossRef] [PubMed]
9. Singh, B.K.; Park, S.H.; Lee, H.B.; Goo, Y.A.; Kim, H.S.; Cho, S.H.; Lee, J.H.; Ahn, G.W.; Kim, J.P.; Kang, S.M.; et al. Kojic acid peptide: A new compound with anti-tyrosinase potential. *Ann. Dermatol.* **2016**, *28*, 555–561. [CrossRef]
10. Orfali, R.; Perveen, S.; Al-Taweel, A.; Ahmed, A.F.; Majrashi, N.; Alluhay, K.; Khan, A.; Luciano, P.; Taglialatela-Scafati, O. Penipyranicins A-C, antibacterial methylpyran polyketides from a hydrothermal spring sediment *Penicillium* sp. *J. Nat. Prod.* **2020**, *83*, 3591–3597. [CrossRef]
11. Orfali, R.; Ebrahim, W.; Perveen, S.; Mejrashi, M.; Alluhayb, K.; Ebada, S.S. Cytotoxic Secondary Metabolites from Mangrove-Rhizosphere-Associated Fungus *Emericella* sp. Strain SWR1718. *J. King Saud Univ. Sci.* **2020**, *32*, 2656–2661. [CrossRef]
12. Orfali, R.; Perveen, S. Secondary metabolites from the *Aspergillus* sp. in the rhizosphere soil of *Phoenix dactylifera* (Palm tree). *BMC Chem.* **2019**, *13*, 103. [CrossRef]
13. Orfali, R.; Perveen, S. New bioactive metabolites from the thermophilic fungus *Penicillium* sp. isolated from Ghamiqa hot spring in Saudi Arabia. *J. Chem.* **2019**, 7162948. [CrossRef]
14. Bhusnure, O.; Mane, J.; Gholve, S.; Thonte, S.; Giram, P.S.; Sangshetti, J. Drug target screening and its validation by zebrafish as a novel tool. *Pharm. Anal. Acta* **2015**, *6*, 1–9. [CrossRef]
15. MacRae, C.A.; Peterson, R.T. Zebrafish as tools for drug discovery. *Nat. Rev. Drug Discov.* **2015**, *14*, 721–731. [CrossRef] [PubMed]
16. Yoganantharjah, P.; Gibert, Y. The use of the zebrafish model to aid in drug discovery and target validation. *Curr. Top. Med. Chem.* **2017**, *17*, 2041–2055. [CrossRef] [PubMed]
17. Suzuki, S.; Murayama, T.; Shiono, Y. Echinolactones C and D: Two illudalane sesquiterpenoids isolated from the cultured mycelia of the fungus *Echinodontium japonicum*. *Z. Naturforsch.* **2006**, *61*, 1295–1298. [CrossRef]
18. Lin, A.; Lu, X.; Fang, Y.; Zhu, T.; Gu, Q.; Zhu, W. Two new 5-hydroxy-2-pyrone derivatives isolated from a marine-derived fungus *Aspergillus flavus*. *J. Antibiot.* **2008**, *61*, 245–249. [CrossRef]
19. Kokubun, T.; Scott-Brown, A.; Kite, G.C.; Simmonds, M.S.J. Protoilludane, illudane, illudalane, and norilludane sesquiterpenoids from *Granulobasidium vellereum*. *J. Nat. Prod.* **2016**, *79*, 1698–1701. [CrossRef] [PubMed]
20. Happi, G.M.; Kouam, S.F.; Talontsi, F.M.; Nkenfou, C.N.; Longo, F.; Zuhlke, S.; Douanla-Meli, C.; Spiteller, M. A new dimeric naphtho-γ-pyrone from an endophytic fungus *Aspergillus niger* AKRN associated with the roots of *Entandrophragma congoënse* collected in Cameroon. *Z. Naturforsch.* **2015**, *70*, 625–630. [CrossRef]
21. Ebrahim, W.; El-Neketi, M.; Lewald, L.I.; Orfali, R.; Lin, W.; Rehberg, N.; Kalscheuer, R.; Daletos, G.; Proksch, P. Metabolites from the fungal endophyte *Aspergillus austroafricanus* in axenic culture and in fungal–bacterial mixed cultures. *J. Nat. Prod.* **2016**, *79*, 914–922. [CrossRef] [PubMed]
22. Ohtani, I.; Kusumi, T.; Kashman, Y.; Kakisawa, H. High-field FT NMR application of Mosher's method. The absolute configurations of marine terpenoids. *J. Am. Chem. Soc.* **1991**, *113*, 4092–4096. [CrossRef]
23. Morisaki, N.; Furukawa, J.; Kobayashi, H.; Iwasaki, S.; Nozoe, S.; Okuda, S. Cyclobutyl cation rearrangements of 6-protoilluden-8α-ol, 7-protoilluden-6-ol and related compounds. *Chem. Pharm. Bull.* **1987**, *35*, 2678–2685. [CrossRef]
24. McMorris, T.C.; Nair, M.S.R.; Singh, P.; Anchel, M. The structure of illudol. *Phytochemistry* **1971**, *10*, 3341–3342. [CrossRef]
25. Nord, C.L.; Menkis, A.; Broberg, A. Cytotoxic illudalane sesquiterpenes from the wood-decay fungus *Granulobasidium vellereum* (Ellis & Cragin) Julich. *Molecules* **2014**, *19*, 14195–14203.
26. Lu, J.; Peng, C.Y.; Cheng, S.; Liu, J.Q.; Ma, Q.G.; Shu, J.C. Four new pterosins from *Pteris cretica* and their cytotoxic activities. *Molecules* **2019**, *24*, 2767. [CrossRef] [PubMed]
27. Kjer, J.; Debbab, A.; Aly, A.; Proksch, P. Methods for isolation of marine-derived endophytic fungi and their bioactive secondary products. *Nat. Protoc.* **2010**, *5*, 479–490. [CrossRef] [PubMed]
28. Finney, D.J. *Probit Analysis: A Statistical Treatment of the Sigmoid Response Curve*; Cambridge University Press: Cambridge, UK, 1952.

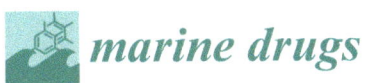

Article

Characteristic Volatile Composition of Seven Seaweeds from the Yellow Sea of China

Pengrui Wang [1], Jiapeng Chen [1], Lujing Chen [1], Li Shi [1] and Hongbing Liu [1,2,*]

[1] Key Laboratory of Marine Drugs, Chinese Ministry of Education, School of Medicine and Pharmacy, Ocean University of China, Qingdao 266003, China; wangpengrui@stu.ouc.edu.cn (P.W.); cjp@stu.ouc.edu.cn (J.C.); clj3855@stu.ouc.edu.cn (L.C.); sl7613@stu.ouc.edu.cn (L.S.)

[2] Laboratory for Marine Drugs and Bioproducts, Pilot National Laboratory for Marine Science and Technology (Qingdao), Qingdao 266237, China

[*] Correspondence: liuhongb@ouc.edu.cn; Tel.: +86-0532-8203-1823

Abstract: Plant volatile organic compounds (VOCs) represent a relatively wide class of secondary metabolites. The VOC profiles of seven seaweeds (*Grateloupia filicina*, *Polysiphonia senticulosa*, *Callithamnion corymbosum*, *Sargassum thunbergii*, *Dictyota dichotoma*, *Enteromorpha prolifera* and *Ulva lactuca*) from the Yellow Sea of China were investigated using multifiber headspace solid phase microextraction coupled with gas chromatography–mass spectrometry (HS-SPME/GC–MS), among them, the VOCs of three red algae Grateloupia filicina, Polysiphonia senticulosa, and Callithamnion corymbosum were first reported. Principal component analysis (PCA) was used to disclose characteristic categories and molecules of VOCs and network pharmacology was performed to predict potential biomedical utilization of candidate seaweeds. Aldehyde was found to be the most abundant VOC category in the present study and (E)-β-ionone was the only compound found to exist in all seven seaweeds. The chemical diversity of aldehydes in *E. prolifera* suggest its potential application in chemotaxonomy and hinted that divinylbenzene/carboxen/polydimethylsiloxane (DVB/CAR/PDMS) fiber is more suitable for aldehyde extraction. VOCs in *D. dichotoma* were characterized as sesquiterpenes and diterpenes and the most relevant pharmacological pathway was the neuroactive ligand–receptor interaction pathway, which suggests that *D. dichotoma* may have certain preventive and therapeutic values in cancer, especially in lung cancer, in addition to neuropsychiatric diseases.

Keywords: volatile organic compounds; seaweeds; characteristic VOCs; chemotaxonomy; biomedical utilization; headspace solid phase microextraction

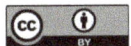

1. Introduction

Plant volatile organic compounds (VOCs) are produced by a range of physiological processes in many different plant tissues and typically occur as a complex mixture of lipophilic compounds with extremely diverse structures [1]. Their low molecular weight and high vapor pressure under ambient conditions allow them to freely exit through cellular membranes and reach the surrounding environment [2].

Plant VOCs have been reported in different geographical conditions ranging from Mediterranean environments [3] and tropical rainforests [4] to various extreme environments [5]. In aquatic ecosystems, algae are the main emitter of VOCs and the extraction of VOCs using headspace solid phase microextraction (HS-SPME) technology has been reported from brown algae [6], red algae [7] and green algae [8]. Algae release an abundance of VOCs to increase their tolerance to abiotic stresses, transfer stress information to homogenate algae to induce defense, play allelopathic roles on heterogeneous algae and aquatic macrophytes for competing nutrients, or protect against predators [9]. In addition, the volatile contaminant in algae caught the interest of environmentalists [10]. Most of the studies on marine algae VOCs have focused on their allelopathy effects, whereas their contributions in other areas have been seldom investigated. VOCs are released under biotic or abiotic stresses and have great significance for plant survival and reproduction. In many cases, evolution has resulted in some plant VOCs acting as metabolic safety valves, protective or defense compounds, or communication cues [1]. VOCs can be divided chemically as aldehydes, alcohols, terpenoids, ketones, halogenated compounds, sulfur compounds and hydrocarbons and exhibit multitudinous functions, such as in being feeding attractants [11], pheromones [12] involved in chemical defenses [13–15] and acting as antimicrobial agents [16].

In the present study, VOC profiles of seven seaweeds blooming in the littoral area of Qingdao (the Yellow Sea of China) were investigated, including the first report of VOCs for three red algae species—*Grateloupia filicina*, *Polysiphonia senticulosa* and *Callithamnion corymbosum*. Characteristic categories and molecules of VOCs are discussed from the point of view of their chemotaxonomic significance and bioactivities are discussed in order to further expand these seaweeds' potential utilities in pharmaceutical areas. Our study provides new insights for the chemotaxonomy of algae and for the biomedical application of *D. dichotoma*.

2. Results and Discussion

2.1. Headspace VOC Composition of Seaweeds

VOC compositions were investigated in seven algae using headspace solid phase microextraction coupled with gas chromatography–mass spectrometry (HS-SPME/GC–MS) and are reported according to their phylum. The number of VOC categories identified in each alga are given in Figure 1.

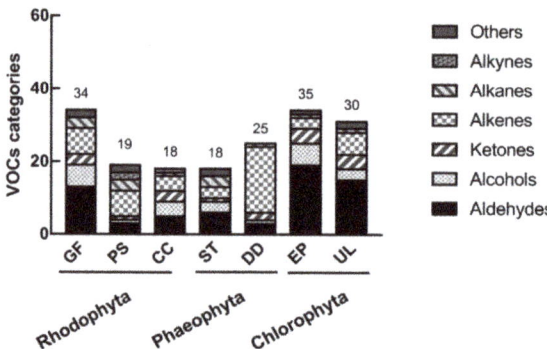

Figure 1. The number of volatile organic compound (VOC) categories identified in seaweeds GF—*Grateloupia filicina*, PS—*Polysiphonia senticulosa*, CC—*Callithamnion corymbosum*, ST—*Sargassum thunbergii*, DD—*Dictyota dichotoma*, EP—*Enteromorpha prolifera* and UL—*Ulva lactuca*.

2.1.1. Headspace VOC Composition of Rhodophyta

There were 34, 19 and 18 compounds identified from *Grateloupia filicina*, *Polysiphonia senticulosa* and *Callithamnion corymbosum*, respectively (Table 1), and, among them, four compounds were common to all three species, including two norisoprenoids (β-cyclocitral and (E)-β-ionone), one alkene (3,5,5-trimethyl-1-hexene) and one alkane (heptadecane). This is the first report on the headspace VOC composition for these three red algae species.

The VOCs of *G. filicina* exhibited the most chemical diversity, with the most abundant being pentadecanal (20.11% in polydimethylsiloxane (PDMS) fiber), tridecanal (19.20% in PDMS fiber), 1-hexen-3-ol (19.58% in divinylbenzene/carboxen/polydimethylsiloxane (DVB/CAR/PDMS) fiber) and 1-octen-3-ol (18.72% in DVB/CAR/PDMS fiber). Wang Xiu-juan et al. [17] analyzed the semi-volatile organic compounds (SVOCs) of *G. filicina* using ethyl acetate as an extraction solvent and found that the main SVOCs were aldehydes, fatty acids and alcohols, with pentadecanal having the highest concentration. Our VOC analysis results are consistent with the results for SVOCs in the literature, suggesting that aldehydes play an important role in the metabolism of G. filicina.

Table 1. VOC composition in Rhodophyta, determined by headspace solid phase microextraction coupled with gas chromatography–mass spectrometry (HS-SPME/GC–MS).

NO.	Compound	Molecular Formula	Compound Class	RI [a]	Area Percentage (%)			Identification
					GF [b]	PS [b]	CC [b]	
1	(E,E,E)-2,4,6-Octatriene [T]	C_8H_{12}	Alkene	<800	1.03 *	0.00	0.00	MS
2	3,5,5-Trimethyl-1-hexene [T]	C_9H_{18}	Alkene	<800	8.24 *	1.74 *	2.74 *	MS
3	3,5-Dimethyl-1-hexene [T]	C_8H_{16}	Alkene	<800	0.36 *	0.00	0.00	MS
4	1-Hexen-3-ol [T]	$C_6H_{12}O$	Alcohol	<800	19.58 *	0.00	4.44 *	MS
5	2-Propyl-furan [T]	$C_7H_{10}O$	Furan derivative	<800	0.30 *	1.02 *	0.00	MS
6	3-Ethyl-1,4-hexadiene [T]	C_8H_{14}	Alkene	846	1.16 *	1.25 *	0.00	MS
7	2-Methylpropylidene-Cyclopentane	C_9H_{16}	Alkene	908	1.48 *	0.00	0.00	MS, RI
8	(Z)-2-Octen-1-ol [T]	$C_8H_{16}O$	Unsaturated alcohol	927	8.5 #	0.00	0.00	MS
9	Isocumene	C_9H_{12}	Others	931	0.00	1.67 *	0.00	MS, RI
10	3-Cyclohexene-1-ethanol	$C_8H_{14}O$	Alcohol	935	2.90 #	0.00	0.00	MS.RI
11	(E)-2-Heptenal	$C_7H_{12}O$	Aldehyde	960	4.78 *	1.51 *	0.00	MS, RI
12	1-Octen-3-ol [S]	$C_8H_{16}O$	Alcohol	980	18.72 #	0.00	2.15 *	MS, RI
13	3,7-Dimethyl-1-octene [T]	$C_{10}H_{20}$	Alkene	985	0.00	0.00	7.81 #	MS
14	2,7-Octadien-1-ol [T]	$C_8H_{14}O$	Unsaturated alcohol	986	8.39 *	0.00	0.00	MS
15	4-Methyl-2-propyl-1-pentanol [T]	$C_9H_{20}O$	Alcohol	990	0.00	0.00	3.59 #	MS
16	5-Methyl-1-undecene [T]	$C_{12}H_{24}$	Alkene	1025	0.00	6.91 *	12.70 *	MS
17	(E)-2-Undecen-1-ol [T]	$C_{11}H_{22}O$	Unsaturated alcohol	1039	0.25 *	1.28 *	0.00	MS
18	(9Z)-1,9-Dodecadiene [T]	$C_{12}H_{22}$	Alkene	1092	0.00	0.00	1.77 #	MS
19	Ectocarpene [T]	$C_{11}H_{16}$	Alkene	1105	0.00	21.83 *, 14.71 #	0.00	MS
20	1-Undecyne	$C_{11}H_{20}$	Alkyne	1108	0.00	2.46 *	8.86 *	MS, RI
21	Dictyoterene D' [T]	$C_{11}H_{18}$	Alkene	1112	0.00	1.74 *, 0.95 #	0.00	MS
22	(Z)-6-Nonenal	$C_9H_{16}O$	Aldehyde	1113	3.25 *	0.00	0.00	MS, RI
23	Decanal	$C_{10}H_{20}O$	Aldehyde	1173	0.07 *	0.00	0.00	MS, RI
24	β-Cyclocitral	$C_{10}H_{16}O$	C_{10}-Norisoprenoid	1192	0.79 *, 0.69 #	1.55 *	0.95 *	MS, RI
25	β-Cyclohomocitral	$C_{11}H_{18}O$	Aldehyde	1236	0.07 *	0.00	0.00	MS, RI
26	2,4-Decadienal	$C_{10}H_{16}O$	Unsaturated aldehyde	1275	0.33 *	0.00	0.00	MS, RI
27	Undecanal	$C_{11}H_{22}O$	Aldehyde	1290	0.47 *, 0.52 #	0.00	0.00	MS, RI
28	(E,E)-2,4-Decadienal	$C_{10}H_{16}O$	Unsaturated aldehyde	1298	0.98 *, 0.66 #	0.69 *	0.00	MS, RI
29	Dodecanal	$C_{12}H_{24}O$	Aldehyde	1400	0.37 *, 0.95 #	0.00	0.00	MS, RI
30	α-Ionone	$C_{13}H_{20}O$	C_{13}-Norisoprenoid	1420	1.50 *, 2.01 #	0.00	1.16 *, 1.60 #	MS, RI
31	Dihydropseudoionone	$C_{13}H_{22}O$	C_{13}-Norisoprenoid	1447	0.15 *, 0.40 #	0.00	0.00	MS, RI
32	(E)-β-Ionone [S]	$C_{13}H_{20}O$	C_{13}-Norisoprenoid	1481	2.65 *, 5.68 #	1.37 #	2.39 *, 4.01 #	MS, RI
33	1-Pentadecene	$C_{15}H_{30}$	Alkene	1484	3.84 *, 2.33 #	1.33 #	0.00	MS, RI
34	Pentadecane [S]	$C_{15}H_{32}$	Alkane	1492	0.57 *, 0.88 #	1.39 #, 11.19#	0.00	MS.RI
35	Tridecanal [S]	$C_{13}H_{26}O$	Aldehyde	1503	5.55 *, 19.20 #	0.00	2.28 *, 5.60 #	MS, RI
36	Cyclopentadecane [T]	$C_{15}H_{30}$	Alkane	1508	0.31 *	1.16 #	0.00	MS
37	Dihydroactinidiolide	$C_{11}H_{16}O_2$	C_{11}-Norisoprenoid	1525	0.06 *	0.00	0.00	MS, RI
38	Tetradecanal [S]	$C_{14}H_{28}O$	Aldehyde	1608	1.75 #	0.00	1.16 #	MS, RI
39	8-Heptadecene	$C_{17}H_{34}$	Alkene	1681	0.10 *	2.85#	0.00	MS, RI
40	Z-11-Pentadecenal [T]	$C_{15}H_{28}O$	Aldehyde	1689	0.26 *, 1.78 #	0.00	1.09 #	MS
41	Heptadecane [S]	$C_{17}H_{36}$	Alkane	1693	1.73 *, 5.76 #	3.19 *, 15.93 #	2.04 *, 3.15 #	MS, RI
42	Pentadecanal	$C_{15}H_{30}O$	Aldehyde	1711	3.23 *, 20.11 #	0.00	11.64 *, 35.43 #	MS, RI
43	Perhydrofarnesyl acetone	$C_{18}H_{36}O$	Ketone	1840	0.00	0.00	0.91 *, 3.14 #	MS, RI
44	1,11-Dodecadiyne [T]	$C_{12}H_{18}$	Alkyne	1845	0.00	0.81 #	0.00	MS
45	(Z,Z)-6,9-Pentadecadien-1-ol [T]	$C_{15}H_{28}O$	Unsaturated alcohol	1889	0.00	0.00	0.46 *, 1.92 #	MS
	Total Identified (%)				90.59 *, 74.10 #	49.61 *, 48.92 #	60.53 *, 62.46 #	

[T] tentatively identified. [S] identified by mass spectra (MS) and retention index (RI) compared with authentic standard. [a] RI: retention index relative to C7-C30 alkanes. [b] GF—*Grateloupia filicina*; PS—*Polysiphonia senticulosa*; CC—*Callithamnion corymbosum*. * data from fiber DVB/CAR/PDMS. # data from fiber PDMS.

Both *P. senticulosa* and *C. corymbosum* are from the same taxonomical order, Ceramiales Oltmanns and were found to contain two common compounds, 5-methyl-1-undecene and 1-undecyne, which were not found in *G. filicina*. Moreover, ectocarpene (21.83% in DVB/CAR/PDMS fiber; 14.71% in PDMS fiber) was a uniquely abundant compound in *P. senticulosa*.

2.1.2. Headspace VOC Composition of Phaeophyta

The VOC compositions of brown algae *Sargassum thunbergia* and *Dictyota dichotoma* are reported in Table 2. Four compounds were commonly found, including one norisoprenoid ((E)-β-Ionone), one alkane (pentadecane) and two aldehydes (tridecanal and pentadecanal).

Table 2. VOC composition in brown algae, determined by headspace solid phase microextraction coupled with gas chromatography–mass spectrometry (HS-SPME/GC–MS).

NO.	Compound	Molecular Formula	Compound Class	RI [a]	Area Percentage (%) ST [b]	Area Percentage (%) DD [b]	Identification
1	2-Propyl-furan [T]	$C_7H_{10}O$	Furan derivative	<800	1.37 *	0.00	MS
2	(E)-2-Hepten-1-ol [T]	$C_7H_{14}O$	Alcohol	830	0.00	4.62 *	MS
3	Sulcatone [T]	$C_8H_{14}O$	C_{13}-Norisoprenoid	852	0.00	5.21 *	MS
4	2-Propyl-1-pentanol [T]	$C_8H_{18}O$	Alcohol	896	0.82 *	0.00	MS
5	Isocumene	C_9H_{12}	Others	931	1.14 *	0.00	MS, RI
6	2,7-Dimethyl-1-octanol [T]	$C_{10}H_{22}O$	Alcohol	1023	0.94 *	0.00	MS
7	(E)-2-Undecen-1-ol [T]	$C_{11}H_{22}O$	Alcohol	1039	1.48 *	0.00	MS
8	Ectocarpene [T]	$C_{11}H_{16}$	Alkene	1105	3.40 *	0.00	MS
9	β-Cyclocitral	$C_{10}H_{16}O$	C_{10}-Norisoprenoid	1192	1.05 *	0.00	MS, RI
10	2,4-Decadienal	$C_{10}H_{16}O$	Unsaturated aldehyde	1275	0.00	0.72 *	MS, RI
11	α-Cubebene	$C_{15}H_{24}$	Sesquiterpene	1338	0.00	0.81 *	MS, RI
12	β-Bourbonene	$C_{15}H_{24}$	Sesquiterpene	1376	0.00	1.07 *, 1.39 #	MS, RI
13	Cedrene	$C_{15}H_{24}$	Sesquiterpene	1418	0.00	0.28 #	MS, RI
14	β-Copaene	$C_{15}H_{24}$	Sesquiterpene	1423	0.00	0.57 *	MS, RI
15	cis-Muurola-3,5-diene	$C_{15}H_{24}$	Sesquiterpene	1441	0.00	0.48 *	MS, RI
16	β-Gurjunene	$C_{15}H_{24}$	Sesquiterpene	1458	0.00	1.72 *	MS, RI
17	γ-Muurolene	$C_{15}H_{24}$	Sesquiterpene	1468	0.00	2.82 *, 0.62 #	MS, RI
18	Germacrene D [S]	$C_{15}H_{24}$	Sesquiterpene	1477	0.00	34.83 *, 62.00 #	MS, RI
19	(E)-β-Ionone [S]	$C_{13}H_{20}O$	C_{13}-Norisoprenoid	1481	1.22 *, 0.93 #	0.52 *, 0.44 #	MS, RI
20	1-Pentadecene	$C_{15}H_{30}$	Alkene	1484	4.31 *, 5.46 #	0.00	MS, RI
21	α-Selinene	$C_{15}H_{24}$	Sesquiterpene	1488	0.00	0.38 #	MS, RI
22	Pentadecane [S]	$C_{15}H_{32}$	Alkane	1492	9.24 *, 13.87 #	5.94 *, 7.98 #	MS,RI
23	Tridecanal [S]	$C_{13}H_{26}O$	Aldehyde	1503	11.46 *, 11.02 #	2.51 *, 1.74 #	MS, RI
24	Cyclopentadecane [T]	$C_{15}H_{30}$	Alkane	1508	2.94 *, 1.51 #	0.00	MS
25	Muurola-4,9-diene	$C_{15}H_{24}$	Sesquiterpene	1510	0.00	3.37 *	MS, RI
26	β-Cadinene	$C_{15}H_{24}$	Sesquiterpene	1518	0.00	0.52 #	MS, RI
27	δ-Cadinene	$C_{15}H_{24}$	Sesquiterpene	1520	0.00	5.28 *	MS, RI
28	1,4-Cadinadiene	$C_{15}H_{24}$	Sesquiterpene	1529	0.00	0.44 *	MS, RI
29	α-Muurolene [T]	$C_{15}H_{24}$	Sesquiterpene	1535	0.00	0.82 *	MS
30	Tetradecanal [S]	$C_{14}H_{28}O$	Aldehyde	1608	0.62 *, 0.48 #	0.00	MS, RI
31	Cubenol	$C_{15}H_{26}O$	Sesquiterpene	1637	0.00	3.69 *, 4.70 #	MS, RI
32	8-Heptadecene	$C_{17}H_{34}$	Alkene	1681	5.97 *, 14.82 #	0.00	MS, RI
33	Heptadecane [S]	$C_{17}H_{36}$	Alkane	1693	1.63 *, 1.59 #	0.00	MS, RI
34	(Z)-11-Pentadecenal [T]	$C_{15}H_{28}O$	Aldehyde	1689	5.49 *, 5.85 #	0.00	MS
35	Pentadecanal	$C_{15}H_{30}O$	Aldehyde	1711	6.86 *, 11.33 #	0.46 #	MS, RI
36	(Z,Z,Z)-7,10,13-Hexadecatrienal [T]	$C_{16}H_{26}O$	Unsaturated aldehyde	1890	0.91 #	0.00	MS
37	1,5,9-Trimethyl-12-(1-methylethyl)-4,8,13-Cyclotetradecatriene-1,3-diol [T]	$C_{20}H_{34}O_2$	Diterpene	1989	0.00	5.70 #	MS
38	Thunbergol	$C_{20}H_{34}O_2$	Diterpene	2089	0.00	3.30 #	MS, RI
39	Geranyl-α-terpinene [T]	$C_{20}H_{32}$	Diterpene	>2100	0.00	1.04 *, 0.99 #	MS
	Total Identified (%)				59.94 *, 67.77 #	76.46 *, 90.51 #	

[T] tentatively identified. [S] identified by mass spectra (MS) and retention index (RI) compared with authentic standard. [a] RI: retention index relative to C7–C30 alkanes. [b] ST—Sargassum thunbergii; DD—Dictyota dichotoma. * data from fiber DVB/CAR/PDMS. # data from fiber PDMS.

The most abundant VOCs in *S. thunbergia* are 8-heptadecene (5.97% in DVB/CAR/PDMS fiber; 14.82% in PDMS fiber), pentadecane (9.24% in DVB/CAR/PDMS fiber; 13.87% in PDMS fiber), pentadecanal (11.33% in PDMS fiber) and tridecanal (11.46% in DVB/CAR/PDMS fiber; 11.02% in PDMS fiber). A low relative content of 8-heptadecene (1.70%) has been reported in *S. thunbergia*, also using the SPME method though the fiber type was not mentioned [18]. Our data suggest that the choice of fiber type in the HS-SPME method has a decisive influence on the study's conclusion. In addition, two types of volatile polyenes were reported to have been found in an essential oil prepared by a simultaneous distillation extraction method from *S. thunbergia* [19], although no polyenes were found in our study.

Fifteen sesquiterpenes were found in *D. dichotoma*, with the predominant one being germacrene D (34.83% in DVB/CAR/PDMS fiber; 62% in PDMS fiber) together with minor ones such as cadinene, muurolene and bourbonene. Compared with the VOC results (PDMS/DVB fiber) from *D. dichotoma* collected from the Adriatic Sea [20], we identified a lower number of sesquiterpenes. The reason for this difference may be that the profile of plant secondary metabolites may vary in different environments, or that different extract fibers have differing abilities to capture sesquiterpenes.

It has been reported that a total of 233 diterpenes were isolated from *Dictyota* species, most of which were from *D. dichotoma* [21]. The present study firstly reports three volatile diterpenes—1,5,9-trimethyl-12-(1-methylethyl)-4,8,13-cyclotetradecatriene-1,3-diol, thunbergol and geranyl-α-terpinene in *Dictyota*. 1,5,9-Trimethyl-12-(1-methylethyl)-4,8,13-cyclotetradecatriene-1,3-diol is a macrocyclic diterpene and is used as a representative flavor compound in tobacco [22]. Geranyl-α-terpinene is distributed in some Compositae plants, as well as existing in the volatiles of beech buds, which act as semiochemical attractants for the beech leaf-mining weevil, *Orchestes fagi* [23].

2.1.3. Headspace VOC Composition of Chlorophyta

The results for two green algae, *Enteromorpha prolifera* and *Ulva lactuca*, are presented in Table 3. In total, 40 VOCs were identified and, among these, 21 were aldehydes.

Table 3. VOC composition in green algae determined by headspace solid phase microextraction coupled with gas chromatography–mass spectrometry (HS-SPME/GC–MS).

NO.	Compound	Molecular Formula	Compound Class	RI [a]	Area Percentage (%)		Identification
					EP [b]	UL [b]	
1	3,5,5-Trimethyl-1-hexene [T]	C_9H_{18}	Alkene	<800	0.00	1.34 *	MS
2	3,5-Dimethyl-1-hexene [T]	C_8H_{16}	Alkene	<800	3.75 *	1.27 *	MS
3	2-Propyl-furan [T]	$C_7H_{10}O$	Furan derivatives	<800	4.61 *	4.74 *, 3.82 #	MS
4	2,4-Octadiene	C_8H_{14}	Alkene	805	0.00	3.06 *	MS, RI
5	3-Ethyl-1,4-hexadiene [T]	C_8H_{14}	Alkene	846	3.59 *	10.17 *	MS
6	(E)-2-Heptenal	$C_7H_{12}O$	Aldehyde	960	9.64 *	4.60 *	MS, RI
7	1,2-Dimethyl-cycloheptene [T]	C_9H_{16}	Alkene	988	3.32 *	3.40 *	MS
8	4-Heptenal [T]	$C_7H_{12}O$	Aldehyde	1001	2.94 *	0.00	MS
9	(4E)-2-Methyl-4-hexen-3-ol [T]	$C_7H_{14}O$	Alcohol	1025	3.08 *	0.00	MS
10	(E)-2-Undecen-1-ol [T]	$C_{11}H_{22}O$	Unsaturated alcohol	1039	3.15 *	1.27 *	MS
11	2,4-Dimethyl-Cyclohexanol	$C_8H_{16}O$	Alcohol	1045	0.80 *	1.90 *	MS, RI
12	3-Cyclohexene-1-carboxaldehyde [T]	$C_8H_{12}O$	Aldehyde	1056	0.50 *	0.00	MS
13	(Z)-6-Nonenal	$C_9H_{16}O$	Aldehyde	1113	0.00	1.94 *	MS, RI
14	2,4-Nonadienal	$C_9H_{14}O$	Unsaturated aldehyde	1180	0.95 *	0.52 *	MS, RI
15	Decanal	$C_{10}H_{20}O$	Aldehyde	1173	1.36 *	0.58 *	MS, RI
16	9-Oxabicyclo [6.1.0]nonan-4-ol [T]	$C_8H_{14}O_2$	Alcohol	1186	0.70 *	0.00	MS
17	β-Cyclocitral	$C_{10}H_{16}O$	C_{10}-Norisoprenoid	1192	0.89 *, 1.05 #	3.05 *, 3.17 #	MS, RI
18	(Z)-2-Decenal	$C_{10}H_{18}O$	Aldehyde	1243	0.70 *	0.00	MS, RI
19	Citral	$C_{10}H_{16}O$	C_{10}-Norisoprenoid	1253	0.32 *	0.00	MS, RI
20	1-Butenylidene-cyclohexane [T]	$C_{10}H_{16}$	Alkane	1260	0.81 *	1.80 *, 1.80 #	MS
21	Undecanal	$C_{11}H_{22}O$	Aldehyde	1290	0.31 *	0.15 *	MS, RI
22	2,4-Decadienal	$C_{10}H_{16}O$	Unsaturated aldehyde	1275	0.00	0.96 *, 0.48 #	MS, RI
23	(E,E)-2,4-Decadienal	$C_{10}H_{16}O$	Unsaturated aldehyde	1298	0.77 *, 1.61 #	3.02 *, 2.59 #	MS, RI
24	4,4,6-Trimethyl-cyclohex-2-en-1-ol	$C_9H_{16}O$	Alcohol	1330	0.28 *	0.00	MS, RI
25	2-Undecenal	$C_{11}H_{20}O$	Aldehyde	1353	0.65 *	0.00	MS, RI
26	(E)-4,5-Epoxydec-2-enal	$C_{10}H_{16}O_2$	Unsaturated Aldehyde	1368	1.70 *, 0.85 #	0.28 *	MS, RI
27	6,10-Dimethyl-2-undecanone	$C_{13}H_{26}O$	Ketone	1395	0.56 *	0.19 *	MS, RI
28	Dodecanal	$C_{12}H_{24}O$	Aldehyde	1400	0.43 *	0.00	MS, RI
29	α-Ionone	$C_{13}H_{20}O$	C_{13}-Norisoprenoid	1420	0.21 *, 0.45 #	2.59 *, 4.24 #	MS, RI
30	(E)-Geranylacetone	$C_{13}H_{22}O$	C_{13}-Norisoprenoid	1447	0.93 *, 1.74 #	0.29 *, 0.48 #	MS, RI
31	(E)-β-Ionone [S]	$C_{13}H_{20}O$	C_{13}-Norisoprenoid	1481	3.53 *, 5.97 #	8.69 *, 18.13 #	MS, RI
32	Tridecanal [S]	$C_{13}H_{26}O$	Aldehyde	1503	1.31 *, 2.37 #	0.37 *, 0.65 #	MS, RI

Table 3. Cont.

NO.	Compound	Molecular Formula	Compound Class	RI [a]	Area Percentage (%) EP [b]	Area Percentage (%) UL [b]	Identification
33	Dihydroactinidiolide	$C_{11}H_{16}O_2$	C_{11}-Norisoprenoid	1525	0.00	0.29 *	MS, RI
34	Tetradecanal [S]	$C_{14}H_{28}O$	Aldehyde	1608	3.34 *, 6.32 #	0.79 #	MS, RI
35	8-Heptadecene	$C_{17}H_{34}$	Alkene	1681	2.72 #	5.32 *, 19.70 #	MS, RI
36	(Z)-11-Pentadecenal [T]	$C_{15}H_{28}O$	Aldehyde	1689	0.40 *, 0.81 #	0.77 *	MS
37	Pentadecanal	$C_{15}H_{30}O$	Aldehyde	1711	8.49 *, 24.40 #	3.83 *, 7.36 #	MS, RI
38	(Z)-11-Hexadecenal	$C_{16}H_{30}O$	Aldehyde	1793	0.59 *, 1.18 #	0.00	MS, RI
39	(Z,Z)-6,9-Pentadecadien-1-ol [T]	$C_{15}H_{28}O$	Unsaturated alcohol	1889	0.83 #	0.54 *, 0.93 #	MS
40	(Z,Z,Z)-7,10,13-Hexadecatrienal [T]	$C_{16}H_{26}O$	Unsaturated aldehyde	1890	0.46 *, 6.13 #	2.83 *, 4.96 #	MS
	Total Identified (%)				65.07 *, 56.43 #	69.79 *, 69.10 #	

[T] tentatively identified. [S] identified by mass spectra (MS) and retention index (RI) compared with authentic standard. [a] RI: retention index relative to C7–C30 alkanes. [b] EP—Enteromorpha prolifera; UL—Ulva lactuca. * data from fiber DVB/CAR/PDMS. # data from fiber PDMS.

The top three compounds with the highest content in *E. prolifera* were aldehydes, consisting of pentadecanal (8.49% in DVB/CAR/PDMS fiber; 24.4% in PDMS fiber), (E)-2-heptenal (9.64% in DVB/CAR/PDMS fiber) and tetradecanal (3.34% in DVB/CAR/PDMS fiber; 6.32% in PDMS fiber). It has been reported that significant differences were observed in the composition and types of VOCs in different harvest seasons for *E. prolifera* [24]. Differently from *E. prolifera*, the top three compounds with the highest content found in *U. lactuca* were not aldehydes, but alkenes and a ketone, including 8-heptadecene (5.32% in DVB/CAR/PDMS fiber; 19.70% in PDMS fiber), (E)-β-ionone (8.69% in DVB/CAR/PDMS fiber; 18.13% in PDMS fiber) and 3-ethyl-1,4-hexadiene (10.17% in DVB/CAR/PDMS fiber).

For *U. lactuca*, 30 VOCs were identified. Among them, 25 compounds also existed in *E. prolifera*, including 11 aldehydes ((E)-2-heptenal, 2,4-nonadienal, decanal, (E,E)-2,4-decadienal, undecanal, (E)-4,5-epoxydec-2-enal, tridecanal, tetradecanal, Z-11-pentadecenal, pentadecanal, (Z,Z,Z)-7,10,13-hexadecatrienal); four norisoprenoids (β-cyclocitral, α-ionone, (E)-geranylacetone, (E)-β-ionone); four alkenes (3,5-dimethyl-1-hexene, 3-ethyl-1,4-hexadiene, 1,2-dimethyl-cycloheptene, 8-heptadecene); two alkanes (1-butenylidene-cyclohexane, heptadecane); three alcohols ((E)-2-undecen-1-ol, 2,4-dimethyl-cyclohexanol, (Z,Z)-6,9-pentadecadien-1-ol); one ketone (6,10-dimethyl-2-undecanone) and one furan derivative (2-propyl-furan). The above common constituents in the two green algae covered almost all the VOC categories, differently from the red and brown algae.

(E)-β-Ionone was the only compound found to existing in all seven algae characterized in this study and it is widely distributed in the plant kingdom. As a C_{13} norisoprenoid, (E)-β-ionone can be produced by secondary metabolism of β-carotene and can also be produced by thermal degradation and photooxidation of carotenoids [25,26]. It has been reported that (E)-β-ionone has a wide range of biological activities, including having a strong anticancer effect [27].

2.2. Characteristic VOC Molecules and Potential Application in Chemotaxonomy

2.2.1. PCA on Total VOCs Variables

Principal component analysis (PCA) on data from fiber DVB/CAR/PDMS exhibited that, except for *D. dichotoma* and *E. prolifera*, the other five seaweeds were clustered together (Figure 2a). The PCA results for fiber PDMS show that *D. dichotoma* was distinct from the other six seaweeds (Figure 2b).

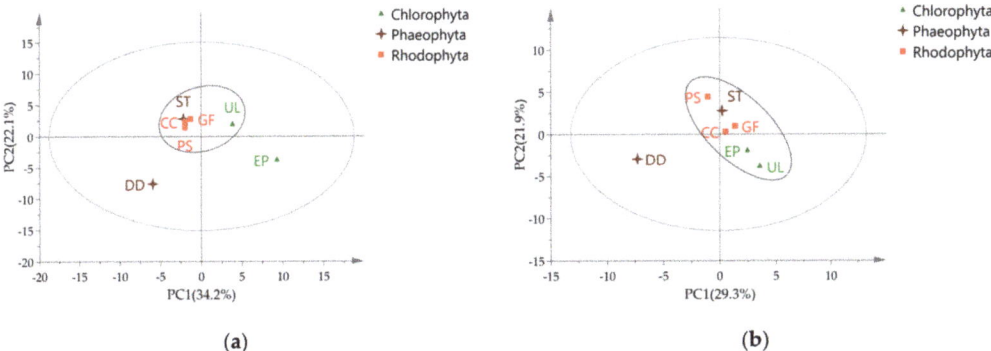

Figure 2. Principal component analysis (PCA) of VOC compositions in seven seaweeds determined by HS-SPME/GC–MS; score plot for (**a**) divinylbenzene/carboxen/polydimethylsiloxane (DVB/CAR/PDMS) fiber; (**b**) polydimethylsiloxane (PDMS) fiber.

D. dichotoma is an outlier in PCA, being very different from the other six seaweeds. The molecules that contributed most to this difference were revealed in the loading plot and are reported in the Supplementary Materials (Figure S1 and Table S1). As expected, the main differences were regarding sesquiterpenes and diterpenes.

Based on the revised biogenetic scheme that is widely cited, *Dictyota* diterpenes can be divided into three groups (I–III), resulting from the first formal cyclization of the geranylgeraniol precursor, which makes them potentially useful as chemotaxonomic and phylogenetic markers [28]. Unfortunately, the number of diterpenes available in *Dictyota* VOCs is very limited, making it difficult for them to be used in chemotaxonomy.

On the other hand, *Dictyota* contains large numbers of sesquiterpenes, distinguishing them from other seaweeds in this study. It is still not clear whether volatile sesquiterpenes can be used as chemotaxonomic markers for species identification of genus *Dictyota*, but it is worth exploring this through the VOC approach.

2.2.2. PCA on Aldehyde Variables

Using all the VOC data as PCA variables, *E. prolifera* was found to be an outlier, as shown in Figure 2a (DVB/CAR/PDMS fiber), but not in Figure 2b (PDMS fiber). Considering that aldehydes are the most abundant VOC categories (Figure 1), aldehydes were used as variables in PCA to reveal chemical differences between species. The results show that *E. prolifera* was separated well from other seaweeds (Figure 3). The aldehydes that contribute the most to species differences are shown in Table 4. There are six aldehydes characteristically distributed in *E. prolifera*.

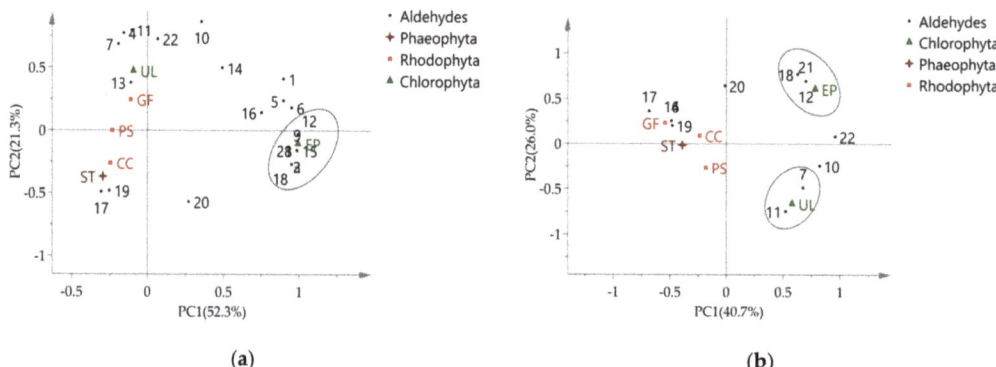

Figure 3. Bi-plot of PCA using aldehydes: (**a**) DVB/CAR/PDMS fiber; (**b**) PDMS fiber.

Table 4. Various aldehydes in PCA loading plot, as shown in Figure 3.

No.	Aldehydes	Molecular Formula	Related Fiber	Algae
2	4-Heptenal	$C_7H_{12}O$	DVB/CAR/PDMS	EP
3	3-Cyclohexene-1-carboxaldehyde	$C_8H_{12}O$	DVB/CAR/PDMS	EP
7	β-Cyclocitral	$C_{10}H_{16}O$	PDMS	EP, UL $^\Delta$, GF, PS, CC, ST
8	(Z)-2-Decenal	$C_{10}H_{18}O$	DVB/CAR/PDMS	EP
9	Citral	$C_{10}H_{16}O$	DVB/CAR/PDMS	EP
11	2,4-Decadienal	$C_{10}H_{16}O$	PDMS	UL $^\Delta$, GF, DD
12	(E)-4,5-Epoxydec-2-enal	$C_{10}H_{16}O_2$	DVB/CAR/PDMS, PDMS	EP $^\Delta$, UL
15	2-Undecenal	$C_{11}H_{20}O$	DVB/CAR/PDMS	EP
18	Tetradecanal	$C_{14}H_{28}O$	DVB/CAR/PDMS, PDMS	EP $^\Delta$, UL, GF, CC, ST
21	(Z)-11-Hexadecenal	$C_{16}H_{30}O$	DVB/CAR/PDMS, PDMS	EP

$^\Delta$ with the highest content.

Aldehydes are substances released by algae under biotic or abiotic stress and some aldehydes may induce the synthesis of a series of oxylipins in algae and therefore act as inducers of metabolic responses [29]. In view of the limited species and numbers of seaweeds in the present study, our data can only suggest that aldehydes may be of important value for the chemotaxonomic significance of *E. prolifera* and that the DVB/CAR/PDMS fiber is more suitable for headspace solid phase microextraction for aldehydes.

The volatile components of red algae *Bangia fuscopurpurea*, *Gelidium latifolium*, *Callithamnion granulatum*, *Ceramium elegans*, *Laurencia papillosa* and *Laurencia coronopus* from Black sea was detected and found that hydrocarbons can be used as chemotaxonomic markers of the two classes Bangiophyceae and Florideophyceae [30]. The chemotaxonomic significance was also discussed according to VOCs detection in two brown algae: *Taonia atomaria* and *Padina pavonica* [6]. The VOCs were used in evolutionary relationship discussion between the algae and liverwort *Fossombronia angulosa* due to the similarity [31].

2.3. Network Pharmacology and Potential Biomedical Application of D. Dichotoma

VOCs in *D. dichotoma* are characterized by sesquiterpenes and diterpenes. It has been reported that a total of 78 structurally diverse diterpenes have been isolated from

D. dichotoma and exhibit multi-biological properties, such as cytotoxic, antitumor, antiviral, antifouling, antioxidant, antibacterial and antifungal activities [21]. In the present study, a network pharmacology method was performed to verify and discover new bioactivities of *D. dichotoma*.

First, the VOCs of *D. dichotoma* were entered into the Traditional Chinese Medicine Systems Pharmacology Database and Analysis Platform (TCMSP) in the "chemical name" search box to obtain relevant targets. The "compound–target" relationships are shown in Figure 4, with 31 nodes (1 alga, 10 compounds and 20 targes). Comparing with the average degree score, 6.07, from network topology analysis, six key compounds were disclosed as cedrene, α-selinene, cubenol, α-muurolene, 2,4-decadienal and γ-muurolene, of which most are sesquiterpenes. The first three compounds are cedrene, α-selinene and cubenol, each of which can act on 10 targets.

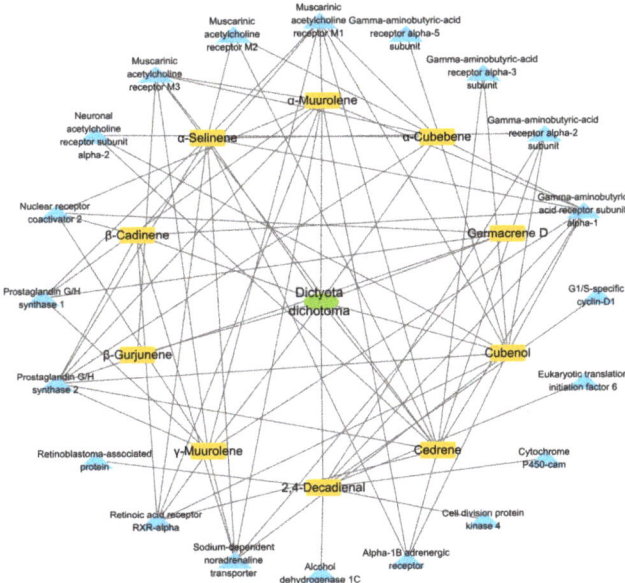

Figure 4. Compound–target interaction network of Dictyota dichotoma.

Next, the Kyoto Encyclopedia of Genes and Genomes (KEGG) enrichment analysis was used to obtain the potential pathway in which VOCs might play a role. The 10 identified pathways ($p < 0.01$) are shown in Figure 5: neuroactive ligand–receptor interaction, small cell lung cancer, retrograde endocannabinoid signaling, nicotine addiction, non-small cell lung cancer, GABAergic synapse, morphine addiction, bladder cancer, PI3K–Akt signaling pathway and the calcium signaling pathway.

According to the literature, the neuroactive ligand–receptor interaction pathway plays an important role in lung cancer etiology [32]. Considering other pathways such as small cell lung cancer, non-small cell lung cancer, retrograde endocannabinoid signaling and PI3K–Akt signaling, we supposed that *D. dichotoma* may have certain preventive and therapeutic value in cancer, especially in lung cancer. The non-polar fractions of *D. dichotoma* exhibit anticancer activity in vitro, including the lung adenocarcinoma cell line (A-549) [33].

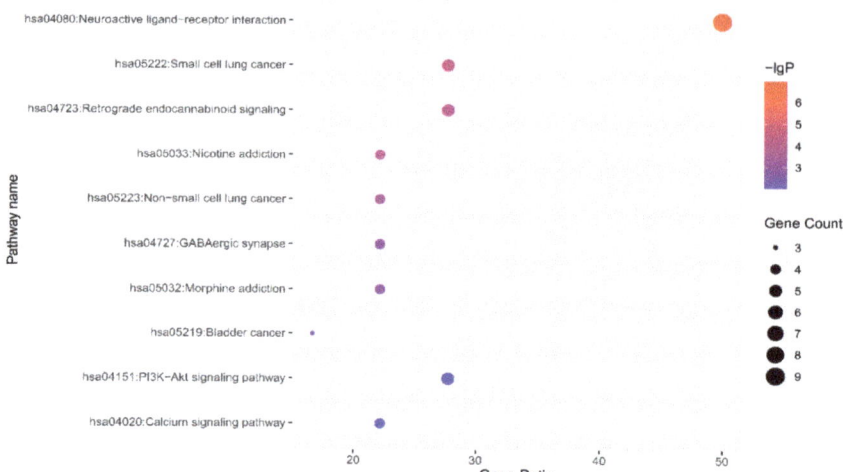

Figure 5. Bubble chart of pathway enrichment information.

In addition, it should be noted that the neuroactive ligand–receptor interaction pathway is the most relevant pathway for VOCs in *D. dichotoma*, with nine target genes involved—CHRM1, CHRM2, CHRM3, CHRNA2, GABRA1, GABRA2, GABRA3, GABRA5 and ADRA1B. The neuroactive ligand–receptor interaction pathway is involved in environmental information processing as well as signaling molecules and interactions and an association has been found with certain neuropsychiatric disorders [34]. Therefore, *D. dichotoma* may have some potential use in the study of some neuropsychiatric diseases.

3. Materials and Methods

3.1. Sample Collection

The samples of seven algae were single-point collected from the coast of Qingdao city (120°20′30″ E, 36°3′43″ N, the Yellow Sea), Shandong Province, China, in July 2019. All of the studied algae are local common species, including *Grateloupia filicina* (Wulfen) C. Agardh, 1822 (Halymeniaceae Bory, Gigartinales Schmitz, Rhodophyceae), *Polysiphonia senticulosa* Harvey,1862 (Rhodomelaceae Areschoug, Ceramiales Oltmanns, Rhodophyceae), *Callithamnion corymbosum* (Smith) Lyngbye, 1819 (Ceramiaceae Dumortier, Ceramiales Oltmanns, Rhodophyceae), *Sargassum thunbergii* (Mertens ex Roth) O'Kuntze, 1893 (Sargassaceae Kuetzing, Fucales Kylin, Phaeophyta), *Dictyota dichotoma* (Hudson) J. V. Lamouroux, 1809a (Dictyotaceae Lamourous ex Dumortier, Dictyotales Kjellman in Engler et Prantl, Phaeophyta), *Enteromorpha prolifera* (O.F.Müller) J. Agardh, 1883 (Ulvales Blackman et Tansley, Ulvaceae Lamourous ex Dumortier, Chlorophyta), *Ulva lactuca* Linneaeus, 1753 (Ulvales Blackman et Tansley, Ulvaceae Lamourous ex Dumortier, Chlorophyta). The voucher specimens have been deposited in the Key Laboratory of Marine Drugs, Chinese Ministry of Education, School of Medicine and Pharmacy, Ocean University of China.

The samples were separately collected and placed in an air-tight plastic bag containing surrounding seawater and were immediately transported to the laboratory. Before extraction, each sample were cut into small pieces and excess water was removed using filter paper.

3.2. Headspace Solid Phase Microextraction (HS-SPME)

HS-SPME was performed with a manual SPME holder. Four types of fibers obtained from Supelco Co. (Bellefonte, PA, USA) were compared for their adsorption properties in pilot experiments and two fibers, divinylbenzene/carboxen/polydimethylsiloxane (DVB/CAR/PDMS, 50/30 μm) and polydimethylsiloxane (PDMS, 100 μm) were finally, chosen. Fibers polyacrylate (PA, 85 μm) and 7 μm PDMS were not used in the present study. The fibers were activated in advance, according to the instructions.

A 1 g amount of prepared sample was placed into 4 mL glass vials and sealed using a cover with a Teflon gasket to provide a closed environment. The vials were placed at 60 °C for 15 min to equilibrate and the fiber was then pushed into the vial and maintained there for 20 min to adsorb the VOCs of the sample. After absorption, the fiber was removed from the vial and inserted into the injector (250 °C) of the GC–MS and kept for 6 min (DVB/CAR/PDMS fiber) or 4 min (PDMS fiber) to realize desorption. HS-SPME was performed in triplicate for each sample.

3.3. Gas Chromatography–Mass Spectrometry (GC–MS) Analyses

GC–MS analyses was performed on a Thermo Trace 1300 ISQ gas chromatography-mass spectrometer (Thermo Fisher Scientific Inc., San Jose, CA, USA) equipped with a TG-5MS capillary column (5% phenyl-methylpolysiloxane, 30 m × 0.25 mm, 0.25 μm, Thermo Fisher Scientific Inc.). For DVB/CAR/PDMS fiber, the oven temperature was initially set at 70 °C and maintained for 1 min, increased at a rate of 3 °C/min to 100 °C and continually increased at a rate of 5 °C/min to 200 °C, followed by a final hold at this temperature for 2 min. For PDMS fiber, the oven temperature was initially maintained at 70 °C for 2 min, increased from 70 to 200 °C at 3 °C/min and then held at 200 °C for 6 min. Helium (99.9% purity) was used as the carrier gas at a flow rate of 1 mL/min. The temperature of the injector, detector transfer line and ion source were 250, 270 and 230 °C, respectively. The MS detector was operated in the full scan mode and the electron energy was 70 eV and the scan range was from *m/z* 30 to 350 amu. All analyses were performed in triplicate.

Visualization, calibration and normalization of the GC–MS data were performed using Xcalibur 2.1 (Thermo Fisher Scientific Inc.). The VOC peaks were identified by comparison of their retention index (RI) and MS data with data in the NIST Chemistry WebBook [35] and NIST 11 MS Data Library, respectively. The RI values of the VOCs were calculated by analyzing the C7–C30 *n*-alkanes (Sigma-Aldrich, St. Louis, MO, USA) under the same GC–MS conditions as samples. Authentic standards included trans-2-nonenal (Shanghai Macklin Biochemical Co., Ltd., Shanghai, China), tridecanal (Shanghai Macklin Biochemical Co., Ltd.), 1-octen-3-ol (Shanghai Macklin Biochemical Co., Ltd.), tetradecanal (Shanghai Aladdin Biochemical Technology Co., Ltd., Shanghai, China), germacrene D (Toronto Research Chemicals, Toronto, ON, Canada) and (*E*)-β-ionone (Xiya Chemical Technology Co., Ltd., Chengdu, China), which were used for confirming VOC identity. All VOC peaks were quantified by area normalization with consistent peak parameters (baseline, area noise and peak noise) prior to data analysis and statistics.

3.4. Chemometrics and Network Pharmacology Analysis

The principal components analysis (PCA) of all VOCs was conducted using SIMCA 14.1. The targets of identified volatile components were obtained from the Traditional Chinese Medicine Systems Pharmacology Database and Analysis Platform (TCMSP, https://tcmspw.com/tcmsp.php, accessed on 21 December 2020) [36], the gene information of the related targets was taken from the Uniport database (https://www.Unitprot.org/, accessed on 21 December 2020) and the String database (https://string-db.org/, accessed on 21 December 2020) [37,38] and KEGG pathway enrichment analysis were accessed through DAVID software (https://david.ncifcrf.gon/, accessed on 21 December 2020) [39] with the corresponding bubble chart realized using the R program. The interactive component–target relationships in algae were visualized using Cytoscape 3.7.2 software.

4. Conclusions

The volatile composition of seven algae from Yellow Sea of China was detected by HS-SPME/GC-MS, the VOCs of three red algae *Grateloupia filicina*, *Polysiphonia senticulosa* and *Callithamnion corymbosum* among them are first reported. The PCA analysis of VOCs reveals the chemotaxonomy significance of aldehydes in green algae *Enteromorpha prolifera* and sesquiterpenes in brown algae *Dictyota dichotoma*, as well as the applicability of DVB/CAR/PDMS fiber in volatile aldehydes. The network pharmacology analysis of *Dictyota dichotoma* indicate the potential biomedical application in fields of lung cancer and neuropsychiatric diseases. Our study exploits the new research value of VOCs in algae from the perspective of chemotaxonomy and network pharmacology.

Supplementary Materials: The following are available online at https://www.mdpi.com/article/10.3390/md19040192/s1, Figure S1: PCA of VOC compositions in seven seaweeds determined by HS-SPME/GC–MS, loading plot with: (a) DVB/CAR/PDMS fiber; (b) PDMS fiber. Table S1: The compounds corresponding to dots with coordinates in the loading plot.

Author Contributions: Conceptualization, H.L. and P.W.; methodology, P.W.; software, P.W., J.C. and L.C.; validation, L.C. and L.S.; formal analysis, P.W.; investigation, P.W.; data curation, P.W.; writing—original draft preparation, P.W.; writing—review and editing, H.L.; project administration, H.L.; funding acquisition, H.L. and P.W. All authors have read and agreed to the published version of the manuscript.

Funding: This research was funded by the National Natural Science Foundation of China, grant number 81973433 (H.-B. Liu), Independent Research Projects for Graduate Students of Ocean University of China (P.-R. Wang).

Institutional Review Board Statement: Not applicable.

Informed Consent Statement: Not applicable.

Data Availability Statement: The data presented in this study are available in the manuscript.

Conflicts of Interest: The authors declare no conflict of interest.

References

1. Penuelas, J.; Llusia, J. Plant VOC emissions: Making use of the unavoidable. *Trends Ecol. Evol.* **2004**, *19*, 402–404. [CrossRef] [PubMed]
2. Pichersky, E.; Noel, J.P.; Dudareva, N. Biosynthesis of plant volatiles: Nature's diversity and ingenuity. *Science* **2006**, *311*, 808–811. [CrossRef]
3. Owen, S.M.; Boissard, C.; Hewitt, C.N. Volatile organic compounds (VOCs) emitted from 40 Mediterranean plant species: VOC speciation and extrapolation to habitat scale. *Atmos. Environ.* **2001**, *35*, 5393–5409. [CrossRef]
4. Kesselmeier, J.; Guenther, A.; Hoffmann, T.; Piedade, M.T.; Warnke, J. Natural volatile organic compound emissions from plants and their roles in oxidant balance and particle formation. In *Amazonia and Global Change*; American Geophysical Union: Washington, DC, USA, 2009; Volume 186, pp. 183–206. [CrossRef]
5. Rinnan, R.; Steinke, M.; McGenity, T.; Loreto, F. Plant volatiles in extreme terrestrial and marine environments. *Plant Cell Environ.* **2014**, *37*, 1776–1789. [CrossRef]
6. Jerkovic, I.; Kranjac, M.; Marijanovic, Z.; Roje, M.; Jokic, S. Chemical diversity of headspace and volatile oil composition of two brown algae (*Taonia atomaria* and *Padina pavonica*) from the Adriatic Sea. *Molecules* **2019**, *24*, 495. [CrossRef]
7. De Alencar, D.B.; Diniz, J.C.; Rocha, S.A.S.; Dos Santos Pires-Cavalcante, K.M.; Freitas, J.O.; Nagano, C.S.; Sampaio, A.H.; Saker-Sampaio, S. Chemical composition of volatile compounds in two red seaweeds, *Pterocladiella capillacea* and *Osmundaria obtusiloba*, using static headspace gas chromatography mass spectrometry. *J. Appl. Phycol.* **2017**, *29*, 1571–1576. [CrossRef]
8. Yamamoto, M.; Baldermann, S.; Yoshikawa, K.; Fujita, A.; Mase, N.; Watanabe, N. Determination of volatile compounds in four commercial samples of Japanese green algae using solid phase microextraction gas chromatography mass spectrometry. *Sci. World J.* **2014**, *2014*, 289780:1–289790:8. [CrossRef]
9. Zuo, Z. Why algae release volatile organic compounds—The emission and roles. *Front. Microbiol.* **2019**, *10*, 491. [CrossRef]
10. Rocha, F.; Homem, V.; Castro-Jimenez, J.; Ratola, N. Marine vegetation analysis for the determination of volatile methylsiloxanes in coastal areas. *Sci. Total Environ.* **2019**, *650*, 2364–2373. [CrossRef]
11. Akakabe, Y.; Kajiwara, T. Bioactive volatile compounds from marine algae: Feeding attractants. *J. Appl. Phycol.* **2008**, *20*, 661–664. [CrossRef]
12. Pohnert, G.; Boland, W. The oxylipin chemistry of attraction and defense in brown algae and diatoms. *Nat. Prod. Rep.* **2002**, *19*, 108–122. [CrossRef]
13. Van Alstyne, K.L.; Houser, L.T. Dimethylsulfide release during macroinvertebrate grazing and its role as an activated chemical defense. *Mar. Ecol. Prog. Ser.* **2003**, *250*, 175–181. [CrossRef]
14. Schnitzler, I.; Pohnert, G.; Hay, M.; Boland, W. Chemical defense of brown algae (Dictyopteris spp.) against the herbivorous amphipod *Ampithoe longimana*. *Oecologia* **2001**, *126*, 515–521. [CrossRef]

15. Wiesemeier, T.; Hay, M.; Pohnert, G. The potential role of wound-activated volatile release in the chemical defence of the brown alga *Dictyota dichotoma*: Blend recognition by marine herbivores. *Aquat. Sci.* **2007**, *69*, 403–412. [CrossRef]
16. Kajiwara, T.; Matsui, K.; Akakabe, Y.; Murakawa, T.; Arai, C. Antimicrobial browning-inhibitory effect of flavor compounds in seaweeds. *J. Appl. Phycol.* **2006**, *18*, 413–422. [CrossRef]
17. Wang, X.J.; Xu, J.L.; Yan, X.J. Analysis of the semivolatile organic compounds of two seaweeds. *Haiyang Kexue* **2010**, *34*, 25–28. (In Chinese)
18. Zhang, M.; Li, R.X.; Hu, C.M.; Yang, L.E.; Tang, J.; Lu, Q.Q.; Zhang, T.; Shen, Z.G.; Shen, S.D.; Xu, P.; et al. The metabolism of 8-heptadecene in *Pyropia* (Bangiaceae, Rhodophyta). *J. Appl. Phycol.* **2014**, *26*, 1181–1187. [CrossRef]
19. Lu, S.J.; Yosemoto, S.; Satomi, D.; Handa, H.; Akakabe, Y. Two types of volatile polyenes in the brown alga *Sargassum thunbergii*. *J. Oleo Sci.* **2018**, *67*, 1463–1471. [CrossRef]
20. Jerkovic, I.; Marijanovic, Z.; Roje, M.; Kus, P.M.; Jokic, S.; Coz-Rakovac, R. Phytochemical study of the headspace volatile organic compounds of fresh algae and seagrass from the Adriatic Sea (single point collection). *PLoS ONE* **2018**, *13*, 1–13. [CrossRef] [PubMed]
21. Chen, J.Y.; Li, H.; Zhao, Z.S.; Xia, X.; Li, B.; Zhang, J.R.; Yan, X.J. Diterpenes from the marine algae of the genus *Dictyota*. *Mar. Drugs* **2018**, *16*, 159. [CrossRef]
22. Roberts, D.L.; Rowland, R.L. Macrocyclic diterpenes. α- and β-4,8,13-Duvatriene-1,3-diols from Tobacco. *J. Org. Chem.* **1962**, *27*, 3989–3995. [CrossRef]
23. Silk, P.J.; Mayo, P.D.; LeClair, G.; Brophy, M.; Pawlowski, S.; MacKay, C.; Hillier, N.K.; Hughes, C.; Sweeney, J.D. Semiochemical attractants for the beech leaf-mining weevil, *Orchestes fagi*. *Entomol. Exp. Appl.* **2017**, *164*, 102–112. [CrossRef]
24. Miao, F.F.; Ding, Y.; Lin, J.L.; He, H.P.; Zhu, W.C.; Su, X.R. Analysis of volatile compounds in *Enteromorpha prolifera* harvested during different seasons by electronic nose and HS-SPME-GC-MS. *Mod. Food Sci. Technol.* **2014**, *30*, 258–263. (In Chinese) [CrossRef]
25. Reese, K.L.; Fisher, C.L.; Lane, P.D.; Jaryenneh, J.D.; Moorman, M.W.; Jones, A.D.; Frank, M.; Lane, T.W. Chemical profiling of volatile organic compounds in the headspace of algal cultures as early biomarkers of algal pond crashes. *Sci. Rep.* **2019**, *9*, 13866. [CrossRef] [PubMed]
26. Zhang, K.J.; Lin, T.F.; Zhang, T.Q.; Li, C.; Gao, N.Y. Characterization of typical taste and odor compounds formed by *Microcystis aeruginosa*. *J. Environ. Sci.* **2013**, *25*, 1539–1548. [CrossRef]
27. Jones, S.; Fernandes, N.V.; Yeganehjoo, H.; Katuru, R.; Qu, H.B.; Yu, Z.L.; Mo, H.B. β-Ionone induces cell cycle arrest and apoptosis in human prostate tumor cells. *Nutr. Cancer* **2013**, *65*, 600–610. [CrossRef]
28. Teixeira, V.L.; Kelecom, A. A chemotaxonomic study of diterpenes from marine brown algae of the genus *Dictyota*. *Sci. Total Environ.* **1988**, *75*, 271–283. [CrossRef]
29. Goulitquer, S.; Ritter, A.; Thomas, F.; Ferec, C.; Salauen, J.P.; Potin, P. Release of volatile aldehydes by the brown algal kelp *Laminaria digitata* in response to both biotic and abiotic stress. *ChemBioChem* **2009**, *10*, 977–982. [CrossRef]
30. Kamenarska, Z.; Ivanova, A.; Stancheva, R.; Stoyneva, M.; Stefanov, K.; Dimitrova-Konaklieva, S.; Popov, S. Volatile compounds from some Black Sea red algae and their chemotaxonomic application. *Bot. Mar.* **2006**, *49*, 47–56. [CrossRef]
31. Ludwiczuk, A.; Nagashima, F.; Gradstein, R.S.; Asakawa, Y. Volatile components from selected Mexican, Ecuadorian, Greek, German and Japanese liverworts. *Nat. Prod. Commun.* **2008**, *3*, 133–140. [CrossRef]
32. Ji, X.M.; Bossé, Y.; Landi, M.T.; Gui, J.; Xiao, X.J.; Qian, D.; Joubert, P.; Lamontagne, M.; Li, Y.F.; Gorlov, I.; et al. Identification of susceptibility pathways for the role of chromosome 15q25.1 in modifying lung cancer risk. *Nat. Commun.* **2018**, *9*, 1–15. [CrossRef]
33. El-Shaibany, A.; Al-Habori, M.; Al-Maqtari, T.; Al-Mahbashi, H. The yemeni brown algae *Dictyota dichotoma* exhibit high in vitro anticancer activity independent of its antioxidant capability. *Biomed Res. Int.* **2020**, 2425693:1–2425693:9. [CrossRef]
34. Adkins, D.E.; Khachane, A.N.; McClay, J.L.; Åberg, K.; Bukszár, J.; Sullivan, P.F.; van den Oord, E.J.C.G. SNP-based analysis of neuroactive ligand–receptor interaction pathways implicates PGE2 as a novel mediator of antipsychotic treatment response: Data from the CATIE study. *Schizophr. Res.* **2012**, *135*, 200–201. [CrossRef]
35. NIST Chemistry WebBook, SRD 69. Available online: https://webbook.nist.gov/chemistry/ (accessed on 1 June 2020).
36. Lab of System Pharmacology. Available online: https://tcmspw.com/tcmsp.php (accessed on 21 December 2020).
37. Unitprot. Available online: https://www.uniprot.org/ (accessed on 21 December 2020).
38. STRING. Available online: https://string-db.org/ (accessed on 21 December 2020).
39. DAVID Bioinformatics Resources 6.8. Available online: https://david.ncifcrf.gov/ (accessed on 21 December 2020).

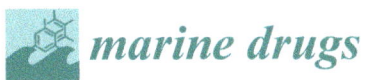

Article

Metabolites with Anti-Inflammatory Activity from the Mangrove Endophytic Fungus *Diaporthe* sp. QYM12

Yan Chen [1,2], Ge Zou [2], Wencong Yang [2], Yingying Zhao [1], Qi Tan [2], Lin Chen [3], Jinmei Wang [1], Changyang Ma [1], Wenyi Kang [1,*] and Zhigang She [2,*]

1. National R & D Center for Edible Fungus Processing Technology, Henan University, Kaifeng 475004, China; chenyan27@mail2.sysu.edu.cn (Y.C.); zhaoyingying@vip.henu.edu.cn (Y.Z.); wangjinmei@henu.edu.cn (J.W.); macaya1024@vip.henu.edu.cn (C.M.)
2. School of Chemistry, Sun Yat-Sen University, Guangzhou 510275, China; zoug5@mail2.sysu.edu.cn (G.Z.); yangwc6@mail2.sysu.edu.cn (W.Y.); tanq27@mail2.sysu.edu.cn (Q.T.)
3. Henan Joint International Research Laboratory of Drug Discovery of Small Molecules, Zhengzhou Key Laboratory of Synthetic Biology of Natural Products, Huanghe Science and Technology College, Zhengzhou 450063, China; lchenchina@hhstu.edu.cn
* Correspondence: kangwenyi@henu.edu.cn (W.K.); cesshzhg@mail.sysu.edu.cn (Z.S.)

Abstract: One new diterpenoid, diaporpenoid A (**1**), two new sesquiterpenoids, diaporpenoids B–C (**2**,**3**) and three new α-pyrone derivatives, diaporpyrones A–C (**4**–**6**) were isolated from an MeOH extract obtained from cultures of the mangrove endophytic fungus *Diaporthe* sp. QYM12. Their structures were elucidated by extensive analysis of spectroscopic data. The absolute configurations were determined by electronic circular dichroism (ECD) calculations and a comparison of the specific rotation. Compound **1** had an unusual 5/10/5-fused tricyclic ring system. Compounds **1** and **4** showed potent anti-inflammatory activities by inhibiting the production of nitric oxide (NO) in lipopolysaccharide (LPS)-induced RAW264.7 cells with IC_{50} values of 21.5 and 12.5 µM, respectively.

Keywords: mangrove endophytic fungus; *Diaporthe* sp.; anti-inflammatory activity

1. Introduction

Mangrove endophytic fungi are the second largest ecological group of the marine fungi [1]. The particular environmental conditions of mangroves allow the activation of unique metabolic pathways in endophytic fungi, enabling the production of novel chemical backbones with diverse biological activities, making them a promising source of drug leads [2–5]. *Diaporthe* is a ubiquitous fungus commonly isolated from most plant hosts [6]. It is known to produce diverse compounds with antibacterial [7], antifungal [6], cytotoxic [8], antitubercular [9], antiparasitic [10] and anticancer [11] activities. With the aim of seeking new bioactive natural products from marine microorganisms, a mangrove endophytic fungus *Diaporthe* sp. QYM12, which was isolated from *Kandelia candel* collected from the South China Sea, was cultured in solid rice medium. As a result, six new metabolites including diaporpenoids A–C (**1**–**3**) and diaporpyrones A–C (**4**–**6**) together with one known analogue, 4-O-methylgermicidin L (**7**) [12], were isolated (Figure 1). Herein, the isolation, structure elucidation and anti-inflammatory activity of all isolated compounds are described.

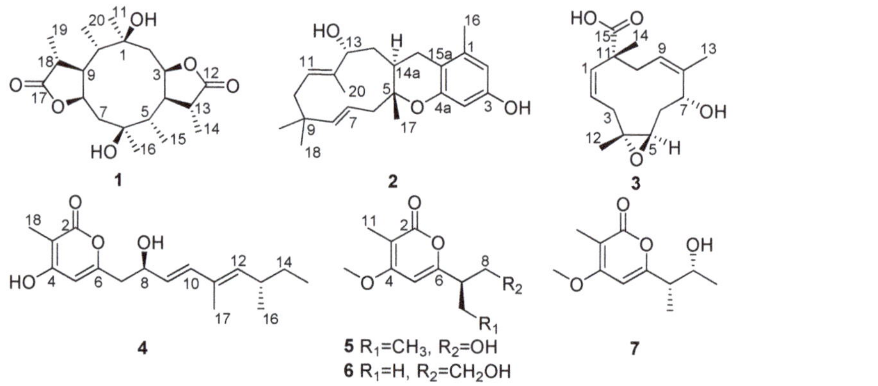

Figure 1. The structures of **1–7**.

2. Results

Compound **1** has a molecular formula of $C_{20}H_{32}O_6$ based on the (+)-HRESIMS (m/z: 391.20900 [M + Na]$^+$), requiring five indices of hydrogen deficiency. The ^{1}H NMR data (Table 1) showed six methyl signals at δ_H 1.20 (s, H$_3$-11), 1.33 (d, J = 7.6 Hz, H$_3$-14), 0.97 (d, J = 7.3 Hz, H$_3$-15), 1.22 (s, H$_3$-16), 1.31 (d, J = 7.3 Hz, H$_3$-19) and 0.99 (d, J = 7.2 Hz, H$_3$-20). Twenty carbon resonances in the ^{13}C NMR data showed six methyls, two sp^3 methylenes, eight sp^3 methines and four quaternary carbons (two carbonyl carbons). These data suggested that **1** may be a tricyclic diterpenoid. The ^{1}H-^{1}H COSY spectrum revealed two spin systems: H$_2$-2/H-3/H-4(/H-5)/H-13/H$_3$-14 and H$_2$-7/H-8/H-9(/H-10)/H-18/H$_3$-19. The HMBC correlations (Figure 2) from H$_3$-11 to C-1, C-2 and C-10, and from H$_3$-16 to C-5, C-6 and C-7 implied the existence of a ten-membered ring core structure. Moreover, the correlations from H-3 to C-12, from H$_3$-14 to C-4 and C-12, from H$_3$-19 to C-9 and C-17, and from H-8 to C-17 were consistent with the existence of two five-membered lactones. The NOESY correlations (Figure 3) from H$_3$-11/ H-3, H$_3$-11/ H-9, H-9/H$_3$-20, H-9/H$_3$-19, H-4/ H$_3$-16, H-4/ H$_3$-15, H-4/ H$_3$-14 and H$_3$-16/H-8 suggested that these protons were cofacial. Thus, the relative configuration of **1** has two possible enantiomers: **1a** (1R, 3S, 4S, 5R, 6R, 8S, 9S, 10R, 13S, 18S) and **1b** (1S, 3R, 4R, 5S, 6S, 8R, 9R, 10S, 13R, 18R). Comparing the experimental and calculated ECD spectra (Figure 4) between **1** and **1b** at the level of B3LYP/DGDZVP determined the absolution configuration of **1** as 1S, 3R, 4R, 5S, 6S, 8R, 9R, 10S, 13R, 18R.

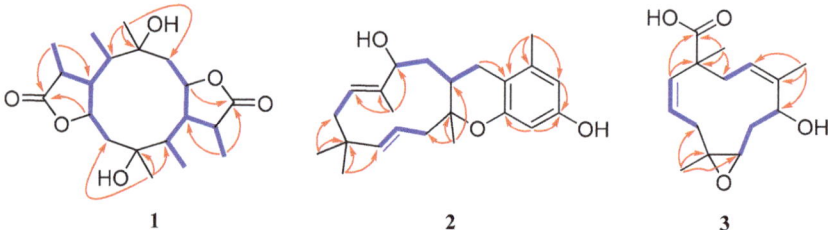

Figure 2. Key HMBC (red arrows) and COSY (blue bold lines) correlations of **1–3**.

Table 1. ^{1}H and ^{13}C NMR data for Compounds **1** and **2** in CDCl$_3$.

No.	1		2	
	δ_C, Type	δ_H (J in Hz)	δ_C, Type	δ_H (J in Hz)
1	80.9, C		137.8, C	
2	46.4, CH$_2$	2.16, m	108.9, CH	6.26, d (2.2)
3	81.5, CH	4.95, td (2.5, 7.3)	154.4, C	
4	54.1, CH	2.16, m	101.4, CH	6.18, d (2.3)
4a			154.5, C	
5	50.6, CH	1.96, dt (6.8, 13.2)	79.4, C	
6α	81.2, C		42.8, CH$_2$	2.51, d (14.5)
6β				2.22, m
7	46.0, CH$_2$	2.21, m	121.3, CH	5.14, m
		2.05, m		
8	81.0, CH	4.86, td (2.5, 6.8)	141.4, CH	5.15, d (2.2)
9	49.6, CH	2.56, dt (7.2, 10.0)	38.5, C	
10	44.0, CH	2.05, m	40.6, CH$_2$	2.23, m
				1.77, m
11	23.7, CH$_3$	1.20, s	123.5, CH	5.17, m
12	181.1, C		138.6, C	
13	42.6, CH	2.72, qd (3.1, 7.6)	78.2, CH	3.99, d (9.6)
14α	18.3, CH$_3$	1.33, d (7.6)	39.7, CH$_2$	1.76, m
14β				1.11, dd (9.3, 13.5)
14a			34.2, CH	1.69, m
15α	15.9, CH$_3$	0.97, d (7.3)	27.3, CH$_2$	2.88, dd (5.6, 16.4)
15β				2.24, m
15a			112.7, C	
16	23.8, CH$_3$	1.22, s	19.3, CH$_3$	2.19, s
17	180.5, C		19.8, CH$_3$	1.06, s
18	38.3, CH	2.90, dq (7.3, 9.9)	24.1, CH$_3$	1.01, s
19	11.6, CH$_3$	1.31, d (7.3)	30.4, CH$_3$	1.06, s
20	15.8, CH$_3$	0.99, d (7.2)	10.6, CH$_3$	1.65, s

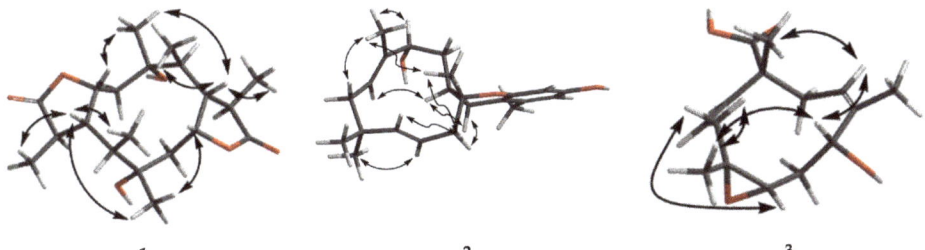

Figure 3. NOESY correlations of **1**–**3**.

Compound **2** was isolated as a colorless oil and had a molecular formula of C$_{23}$H$_{32}$O$_3$ via HRESIMS. The NMR data of **2** were similar to those of pughiinin A [13]. It was confirmed that **2** had the same planar structure as pughiinin A by analyzing the COSY and HMBC correlations (Figure 2). The main difference was the 11*E*-configuration of the double bond between C-11 and C-12, which was confirmed by the NOESY correlation (Figure 3) from Hα-10/H$_3$-20. The chemical shift at C-20 (δ_C 10.6) in **2** further supported the 11*E*-configuration [14]. The relative configuration of **2** was elucidated by the NOESY correlations from H-13/H$_3$-20, H$_3$-20/H$_3$-17, H$_3$-17/H-6β, H-6α/H-15α and H-15α/H-14a. Thus, the structure of **2** was defined as shown in Figure 1.

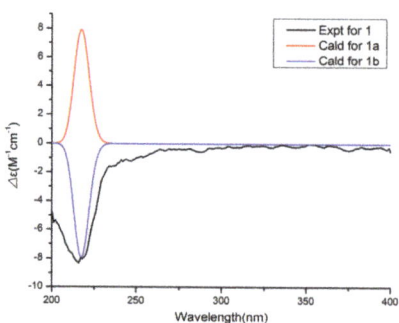

Figure 4. Comparison of the experimental and calculated ECD spectra of **1**.

The HRESIMS data of **3** suggested a molecular formula of $C_{15}H_{22}O_4$. The ^{13}C NMR data (Table 2) showed 15 carbon resonances, including three methyls, three sp^3 methylenes, five methines (two oxygen-bearing and three olefinic) and four quaternary carbons (one olefinic and one carbonyl). The COSY correlations (Figure 2) revealed the presence of three spin systems from H-1/H-2/H$_2$-3, H-5/H$_2$-6/H-7 and H-9/H$_2$-10. The HMBC correlations from H$_3$-12 to C-3, C-4 and C-5, H$_3$-13 to C-7, C-8 and C-9, H$_3$-14 to C-10, C-11 and C-15, and H-1 to C-11 and C-15 established the 11-membered ring core structure. The presence of a 4,5-oxirane ring was determined by the chemical shift values of C-4 (δ_C 64.6) and C-5 (δ_C 60.7). The NOESY correlations (Figure 3) from Ha-3/H-5, Hb-3/H$_3$-12, H$_3$-12/H-7, H-7/H-9 and H-9/H$_3$-14 indicated the relative configuration as 4R^*, 5R^*, 7R^*, 11R^*. The limited quantity did not allow one to define the absolute configuration of **3** through the modified Mosher's method.

Table 2. ^{1}H and ^{13}C NMR data for **3** and **4** in MeOH-d_4.

No.	3		No.	4	
	δ_C, Type	δ_H (J in Hz)		δ_C, Type	δ_H (J in Hz)
1	138.8, CH	5.50, d (15.8)	2	167.7, C	
2	124.6, CH	5.45, ddd (4.7, 10.6, 15.8)	3	97.8, C	
3α	44.1, CH$_2$	2.60, dd (4.7, 11.9)	4	166.4, C	
3β		1.57, dd (10.6, 11.9)	5	101.7, CH	6.06, s
4	64.6, C		6	160.0, C	
5	60.7, CH	2.45, dd (5.2, 9.7)	7	41.4, CH$_2$	2.65, m
6α	34.4, CH$_2$	2.19, ddd (5.1, 10.0, 13.3)	8	69.8, CH	4.47, d (6.5)
6β		1.61, m	9	127.7, CH	5.58, dd (6.8, 15.6)
7	76.4, CH	4.10, dd (6.6, 10.1)	10	135.8, CH	6.25, d (15.6)
8	137.3, C		11	131.6, C	
9	126.5, CH	5.16, brd (11.4)	12	139.6, CH	5.23, d (10.0)
10α	36.4, CH$_2$	2.71, dd (12.2, 13.3)	13	34.2, CH	2.40, m
10β		2.08, brd (12.2)	14α	30.1, CH$_2$	1.38, m
11	49.1, C		14β		1.24, m
12	17.0, CH$_3$	1.34, s	15	10.9, CH$_3$	0.83, t (7.4)
13	10.8, CH$_3$	1.64, s	16	19.6, CH$_3$	0.94, d (6.6)
14	19.7, CH$_3$	1.39, s	17	11.5, CH$_3$	1.74, s
15	181.5, C		18	6.8, CH$_3$	1.85, s

Compound **4** was assigned the molecular formula $C_{17}H_{24}O_4$ by the HRESIMS (*m/z*: 291.16021 [M − H]$^-$). The ^{1}H NMR data (Table 2) exhibited the presence of four methyl signals at δ_H 0.83 (t, *J* = 7.4 Hz, 3H), 0.94 (d *J* = 6.6 Hz, 3H), 1.74 (s, 3H) and 1.85 (s, 3H), and four olefinic proton signals at δ_H 6.06 (s, 1H), 5.58 (dd, *J* = 6.8, 15.6 Hz, 1H), 6.25 (d, *J* = 15.6 Hz, 1H) and 5.23 (d, *J* = 10.0 Hz, 1H). The ^{13}C NMR data revealed 17 carbon resonances including four methyls, two methylenes, six methines (four olefinic carbons) and five other carbons (one carbonyl carbon and two olefinic carbons). Similar NMR data suggested that the structure of **4** was similar to that of proasperfuranone B [15]. The main difference was that the ketone carbonyl group in proasperfuranone B was reduced to a hydroxyl group in **4**. The deduction was confirmed by the HMBC correlations from H-8 to C-6, C-7 and C-9 (Figure 5). Thus, the planar structure of **4** was established. The calculated ECD spectrum fit the experimental spectrum perfectly well (Figure 6) at the BVP86/LANL2MB level in methanol; the absolute configuration of C-8 was determined as 8*R*.

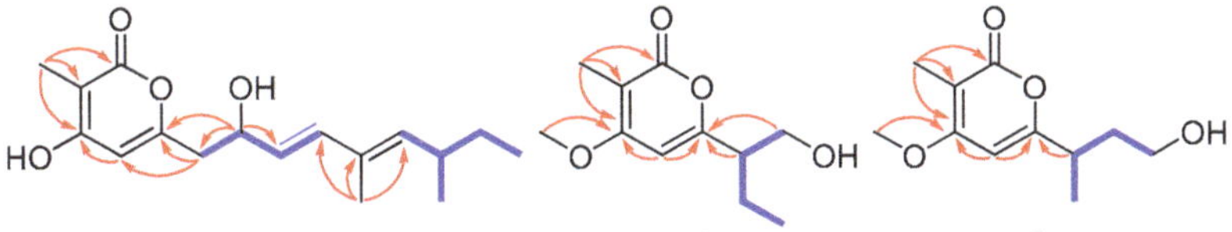

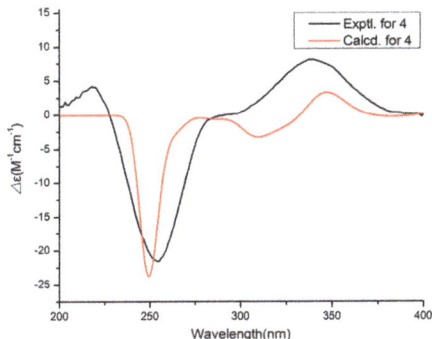

Figure 5. Key HMBC (red arrows) and COSY (blue bold lines) correlations of **4–6**.

Figure 6. Experimental and calculated ECD spectra of **4**.

Compound **5**, isolated as a colorless oil, gave a molecular formula of $C_{11}H_{16}O_4$ by HRESIMS data. The ^{1}H NMR data (Table 3) exhibited the presence of three methyl signals at δ_H 0.92 (t, *J* = 7.4 Hz, 3H), 1.91 (s, 3H) and 3.90 (s, 3H), and one olefinic proton at δ_H 6.10 (s, 1H). The ^{13}C NMR data showed 11 carbon resonances assigned to two methyls (δ_C 8.5, 11.7), one methoxy (δ_C 56.2), two methylenes (δ_C 63.6, 22.1), two methines (δ_C 96.2, 49.4) and four nonprotonated carbons (δ_C 165.6, 101.3, 163.9 and 165.5). The HMBC correlations from H$_3$-11 to C-2, C-3 and C4, and H-5 to C-4 and C-6 revealed the presence of the α-pyrone moiety. The correlations from H-7 and H-8 to C-6, as well as the ^{1}H-^{1}H COSY cross-peaks of H$_2$-8/H-7/H$_2$-9/H$_3$-10 (Figure 5) indicated the side chain attached to C-6. Thus, the planar structure of **5** was established. By comparing the specific rotation value of **5** ($[\alpha]_D^{25}$ −32, *c* 0.28, MeOH) with 4-deoxyphomapyrone C ($[\alpha]_D^{25}$ −40, *c* 0.37, MeOH) [16] and germicidin C ($[\alpha]_D^{25}$ +21, *c* 0.36, MeOH) [17], the absolute configuration of **5** was assigned as 7*R*.

Table 3. ^{1}H and ^{13}C NMR data for **5–7** in CDCl$_3$.

No.	5		6	
	δ_C, Type	δ_H (J in Hz)	δ_C, Type	δ_H (J in Hz)
2	165.6, C		166.2, C	
3	101.3, C		101.2, C	
4	163.9, C		166.2, C	
5	96.2, CH	6.10, s	93.8, CH	6.25, s
6	165.5, C		167.6, C	
7	49.4, CH	2.56, m	35.5, CH	2.82, dq (6.8, 13.7)
8	63.6, CH$_2$	3.88, m	37.4, CH$_2$	1.93, m
				1.75, dt (6.1, 13.6)
9	22.1, CH$_2$	1.65, m	60.3, CH$_2$	3.63, m
10	11.7, CH$_3$	0.92, t (7.4)	18.7, CH$_3$	1.25, d (6.9)
11	8.5, CH$_3$	1.91, s	8.5, CH$_3$	1.87, s
12	56.2, CH$_3$	3.90, s	56.4, CH$_3$	3.86, s

Compound **6** was obtained as a colorless oil and had a molecular formula of $C_{11}H_{16}O_4$ by HRESIMS. The ^{1}H and ^{13}C NMR data (Table 3) of **6** were similar to those of **5**, revealing an α-pyrone derivative. Moreover, the planar structure of **6** was established by the spin system of H$_3$-10/H-7/H$_2$-8/H$_2$-9 from ^{1}H-^{1}H COSY spectra together with the HMBC correlations (Figure 5) from H-7 and H$_2$-8 to C-6. Meanwhile, the planar structure of **6** was identified as being the same as phomopyronol [18]. Finally, the calculated ECD spectrum and the experimental data (Figure 7) were well matched, indicating the 7R configuration of **6**.

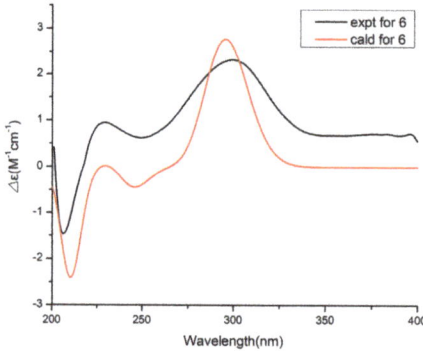

Figure 7. Experimental and calculated ECD spectra of compound **6**.

Compound **7** was identified as 4-O-methylgermicidin L (**7**) [12] by a comparison of the spectroscopic data with the literature.

Nitric oxide (NO) is a key biological signaling molecule regulating the variety of physiological functions [19]. The excessive production of NO could induce tissue damage, and it is essential to find new effective NO inhibitors to treat inflammatory diseases and related disorders. Thus, the anti-inflammatory activity of isolated compounds was evaluated against nitric oxide (NO) production in lipopolysaccharide (LPS)-stimulated mouse macrophage RAW 264.7 cells. The results (Table 4 and Table S1) showed that **4** exhibited a potent inhibitory activity with an IC$_{50}$ value of 12.5 μM. Compounds **1–2** showed a moderate activity with IC$_{50}$ values of 21.5 and 36.8 μM, respectively, when compared to the positive control (L-NMMA, IC$_{50}$: 15.0 μM). All the tested compounds were nontoxic at the tested concentration.

Table 4. The anti-inflammatory activities of compounds 1–8.

Compound	1	2	3	4	5	6	7	L-NMMA [a]
IC$_{50}$ (μM)	21.5	36.8	50.0	12.5	-	-	50.0	15.0

- not tested. [a] positive control.

3. Experimental Section

3.1. General Experimental Procedures

Specific rotations were taken on a MCP 300 (Anton Paar) polarimeter at 28 °C. UV spectra were recorded in MeOH using a PERSEE TU-1900 spectrophotometer, and ECD data were measured on a Chirascan CD spectrometer (Applied Photophysics). IR spectra were obtained on a Nicolet Nexus 670 spectrophotometer, in KBr discs. All NMR experiments were performed on a Bruker Avance 500 spectrometer at room temperature. HRESIMS spectra were obtained on a Thermo Fisher Scientific Q-TOF mass spectrometer. Column chromatography (CC) was conducted using silica gel (200–300 mesh, Qingdao Marine Chemical Factory) and Sephadex LH-20 (Amersham Pharmacia). Semipreparative HPLC was carried out using a C18 column (ODS, 250 × 10 mm, 5 μm). Thin-layer chromatography (TLC) was performed on silica gel plates (Qingdao Huang Hai Chemical Group Co., G60, F-254).

3.2. Fungal Material, Fermentation and Isolation

The strain QYM12 was isolated from the healthy leaves of *Kandelia candel*, which were collected in June 2017 from the South China Sea, Dongzhai Harbor Mangrove Nature Reserve Area, Hainan Province, China. Fungal identification was achieved using a molecular biological protocol by DNA amplification and ITS sequence [20]. The sequence was the most similar (99%) to the sequence of *Diaporthe* sp. (GU066666.1) via BLAST research. The sequence data of the strain has been deposited at GenBank with the accession number MW332459. The fungus was preserved at Sun Yat-Sen University, China. The strain was cultured on PDA medium for four days. Then, the seed culture was prepared by the mycelia of the fungus being inoculated into 500 mL of PDB medium for five days. Thereafter, the seed culture was transferred into solid rice medium (800 × 1000 Erlenmeyer flasks each containing 80 g of raw rice and 70 mL of 0.3% seawater) at 28 °C for 30 days.

Thereafter, the fermented material was extracted with MeOH three times, and organic phases were combined and evaporated under reduced pressure to yield an extract of 25.0 g. Then, the residue was fractionated by silica gel column chromatography with a gradient of petroleum ether/EtOAc from 10:0 to 0:10 to give eight fractions (Fr.1-Fr.8, per 10 mL). Fr.3 (380.0 mg) was subjected to Sephadex LH-20 CC (CH$_2$Cl$_2$/MeOH v/v, 1:1) to yield three fractions (3.1–3.3). Fr.3.1 (10.0 mg) was purified by silica gel CC (CH$_2$Cl$_2$/MeOH v/v, 75:1) to yield compound **1** (3.5 mg). Fr.4 (565.0 mg) was subjected to Sephadex LH-20 CC (CH$_2$Cl$_2$/MeOH v/v, 1:1) to yield two fractions (4.1 and 4.2). Fr.4.1 (36.5 mg) was purified by semipreparative reversed-phase HPLC (MeOH-H$_2$O, 50:1) to yield compound **7** (3.1 mg). Fr.4.2 (46.2 mg) was subjected to silica gel CC (CH$_2$Cl$_2$/MeOH v/v, 95:5) to yield compounds **2** (2.0 mg) and **5** (5.6 mg). Fr.5 (522.0 mg) was purified by Sephadex LH-20 CC (CH$_2$Cl$_2$/MeOH v/v, 1:1) to afford three fractions (5.1–5.3). Fr.5.1 (7.6 mg) was subjected to silica gel CC (CH$_2$Cl$_2$/MeOH v/v, 25:1) to give compound **3** (2.0 mg). Fr.6 (650.0 mg) was subjected to Sephadex LH-20 CC (CH$_2$Cl$_2$/MeOH v/v, 1:1) to give four fractions (6.1–6.4). Fr.6.1 (38.0 mg) was purified by silica gel CC (CH$_2$Cl$_2$/MeOH v/v, 10:1) to yield compound **6** (6.8 mg). Fr.6.2 (15.0 mg) was subjected to silica gel CC (CH$_2$Cl$_2$/MeOH v/v, 17:3) to yield compound **4** (3.3 mg).

Diaporpenoid A (**1**): colorless oil; $[\alpha]_D^{25}$ −32 (c 0.46, MeOH); UV (MeOH) λ_{max} (log ε): 215 (2.52) nm; IR (KBr) v_{max}: 3376, 2910, 2896, 1685, 1413, 1352, 1206, 1026 cm^{-1}; ^{1}H and ^{13}C NMR (500 MHz, CDCl$_3$) data, Table 1; HRESIMS m/z 391.20900 [M + Na]$^+$ (calcd for C$_{20}$H$_{32}$O$_6$Na, 391.20911).

Diaporpenoid B (**2**): colorless oil; $[\alpha]_D^{25}$ +28 (c 0.06, CDCl$_3$); UV (MeOH) λ_{max} (log ε): 209 (1.86), 281 (3.02) nm; IR (KBr) ν_{max}: 3422, 3268, 2798, 1632, 1590, 1330, 1215, 1063 cm^{-1}; ^{1}H and ^{13}C NMR (500 MHz, CDCl$_3$) data, see Table 1; HRESIMS m/z 357.24244 [M + H]$^+$ (calcd for C$_{20}$H$_{32}$O$_6$, 357.24242).

Diaporpenoid C (**3**): colorless oil; $[\alpha]_D^{25}$ +18 (c 0.04, MeOH); UV (MeOH) λ_{max} (log ε): 220 (2.52) nm; IR (KBr) ν_{max}: 3320, 1762, 1525, 1376, 1356, 1132, 1010 cm^{-1}; ^{1}H and ^{13}C NMR (500 MHz, MeOH-d_4) data, see Table 2; HRESIMS m/z 265.14401 [M − H]$^-$ (calcd for C$_{15}$H$_{22}$O$_4$, 265.14453).

Diaporpyrane A (**4**): colorless oil; $[\alpha]_D^{25}$ +12 (c 0.07, MeOH); UV (MeOH) λ_{max} (log ε): 212 (3.22), 240 (3.53) nm; IR (KBr) ν_{max}: 3420, 2986, 2855, 1762, 1727, 1612, 1344, 1235, 1086 cm^{-1}; ^{1}H and ^{13}C NMR (500 MHz, MeOH-d_4) data, see Table 2; HRESIMS m/z 291.16021 [M − H]$^-$ (calcd for C$_{17}$H$_{24}$O$_4$, 291.16018).

Diaporpyrane B (**5**): colorless oil; $[\alpha]_D^{25}$ −32, (c 0.28, MeOH); UV (MeOH) λ_{max} (log ε): 212 (3.45), 283 (3.62) nm; IR (KBr) ν_{max}: 3176, 2965, 1647, 1580, 1421 cm^{-1}; ^{1}H and ^{13}C NMR (500 MHz, CDCl$_3$) data, see Table 3; HRESIMS m/z 213.11221 [M + H]$^+$ (calcd for 213.11214, C$_{11}$H$_{17}$O$_4$).

Diaporpyrane C (**6**): colorless oil; $[\alpha]_D^{25}$ −65 (c 0.85, MeOH); UV (MeOH) λ_{max} (log ε): 205(3.32), 300 (3.67) nm; IR (KBr) ν_{max}: 3445, 2962, 1735, 1675, 1363, 1256, 1218 cm^{-1}; ^{1}H and ^{13}C NMR (500 MHz, CDCl$_3$) data, see Table 3; HRESIMS m/z 213.1116 [M + H]$^+$ (calcd for C$_{11}$H$_{17}$O$_4$, 213.1117).

3.3. ECD Calculation Methods

The calculation was accomplished according to the method described previously [21]. The conformers of compounds **1**, **4** and **6** were first optimized by DFT methods at the B3LYP/6-31G (d) level in the Gaussian 05 program. Then, the theoretical calculation was performed using the time-dependent density functional theory (TD-DFT) at the level of B3LYP/DGDZVP, BVP86/LANL2MB and B3LYP/DGTZVP, respectively.

3.4. Anti-Inflammatory Assay

The RAW264.7 cells were purchased from Macrophage Resource Center, Shanghai Institute of Life Sciences, Chinese Academy of Sciences (Shanghai, China). The method for the assay of the anti-inflammatory activity was conducted according to a previously published paper [20]. The detailed process is described in the Supplementary Materials.

4. Conclusions

In summary, the strain *Diaporthe* sp. QYM12, which was isolated from *Kandelia candel*, Dongzhai Harbor Mangrove Nature Reserve Area, was cultured in solid rice medium, leading to the identification of six new metabolite diaporpenoids A-C (**1–3**) and diaporpyrones A-C (**4–6**). Compound **1** was a macrocyclic diterpenoid featuring a rare 5/10/5-fused tricyclic ring system, and compounds **2,3** were macrocyclic sesquiterpenoids possessing a hendecane core. Macrocyclic sesquiterpenoids and diterpenoids are a functionally diverse group of natural products with versatile bioactivities [22]. For instance, junceellolide C showed an anti-HBV activity [23], flaccidenol A displayed a cytotoxic activity [24], antipacid B exhibited an anti-inflammatory activity [25], and euphorbesulins A revealed an antimalarial activity [26]. The anti-inflammatory assay suggested that compound **1** showed a moderate activity with an IC$_{50}$ value of 21.5 µM. Compound **4** exhibited a potent inhibitory activity with an IC$_{50}$ value of 12.5 µM. Proinflammatory enzymes, including nitric oxide synthase (iNOS) and cyclooxygenase-2 (COX-2), were reported to play key roles in inflammatory processes [27]. Thus, further research is required to clarify the underlying mechanisms of the active compounds. This study has suggested that these macrocyclic sesquiterpenoids and α-pyrone derivatives have the potential to develop lead compounds for anti-inflammatory agents.

Supplementary Materials: The following are available online at https://www.mdpi.com/1660-3397/19/2/56/s1. Figure S1: ^{1}H NMR spectrum of compound **1** (500 MHz, CDCl$_3$). Figure S2: ^{13}C NMR spectrum of compound **1** (125 MHz, CDCl$_3$). Figure S3: HSQC spectrum of compound **1**. Figure S4: ^{1}H-^{1}H COSY spectrum of compound **1**. Figure S5: HMBC spectrum of compound **1**. Figure S6: HRESIMS spectrum of compound **1**. Figure S7: NOESY spectrum of compound **1**. Figure S8: ^{1}H NMR spectrum of compound **2** (500 MHz, CDCl$_3$). Figure S9: ^{13}C NMR spectrum of compound **2** (125 MHz, CDCl$_3$). Figure S10: HSQC spectrum of compound **2**. Figure S11: ^{1}H-^{1}H COSY spectrum of compound **2**. Figure S12: HMBC spectrum of compound **2**. Figure S13: NOESY spectrum of compound **2**. Figure S14: HRESIMS spectrum of compound **2**. Figure S15: ^{1}H NMR spectrum of compound **3** (500 MHz, MeOH-d_4). Figure S16: ^{13}C NMR spectrum of compound **3** (125 MHz, MeOH-d_4). Figure S17: HSQC spectrum of compound **3**. Figure S18: ^{1}H-^{1}H COSY spectrum of compound **3**. Figure S19: HMBC spectrum of compound **3**. Figure S20: NOESY spectrum of compound **3**. Figure S21: HRESIMS spectrum of compound **3**. Figure S22: ^{1}H NMR spectrum of compound **4** (500 MHz, MeOH-d_4). Figure S23: ^{13}C NMR spectrum of compound **4** (125 MHz, MeOH-d_4). Figure S24: HSQC spectrum of compound **4**. Figure S25: ^{1}H-^{1}H COSY spectrum of compound **4**. Figure S26: HMBC spectrum of compound **4**. Figure S27: HRESIMS spectrum of compound **4**. Figure S28: ^{1}H NMR spectrum of compound **5** (500 MHz, CDCl$_3$). Figure S29: ^{13}C NMR spectrum of compound **5** (125 MHz, CDCl$_3$). Figure S30: HSQC spectrum of compound **5**. Figure S31: ^{1}H-^{1}H COSY spectrum of compound **5**. Figure S32: HMBC spectrum of compound **5**. Figure S33: HRESIMS spectrum of compound **5**. Figure S34: ^{1}H NMR spectrum of compound **6** (500 MHz, CDCl$_3$). Figure S35: ^{13}C NMR spectrum of compound **6** (125 MHz, CDCl$_3$). Figure S36: HSQC spectrum of compound **6**. Figure S37: ^{1}H-^{1}H COSY spectrum of compound **6**. Figure S38: HMBC spectrum of compound **6**. Figure S39: HRESIMS spectrum of compound **6**.

Author Contributions: Y.C. performed the experiments and wrote the paper; G.Z., W.Y. and Q.T. participated in the experiments; Y.Z., C.M., J.W. and L.C. analyzed the data and discussed the result; W.K. and Z.S. reviewed the manuscript; Z.S. designed and supervised the experiments. All authors have read and agreed to the published version of the manuscript.

Funding: This research was funded by the National Natural Science Foundation of China (U20A2001, 21877133), Key Project of Natural Science Foundation of Guangdong Province (2016A030311026) and Key Project in Science and Technology Agency of Henan Province (212102311029) through their generous support.

Institutional Review Board Statement: Not applicable.

Data Availability Statement: Data is contained within the article and Supplementary Material.

Conflicts of Interest: The authors declare no conflict of interest.

References

1. Cheng, Z.S.; Pan, J.H.; Tang, W.C.; Chen, Q.J.; Lin, Y.C. Biodiversity and biotechnological potential of mangrove-associated fungi. *J. For. Res.* **2009**, *20*, 63–72. [CrossRef]
2. Sebastianes, F.L.S.; Cabedo, N.; Aouad, N.E. 3-Hydroxypropionic Acid as an Antibacterial Agent from Endophytic Fungi *Diaporthe phaseolorum*. *Curr. Microbiol.* **2012**, *65*, 622–632. [CrossRef] [PubMed]
3. Zhu, F.; Lin, Y.C. Marinamide, a novel alkaloid and its methyl ester produced by the application of mixed fermentation technique to two mangrove endophytic fungi from the South China Sea. *Chin. Sci. Bull.* **2006**, *51*, 1426–1430. [CrossRef]
4. Rosario, N.; Maria, S.; Anna, A. Secondary Metabolites of Mangrove-Associated Strains of *Talaromyces*. *Mar. Drugs* **2018**, *16*, 12.
5. Deshmukh, S.K.; Gupta, M.K.; Prakash, V. Mangrove-Associated Fungi: A Novel Source of Potential Anticancer Compounds. *J. Fungi* **2018**, *4*, 101. [CrossRef]
6. Carvalho, C.R.D.; Ferreira-D'Silva, A.; Wedge, D.E. Antifungal activities of cytochalasins produced by *Diaporthe miriciae*, an endophytic fungus associated with tropical medicinal plants. *Can. J. Microbiol.* **2018**, *64*, 835–843. [CrossRef]
7. Sousa, J.P.B.; Aguilar-Pérez, M.M.; Arnold, A.E. Chemical constituents and their antibacterial activity from the tropical endophytic fungus *Diaporthe* sp. F2934. *J. Appl. Microbiol.* **2016**, *120*, 1501–1508. [CrossRef]
8. Yang, X.; Wu, P.; Xue, J. Cytochalasans from endophytic fungus *Diaporthe* sp. SC-J0138. *Fitoterapia* **2020**, *145*, 104611. [CrossRef]
9. Dettrakul, S.; Kittakoop, P.; Isaka, M. Antimycobacterial pimarane diterpenes from the Fungus *Diaporthe* sp. *Bioorg. Med. Chem. Lett.* **2003**, *13*, 1253–1255. [CrossRef]
10. Chepkirui, C.; Stadler, M. The genus *Diaporthe*: A rich source of diverse and bioactive metabolites. *Mycol. Prog.* **2017**, *16*, 477–494. [CrossRef]

11. Kumaran, R.S.; Hur, B.K. Screening of species of the endophytic fungus *Phomopsis* for the production of the anticancer drug taxol. *Biotechnol. Appl. Bioc.* **2011**, *54*, 21–30. [CrossRef] [PubMed]
12. Du, Y.; Sun, J.; Gong, Q. New α-Pyridones with Quorum Sensing Inhibitory Activity from Diversity-Enhanced Extracts of a Marine Algae-Derived *Streptomyces* sp. *J. Agric. Food Chem.* **2018**, *66*, 1807–1812. [CrossRef] [PubMed]
13. Pittayakhajonwut, P.; Theerasilp, M.; Kongsaeree, P.; Pughiinin, A. A Sesquiterpene from the Fungus *Kionochaeta pughii* BCC 3878. *Planta Med.* **2002**, *68*, 1017–1019. [CrossRef] [PubMed]
14. Cai, P.; Smith, D.; Cunningham, B. Epolones: Novel Sesquiterpene-Tropolones from Fungus OS-F69284 That Induce Erythropoietin in Human Cells. *J. Nat. Prod.* **1998**, *61*, 791–795. [CrossRef] [PubMed]
15. Chiang, Y.M.; Oakley, C.E.; Ahuia, M. An efficient system for heterologous expression of secondary metabolite genes in *Aspergillus nidulans*. *J. Am. Chem. Soc.* **2013**, *135*, 7720–7731. [CrossRef] [PubMed]
16. Zhang, H.; Saurav, K.; Yu, Z. alpha-Pyrones with Diverse Hydroxy Substitutions from Three Marine-Derived *Nocardiopsis* Strains. *J. Nat. Prod.* **2016**, *79*, 1610–1618. [CrossRef] [PubMed]
17. Aoki, Y.; Matsumoto, D.; Kawaide, H. Physiological role of germicidins in spore germination and hyphal elongation in *Streptomyces coelicolor* A3(2). *J. Antibiot.* **2011**, *64*, 607–611. [CrossRef]
18. Weber, D.; Gorzalczany, S.; Martino, V. Metabolites from Endophytes of the Medicinal Plant Erythrina crista-galli. *Z. Naturforsch. C. Biosci.* **2005**, *60*, 5–6. [CrossRef]
19. Iadecola, C.; Pelligrino, D.A.; Moskowitz, M.A. Nitric oxide synthase inhibition and cerebrovascular regulation. *J. Cereb. Blood Flow Metab.* **1994**, *14*, 175–192. [CrossRef]
20. Chen, Y.; Liu, Z.M.; Liu, H.J. Dichloroisocoumarins with Potential Anti-Inflammatory Activity from the Mangrove Endophytic Fungus *Ascomycota* sp. CYSK-4. *Mar. Drugs* **2018**, *16*, 54. [CrossRef]
21. Chen, Y.; Liu, Z.M.; She, Z.G. Ascomylactams A-C, Cytotoxic 12- or 13-Membered-Ring Macrocyclic Alkaloids Isolated from the Mangrove Endophytic Fungus *Didymella* sp. CYSK-4, and Structure Revisions of Phomapyrrolidones A and C. *J. Nat. Prod.* **2019**, *82*, 1752–1758. [CrossRef] [PubMed]
22. Thomas, B.; Robert, K.; Bernhard, L. Production of Macrocyclic Sesqui- and Diterpenes in Heterologous Microbial Hosts: A Systems Approach to Harness Nature's Molecular Diversity. *Chemcatchem* **2014**, *6*, 1142–1165.
23. Wu, J.R.; Li, X.D.; Lin, W.H. Briarane-type diterpenoids from a gorgonian coral *Ellisella* sp. with anti-HBV activities. *Bioorg. Chem.* **2020**, *105*, 104423. [CrossRef] [PubMed]
24. Tseng, W.-R.; Ahmed, A.F.; Huang, C.-Y.; Tsai, Y.-Y.; Tai, C.-J.; Orfali, R.S.; Hwang, T.-L.; Wang, Y.-H.; Dai, C.-F.; Sheu, J.-H. Bioactive Capnosanes and Cembranes from the Soft Coral *Klyxum flaccidum*. *Mar. Drugs* **2019**, *17*, 461. [CrossRef] [PubMed]
25. Chang, Y.C.; Chiang, C.C.; Chang, Y.S.; Chen, J.J. Novel Caryophyllane-Related Sesquiterpenoids with Anti-Inflammatory Activity from *Rumphella antipathes* (Linnaeus, 1758). *Mar. Drugs* **2020**, *18*, 554. [CrossRef]
26. Zhou, B.; Wu, Y.; Yue, J.M. Euphorbesulins A–P, Structurally Diverse Diterpenoids from *Euphorbia esula*. *J. Nat. Prod.* **2016**, *79*, 1952–1961. [CrossRef]
27. Lee, S.J.; Lee, I.S.; Mar, W. Inhibition of inducible nitric oxide synthase and cyclooxygenase-2 activity by 1,2,3,4,6-penta-O-galloyl-beta-D-glucose in murine macrophage cells. *Arch. Pharm. Res.* **2003**, *26*, 832–839. [CrossRef]

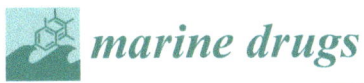

Article

Preparation, COX-2 Inhibition and Anticancer Activity of Sclerotiorin Derivatives

Tao Chen [1], Yun Huang [2,3], Junxian Hong [1], Xikang Wei [1], Fang Zeng [1], Jialin Li [1], Geting Ye [1], Jie Yuan [2,*] and Yuhua Long [1,*]

1. School of Chemistry, Guangzhou Key Laboratory of Analytical Chemistry for Biomedicine, South China Normal University, Guangzhou 510006, China; ct2020@m.scnu.edu.cn (T.C.); hjx2020@m.scnu.edu.cn (J.H.); xk20192421139@m.scnu.edu.cn (X.W.); zengfang@m.scnu.edu.cn (F.Z.); jialinli@m.scnu.edu.cn (J.L.); yegeting@m.scnu.edu.cn (G.Y.)
2. Department of Biochemistry, Zhongshan School of Medicine, Sun Yat-sen University, Guangzhou 510080, China; huangyun11910173@i.smu.edu.cn
3. School of Basic Medical Sciences, Southern Medical University, Guangzhou 510515, China
* Correspondence: yuanjie@mail.sysu.edu.cn (J.Y.); longyh@scnu.edu.cn (Y.L.)

Abstract: The latest research has indicated that anti-tumor agents with COX-2 inhibitory activity may benefit their anti-tumor efficiency. A series of sclerotiorin derivatives have been synthesized and screened for their cytotoxic activity against human lung cancer cells A549, breast cancer cells MDA-MB-435 using the MTT method. Among them, compounds **3, 7, 12, 13, 15, 17** showed good cytotoxic activity with IC_{50} values of 6.39, 9.20, 9.76, 7.75, 9.08, and 8.18 μM, respectively. In addition, all compounds were tested in vitro the COX-2 inhibitory activity. The results disclosed compounds **7, 13, 25** and sclerotiorin showed moderate to good COX-2 inhibition with the inhibitory ratios of 58.7%, 51.1%, 66.1% and 56.1%, respectively. Notably, compound **3** displayed a comparable inhibition ratio (70.6%) to the positive control indomethacin (78.9%). Furthermore, molecular docking was used to rationalize the potential of the sclerotiorin derivatives as COX2 inhibitory agents by predicting their binding energy, binding modes and optimal orientation at the active site of the COX-2. Additionally, the structure-activity relationships (SARS) have been addressed.

Keywords: sclerotiorin derivatives; cytotoxic activity; COX-2 inhibition; molecular docking

1. Introduction

Cancer has become one of the most important factors affecting human life and health in terms of incidence, mortality, and prevalence. In 2018, estimates for global statistics on cancer rates show that there were 18.1 million new cases and 9.6 million deaths. Lung cancer is the most frequent cancer and the leading cause of cancer death among males, followed by prostate and colorectal cancer. Among females, breast cancer is the most commonly diagnosed cancer and the leading cause of cancer death [1]. Cancer metastasis is the major reason of treatment failure and death [2,3]. As the research moves along, authoritative studies have shown that an inflammatory environment plays an important role in various stages of tumor development and affects the body response to chemotherapeutic agents [4,5]. Chronic inflammation is associated with tumor development, and inflammatory mediators are present in the tumor microenvironment, including cytokines, growth factors, reactive oxygen species and reactive nitrogen species [6–8]. These mediators also activate signaling molecules involved in inflammation and carcinogenesis, including nuclear transcription factor, inducible nitric oxide synthase and cyclooxygenase-2. All these factors together result in tumor initiation by increasing cell cycling, inhibiting tumor suppressor pathways and activating oncogenes [8–10].

COX-2 is a member of the cyclooxygenase family, and has long been a research focus in the treatment of inflammation. It is the key enzyme in the conversion of arachidonic

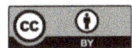

acid to prostanoids, lipid mediators' participation in multifarious physiological and pathological processes. COX-2 is known as an important enzyme in the inflammation process that has tumorigenesis function, and can promote cancer cells proliferation, migration and invasion [11,12]. Zoological and epidemiological studies have shown that COX-2 is closely associated with malignant tumors in recent years [13–15]. COX-2 over expression has been detected in lung cancer, colon cancer, stomach cancer, breast cancer and other tumors [16–18]. In lung cancer, studies show that COX-2 was highly expressed in all stages of NSCLS (non-small-cell lung cancer). Meanwhile, most of invasive and non-invasive lesions have shown elevated COX-2 expression when compared with nonmalignant tissue [19]. Concerning to colorectal cancer, studies have reported that COX-2 was over expressed in 85% and 50% of human colorectal carcinomas and adenomas, respectively. Immunohistochemical studies showed that COX-1 and trace COX-2 is expressed in normal smooth muscle cell and intestinal mucosal epithelial cell. However, COX-2 expression is dramatically increased in cancerous colorectal tissue compared with adjacent normal mucosa [20]. Studies indicated that COX-2 inhibitors aspirin and celecoxib can abrogate the stimulatory effects on lung cancer cell proliferation and migration by inhibition of COX-2 [21]. Moreover, celecoxib has been proved to inhibit growth and induce apoptosis of lung cancer cells [22]. Epidemiologic data demonstrated a role for aspirin in suppressing prostate carcinogenesis and suggested that inhibition of COX-2 via pharmacological means or regulation of its expression can limit the development of human prostate cancer [23]. Therefore, targeting the inhibition of COX-2 and its downstream pathways could be helpful for cancer therapy.

Marine creatures are natural treasures and have played important roles as sources of natural medicinal products [24,25]. Scientific researches showed that marine organisms derived marine natural products (MNPs) exhibited great potential for biological activities such as antifouling, antimalarial and anticancer, etc. [26–28]. Sclerotiorine was first isolated and identified from the mycelium of *Penicillium multicolor* G.M.P. in 1952 [29]. Its wide broad bioactivity makes it bound to get much more attention. Sclerotiorine and other azaphilones isolated from *Penicillium sclerotiorum* OUCMDZ-3839 displayed significant inhibitory activity against α-glycosidase and moderate bioactivity against H1N1 virus [30]. A series of sclerotioramine derivatives were synthesized and showed potent antifouling activity against the larval settlement of the barnacle *Balanus amphitrite* [31]. It is reported that sclerotiorin could substantially decrease the mycobacterial growth inside macrophages and with no cytotoxicity, suggesting that it has potential to supplement antibiotic therapy for tuberculosis (TB) [32]. Recently, evidence showed that sclerotiorin can provide clues for further searching on safer and effective entity against Alzheimer's disease (AD) [33].

During our continuous search for biologically active marine natural compounds, we found an endophytic fungus SCNU-0016 from marine mangrove plant *Acanthus ilicifolius L.* could produce sclerotiorin in high productivity. Our primary research indicated sclerotiorin possesses COX-2 inhibition activity. The literature retrieval showed azaphilones can be antitumor agents [34]. In order to obtain dual targeted pharmaceutical compounds, since COX-2 selective inhibitors can both be anti-inflammatory candidates and benefit antitumor activity, we did the modification of sclerotiorin to afford the cytotoxic compounds with COX-2 inhibitory activity. Herein, we report synthesis, antitumor activity and COX-2 inhibition of a series of sclerotiorin derivatives.

2. Results and Discussion
2.1. Chemistry

The parent compound sclerotiorin was extracted from the fungal *Penicillium sclerotiorum* SCNU-0016. The synthetic route of sclerotiorin derivatives **1–27** was shown in Schemes 1 and 2. Twenty-four amide-derivatives (**1–24**) have been successfully synthesized by one-step reaction of sclerotiorin with various amines in high yields (up to 90%). The derivative **25** was obtained by hydrolysis of sclerotiorin (yields up to 85%). Followed by esterification reaction of propionic anhydride and glutaric anhydride produced **26** and **27** in 82% and 78% yields, respectively. The resulting extract was subjected to silica gel column chromatography to obtain the pure products. The structures of target compounds **1–27** were confirmed by extensive spectroscopic methods including ^{1}H NMR, ^{13}C NMR, MS and HRMS.

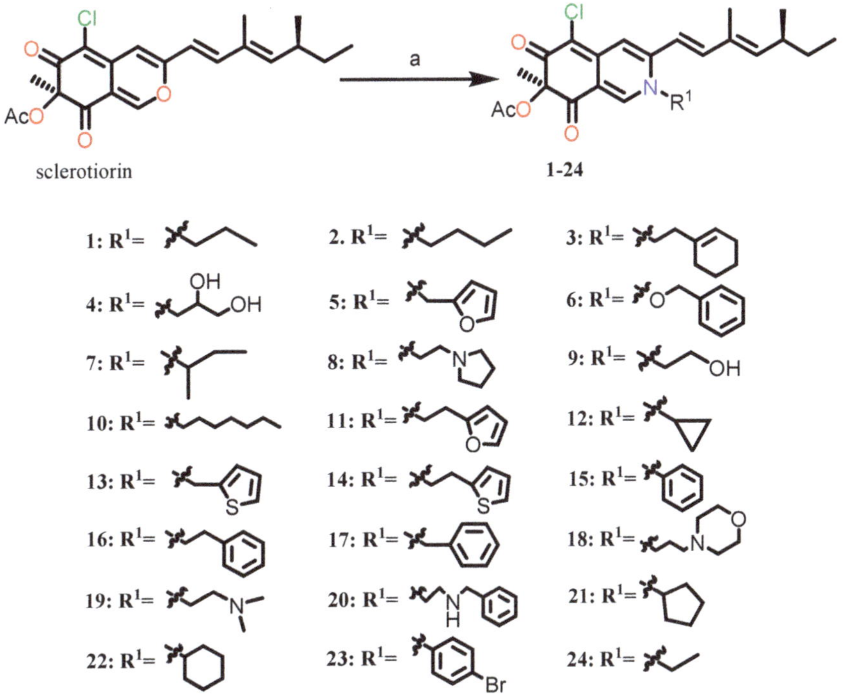

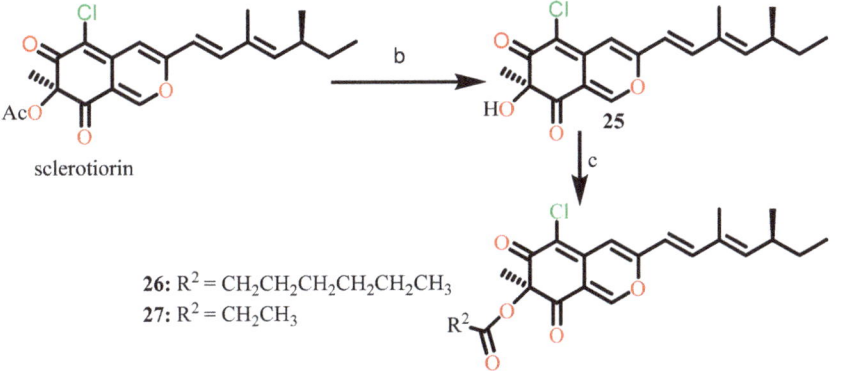

Scheme 1. Reagents and conditions: (a) amine, DCM, r.t.

26: $R^2 = CH_2CH_2CH_2CH_2CH_2CH_3$
27: $R^2 = CH_2CH_3$

Scheme 2. Reagents and conditions: (b) CH$_3$ONa, CH$_3$OH, 40 °C. (c) Pyridine, anhydride, 90 °C.

2.2. Biological Studies

2.2.1. Cytotoxic Activity of Sclerotiorin Derivatives

The cytotoxic activity of all compounds was evaluated against A549 (human lung cancer) and MDA-MB-435 (breast cancer cells) by using the MTT method as described previously.

As shown in Table 1, the four yellow pigments, sclerotiorin and the other three acyl changed derivatives **25, 26, 27,** present no cytotoxic activity on both cancer cell lines (IC_{50} > 50 μM). Compared with sclerotiorin, most of the amine modified sclerotiorin derivatives except **1** and **2** displayed moderate to fine cytotoxic activities against the MDA-MB-435 and A549 cell lines. Particularly noteworthy, compounds **3, 7, 12, 13, 15** and **17** showed excellent cytotoxic activities with IC_{50} values of 6.39, 9.20, 9.76, 7.75, 9.08 and 8.18 μM, respectively. Further SAR analysis can give the following clues: (1) a vinylogous γ-pyridone formed by the corresponding nitrogen atom substituted pyran nucleus of sclerotiorin increase the cytotoxicity; (2) a certain suitable bulky structure can obtain high cytotoxic activity, which was disclosed by comparing the IC_{50} values of compounds **1, 2, 24** to those of **7, 10, 12**; (3) from the observation of compounds **13, 14, 15, 16, 17**, we can conclude one methylene connected aryl side chain have good effect on cytotoxic activity. In order to illustrate the underlying mechanisms for the cytotoxicity of these compounds, several rational deduces are summed up. Firstly, the amine modified sclerotiorin derivatives may be more efficiently served as a basic factor to change the acidic tumor microenvironment. In this respect, we can explain why the nitrogen substituted structures are more cytotoxic to tumor cells. Secondly, sclerotiorin derivatives possess α, β-unsaturated ketone skeleton and could be Michael receptor. Cytotoxic activity of these compounds may be attributed to the Michael addition reactions of sclerotiorin derivatives with active nucleophilic group in the biomolecules, such as amino acids, nucleic acids and other compounds in the tumor cells to irreversibly affect the functions of the biomolecules or regulate the cellular signal pathway. Thirdly, the literature addressing tumor cells always showed some high expression of cellular factors, the sclerotiorin derivatives may exhibit cytotoxicity by inhibiting some of them, such as the COX-2. Further COX-2 inhibitory activity for these compounds was conducted as following.

Table 1. Cytotoxic activity of sclerotiorin derivatives.

Compd.	MDA-MB-435 IC_{50} (μM)	A549 IC_{50} (μM)	Compd.	MDA-MB-435 IC_{50} (μM)	A549 IC_{50} (μM)
1	>50	40.29	2	>50	>50
3	6.39	22.75	4	35.49	>50
5	20.93	20.27	6	44.27	>50
7	9.20	21.47	8	23.52	21.16
9	38.74	40.35	10	11.76	20.19
11	11.13	25.46	12	9.76	25.98
13	7.75	14.08	14	15.66	21.07
15	9.08	22.70	16	21.29	15.06
17	8.18	14.15	18	26.21	32.05
19	16.34	25.29	20	15.71	23.35
21	22.42	28.18	22	16.26	16.53
23	10.23	23.75	24	42.92	21.46
25	>50	>50	26	>50	>50
27	>50	>50	Sclerotiorin	>50	>50
EPI	0.15	0.37			

2.2.2. In Vitro Primary Screen COX-2 Inhibitory Activity

In recent years, COX-2 inhibitors become a new target and hotspot for anticancer drug research and get a lot of attention. For further investigations the biological activity of semi-synthetic analogs of sclerotiorin, all compounds were primarily screened the COX-2 inhibitory activity at a concentration of 20 μM in vitro.

As shown in Figure 1, most of semi-synthetic derivatives and parent compound sclerotiorin displayed good inhibitory activity for COX-2. Among all the derivatives, compound **3** displayed perfect COX-2 inhibition with a ratio of 70.6%, which is comparable to the positive control indomethacin (78.9%). Furthermore, compounds **7**, **13**, **15**, **17**, **25** and sclerotiorin showed moderate COX-2 inhibitory ratio of 58.7%, 51.1%, 46.7%, 47.3%, 66.1% and 56.1%, respectively. More interestingly, compared to the parent compound sclerotiorin, the inhibitory activity of the esterlysis derivative **25** increased from 56.1% to 66.1%. However, **26** and **27**, the esterification product of **25**, displayed low COX-2 inhibitory ratio of 42.8%, 35.1%, respectively.

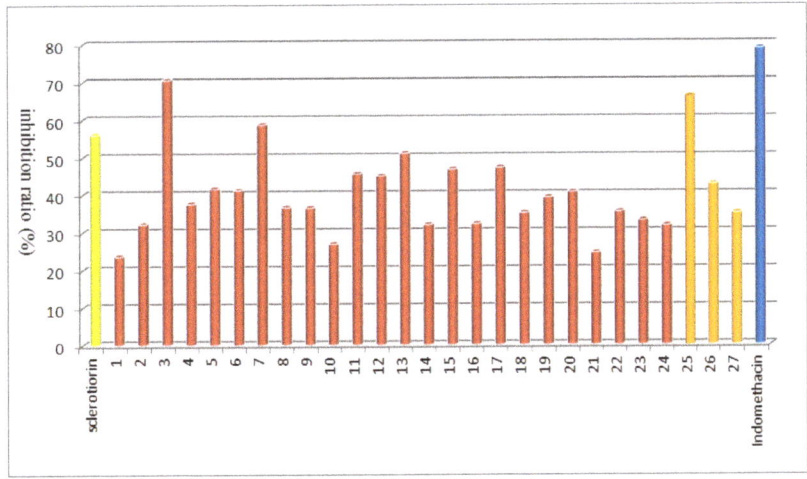

Figure 1. Inhibition ratio of compounds **1–27** to COX-2 in vitro.

Based on the above results, observation was that the COX-2 inhibitory activity of sclerotiorin derivatives were associated with the cytotoxic activity. Overall, the cytotoxic activity of the compounds were positively correlated with the inhibitory activity of COX-2. Out of 28 tested compounds, **3**, **7**, **13**, **15** and **17** showed both cytotoxic activity against two cancer cell lines and potential COX-2 inhibitory activity. Particularly, compound **3** was found to be most potent derivative with high cytotoxic activity against the breast cancer cells and superior COX-2 inhibitory activity. Otherwise, compounds **25**, **26**, **27** and parent compound sclerotiorin were exhibiting good COX-2 inhibitory activity, but almost have no cytotoxic activity. This find suggests sclerotiorin and its esterlysis product **25** deserve intensive investigation on anti-inflammatory activity based on COX-2 inhibition selectivity.

2.2.3. Molecular Docking Studies

The COX-2 inhibitory effects of compound **3** led us to perform molecular docking studies to insight understand the ligand-protein interactions in detail, and dock simulations in COX-2 (PDB ID: 5GMN) [35] were carried out in AutoDock4.2.6 [36]. Docking procedure was validated by docking of 949 (the co-crystallized ligand of COX-2 protein) in the active site of COX-2 and root-mean-square deviation (RMSD) of 0.13 Å to the X-ray structure (Figure 2).

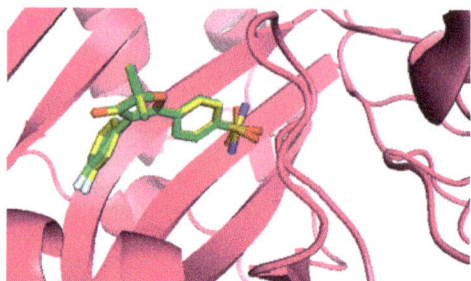

Figure 2. Comparison between the docked pose of 949 (yellow) as produced by docking experiment and the co-crystallized ligand of this inhibitor within COX-2 (green).

Compound **3** was docked into the active site of COX-2 and the interaction energy of 8.24 kcal/mol was obtained. One hydrogen bonding interaction between the ester group of compound **3** with Gln92 (2.96 Å) of COX-2 active site was observed (Figure 3). It is clearly visible in Figure 4 that arachidonic acid and compound **3** were located deeply inside the same pocket of COX-2. Three hydrogen bonding interactions between carboxyl of arachidonic acid with Thr198 (2.92 Å, 2.95 Å) and Thr199 (2.85 Å) of COX-2 active site were observed respectively (Figure 5). The hydrophilic groups of compound **3** including carbonyl and ester group were inclined to via a hydrogen bonding interactions with the hydrophilic amino acid of the outside of the COX-2 protein active pocket. However, alkyl chain and cyclohexene of compound **3** is easier access to the interior of hydrophobic pocket by means of hydrophobic action, which is blocking the binding site of arachidonic acid in COX-2 enzyme to some extent. This may be the reason why the compound **3** showed a perfect inhibitory activity to COX-2 cyclooxygenase (Figure 5).

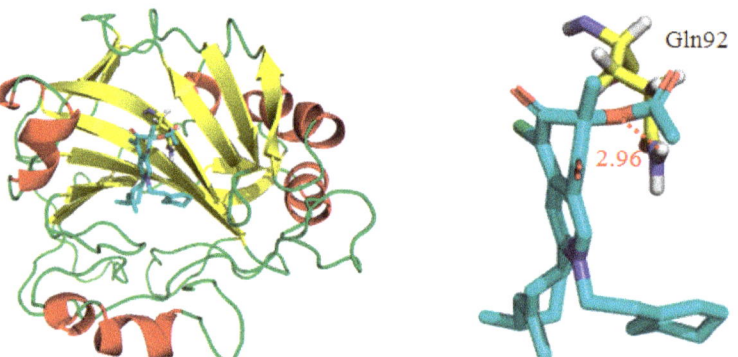

Figure 3. Compound **3** (cyan) docked into the active site of COX-2.

Compound **25** was docked into the active site of COX-2 and the interaction energy of 7.66 kcal/mol was obtained. Unexpectedly, it displayed no H-bonding interaction with the amino acid residue of COX-2 protein. Compound **26** was docked into the active site of COX-2 and the interaction energy of 6.26 kcal/mol was obtained. Three hydrogen bonding interactions between ester group of **26** with His4 (3.40 Å) and Trp5 (2.53 Å, 2.74 Å) of COX-2 active site was observed. One hydrogen bonding interaction between carbonyl group of **26** with Lys169 (3.15 Å) of COX-2 active site was observed. Additionally, Compound **26** showed H-bond interactions of 3.31 Å between its oxygen atom in the ring and Glu238 residues of the COX-2 active site (Figure 6A). However, we found that compound **26** did not located deeply inside the hydrophobic pocket of COX-2 protein as compound **25** did, but docked on the surface of the protein by hydrogen bonding (Figure 6B). Consequently, we deduce that the presence of ester group can resulted in lower activity of compound **26**.

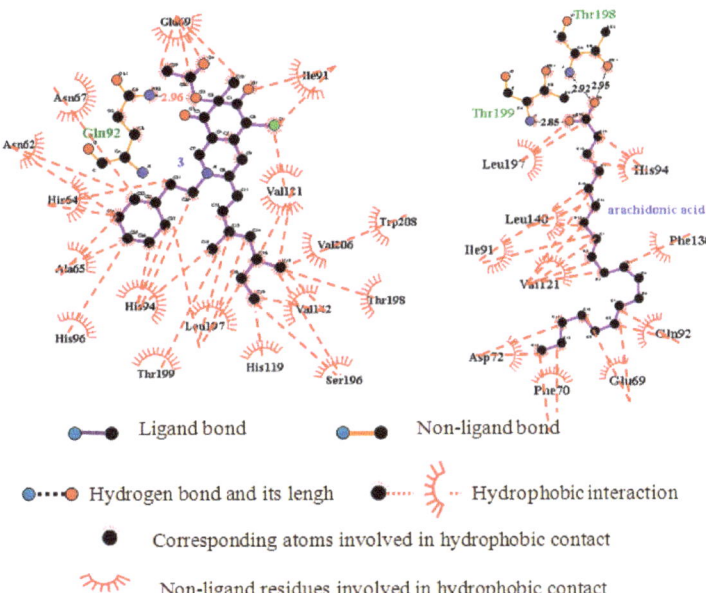

Figure 4. Two-dimensional (2D) diagram of the binding pose of **3** and arachidonic acid in the active site of COX-2.

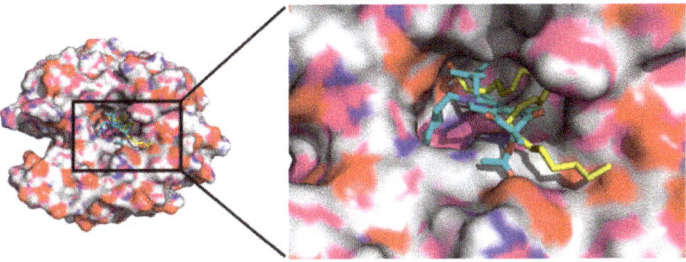

Figure 5. Model showing the placement of **3** (cyan) and arachidonic acid (yellow) in the active site pocket of COX-2.

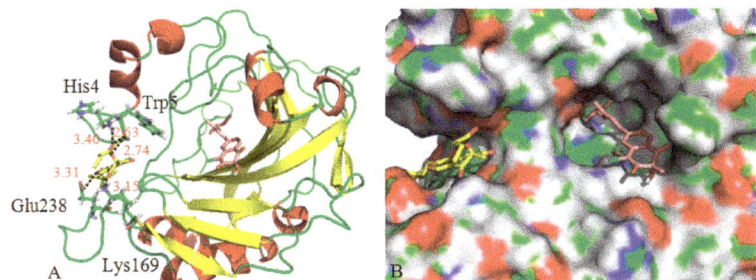

Figure 6. (**A**) 3D diagram of the binding model of **25** (brown) and **26** (yellow) in the active site of COX-2. (**B**) Model showing the placement of **25** (brown) and **26** (yellow) in the active site pocket of COX-2.

3. Materials and Methods

3.1. Chemistry

3.1.1. General Information

Proton and carbon NMR spectra were recorded on Bruker AVANCE NEO 600 MHz spectrometer (Bruker BioSpin, Switzerland). The spectra obtained in CDCl$_3$ were referenced to the residual solvent peak. Chemical shifts (d) are reported in parts per million (ppm) relative to residual undeuterated solvent as an internal reference. HR-ESI-MS data were measured on a Thermo Fisher Scientific Q-TOF mass spectrometer (Thermo Fisher Scientific, Waltham, MA, USA). Silica gel (100–200 and 200–300 mesh) (Qingdao Haiyang Chemical Co., Ltd., Qingdao, China) was used for column chromatography. TLC silica gel GF254 plates (Yantai Zi Fu Chemical Co., Ltd., Yantai, China) and TLC silica gel 60 F254 (MERCK CHEMICALS (SHANGHAI) CO, LTD) were used for thin layer chromatography.

3.1.2. Fungal Materials.

The fungus SCNU-0016 used in the study was isolated from fresh fruit of the mangrove plant *Acanthus ilicifolius L*, which was collected in October 2019 from Hailing island Mangrove Nature Reserve in Guangdong province, China. The fungal isolation was conducted as following. Initially, the plant fruit was washed with sterile water and surface-sterilized in a 100 mL beaker with 75% ethanol for 1 min. This was followed by dipping the sample into 5% sodium hypochlorite for 1 min, then the plant parts were rinsed with sterile water and cut into 3 mm sections and plated on potato dextrose agar (PDA, potatoes 300 mg/mL, dextrose 20 mg/mL, agar 15 mg/mL, chloramphenicol 1 mg/mL) with penicillin (100 units/mL) and streptomycin (0.8 mg/ mL). The plates were incubated at 25 ± 1 °C. The endophytic fungal strains were isolated by routine microbiological. The fungal isolates were numbered and stored at 4 °C in triplicate on PDA slants. Fungal identification was carried out using a molecular biological protocol by DNA amplification and sequencing of the ITS region [37]. The sequence data of the fungal strain have been deposited at Gen Bank with accession no. MW-309502. A BLAST search result showed that the sequence was the most similar (100%) to the sequence of *P. sclerotiorum*. A voucher strain was deposited in School of Chemistry, South China Normal University, Guangzhou, China, with the access code SCNU-F0016.

3.1.3. Fungal Culture and Sclerotiorin Extraction

The fungal strain *P. sclerotiorum* SCNU-0016 was cultured on autoclaved potato liquid-substrate media (one-hundred Erlenmeyer flasks (1000 mL); each containing 400 mL of potato liquid medium, 8 g of glucose and 1.2 g artificial sea salts) at room temperature under static conditions and daylight for 28 days. Following incubation, pancake thallus grew on top of the potato liquid media. Then the air dried fungal were soaked in the solvent MeOH/CH$_2$Cl$_2$ (v:v, 1:1). Extracts were filtered and concentrated under reduced pressure to yield 820 g of residue. The residue was fractionated by column chromatography on silica gel by eluting with a gradient of EtOAc/petroleum ether from 1:10 to 1:1 give five fractions (Fr.1-Fr.5). sclerotiorin was extracted successfully by elution with EtOAc/petroleum ether (v:v, 1:10). sclerotiorin appear good solubility in the EtOAc/petroleum ether solution. Then removal of the solvent afforded 7.82 g of yellow powder.

3.1.4. General Procedure for Synthesis of Sclerotioramine Derivatives 1–24

A mixture of sclerotiorin (39 mg, 0.10 mmol) and varied amines (0.12 mmol) in anhydrous dichloromethane (2 mL) was stirred at room temperature until the sclerotiorin was disappeared. The resulting mixture was extracted with EtOAc (3 × 5 mL) and the organic phase was washed with saturated brine (3 × 15 mL). Then the organic phase was dried with MgSO$_4$ and concentrated in vacuo. The crude product was purified by column chromatography with eluent of EA/PE (5:1, v/v) to give the pure compound. All the synthesized compounds were identified by MS and NMR spectra, please see Figures S1–S79 in the supplementary materials.

Compound 1

(R)-5-chloro-3-((S, 1E, 3E)-3,5-dimethylhepta-1, 3-dien-1-yl)-7-methyl-6, 8-dioxo-2-propyl-2, 6, 7, 8-tetrahydroisoquinolin-7-yl acetate. Red solid, the yield of 90%; m.p. 230.1–232.2 °C. $[\alpha]_D^{25}$ +13.2 (c 0.02, MeOH); UV (MeOH) λmax (log ε): 234 (3.13), 376 (3.03), 488 (1.68) nm; IR (KBr) ν_{max}: 2956, 2922, 1743, 1708, 1590, 1491, 1368, 1251, 1190, 1092, 853 cm^{-1}. ^{1}H NMR (600 MHz, CDCl$_3$) δ_H 7.75 (s, 1H), 7.02 (s, 1H), 6.96(d, J = 15.4 Hz, 1H), 6.12 (d, J = 15.4 Hz, 1H), 5.70 (d, J = 9.7 Hz, 1H), 3.89–3.72 (m, 2H), 2.59–2.34 (m, 1H), 2.16 (s, 3H), 1.85 (s, 3H), 1.80 (dd, J = 14.9, 7.4 Hz, 2H), 1.55 (s, 3H), 1.48–1.40 (m, 1H), 1.39–1.31 (m, 1H), 1.01 (dd, J = 15.3 7.2 Hz, 6H), 0.88 (t, J = 7.4 Hz, 3H). ^{13}C NMR (150 MHz, CDCl$_3$) δ_C 193.9, 184.2, 170.1, 148.2, 147.8, 145.0, 144.6, 141.1, 131.6, 114.6, 114.5, 111.7, 102.2, 84.8, 55.8, 35.1, 30.0, 23.6, 23.2, 20.3, 20.2, 12.6, 12.0, 10.9. LRMS (EI) m/z 432 [M]$^+$.

Compound 2

(R)-2-butyl-5-chloro-3-((S, 1E, 3E)-3,5-dimethylhepta-1, 3-dien-1-yl)-7-methyl-6, 8-dioxo-2, 6, 7, 8-tetrahydroisoquinolin-7-yl acetate. Red solid, the yield of 92%; m.p. 216.3–218.5 °C. $[\alpha]_D^{25}$ +13.6 (c 0.02, MeOH); UV (MeOH) λmax (log ε): 238 (3.10), 378 (3.09), 485 (1.78) nm; IR (KBr) ν_{max}: 2953, 2921, 1743, 1708, 1590, 1493, 1368, 1252, 1190, 1092, 851 cm^{-1}. ^{1}H NMR (600 MHz, CDCl$_3$) δ_H 7.74 (s, 1H), 7.02 (s, 1H), 6.96 (d, J = 15.4 Hz, 1H), 6.13 (d, J = 15.4 Hz, 1H), 5.70 (d, J = 9.7 Hz, 1H), 3.94–3.76 (m, 2H), 2.59–2.39 (m, 1H), 2.16 (s, 3H), 1.84 (s, 3H) 1.74 (s, 2H), 1.54 (s, 3H), 1.48–1.31 (m, 4H), 1.02 (d, J = 6.6 Hz, 3H), 0.98 (t, J = 7.4 Hz, 3H), 0.88 (t, J = 7.4 Hz, 3H). ^{13}C NMR (150 MHz, CDCl$_3$) δ_C 194.1, 184.3, 170.2, 148.3, 147.9, 145.1, 144.7, 141.2, 131.7, 114.8, 114.6, 111.8, 102.3, 84.9, 54.2, 35.2, 32.3, 30.2, 23.4, 20.4, 20.4, 19.8, 13.7, 12.7, 12.1. LRMS (EI) m/z 446 [M]$^+$.

Compound 3

(R)-5-chloro-2-(2-(cyclohex-1-en-1-yl)ethyl)-3-((S, 1E, 3E)-3,5-dimethylhepta-1, 3-dien-1-yl)-7-methyl-6, 8-dioxo-2, 6, 7, 8-tetrahydroisoquinolin-7-yl acetate. Red solid, the yield of 92%; m.p. 180.6–182.8 °C. $[\alpha]_D^{25}$ +14.2 (c 0.02, MeOH); UV (MeOH) λmax (log ε): 235 (3.11), 382 (3.28), 491 (1.66) nm; IR (KBr) ν_{max}: 2965, 2920, 1743, 1703, 1600, 1491, 1368, 1288, 1248, 1180, 1089, 953 cm^{-1}. ^{1}H NMR (600 MHz, CDCl$_3$) δ_H 7.64 (s, 1H), 7.01 (s, 1H), 6.96 (d, J = 15.4 Hz, 1H), 6.16 (d, J = 15.4 Hz, 1H), 5.70 (d, J = 9.7 Hz, 1H), 5.41 (s, 1H), 4.05–3.74 (m, 2H), 2.56–2.38 (m, 1H), 2.31 (t, J = 7.1 Hz, 2H), 2.16 (s, 3H), 2.00–1.87 (m, 4H), 1.85 (s, 3H), 1.63 (dd, J = 10.1, 4.1 Hz, 2H), 1.56–1.48 (m, 5H), 1.47–1.40 (m, 1H), 1.35 (dd, J = 14.3, 6.9, 1H), 1.02 (d, J = 6.6 Hz, 3H), 0.88 (t, J = 7.4 Hz, 3H). ^{13}C NMR (150 MHz, CDCl$_3$) δ_C 194.0, 184.3, 170.1, 148.2, 147.8, 145.1, 144.7, 141.5, 131.9, 131.7, 127.0, 114.7, 114.4, 111.7, 102.1, 84.9, 53.1, 38.6, 35.2, 30.2, 28.4, 25.4, 23.4, 22.7, 22.0, 20.4, 20.4, 12.7, 12.1. HRMS (ESI) for [M + H]$^+$: calcd for C$_{29}$H$_{37}$ClNO$_4$: 498.23332. Found: 498.24115.

Compound 4

(7R)-5-chloro-2-(2, 3-dihydroxypropyl)-3-((S, 1E, 3E)-3,5-dimethylhepta-1, 3-dien-1-yl)-7-methyl-6, 8-dioxo-2, 6, 7, 8-tetrahydroisoquinolin-7-yl acetate. Red solid, the yield of 88%; m.p. 152.8–154.3 °C. $[\alpha]_D^{25}$ +14.5 (c 0.02, MeOH); UV (MeOH) λmax (log ε): 236 (3.09), 379 (3.10), 488 (1.64) nm; IR (KBr) ν_{max}: 3537, 2958, 2926, 1733, 1701, 1581, 1489, 1242, 1154, 858 cm^{-1}. ^{1}H NMR (600 MHz, CD$_3$OD) δ_H 8.15 (s, 1H), 7.20 (s, 1H), 7.11 (d, J = 15.4 Hz, 1H), 6.64 (d, J = 15.4 Hz, 1H), 5.79 (d, J = 9.7 Hz, 1H), 4.46 (dd, J = 14.4, 2.5 Hz, 1H), 3.94 (dd, J = 14.4, 9.2 Hz, 1H), 3.91–3.84 (m, 1H), 3.63 (dd, J = 11.1, 4.7 Hz, 1H), 3.53 (dd, J = 11.1, 6.7 Hz, 1H), 2.56–2.38 (m, 1H), 2.13 (d, J = 20 Hz, 3H), 1.92 (d, J = 0.9 Hz, 3H), 1.51 (d, J = 5.2 Hz, 3H), 1.50–1.46 (m, 1H), 1.41–1.34 (m, 1H), 1.05 (dd, J = 6.7, 2.1 Hz, 3H), 0.91 (t, J = 7.4 Hz, 3H). ^{13}C NMR (150 MHz, CD$_3$OD) δ_C 195.1, 185.5, 171.6, 151.8, 148.7, 148.3, 146.5, 144.9, 134.0, 117.4, 116.1, 112.3, 101.2, 86.2, 71.7, 64.5, 58.3, 36.2, 31.2, 23.8, 20.6, 20.2, 12.8, 12.4. HRMS (ESI) for [M − H]$^-$: calcd for C$_{24}$H$_{29}$ClNO$_6$: 462.17617. Found: 462.16899.

Compound 5

(R)-5-chloro-3-((S, 1E, 3E)-3,5-dimethylhepta-1, 3-dien-1-yl)-2-(furan-2-ylmethyl)-7-methyl-6, 8-dioxo-2, 6, 7, 8-tetrahydroisoquinolin-7-yl acetate. Red solid, the yield of 96%; m.p. 160.0–161.5 °C. $[\alpha]_D^{25}$ +16.6 (c 0.02, MeOH); UV (MeOH) λmax (log ε): 240 (3.16), 380 (3.06), 496 (1.66) nm; IR (KBr) ν_{max}: 2960, 2928, 1735, 1703, 1595, 1497, 1371, 1256, 1144,

1104, 1083, 860 cm^{-1}. ^{1}H NMR (600 MHz, CDCl$_3$) δ$_H$ 7.84 (s, 1H), 7.45–7.41 (m, 1H), 6.97 (s, 1H), 6.90 (d, J = 15.3Hz, 1H), 6.42–6.37 (m, 2H), 6.33 (d, J = 15.4 Hz, 1H), 5.67 (d, J = 9.8 Hz, 1H), 4.97 (d, J = 4.8 Hz, 2H), 2.52–2.40 (m, 1H), 2.14 (s, 3H), 1.84 (d, J = 0.9 Hz, 3H), 1.53 (s, 3H), 1.46–1.40 (m, 1H), 1.36–1.28 (m, 1H), 1.01 (d, J = 6.7 Hz, 3H), 0.87 (t, J = 7.4 Hz, 3H). ^{13}C NMR (150 MHz, CDCl$_3$) δ$_C$ 193.8, 184.5, 170.2, 148.3, 148.1, 147.0, 145.1, 144.5, 144.2, 141.1, 131.9, 115.1, 115.0, 111.6, 111.1, 110.6, 102.7, 85.0, 50.3, 35.1, 30.1, 23.3, 20.4, 20.3, 12.7, 12.1. HRMS (ESI) for [M + H]$^+$: calcd for C$_{26}$H$_{29}$ClNO$_5$: 470.16560. Found: 470.17326.

Compound 6

(R)-2-(benzyloxy)-5-chloro-3-((S, 1E, 3E)-3,5-dimethylhepta-1, 3-dien-1-yl)-7-methyl-6, 8-dioxo-2, 6, 7, 8-tetrahydroisoquinolin-7-yl acetate. Red solid, the yield of 96%; m.p. 166.6–168.3 °C. [α]$_D^{25}$ +14.3 (c 0.02, MeOH); UV (MeOH) λmax (log ε): 248 (3.09), 386 (3.06), 491 (1.67) nm; IR (KBr) ν_{max}: 3080, 2964, 2929, 1723, 1703, 1611, 1487, 1375, 1252, 1221, 1148, 1080, 952, 781 cm^{-1}. ^{1}H NMR (600 MHz, CDCl$_3$) δ$_H$ 7.82 (s, 1H), 7.44 (d, J = 7.1 Hz, 3H), 7.36 (dd, J = 7.6, 1.7 Hz, 2H), 7.08 (d, J = 15.9 Hz, 1H), 7.00 (s, 1H), 6.29 (d, J = 15.9 Hz, 1H), 5.74 (d, J = 9.7 Hz, 1H), 5.06 (dd, J = 25.6, 10.1 Hz, 2H), 258–2.43 (m, 1H), 2.17 (s, 3H), 1.83 (d, J = 0.7 Hz, 3H), 1.53 (s, 3H), 1.48–1.40 (m, 1H), 1.38–1.34 (m, 1H), 1.03 (d, J = 6.6 Hz, 3H), 0.90 (d, J = 7.4 Hz, 3H). ^{13}C NMR (150 MHz, CDCl$_3$) δ$_C$ 193.15, 184.41, 170.22, 149.11, 145.86, 144.88, 143.54, 137.20, 132.12, 131.62, 130.58, 130.27, 129.37, 128.98, 113.77, 112.08, 109.43, 103.14, 84.74, 81.96, 65.71, 35.28, 30.17, 29.83, 23.29, 20.35, 12.63, 12.13. HRMS (ESI) for [M + H]$^+$: calcd for C$_{28}$H$_{31}$ClNO$_5$: 496.18125. Found: 496.18889.

Compound 7

(R)-5-chloro-3-((S, 1E, 3E)-3,5-dimethylhepta-1, 3-dien-1-yl)-7-methyl-6, 8-dioxo-2-(2-(pyrrolidin-1-yl)ethyl)-2, 6, 7, 8-tetrahydroisoquinolin-7-yl acetate. Red solid, the yield of 96%; m.p. 145.5–147.6 °C. [α]$_D^{25}$ +16.1 (c 0.02, MeOH); UV (MeOH) λmax (log ε): 246 (3.09), 379 (3.00), 488 (1.64) nm; IR (KBr) ν_{max}: 2958, 2922, 1748, 1708, 1591, 1491, 1365, 1252, 1190, 1092, 860 cm^{-1}. ^{1}H NMR (600 MHz, CDCl$_3$) δ$_H$ 7.78 (s, 1H), 7.00 (s, 1H), 6.95 (d, J = 15.3 Hz, 1H), 6.23 (d, J = 15.3 Hz, 1H), 5.70 (d, J = 9.8 Hz, 1H), 3.98 (s, 2H), 2.84 (s, 2H), 2.61 (s, 4H), 2.53–2.43 (m, 1H), 2.17 (s, 3H), 1.86 (s, 3H), 1.81 (s, 4H), 1.54 (s, 3H), 1.49–1.40 (m, 1H), 1.38–1.34 (m, 1H), 1.03 (d, J = 6.6 Hz, 3H), 0.90 (d, J = 7.4 Hz, 3H). ^{13}C NMR (150 MHz, CDCl$_3$) δ$_C$ 194.0, 184.4, 170.2, 149.2, 147.6, 145.0, 144.5, 136.5, 131.6, 115.4, 115.3, 112.7, 102.3, 84.9, 58.8, 35.1, 30.1, 30.0, 23.3, 20.9, 20.7, 20.4, 20.3, 12.7, 12.1, 10.8, 10.8. HRMS (ESI) for [M + H]$^+$: calcd for C$_{27}$H$_{36}$ClN$_2$O$_4$: 487.22854. Found: 487.23595.

Compound 8

(7R)-2-(sec-butyl)-5-chloro-3-((S, 1E, 3E)-3,5-dimethylhepta-1, 3-dien-1-yl)-7-methyl-6, 8-dioxo-2, 6, 7, 8-tetrahydroisoquinolin-7-yl acetate. Red solid, the yield of 93%; m.p. 164.4–466.8 °C. [α]$_D^{25}$ +16.8 (c 0.02, MeOH); UV (MeOH) λmax (log ε): 256 (3.05), 386 (2.98), 498 (1.53) nm; IR (KBr) ν_{max}: 2964, 2920, 1736, 1701, 1599, 1497, 1370, 1252, 1200, 1141, 1084, 861 cm^{-1}. ^{1}H NMR (600 MHz, CDCl$_3$) δ$_H$ 7.83 (s, 1H), 6.95 (s, 1H), 6.87 (d, J = 15.3 Hz, 1H), 6.13 (d, J = 15.3 Hz, 1H), 5.67 (d, J = 9.7 Hz, 1H), 4.23 (dd, J = 13.8, 6.9 Hz, 1H), 2.53–2.41 (m, 1H), 2.17 (s, 3H), 1.85 (s,3H), 1.80 (dd, J = 14.8, 7.4 Hz, 2H), 1.56 (s, 3H), 1.47–1.42 (m, 4H), 1.38–1.33 (m, 1H), 1.02 (d, J = 6.6 Hz, 3H), 0.93 (t, J = 7.3 Hz, 3H), 0.88 (t, J = 7.4 Hz, 3H). ^{13}C NMR (150 MHz, CDCl$_3$) δ$_C$ 194.0, 184.5, 170.2, 148.4, 147.9, 145.1, 144.6, 142.2, 131.7, 114.6, 114.4, 111.7, 102.3, 84.9, 54.0, 53.4, 51.5, 35.2, 30.1, 29.8, 23.4, 20.4, 20.3, 12.8, 12.1. HRMS (ESI) for [M + H]$^+$: calcd for C$_{25}$H$_{33}$ClNO$_4$: 446.20199. Found: 446.20947.

Compound 9

(R)-5-chloro-3-((S, 1E, 3E)-3, 5-dimethylhepta-1, 3-dien-1-yl)-2-(2-hydroxyethyl)-7-methyl-6, 8-dioxo-2, 6, 7, 8-tetrahydroisoquinolin-7-yl acetate. Red solid, the yield of 88%; m.p. 180.2–182.8 °C. [α]$_D^{25}$ +15.8 (c 0.02, MeOH); UV (MeOH) λmax (log ε): 233 (3.06), 389 (3.18), 498 (1.64) nm; IR (KBr) ν_{max}: 3535, 2950, 2926, 1733, 1706, 1581, 1484, 1242, 1155, 866 cm^{-1}. ^{1}H NMR (600 MHz, CDCl$_3$) δ$_H$ 7.93 (s, 1H), 7.05 (s, 1H), 6.94 (d, J = 15.3 Hz, 1H), 6.28 (d, J = 15.4 Hz, 1H), 5.70 (d, J = 9.7 Hz, 1H), 4.04 (d, J = 5.4 Hz, 2H), 3.91 (d, J = 4.6 Hz, 2H), 2.46 (d, J = 8.6 Hz, 1H), 2.14 (s, 3H), 1.84 (s, 3H), 1.53 (s, 3H), 1.46–1.42 (m, 1H), 1.36–1.30 (m, 1H), 1.01 (d, J = 6.6 Hz, 3H), 0.87 (t, J = 7.4 Hz, 3H). LRMS (EI) m/z 434 [M]$^+$.

Compound 10

(R)-5-chloro-3-((S, 1E, 3E)-3, 5-dimethylhepta-1, 3-dien-1-yl)-2-heptyl-7-methyl-6, 8-dioxo-2, 6, 7, 8-tetrahydroisoquinolin-7-yl acetate. Red solid, the yield of 93%; m.p. 95.6–97.3 °C. $[\alpha]_D^{25}$ +13.9 (c 0.02, MeOH); UV (MeOH) λmax (log ε): 246 (3.05), 389 (3.20), 488 (1.64) nm; IR (KBr) ν_{max}: 2966, 2928, 1748, 1705, 1591, 1493, 1368, 1252, 1190, 1093, 862 cm^{-1}. ^{1}H NMR (600 MHz, CDCl$_3$) δ$_H$ 7.74 (s, 1H), 7.01 (s, 1H), 6.95 (d, J = 15.3 Hz, 1H), 6.12 (d, J = 15.4 Hz, 1H), 5.70 (d, J = 9.8 Hz, 1H), 3.82 (td, J = 7.2, 2.9 Hz, 2H), 2.52–2.37 (m, 1H), 2.16 (s, 3H), 1.84 (s, 3H), 1.77–1.72 (m, 2H), 1.54 (s, 3H), 1.46–1.42 (m, 1H), 1.37–1.25 (m, 9H), 1.02 (d, J = 6.7 Hz, 3H), 088 (t, J = 7.3 Hz, 6H). ^{13}C NMR (150 MHz, CDCl$_3$) δ$_C$ 194.1, 184.4, 170.2, 148.2, 147.9, 145.0, 144.7, 141.1, 131.7, 114.8, 114.7, 111.8, 102.2, 84.9, 54.5, 35.2, 31.6, 30.3, 30.1, 28.8, 26.4, 23.4, 22.6, 20.4, 20.3, 14.1, 12.7, 12.1. HRMS (ESI) for [M + H]$^+$: calcd for C$_{28}$H$_{39}$ClNO$_4$: 488.24894. Found: 488.25679.

Compound 11

(R)-5-chloro-3-((S, 1E, 3E)-3, 5-dimethylhepta-1, 3-dien-1-yl)-2-(2-(furan-2-yl)ethyl)-7-methyl-6, 8-dioxo-2, 6, 7, 8-tetrahydroisoquinolin-7-yl acetate. Red solid, the yield of 90%; m.p. 130.3–132.8 °C. $[\alpha]_D^{25}$ +15.9 (c 0.02, MeOH); UV (MeOH) λmax (log ε): 256 (3.03), 379 (3.16), 493 (1.54) nm; IR (KBr) ν_{max}: 2966, 2923, 1738, 1703, 1595, 1497, 1372, 1256, 1148, 1104, 1083, 869 cm^{-1}. ^{1}H NMR (600 MHz, CDCl$_3$) δ$_H$ 7.59 (s, 1H), 7.33 (d, J = 1.6 Hz, 1H), 6.96 (d, J = 15.3 Hz, 1H), 6.91 (d, J = 15.3 Hz, 1H), 6.28 (dd, J = 2.9, 2.0 Hz, 1H), 6.09 (d, J = 3.1 Hz, 1H), 5.98 (d, J = 15.3 Hz, 1H), 5.68 (d, J = 9.7 Hz, 1H), 4.17–4.05 (m, 2H), 3.22–2.98 (m, 2H), 2.47 (dt, J = 8.0, 7.3 Hz, 1H), 2.16 (s, 3H), 1.83 (s, 3H), 1.53 (s, 3H), 1.46–1.42 (m, 1H), 1.37–1.31 (m, 1H), 1.02 (d, J = 6.6 Hz, 3H), 0.88 (t, J = 7.4 Hz, 3H). ^{13}C NMR (150 MHz, CDCl$_3$) δ$_C$ 193.8, 184.5, 170.2, 149.4, 148.1, 148.0, 145.2, 144.5, 142.7, 141.0, 131.8, 114.9, 114.5, 111.5, 110.9, 108.6, 102.5, 84.9, 52.8, 35.2, 30.2, 29.0, 23.3, 20.4, 20.4, 12.7, 12.1. HRMS (ESI) for [M + H]$^+$: calcd for C$_{27}$H$_{31}$ClNO$_5$: 484.18125. Found: 484.18897.

Compound 12

(R)-5-chloro-2-cyclopropyl-3-((S, 1E, 3E)-3, 5-dimethylhepta-1, 3-dien-1-yl)-7-methyl-6, 8-dioxo-2, 6, 7, 8-tetrahydroisoquinolin-7-yl acetate. Red solid, the yield of 91%; m.p. 172.3–174.4 °C. $[\alpha]_D^{25}$ +15.6 (c 0.02, MeOH); UV (MeOH) λmax (log ε): 251 (3.01), 388 (3.31), 489 (1.66) nm; IR (KBr) ν_{max}: 2968, 2921, 1743, 1708, 1610, 1491, 1369, 1288, 1245, 1180, 1089, 955 cm^{-1}. ^{1}H NMR (600 MHz, CDCl$_3$) δ$_H$ 7.90 (s, 1H), 7.07 (s, 1H), 6.98 (d, J = 15.6 Hz, 1H), 6.55 (d, J = 15.6 Hz, 1H), 5.72 (d, J = 9.8 Hz, 1H), 3.27 (dd, J = 6.8, 3.3 Hz, 1H), 2.68–2.39 (m, 1H), 2.16 (s, 3H), 1.86 (s, 3H), 1.53 (s, 3H), 1.48–1.40 (m, 1H), 1.37–1.31 (m, 1H), 1.22 (d, J = 6.8 Hz, 2H), 1.05 (dd, J = 15.1, 2.5 Hz, 2H), 1.02 (d, J = 6.7 Hz, 3H), 0.88 (t, J = 7.4 Hz, 3H). LRMS (EI) m/z 431 [M]$^+$.

Compound 13

(R)-5-chloro-3-((S, 1E, 3E)-3, 5-dimethylhepta-1, 3-dien-1-yl)-7-methyl-6, 8-dioxo-2-(thiophen-2-ylmethyl)-2, 6, 7, 8-tetrahydroisoquinolin-7-yl acetate. Red solid, the yield of 89%; m.p. 106.5–108.4 °C. $[\alpha]_D^{25}$ +13.3 (c 0.02, MeOH); UV (MeOH) λmax (log ε): 244 (3.00), 381 (3.10), 497 (1.68) nm; IR (KBr) ν_{max}: 2960, 2924, 1735, 1704, 1591, 1499, 1371, 1256, 1140, 1080, 1008, 860 cm^{-1}. ^{1}H NMR (600 MHz, CDCl$_3$) δ$_H$ 7.86 (s, 1H), 7.35 (dd, J = 3.9, 2.4 Hz, 1H), 7.10–6.98 (m, 3H), 6.92 (d, J = 15.3 Hz, 1H), 6.22 (dd, J = 15.3 Hz, 1H), 5.68 (d, J = 9.8 Hz, 1H), 5.17 (q, J = 16.2 Hz, 2H), 2.54–2.41 (m, 1H), 2.15 (s, 3H), 1.80 (d, J = 10.7 Hz, 3H), 1.54 (s, 3H), 1.46–1.40 (m, 1H), 1.37–1.29 (m, 1H), 1.01 (d, J = 6.7 Hz, 3H), 0.87 (t, J = 7.4 Hz, 3H). ^{13}C NMR (150 MHz, CDCl$_3$) δ$_C$ 193.8, 184.4, 170.3, 148.3, 148.0, 145.3, 144.4, 140.9, 136.3, 131.9, 127.8, 127.5, 127.2, 115.1, 114.9, 111.7, 103.0, 85.0, 52.6, 35.2, 30.1, 23.3, 20.4, 20.3, 12.7, 12.1. HRMS (ESI) for [M + H]$^+$: calcd for C$_{26}$H$_{29}$ClNO$_5$S: 486.14276. Found: 486.15086.

Compound 14

(R)-5-chloro-3-((S, 1E, 3E)-3,5-dimethylhepta-1, 3-dien-1-yl)-7-methyl-6, 8-dioxo-2-(2-(thiophen-2-yl)ethyl)-2, 6, 7, 8-tetrahydroisoquinolin-7-yl acetate. Red solid, the yield of 91%; m.p. 100.2–102.0 °C. $[\alpha]_D^{25}$ +16.2 (c 0.02, MeOH); UV (MeOH) λmax (log ε): 251 (3.09), 389 (3.00), 501 (1.55) nm; IR (KBr) ν_{max}: 2966, 2920, 1735, 1708, 1591, 1489, 1371, 1258, 1140, 1088, 1008, 849 cm^{-1}. ^{1}H NMR (600 MHz, CDCl$_3$) δ$_H$ 7.59 (s, 1H), 7.19 (dd, J = 5.1, 1.1 Hz, 1H), 6.97 (s, 1H), 6.95–6.88 (m, 2H), 6.78 (d, J = 3.3 Hz, 1H), 5.98 (d, J = 15.3 Hz, 1H), 5.68

(d, J = 9.7 Hz, 1H), 4.08 (ddt, J = 78.5, 14.6, 7.2 Hz, 2H), 3.34–3.13 (m, 2H), 2.52–2.39 (m, 1H), 2.16 (s, 3H), 1.82 (d, J = 1.0 Hz, 3H), 1.52 (s, 3H), 1.49–1.39 (m, 1H), 1.38–1.31 (m,1H), 1.02 (d, J = 6.7 Hz, 3H), 0.88 (t, J = 7.4 Hz, 3H). ^{13}C NMR (150 MHz, CDCl$_3$) δ_C 193.8, 184.4, 170.2, 148.3, 147.9, 145.2, 144.4, 140.9, 137.4, 131.8, 127.8, 126.9, 125.4, 114.8, 114.5, 111.6, 102.6, 85.0, 55.5, 35.2, 30.6, 30.2, 23.4, 20.4, 20.4, 12.7, 12.1. HRMS (ESI) for [M + H]$^+$: calcd for C$_{27}$H$_{31}$ClNO$_5$S: 500.15841. Found: 500.16563.

Compound **15**

(*R*)-5-chloro-3-((*S*, 1*E*, 3*E*)-3, 5-dimethylhepta-1, 3-dien-1-yl)-7-methyl-6, 8-dioxo-2-phenyl-2, 6, 7, 8-tetrahydroisoquinolin-7-yl acetate. Red solid, the yield of 93%; m.p. 190.2–192.1 °C. $[\alpha]_D^{25}$ +16.5 (*c* 0.02, MeOH); UV (MeOH) λmax (log ε): 241 (3.19), 379 (3.12), 506 (1.53) nm; IR (KBr) ν_{max}: 3088, 2964, 2916, 1731, 1707, 1611, 1591, 1495, 1363, 1275, 1204, 1130, 1084, 1020, 856, 773 cm^{-1}. ^{1}H NMR (600 MHz, CDCl$_3$) δ_H 7.83 (s, 3H), 7.59–7.47 (m, 3H), 7.32–7.27 (m, 2H), 7.15 (s, 1H), 6.96 (d, J = 15.6 Hz), 5.65 (d, J = 9.7 Hz, 1H), 5.58 (d, J = 15.6 Hz, 1H), 2.46–2.30 (m, 1H), 2.17 (s, 3H), 1.58 (s, 3H), 1.49 (d, J = 0.9 Hz, 3H), 1.45–1.36 (m, 1H), 1.33–1.28 (m, 1H), 0.97 (d, J = 6.6 Hz, 3H), 0.84 (t, 7.4 Hz, 3H). ^{13}C NMR (150 MHz, CDCl$_3$) δ_C 193.9, 184.8, 170.3, 148.0, 147.6, 144.2, 143.3, 141.3, 140.5, 131.9, 130.3, 130.3, 130.2, 126.7, 126.7, 116.3, 114.5, 109.9, 103.4, 84.9, 35.1, 30.1, 23.3, 20.4, 20.3, 12.3, 12.1. LRMS (EI) *m/z* 467 [M]$^+$.

Compound **16**

(*R*)-5-chloro-3-((*S*, 1*E*, 3*E*)-3,5-dimethylhepta-1, 3-dien-1-yl)-7-methyl-6, 8-dioxo-2-phenethyl-2, 6, 7, 8-tetrahydroisoquinolin-7-yl acetate. Red solid, the yield of 91%; m.p. 180.2–181.0 °C. $[\alpha]_D^{25}$ +15.3 (*c* 0.02, MeOH); UV (MeOH) λmax (log ε): 243 (3.06), 386 (3.14), 498 (1.55) nm; IR (KBr) ν_{max}: 3080, 2962, 2916, 1731, 1715, 1611, 1588, 1495, 1366, 1275, 1212, 1130, 1084, 1022, 856, 780 cm^{-1}. ^{1}H NMR (600 MHz, CDCl$_3$) δ_H 7.51 (s, 1H), 7.30 (dd, J = 10.2, 4.6 Hz, 2H), 7.26–7.22 (m, 1H), 7.15- 7.01 (m, 2H), 6.94 (s, 1H), 6.88 (d, J = 15.2 Hz, 1H), 5.99 (d, J = 15.4 Hz, 1H), 5.67 (d, J = 9.7 Hz, 1H), 4.32–3.89 (m, 2H), 3.28–2.84 (m, 2H), 2.53–2.40 (m, 1H), 2.14 (s, 3H), 1.80 (d, J = 1.0 Hz, 3H), 1.50 (s, 3H), 1.48–1.40 (m, 1H), 1.38–1.31 (m, 1H), 1.02 (d, J = 6.7 Hz, 3H), 0.88 (t, J = 7.4 Hz, 3H). ^{13}C NMR (150 MHz, CDCl$_3$) δ_C 193.8, 184.4, 170.1, 148.1, 148.0, 145.1, 144.5, 141.1, 135.9, 131.8, 129.3, 129.3, 128.9, 128.9, 127.8, 114.7, 114.7, 111.5, 102.3, 85.0, 55.6, 36.7, 35.1, 30.1, 23.4, 20.4, 20.3, 12.7, 12.1. LRMS (EI) *m/z* 495 [M]$^+$.

Compound **17**

(*R*)-2-benzyl-5-chloro-3-((*S*, 1*E*, 3*E*)-3,5-dimethylhepta-1, 3-dien-1-yl)-7-methyl-6, 8-dioxo-2, 6, 7, 8-tetrahydroisoquinolin-7-yl acetate. Red solid, the yield of 92%; m.p. 188.8–190.2 °C. $[\alpha]_D^{25}$ +13.9 (*c* 0.02, MeOH); UV (MeOH) λmax (log ε): 259 (3.06), 399 (3.10), 499 (1.65) nm; IR (KBr) ν_{max}: 3082, 2964, 2918, 1731, 1710, 1611, 1591, 1495, 1363, 1276, 1204, 1130, 1084, 1020, 858, 773 cm^{-1}. ^{1}H NMR (600 MHz, CDCl$_3$) δ_H 7.86 (s, 1H), 7.45–7.33 (m, 3H), 7.18 (d, J = 7.2 Hz, 2H), 7.04 (s, 1H), 6.89 (d, J = 15.4 Hz, 1H), 6.02 (d, J = 15.4 Hz, 1H), 5.64 (d, J = 9.8 Hz, 1H), 5.19–4.88 (m, 2H), 2.54–2.30 (m, 1H), 2.16 (s, 3H), 1.66 (d, J = 1.0 Hz, 3H), 1.57 (s, 3H), 1.46–1.40 (m, 1H), 1.34–1.28 (s, 1H), 0.98 (d, J = 6.7 Hz, 3H), 0.84 (t, J = 6.7 Hz, 3H). ^{13}C NMR (150 MHz, CDCl$_3$) δ_C 194.0, 184.6, 170.3, 148.4, 148.2, 145.0, 144.5, 141.7, 134.2, 131.8, 129.7, 129.7, 129.1, 126.6, 126.6, 115.2, 114.9, 111.7, 102.9, 84.9, 57.9, 35.1, 30.1, 23.4, 20.4, 20.3, 12.6, 12.1. HRMS (ESI) for [M + H]$^+$: calcd for C$_{28}$H$_{31}$ClNO$_4$: 480.1863. Found: 480.1935.

Compound **18**

(*R*)-5-chloro-3-((*S*, 1*E*, 3*E*)-3, 5-dimethylhepta-1, 3-dien-1-yl)-7-methyl-2-(3-morpholinopropyl) -6, 8-dioxo-2, 6, 7, 8-tetrahydroisoquinolin-7-yl acetate. Red solid, the yield of 96%; m.p. 110.2–112.6 °C. $[\alpha]_D^{25}$ +16.6 (*c* 0.02, MeOH); UV (MeOH) λmax (log ε): 245 (3.19), 376 (3.00), 505 (1.63) nm; IR (KBr) ν_{max}: 2960, 2920, 1727, 1706, 1595, 1499, 1371, 1248, 1208, 1148, 1080, 864 cm^{-1}. ^{1}H NMR (600 MHz, CDCl$_3$) δ_H 7.93 (s, 1H), 7.01 (s, 1H), 6.96 (d, J = 15.4 Hz, 1H), 6.18 (d, J = 15.4 Hz, 1H), 5.71 (d, J = 9.7 Hz, 1H), 4.01 (s, 2H), 3.75 (s, 4H), 2.68–2.24 (m, 7H), 2.16 (s, 3H), 1.98 (dd, J = 28.3, 21.6 Hz, 2H), 1.86 (s, 3H), 1.54 (s, 3H), 1.46–1.40 (m, 1H), 1.37–1.32 (m, 1H), 1.02 (d, J = 6.6 Hz, 3H), 0.88 (t, J = 7.4 Hz, 3H). ^{13}C NMR (150 MHz, CDCl$_3$) δ_C 194.1, 184.5, 170.2, 148.4, 147.9, 145.1, 144.6, 142.2, 131.7,

114.6, 114.4, 111.7, 102.3, 84.9, 54.0, 53.4, 51.5, 35.2, 30.1, 29.8, 23.4, 20.4, 20.3, 12.8, 12.1. 10.9, 10.8. HRMS (ESI) for [M + H]$^+$: calcd for $C_{28}H_{38}ClN_2O_5$: 517.22345. Found:517.24647.

Compound 19

(R)-5-chloro-2-(2-(dimethylamino)ethyl)-3-((S, 1E, 3E)-3,5-dimethylhepta-1, 3-dien-1-yl)-7-methyl-6, 8-dioxo-2, 6, 7, 8-tetrahydroisoquinolin-7-yl acetate. Red solid, the yield of 92%; m.p. 185.6–187.2 °C. $[\alpha]_D^{25}$ +14.8 (c 0.02, MeOH); UV (MeOH) λmax (log ε): 236 (3.01), 371 (3.23), 487 (1.45) nm; IR (KBr) ν_{max}: 2960, 2923, 1731, 1706, 1595, 1499, 1371, 1251, 1209, 1140, 1080, 866 cm^{-1}. ^{1}H NMR (600 MHz, CDCl$_3$) δ$_H$ 7.77 (s, 1H), 7.00 (s, 1H), 6.94 (d, J = 15.3 Hz, 1H), 6.21 (d, J = 15.4 Hz, 1H), 5.70 (d, J = 9.70 Hz, 1H), 3.93 (s, 2H), 2.64 (s, 2H), 2.53–2.41 (m, 1H), 2.31 (s, 6H), 2.16 (s, 3H), 1.85 (d, J = 0.8 Hz, 3H), 1.54 (s, 3H), 1.46–1.40 (m, 1H), 1.39–1.31 (m, 1H), 1.02 (d, J = 6.6 Hz, 3H), 0.88 (t, J = 7.4 Hz, 3H). ^{13}C NMR (150 MHz, CDCl$_3$) δ$_C$ 193.9, 184.4, 170.1, 148.1, 148.0, 145.1, 144.5, 141.5, 131.7, 114.8, 114.6, 111.6, 102.3, 84.9, 58.5, 51.8, 45.6, 35.1, 30.0, 29.3, 23.3, 20.3, 20.2, 12.6, 12.0. HRMS (ESI) for [M + H]$^+$: calcd for $C_{25}H_{34}ClN_2O_4$: 461.26289. Found: 461.22027.

Compound 20

(R)-2-(2-(benzylamino)ethyl)-5-chloro-3-((S, 1E, 3E)-3, 5-dimethylhepta-1, 3-dien-1-yl)-7-methyl-6, 8-dioxo-2, 6, 7, 8-tetrahydroisoquinolin-7-yl acetate. Red solid, the yield of 91%; m.p. 160.1–161.8. $[\alpha]_D^{25}$ +14.3 (c 0.02, MeOH); UV (MeOH) λmax (log ε): 251 (3.03), 381 (3.26), 497 (1.55) nm; IR (KBr) ν_{max}: 3412, 2963, 2924, 1737, 1703, 1589, 1495, 1369, 1249, 1145, 1082, 1007, 965, 861 cm^{-1}. ^{1}H NMR (600 MHz, CDCl$_3$) δ$_H$ 7.81 (s, 1H), 7.32–7.27 (m, 2H), 7.24 (td, J = 7.6, 2.1 Hz, 3H), 6.94 (s, 1H), 6.83 (d, J = 15.3 Hz, 1H), 6.16 (d, J = 15.4 Hz, 1H), 5.66 (d, J = 9.7 Hz, 1H), 4.09–3.80 (m, 2H), 3.79 (s, 2H), 3.12–2.77 (m, 2H), 2.53–2.37 (m, 1H), 2.16 (s, 3H), 1.80 (d, J = 1.0 Hz, 3H), 1.55 (s, 3H), 1.49–1.41 (m, 1H), 1.37–1.32 (m, 1H), 1.01 (d, J = 6.7 Hz, 3H), 0.88 (t, J = 7.4 Hz, 3H). ^{13}C NMR (150 MHz, CDCl$_3$) δ$_C$ 194.1, 184.5, 170.2, 148.1, 148.0, 145.1, 144.8, 142.1, 131.8, 128.8, 128.8, 128.8, 128.3, 128.3, 127.6, 114.9, 114.4, 111.8, 102.2, 85.0, 54.1, 53.6, 47.5, 35.13, 30.2, 23.4, 20.5, 20.4, 12.7, 12.1. HRMS (ESI) for [M + H]$^+$: calcd for $C_{30}H_{36}ClN_2O_5$: 523.22854. Found: 523.23594.

Compound 21

(R)-5-chloro-2-cyclopentyl-3-((S, 1E, 3E)-3, 5-dimethylhepta-1, 3-dien-1-yl)-7-methyl-6, 8-dioxo-2, 6, 7, 8-tetrahydroisoquinolin-7-yl acetate. Red solid, the yield of 95%; m.p. 132.3–133.5 °C. $[\alpha]_D^{25}$ +15.3 (c 0.02, MeOH); UV (MeOH) λmax (log ε): 233 (3.09), 369 (3.13), 499 (1.65) nm; IR (KBr) ν_{max}: 2971, 2925, 1743, 1700, 1600, 1491, 1368, 1288, 1246, 1180, 1089, 955 cm^{-1}. ^{1}H NMR (600 MHz, CDCl$_3$) δ$_H$ 7.88 (s, 1H), 6.95 (s, 1H), 6.87 (d, J = 15.3 Hz, 1H), 6.19 (d, J = 15.3 Hz, 1H), 5.67 (d, J = 9.7 Hz, 1H), 4.53 (p, J = 7.4 Hz, 1H), 2.55–2.38 (m, 1H), 2.29–2.12 (m, 5H), 1.91 (ddd, J = 16.4, 8.5, 5.0 Hz, 2H), 1.85 (d, J = 1.0 Hz, 3H), 1.84–1.70 (m, 4H), 1.54 (s, 3H), 1.46–1.39 (m,1H), 1.38–1.30 (m, 1H), 1.01 (d, J = 6.7 Hz, 3H), 0.88 (t, J = 7.4 Hz, 3H). ^{13}C NMR (150 MHz, CDCl$_3$) δ$_C$ 194.1, 184.4, 170.2, 149.1, 147.7, 144.9, 144.5, 136.9, 131.7, 115.6, 115.3, 112.7, 102.2, 84.9, 62.7, 35.1, 33.3, 33.2, 30.1, 24.3, 24.3, 23.4, 20.4, 20.4, 12.8, 12.1. HRMS (ESI) for [M + H]$^+$: calcd for $C_{26}H_{33}ClNO_4$: 458.20199. Found: 458.20981.

Compound 22

(R)-5-chloro-2-cyclohexyl-3-((S, 1E, 3E)-3, 5-dimethylhepta-1, 3-dien-1-yl)-7-methyl-6, 8-dioxo-2, 6, 7, 8-tetrahydroisoquinolin-7-yl acetate. Red solid, the yield of 95%; m.p. 136.2–138.1 °C. $[\alpha]_D^{25}$ +16.5 (c 0.02, MeOH); UV (MeOH) λmax (log ε): 248 (3.08), 379 (3.16), 503 (1.51) nm; IR (KBr) ν_{max}: 2955, 2918, 1743, 1705, 1600, 1491, 1368, 1286, 1248, 1180, 1089, 923 cm^{-1}. ^{1}H NMR (600 MHz, CDCl$_3$) δ$_H$ 7.90 (s, 1H), 6.96 (s, 1H), 6.88 (d, J = 15.2 Hz, 1H), 6.14 (d, J = 15.3 Hz, 1H), 5.68 (d, J = 9.7 Hz, 1H), 3.97 (tt, J = 12.0, 3.2 Hz, 1H), 2.65–2.34 (m, 1H), 2.16 (s, 3H), 1.98 (dd, J = 23.3, 12.1 Hz, 5H), 1.85 (d, J = 1.0 Hz, 3H), 1.77 (d, J = 13.3 Hz, 1H), 1.64 (tt, 12.4, 6.3 Hz, 2H), 1.47–1.31 (m, 4H), 1.29–1.16 (m, 3H), 1.02 (d, J = 6.7 Hz, 3H), 0.88 (t, J = 7.4 Hz, 3H). ^{13}C NMR (150 MHz, CDCl$_3$) δ$_C$ 194.1, 184.4, 170.2, 148.6, 147.7, 145.1, 144.6, 136.9, 131.6, 115.1, 115.0, 112.9, 102.1, 84.9, 61.2, 35.1, 33.3, 33.1, 30.1, 25.8, 25.8, 25.0, 23.4, 20.4, 20.4, 12.7, 12.1. LRMS (EI) m/z 472 [M]$^+$.

Compound **23**

(*R*)-2-(4-bromophenyl)-5-chloro-3-((*S*, 1*E*, 3*E*)-3, 5-dimethylhepta-1, 3-dien-1-yl)-7-methyl-6, 8-dioxo-2, 6, 7, 8-tetrahydroisoquinolin-7-yl acetate. Red solid, the yield of 91%; m.p. 190.0–192.3 °C. $[\alpha]_D^{25}$ +16.8 (*c* 0.02, MeOH); UV (MeOH) λmax (log ε): 236 (3.03), 377 (3.25), 493 (1.48) nm; IR (KBr) ν_{max}: 3101, 2959, 2919, 1735, 1707, 1601, 1508, 1487, 1365, 1268, 1250, 1207, 1129, 1080, 960 cm^{-1}. ^{1}H NMR (600 MHz, CDCl$_3$) δ_H 7.76 (s, 1H), 7.73–7.63 (m, 2H), 7.24–7.15 (m, 2H), 7.12 (s, 1H), 6.96 (d, *J* = 15.5 Hz, 1H), 5.67 (d, *J* = 9.7 Hz, 1H), 5.55 (d, *J* = 15.5 Hz, 1H), 2.53–2.32 (m, 1H), 2.17 (s, 3H), 1.63–1.49 (m, 6H), 1.46–1.40 (m, 1H), 1.39–1.31 (m, 1H), 0.99 (d, *J* = 6.6 Hz, 3H), 0.85 (t, *J* = 7.4 Hz, 3H). ^{13}C NMR (150 MHz, CDCl$_3$) δ_C 193.7, 184.9, 170.3, 148.3, 147.2, 143.8, 143.6, 140.9, 139.5, 133.6, 133.6, 131.9, 128.3, 128.3, 124.3, 116.0, 114.7, 110.1, 104.0, 84.8, 35.1, 30.1, 23.2, 20.4, 20.3, 12.5, 12.1. HRMS (ESI) for [M + H]$^+$: calcd for C$_{27}$H$_{28}$ClBrNO$_4$: 544.08120. Found: 544.08855.

Compound **24**

(*R*)-5-chloro-3-((*S*, 1*E*, 3*E*)-3, 5-dimethylhepta-1, 3-dien-1-yl)-2-ethyl-7-methyl-6, 8-dioxo-2, 6, 7, 8-tetrahydroisoquinolin-7-yl acetate. Red solid, the yield of 91%; m.p. 250.0–251.1 °C. $[\alpha]_D^{25}$ +15.5 (*c* 0.02, MeOH); UV (MeOH) λmax (log ε): 238 (3.12), 385 (3.33), 499 (1.47) nm; IR (KBr) ν_{max}: 2955, 2922, 1748, 1712, 1591, 1491, 1368, 1252, 1190, 1093, 853 cm^{-1}. ^{1}H NMR (600 MHz, CDCl$_3$) δ_H 7.78 (s, 1H), 6.99 (s, 1H), 6.95 (d, *J* = 15.3 Hz, 1H), 6.14 (d, *J* = 15.4 Hz, 1H), 5.69 (d, *J* = 9.7 Hz, 1H), 3.92 (q, *J* = 7.3 Hz, 2H), 2.52–2.36 (m, 1H), 2.14 (s, 3H), 1.84 (d, *J* = 0.9 Hz, 3H), 1.52 (s, 3H), 1.46–1.36 (m, 4H), 1.36–1.27 (m, 1H), 1.00 (d, *J* = 6.7 Hz, 3H), 0.86 (t, *J* = 7.4 Hz, 3H). ^{13}C NMR (150 MHz, CDCl$_3$) δ_C 193.9, 184.3, 170.2, 148.2, 147.9, 145.1, 144.8, 140.8, 131.7, 115.0, 114.5, 111.7, 102.0, 84.9, 49.5, 35.1, 30.1, 23.2, 20.4, 20.3, 15.7, 12.7, 12.1. HRMS (ESI) for [M + H]$^+$: calcd for C$_{23}$H$_{29}$ClNO$_4$: 418.17069. Found: 418.17845.

3.1.5. General Procedure for Synthesis of 25

To a solution of sclerotiorin (39 mg, 0.10 mmol) in anhydrous dichloromethane (2 mL), the CH$_3$ONa (54 mg, 10 mmol) was add. The resulting reaction mixture was stirred at 40 °C until the sclerotiorin was disappeared. 12 mL HCl (2M) was added to the mixture to regulate the pH to 2. The mixture was extracted with EtOAc (3 × 5 mL) and the organic phase was washed with saturated brine (3 × 15 mL). Then the organic phase was dried with MgSO$_4$ and concentrated in vacuo. The crude product was purified by column chromatography with eluent of EA/PE (2:1, *v*/*v*) to give the pure compound.

Compound **25**

(*R*)-5-chloro-3-((*S*, 1*E*, 3*E*)-3, 5-dimethylhepta-1, 3-dien-1-yl)-7-hydroxy-7-methyl-6*H*-isochromene-6, 8 (7*H*)-dione. Yellow solid, the yield of 88%; m.p. 130.5–132.1 °C. $[\alpha]_D^{25}$ +221.7 (*c* 0.6, MeOH); UV (MeOH) λmax (log ε): 234 (3.01), 344 (3.13) nm; IR (KBr) ν_{max}: 3537, 2949, 1625, 1510, 1183, 1154, 1131, 1079, 966 cm^{-1}. ^{1}H NMR (600 MHz, CD$_3$OD) δ_H 8.13 (s,1H), 7.17 (d, *J* = 15.7 Hz, 1H), 6.81 (s, 1H), 6.36 (d, *J* = 15.7 Hz, 1H), 5.74 (d, *J* = 9.8 Hz, 1H), 2.63–2.42 (m, 1H), 1.90 (d, *J* = 1.1 Hz, 3H), 1.52 (s, 3H), 1.49–1.46 (m, 1H), 1.38–1.34 (m, 1H), 1.00 (d, *J* = 6.7 Hz, 3H), 0.86 (t, *J* = 7.4 Hz, 3H). ^{13}C NMR (150 MHz, CD$_3$OD) δ_C 196.8, 191.8, 160.2, 153.6, 149.2, 143.8, 141.4, 133.8, 117.5, 116.4, 110.4, 107.0, 84.9, 36.3, 31.2, 27.7, 20.6, 12.5, 12.3. HRMS (ESI) for [M + H]$^+$: calcd for C$_{19}$H$_{22}$ClO$_4$: 349.1128. Found: 349.1212.

3.1.6. General Procedure for Synthesis of 26 and 27

A solution of **25** (39 mg, 0.11 mmol) and anhydride (1.10 mmol) in anhydrous pyridine (3 mL) was refluxed at 90 °C until the **25** disappeared. After being cooled to room temperature, 2 mL HCl (2M) was added to the mixture to regulate the pH to 2. The resulting mixture was extracted with EtOAc (3 × 5 mL) and the organic phase was washed with saturated brine (3 × 15 mL). Then the organic phase was dried with MgSO$_4$ and concentrated in vacuo. The crude product was purified by column chromatography with eluent of EA/PE (1:10, *v*/*v*) to give the pure compound.

Compound 26

(R)-5-chloro-3-((S, 1E, 3E)-3, 5-dimethylhepta-1, 3-dien-1-yl)-7-methyl-6, 8-dioxo-7, 8-dihydro-6H-isochromen-7-yl butyrate. Yellow oil, the yield of 78%. $[\alpha]_D^{25}$ +42.8 (c 0.2, MeOH); UV (MeOH) λmax (log ε): 241 (3.08), 348 (3.15) nm; IR (KBr) ν_{max}: 2949, 1737, 1625, 1509, 1180, 1135, 1079, 958 cm^{-1}. ^{1}H NMR (600 MHz, CD$_3$OD) δ$_H$ 8.19 (s, 1H), 7.19 (d, J = 15.7 Hz, 1H), 6.87 (s, 1H), 6.38 (d, J = 15.7 Hz, 1H), 5.75 (d, J = 9.8 Hz, 1H), 2.63-2.51 (m, 1H), 2.43 (t, J = 7.4 Hz, 2H), 1.90 (d, J = 1.1 Hz, 3H), 1.64 (ddd, J = 7.1, 5.0, 2.5 Hz, 2H), 1.55 (s, 3H), 1.51–1.44 (m, 1H), 1.38-1.34 (m, 5H), 1.04 (d, J = 6.7 Hz, 3H), 0.94 (t, J = 7.1HZ, 3H), 0.90 (t, J = 7.4 Hz, 3H). ^{13}C NMR (150 MHz, CD$_3$OD) δ$_C$ 192.9, 188.1, 174.2, 160.5, 155.1, 149.4, 144.1, 141.5, 133.9, 117.4, 115.8, 110.7, 107.3, 86.0, 36.3, 34.0, 32.2, 31.2, 25.5, 23.4, 22.9, 20.6, 14.2, 12.5, 12.4. HRMS (ESI) for [M + H]$^+$: calcd for C$_{22}$H$_{32}$ClO$_5$: 447.1600. Found: 447.1936.

Compound 27

(R)-5-chloro-3-((S, 1E, 3E)-3, 5-dimethylhepta-1, 3-dien-1-yl)-7-methyl-6, 8-dioxo-7, 8-dihydro-6H-isochromen-7-yl propionate. yellow oil, the yield of 83%. $[\alpha]_D^{25}$ +37.2 (c 0.2, MeOH); UV (MeOH) λmax (log ε): 238 (3.11), 340 (3.08) nm; IR (KBr) ν_{max}: 2959, 1738, 1625, 1506, 1180, 1135, 1079, 962 cm^{-1}. ^{1}H NMR (600 MHz, CD$_3$OD) δ$_H$ 8.20 (s, 1H), 7.19 (d, J = 15.7 Hz, 1H), 6.88 (s, 1H), 6.38 (d, J = 15.7 Hz, 1H), 5.76 (d, J = 9.8 Hz, 1H), 2.59–2.51 (m, 1H), 2.49-2.45 (m, 2H), 1.90 (d, J = 1.0 Hz, 3H), 1.56 (s, 3H), 1.51–1.44 (m, 1H), 1.39–1.34 (m, 1H), 1.14 (t, J = 7.6 Hz, 3H), 1.04 (d, J = 6.6 Hz, 3H), 0.90 (t, J = 7.4 Hz, 3H). ^{13}C NMR (150 MHz, CD$_3$OD) δ$_C$ 192.9, 188.1, 174.9, 160.5, 155.1, 149.5, 144.1, 141.5, 133.9, 117.4, 115.8, 110.7, 107.3, 86.1, 36.3, 31.2, 27.5, 22.9, 20.6, 12.5, 12.3, 9.1. HRMS (ESI) for [M + H]$^+$: calcd for C$_{22}$H$_{26}$ClO$_5$: 405.1391. Found: 405.1465.

3.2. Cytotoxic Activity

The test compounds at a serial final concentration of 50, 25, 12.5, 6.25, and 3.125 μM were evaluated against A549 (human lung cancer cells), MDA-MB-435 (breast cancer cells) using the MTT method. Human breast cancer cell lines MDA-MB-435, human lung cancer cell line A549 were obtained from Keygen Biotech (Nanjing, China) and cultuRed in Dulbecco's modified Eagle's medium (DMEM) (Invitrogen, Carlsbad, CA, USA) supplemented with 5% fetal bovine serum (Hyclone, Logan, UT, USA), 2 mM l-glutamine, 100 mg/mL streptomycin, and 100 units/mL penicillin (Invitrogen). The cultures were maintained at 37 °C in a humidified atmosphere of 5% CO$_2$.

3.3. COX-2 Inhibitory Activity

The in vitro inhibitory of the compounds were evaluated by using COX-2 (human) inhibitor screening assay kit (Item NO:701080) supplied by Cayman chemicals USA. Indomethacin was used as a positive control and the tested compounds was dissolved in DMSO.

Each compound was tested in triplicate at 20 μM, and the percent inhibition for COX-2 was obtained for each experiment. The amount of prostaglandins produced by enzyme in the presence of the test compounds was measured and compared with the control experiments (also performed in triplicate) with enzyme inhibition = 1/concentration of prostaglandin in each enzymatic reaction (The percent inhibition of test compound was inversely proportional to the amount of prostaglandins produced by each wells). Finally, the calculations were performed as per the kit guidelines.

3.4. Molecular Docking

The X-ray crystal structure of COX-2 cyclooxygenase (PDB ID: 5GMN) enzyme was obtained from protein data bank in PDB format as initialing point. The crystal original ligand was extracted from the crystal structure prior to docking. Then, all waters were removed in the crystal structure. Hydrogens addition and Gasteiger charges were executed in turn. The protein was regarded as rigid and the conformation of the ligand was regarded as changeable. The parameter of grid box was set as 100 × 100 × 100 points and center on the protein. The Lamarckian genetic algorithm was used to dock algorithm and number of GA runs was 100. PyMOL [38] and LigPolt [39] were used to visualize and analyze results.

4. Conclusions

In summary, a novel series of sclerotiorin derivatives were synthesized. All compounds have been screened for their cytotoxic activity in vitro. Most of sclerotiorin derivatives showed good to great cytotoxic activity. In addition, the COX-2 inhibitory results disclosed that most of the derivatives displayed considerable inhibition of COX-2. Particularly, compound **3** displayed superior inhibitory ratio of 70.6%, a comparable inhibition ratio to positive indomethacin (78.9%) in 20 μM. Moreover, both in vitro and in silico studies showed that some of the new compounds act as promising COX-2 inhibitors. The results of this research will provide useful information for the design of novel series of anticancer agents with COX-2 inhibitory activity.

Supplementary Materials: The following are available online at https://www.mdpi.com/1660-3397/19/1/12/s1. Figure S1. MS spectrum of compound 1; Figures S2 and S3: NMR (in CDCl3) spectra of compound 1; Figure S4: MS spectrum of compound 2; Figures S5 and S6: NMR (in CDCl3) spectra of compound 2; Figure S7: HRMS spectrum of compound 3; Figures S8 and S9: NMR (in CDCl3) spectra of compound 3; Figure S10. HRMS spectrum of compound 4; Figures S11 and S12: NMR (in CD3OD) spectra of compound 4; Figure S13: HRMS spectrum of compound 5; Figures S14 and S15: NMR (in CDCl3) spectra of compound 5; Figure S16: HRMS spectrum of compound 6; Figures S17 and S18: NMR (in CDCl3) spectra of compound 6; Figure S19: HRMS spectrum of compound 7; Figures S20 and S21: NMR (in CDCl3) spectra of compound 7; Figure S22: HRMS spectrum of compound 8; Figures S23 and S24: NMR (in CDCl3) spectra compound 8; Figure S25: MS spectrum of compound 9; Figures S26 and S27: NMR (in CDCl3) spectrum of compound 9; Figure S27: HRMS spectrum of compound 10; Figures S28 and S29: NMR (in CDCl3) spectra of compound 10; Figure S30: HRMS spectrum of compound 11; Figures S31 and S32: NMR (in CDCl3) spectra of compound 11; Figure S33: MS spectrum of compound 12; Figure S34: ^{1}H NMR (in CDCl3) spectra of compound 12; Figure S35: HRMS spectrum of compound 13; Figures S36 and S37: NMR (in CDCl3) spectra of compound 13; Figure S38: HRMS spectrum of compound 14; Figures S39 and S40: NMR (in CDCl3) spectra of compound 14; Figure S41: MS spectrum of compound 15; Figures S42 and S43: NMR (in CDCl3) spectra of compound 15; Figure S44: MS spectrum of compound 16; Figures S45 and S46: NMR (in CDCl3) spectra of compound 16; Figure S47: HRMS spectrum of compound 17; Figures S48 and S49: NMR (in CDCl3) spectra of compound 17; Figure S50: HRMS spectrum of compound 18; Figures S51 and S52: NMR (in CDCl3) spectra of compound 18; Figure S53: HRMS spectrum of compound 19; Figures S54 and S55: NMR (in CDCl3) spectra of compound 19; Figure S56: HRMS spectrum of compound 20; Figures S57 and S58: NMR (in CDCl3) spectra of compound 20; Figure S59: HRMS spectrum of compound 21; Figures S60 and S61: NMR (in CDCl3) spectra of compound 21; Figure S62: MS spectrum of compound 22; Figures S63 and S64: NMR (in CDCl3) spectra of compound 22; Figure S65: HRMS spectrum of compound 23; Figures S66 and S67: NMR (in CDCl3) spectra of compound 23; Figure S68c: HRMS spectrum of compound 24; Figures S69 and S70: NMR (in CDCl3) spectra of compound 24; Figure S71: HRMS spectrum of compound 25; Figures S72 and S73: NMR (in CDCl3) spectra of compound 25; Figure S74: HRMS spectrum of compound 26; Figures S75 and S76: NMR (in CDCl3) spectra of compound 26; Figure S77: HRMS spectrum of compound 27; Figures S78 and S79: NMR (in CDCl3) spectra of compound 27.

Author Contributions: Conceptualization, Y.L.; methodology, T.C., Y.H., J.Y.; software, T.C.; formal analysis, Y.L., J.Y.; investigation, T.C., Y.H., J.H., X.W., F.Z., J.L., G.Y.; resources, Y.L., J.Y.; data curation, Y.L., J.Y.; writing—original draft preparation, T.C.; writing—review and editing, T.C., Y.L.; visualization, T.C., Y.H., J.H., X.W., F.Z., J.L., G.Y., Y.L., J.Y.; supervision, Y.L.; project administration, Y.L.; funding acquisition, Y.L. All authors have read and agreed to the published version of the manuscript.

Funding: This research received no external funding.

Data Availability Statement: The data presented in this study are available in the Supplementary Materials.

Acknowledgments: The authors thank Idrees Sumra (South China Normal University) for her help in language polish of this paper and gratefully acknowledge grants from the National Natural Science Foundation of China (41876153), the Key Project of Natural Science Foundation of Guangdong Province (2016A030311026) and the Guangdong MEPP Fund (GDOE [2019]A21).

Conflicts of Interest: The authors declare no conflict of interest

References

1. Bray, F.; Ferlay, J.; Soerjomataram, I.; Siegel, R.L.; Torre, L.A.; Jemal, A. Global cancer statistics 2018: Globocan estimates of incidence and mortality worldwide for 36 cancers in 185 countries. *CA A Cancer J. Clin.* **2018**, *68*, 394–424. [CrossRef] [PubMed]
2. Eckhardt, B.L.; Cao, Y.; Redfern, A.D.; Chi, L.H.; Anderson, R.L. Activation of canonical bmp4-smad7 signaling suppresses breast cancer metastasis. *Cancer Res.* **2020**, *80*, 1304–1315. [CrossRef] [PubMed]
3. Nguyen, D.X.; Massagué, J. Genetic determinants of cancer metastasis. *Nat. Rev. Genet.* **2007**, *8*, 341–352. [CrossRef] [PubMed]
4. Shi, X.; Fang, H.; Guo, Y.; Yuan, H.; Guo, Z.; Wang, X. Anticancer copper complex with nucleus, mitochondrion and cyclooxygenase-2 as multiple targets. *J. Inorg. Biochem.* **2019**, *190*, 38–44. [CrossRef] [PubMed]
5. Gomes, R.N.; Souza, F.C.; Colquhoun, A. Eicosanoids and cancer. *Clinics* **2018**, *73*, e530s. [CrossRef]
6. Moore, M.M.; Chua, W.; Charles, K.A.; Clarke, S.J. Inflammation and cancer: Causes and consequences. *Clin. Pharmacol Ther.* **2010**, *87*, 504–508. [CrossRef]
7. Wu, Y.; Antony, S.; Meitzler, J.L.; Doroshow, J.H. Molecular mechanisms underlying chronic inflammation-associated cancers. *Cancer Lett.* **2014**, *345*, 164–173. [CrossRef]
8. Wilson, G.S.; George, J. Physical and chemical insults induce inflammation and gastrointestinal cancers. *Cancer Lett.* **2014**, *345*, 190–195. [CrossRef]
9. Ohshima, H.; Tazawa, H.; Sylla, B.S.; Sawa, T. Prevention of human cancer by modulation of chronic inflammatory processes. *Mutat. Res. Fund. Mol. Mech.* **2005**, *591*, 110–122. [CrossRef]
10. Hanahan, D.; Weinberg, R.A. Hallmarks of cancer: The next generation. *Cell* **2011**, *144*, 646–674. [CrossRef]
11. Mishan, M.A.; Tabari, M.A.K.; Zargari, M.; Bagheri, A. Micrornas in the anticancer effects of celecoxib: A systematic review. *Eur. J. Pharmacol.* **2020**, *882*, 173325. [CrossRef] [PubMed]
12. Goradel, N.H.; Najafi, M.; Salehi, E.; Farhood, B.; Mortezaee, K. Cyclooxygenase-2 in cancer: A review. *J. Cell. Physiol.* **2019**, *234*, 5683–5699. [CrossRef] [PubMed]
13. Moon, H.; White, A.C.; Borowsky, A.D. New insights into the functions of Cox-2 in skin and esophageal malignancies. *Exp. Mol. Med.* **2020**, *52*, 538–547. [CrossRef] [PubMed]
14. Sminia, P.; Kuipers, G.K.; Geldof, A.; Lafleur, V.; Slotman, B. COX-2 inhibitors act as radiosensitizer in tumor treatment. *Biomed. Pharmacother.* **2005**, *59*, 272–275. [CrossRef]
15. Han, Y.; Guo, W.; Ren, T.; Wang, S.; Liu, K.; Zheng, B.; Yang, K.; Zhang, H.; Liang, X. Tumor-associated macrophages promote lung metastasis and induce epithelial-mesenchymal transition in osteosarcoma by activating the COX-2/STAT3 axis. *Cancer Lett.* **2019**, *18*, 116–125. [CrossRef] [PubMed]
16. Patti, R.; GumiRed, K.; Reddanna, P.; Sutton, L.N.; Phillips, P.C.; Reddy, C.D. Overexpression of cyclooxygenase-2 (COX-2) in human primitive neuroectodermal tumors: Effect of celecoxib and rofecoxib. *Cancer Lett.* **2002**, *180*, 13–21. [CrossRef]
17. Joanna, B.; Jolanta, B.; Agnieszka, G.; Diana, H.Z.; Krystyna, S. Vitamin, D. linoleic acid, arachidonic acid and COX-2 in colorectal cancer patients in relation to disease stage, tumour localisation and disease progression. *Arab J. Gastroenterol.* **2019**, *20*, 121–126. [CrossRef]
18. Xuan, Y.; Wang, J.; Ban, L.; Lu, J.-J.; Yi, C.; Li, Z.; Yu, W.; Li, M.; Xu, T.; Yang, W.; et al. hnRNPA2/B1 activates cyclooxygenase-2 and promotes tumor growth in human lung cancers. *Mol. Oncol.* **2016**, *10*, 610–624. [CrossRef]
19. Koki, A.T.; Masferrer, J.L. Celecoxib: A specific COX-2 inhibitor with anticancer properties. *Cancer Control.* **2002**, *9*, 28–35. [CrossRef]
20. Brown, J.R.; Dubois, R.N. COX-2: A molecular target for colorectal cancer prevention. *J. Clin.Oncol.* **2005**, *23*, 2840–2855. [CrossRef]
21. Wang, L.; Zhang, L.-F.; Wu, J.; Xu, S.-J.; Xu, Y.-Y.; Li, D.; Lou, J.-T.; Liu, M.-F. IL-1b-mediated repression of microRNA-101 is crucial for inflammation-promoted lung tumorigenesis. *Cancer Res.* **2014**, *74*, 4720–4730. [CrossRef] [PubMed]
22. Zhang, M.; Xu, Z.-G.; Shi, Z.; Shao, D.; Li, O.; Li, W.; Li, Z.-J.; Wang, K.-Z.; Chen, L. Inhibitory effect of celecoxib in lung carcinoma by regulation of cyclooxygenase-2/cytosolic phospholipase A_2 and peroxisome proliferator-activated receptor gamma. *Mol. Cell. Biochem.* **2011**, *355*, 233–240. [CrossRef] [PubMed]
23. Gallego, G.A.; Prado, S.D.; Fonseca, P.J.; Campelo, R.G.; Espinosa, J.C.; Aparicio, L.M.A. Cyclooxygenase-2 (COX-2): A molecular target in prostate cancer. *Clin. Transl. Oncol.* **2007**, *9*, 694–702. [CrossRef] [PubMed]
24. Jimenez, C. Marine natural products in medicinal chemistry. *ACS Med. Chem. Lett.* **2018**, *9*, 959–961. [CrossRef]
25. Kiuru, P.; D'auria, M.V.; Muller, C.; Muller, C.D.; Tammela, P.; Vuorela, H.; Kauhaluoma, J.Y. Exploring marine resources for bioactive compounds. *Planta Med.* **2014**, *80*, 1234–1246. [CrossRef]
26. Kwong, T.F.N.; Miao, L.; Li, X.; Qian, P.Y. Novel antifouling and antimicrobial compound from a marine-derived fungus *Ampelomyces* sp. *Mar. Biotechnol.* **2006**, *8*, 634–640. [CrossRef]
27. Laurent, D.; Pietra, F. Antiplasmodial marine natural products in the perspective of current chemotherapy and prevention of malaria. A review. *Mar. Biotechnol.* **2006**, *8*, 433–447. [CrossRef]

28. Fan, M.; Nath, A.K.; Tang, Y.; Choi, Y.J.; Debnath, T.; Choi, E.J.; Kim, E.K. Investigation of the anti-prostate cancer properties of marine-derived compounds. *Mar. Drugs* **2018**, *16*, 160. [CrossRef]
29. Watanabe, H. On the structure of sclerotiorine (1). *Yakugaku Zasshi* **1952**, *72*, 807–811. [CrossRef]
30. Jia, Q.; Du, Y.; Wang, C.; Wang, Y.; Zhu, T.; Zhu, W. Azaphilones from the marine sponge-derived fungus *Penicillium sclerotiorum* OUCMDZ-3839. *Mar. Drugs* **2019**, *17*, 260. [CrossRef]
31. Wei, M.-Y.; Wang, C.-F.; Wang, K.-L.; Qian, P.-Y.; Wang, C.-Y.; Shao, C.-L. Preparation, structure, and potent antifouling activity of sclerotioramine derivatives. *Mar. Biotechnol.* **2017**, *19*, 372–378. [CrossRef] [PubMed]
32. Chen, D.; Ma, S.; He, L.; Yuan, P.; She, Z.; Lu, Y. Sclerotiorin inhibits protein kinase g from mycobacterium tuberculosis and impairs mycobacterial growth in macrophages. *Tuberculosis* **2017**, *103*, 37–43. [CrossRef] [PubMed]
33. Wiglenda, T.; Groenke, N.; Hoffmann, W.; Manz, L.D.; Buntru, A.; Brusendorf, L.; Neuendorf, N.; Schnoegl, S.; Heaning, C.; Schmieder, P.; et al. Sclerotiorin stabilizes the assembly of nonfibrillar abeta42 oligomers with low toxicity, seeding activity, and beta-sheet content. *J. Mol. Biol.* **2020**, *432*, 2080–2098. [CrossRef] [PubMed]
34. Gao, J.-M.; Yang, S.-X.; Qin, J.-C. Azaphilones: Chemistry and biology. *Chem. Rev.* **2013**, *113*, 4755–4811. [CrossRef] [PubMed]
35. Lucido, M.J.; Orlando, B.J.; Vecchio, A.J.; Malkowski, M.G. Crystal structure of aspirin-acetylated human cyclooxygenase-2: Insight into the formation of products with reversed stereochemistry. *Biochemistry* **2016**, *55*, 1226–1238. [CrossRef] [PubMed]
36. Morris, G.M.; Huey, R.; Lindstrom, W.; Sanner, M.F.; Olson, A.L. AutoDock4 and AutoDockTools4: Automated docking with selective receptor flexibility. *J. Comp. Chem.* **2009**, *30*, 2785–2791. [CrossRef]
37. Liu, Y.; Yang, Q.; Xia, G.; Huang, H.; Li, H.; Ma, L.; Lu, Y.; He, L.; Xia, X.; She, Z. Polyketides with α-glucosidase inhibitory activity from a mangrove endophytic fungus, *Penicillium* sp. HN29-3B1. *J. Nat. Prod.* **2015**, *78*, 1816–1822. [CrossRef]
38. DeLano, W.L. The PyMOL Molecular Graphics System. 2002. Available online: http://www.pymol.org (accessed on 30 August 2020).
39. Wallace, A.C.; Laskowski, R.A.; Thornton, J.M. LIGPLOT: A program to generate schematic diagrams of protein-ligand interactions. *Protein Eng.* **1995**, *8*, 127–134. [CrossRef]

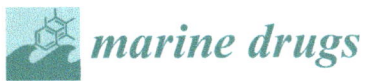

Article

Phenylhydrazone and Quinazoline Derivatives from the Cold-Seep-Derived Fungus *Penicillium oxalicum*

Ya-Ping Liu [1,2], Sheng-Tao Fang [1], Zhen-Zhen Shi [1], Bin-Gui Wang [3], Xiao-Nian Li [4] and Nai-Yun Ji [1,*]

1. Yantai Institute of Coastal Zone Research, Center for Ocean Mega-Science, Chinese Academy of Sciences, Yantai 264003, China; ypliu@yic.ac.cn (Y.-P.L.); stfang@yic.ac.cn (S.-T.F.); zzshi@yic.ac.cn (Z.-Z.S.)
2. University of Chinese Academy of Sciences, Beijing 100049, China
3. Laboratory of Marine Biology and Biotechnology of the Qingdao National Laboratory for Marine Science and Technology, Key Laboratory of Experimental Marine Biology at the Institute of Oceanology, Center for Ocean Mega-Science, Chinese Academy of Sciences, Qingdao 266071, China; wangbg@ms.qdio.ac.cn
4. Kunming Institute of Botany, Chinese Academy of Sciences, Kunming 650201, China; lixiaonian@mail.kib.ac.cn
* Correspondence: nyji@yic.ac.cn; Tel.: +86-535-210-9176

Abstract: Three new phenylhydrazones, penoxahydrazones A–C (compounds **1**–**3**), and two new quinazolines, penoxazolones A (compound **4**) and B (compound **5**), with unique linkages were isolated from the fungus *Penicillium oxalicum* obtained from the deep sea cold seep. Their structures and relative configurations were assigned by analysis of 1D/2D NMR and mass spectroscopic data, and the absolute configurations of **1**, **4**, and **5** were established on the basis of X-ray crystallography or ECD calculations. Compound **1** represents the first natural phenylhydrazone-bearing steroid, while compounds **2** and **3** are rarely occurring phenylhydrazone tautomers. Compounds **4** and **5** are enantiomers that feature quinazoline and cinnamic acid units. Some isolates exhibited inhibition of several marine phytoplankton species and marine-derived bacteria.

Keywords: *Penicillium oxalicum*; deep sea; cold seep; phenylhydrazone; quinazoline

1. Introduction

Microorganisms of different origin may possess unique genomes and potentials that enable them to produce rare metabolites [1,2]. As an important class of microorganisms, fungi are substantial sources of striking secondary metabolites with diverse structures and bioactivities. The fungal species *Penicillium oxalicum* is widespread in terrestrial and marine environments, and its secondary metabolites are abundant. In the investigation towards terrestrial-derived *P. oxalicum*, an azo compound [3], a diterpene [4], a diphenylmethanone [5], a spiro-oxindole alkaloid [6], isochroman carboxylic acids [3], and polyketides [7] were obtained from soil-derived isolates, several limonoids [8], butyrolactones [9], and isocoumarins [10] were discovered from plant-derived isolates, and alkaloids with 1,3-thiazole and 1,2,4-thiadiazole units [11] were separated from an animal-derived isolate. On the other hand, more and more marine-derived *P. oxalicum* strains were chemically examined. A variety of metabolites including chromones [12–15] from marine-animal-derived strains, phenolic enamides [16], meroterpenoids [16], and alkaloids [17,18] from marine-plant-derived strains, and secalonic acids [19–21], anthraquinones [22], alkaloids [23], and a diphenylmethanone [21] from marine-sediment-derived strains were characterized. It is obvious that the metabolic profiles of *P. oxalicum* strains varied with their habitats. Secondary metabolite biosynthesis genes from fungi have been found to be expressed in deep sea sediments [24,25]. However, chemical surveys were rarely performed on deep-sea-derived *P. oxalicum* strains, especially cold-seep-derived ones.

2. Results and Discussion

Penicillium oxalicum 13–37 was isolated from the deep sea cold seep sediments. After static fermentation at room temperature for 30 days, the cultures were extracted with organic solvents and then purified by repeated column chromatography on silica gel, RP-18, and Sephadex LH-20 as well as semipreparative HPLC to yield penoxahydrazones A–C (**1–3**), penoxazolones A (**4**) and B (**5**), and dankasterone A (Figure 1). The structures of these compounds were identified by extensive 1D/2D NMR and mass spectrometric data, X-ray crystallographic analysis or ECD calculations.

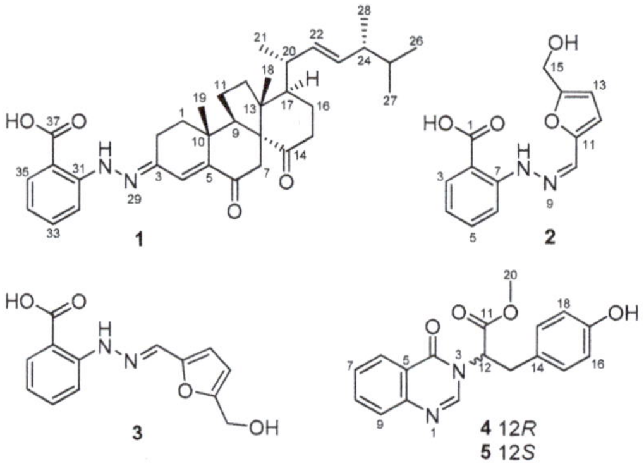

Figure 1. Chemical structures of compounds **1–5**.

Penoxahydrazone A (**1**) was purified as yellow crystals. The molecular formula $C_{35}H_{46}N_2O_4$ was determined by interpretation of HRESIMS data. In combination with HSQC correlations, the ^{1}H NMR spectrum (Table 1) displayed four methyl doublets, two methyl singlets, two double doublets and one singlet ascribable to three olefinic protons, two double doublets and two doublets attributable to four aromatic protons, and a range of signals at δ_H 1.3–2.9 for seven methylenes and five methines. The ^{13}C NMR spectrum (Table 1) exhibited 35 resonances, classified into six methyls, seven methylenes, twelve methines, and ten non-protonated carbons by DEPT experiments. The above NMR data partially resembled those for co-isolated dankasterone A [26]. Replacing the signal at δ_C 199.1 for the C-3 carbonyl group in dankasterone A, a signal at δ_C 144.4 appeared in the ^{13}C NMR spectrum of **1**, and this carbon atom was located at C-3 by its heteronuclear multiple bond correlation (HMBC) with H-1a. Additionally, the remaining NMR data corresponded to an ortho-substituted benzoic acid unit [27], as supported by the ^{1}H-^{1}H chemical shift correlation spectroscopy (COSY) correlations from H-32 thoroughly to H-35 and the HMBC correlations from H-32 to C-36, from H-33 to C-31 and C-35, and from H-35 to C-33 and C-37. To satisfy the elemental composition, an azo unit was situated between C-3 and C-31, which was supported by the HMBC correlations from H-30 to C-3, C-31, C-32, and C-36. Thus, the whole connectivity of **1** was established, which was further validated by other COSY and HMBC correlations (Figure 2). The absolute configuration was determined by X-ray crystallographic analysis (Figure 3). A suitable single crystal was obtained from a solution of EtOH with a drop of water and then subjected to the X-ray diffraction analysis using Cu Kα radiation [28]. Consequently, the absolute configuration of **1** was assigned to be 8R, 9R, 10R, 13R, 17R, 20R, and 24R. Although more than 200 natural molecules with a nitrogen–nitrogen bond have been found so far, phenylhydrazone derivatives rarely occurred [27,29]. Furthermore, **1** represents the first natural phenylhydrazone-bearing steroid.

Table 1. ^{1}H and ^{13}C NMR data for compound **1** (in CDCl$_3$, 500 MHz).

Pos	δ_c, Type	δ_H (J in Hz)
1a	37.6, CH$_2$	1.98, m
1b		1.90, m
2a	20.9, CH$_2$	2.60, m
2b		2.40, m
3	144.4, C	
4	131.7, CH	7.08, s
5	141.6, C	
6	199.2, C	
7a	41.3, CH$_2$	2.61, d (16.1)
7b		2.53, d (16.1)
8	62.8, C	
9	49.5, CH	2.85, t (9.4)
10	35.6, C	
11a	25.6, CH$_2$	1.92, m
11b		1.81, m
12a	39.2, CH$_2$	1.75, m
12b		1.62, dt (12.5, 8.1)
13	53.8, C	
14	215.9, C	
15a	38.2, CH$_2$	2.56, m
15b		2.46, m
16a	23.2, CH$_2$	1.86, m
16b		1.74, m
17	50.8, CH	1.39, br d (12.7)
18	17.3, CH$_3$	1.00, s
19	24.5, CH$_3$	1.16, s
20	37.5, CH	2.39, m
21	23.6, CH$_3$	1.07, d (7.0)
22	132.8, CH	5.25, dd (15.5, 4.6)
23	135.0, CH	5.28, dd (15.5, 5.0)
24	43.4, CH	1.87, m
25	33.2, CH	1.47, octet (6.8)
26	19.8, CH$_3$	0.82, d (6.8)
27	20.2, CH$_3$	0.84, d (6.8)
28	17.8, CH$_3$	0.92, d (6.8)
30		11.07, s
31	147.3, C	
32	114.1, CH	7.66, d (8.5)
33	135.8, CH	7.45, dd (8.5, 7.1)
34	119.1, CH	6.84, dd (7.8, 7.1)
35	131.7, CH	7.98, d (7.8)
36	109.4, C	
37	172.4, C	

Penoxahydrazones B(**2**) and C(**3**) were obtained as a brown powder. During the purification process, **2** could gradually turn to **3** and vice versa. The sodium adducts ion peaks at m/z 283.0695 and m/z 283.0691 determined by high performance liquid chromatography-electrospray mass spectrometry (HPLC-ESIMS) suggested that **2** and **3** feature the same molecular formula C$_{13}$H$_{12}$N$_2$O$_4$. On the basis of these characteristics, it is inferred that these two compounds should be a pair of tautomers. The ^{1}H and ^{13}C NMR spectra (Table 2) showed two sets of signals with a ratio of 2:1. Aided by HSQC data, they indicated the presence of one oxymethylene, 11 aromatic/olefinic methines, and one carboxyl in each compound. Similar to the analysis of the structure of compound **1**, an ortho-substituted benzoic acid unit was deduced to be present in both **2** and **3** based on their NMR data [27], which was further supported by the COSY and the HMBC correlations (Figure 2). Compared to the NMR data of δ-hydroxymethyl-α-vinylfuran [30], the remaining carbon signals could be assigned to δ-hydroxymethyl furan attached by an olefinic methine group at α position, which was verified by the COSY correlation between H-12 and H-13 and the HMBC correlations from H-10 to C-11 and C-12 and from H$_2$-15 to C-13 and C-14. To match the molecular formula, these two moieties were linked via an azo unit, as seen from the HMBC correlation from the de-shielded exchangeable proton to C-7 and C-10 in **2**. Although this HMBC correlation was not detected for **3**, the similarities of NMR data for C-7 and C-10 between **2** and **3** suggested the same connectivity of them. Through analysis of the whole structures of **2** and **3**, their tautomerization probably arose from the geometric isomerization of the double bond between N-9 and C-10. The ^{13}C NMR data of 9Z and 9E isomers were computed using the gauge-independent atomic orbital (GIAO) method at the B3LYP/6-31+G(d,p) level via Gaussian 09 software [31] and then were input into Sarotti's DP4+ sheet (https://sarotti-nmr.weebly.com) [32]. According to the DP4+ probabilities for ^{1}H (100% between 9Z isomer and **2**, 100% between 9E isomer and **3**, Tables S1 and S2) and ^{13}C NMR data (99.99% between 9Z isomer and **2**, 98.80% between 9E isomer and **3**, Tables S3 and S4), **2** and **3** were proposed to possess 9Z and 9E configurations, respectively. These two tautomers are possibly formed by the reaction between 2-hydrazinylbenzoic acid and 5-hydroxymethylfurfural, and the latter is a valuable platform chemical produced mainly by the hydrolysis of saccharides [30].

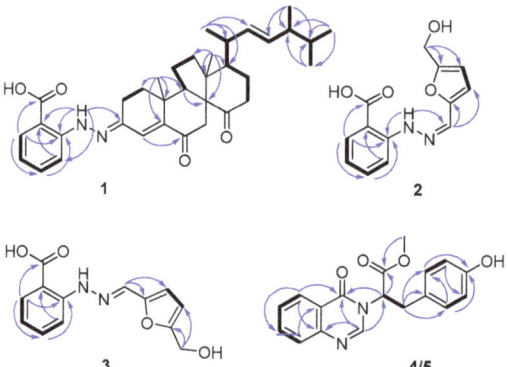

Figure 2. Key COSY (bold lines) and HMBC (arrows) correlations of compounds **1–5**.

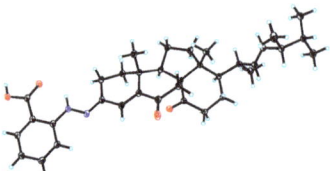

Figure 3. X-ray crystallographic structure of compound **1**.

Penoxazolones A (**4**) and B (**5**) were originally purified as a colorless oil by a series of achiral isolation. HRESIMS analysis gave the molecular formula C$_{18}$H$_{16}$N$_2$O$_4$. In accordance with the molecular formula, the ^{1}H and ^{13}C NMR spectra (Table 3) displayed just one set of signals assignable to one methyl, one methylene, ten methines, and six non-protonated carbons aided by DEPT and HSQC data. A detailed comparison of NMR data revealed the presence of a quinazolin-4(3H)-one unit [33], which was supported by the COSY correlations from H-6 thoroughly to H-9 and the HMBC correlations from H-2 to C-4 and C-10, from H-6 to C-4, C-8, and C-10, from H-8 to C-6 and C-10, and from H-9 to C-5. However, the signal for an exchangeable proton (H-3) in quinazolin-4(3H)-one was missing. The remaining NMR data corresponded to methyl 3-(4-hydroxyphenyl) propanoate [34], except for the presence of signals for a de-shielded methine group and the lack of signals for a methylene group. This methine group was adjacent to the ester carbonyl group as seen from their HMBC correlation, and it was bonded to N-3 of the quinazolin-4(3*H*)-one moiety on the basis of its HMBC correlations with C-2 and C-4. Thus, the planar structure was established, validated by other COSY and HMBC correlations (Figure 2). Before assignment of the absolute configuration, a chiral HPLC was used to detect the enantiomeric purity due to the presence of a stereogenic carbon atom (C-12). As a result, enantiomers **4** and **5** with a ratio of 1:2 were obtained (Figure S26), and they exhibited opposite optical rotations. To ascertain the absolute configurations of **4** and **5**, their ECD spectra were determined in MeOH and simulated via the time-dependent density function theory method with the same solvent. Based on the similarities between experimental and calculated ECD spectra (Figure 4), the absolute configurations of **4** and **5** were proposed as 12R and 12S, respectively. These two enantiomers might be yielded by adding quinazolin-4(3H)-one to methyl 3-(4-hydroxyphenyl)acrylate through a carbocation intermediate.

Table 2. ^{1}H and ^{13}C NMR data for compounds **2** and **3** (in DMSO-d_6).

Pos	2		3	
	δ_C, Type	δ_H (J in Hz)	δ_C, Type	δ_H (J in Hz)
1	169.6, C		169.5, C	
2	111.0, C		110.1, C	
3	131.3, CH	7.89, dd (7.9, 1.3)	131.2, CH	7.84, dd (7.9, 1.4)
4	118.3, CH	6.84, br dd (7.9, 7.1)	117.6, CH	6.79, dd (7.9, 7.1)
5	134.4, CH	7.48, br dd (8.4, 7.1)	134.4, CH	7.48, br dd (8.4, 7.1)
6	112.9, CH	7.68, br d (8.4)	113.1, CH	7.59, br d (8.4)
7	147.1, C		146.9, C	
8		12.33, br s		11.23, br s
10	125.4, CH	7.27, s	131.4, CH	8.03, s
11	146.8, C		149.4, C	
12	113.7, CH	7.01, d (3.3)	112.0, CH	6.65, d (3.3)
13	108.9, CH	6.54, d (3.3)	109.2, CH	6.40, d (3.3)
14	157.2, C		156.7, C	
15	56.0, CH$_2$	4.57, s	55.8, CH$_2$	4.44, s

Table 3. ^{1}H and ^{13}C NMR data for compounds **4** and **5** (in DMSO-d_6).

Pos	δ_C, Type	δ_H (J in Hz)
2	147.2, CH	8.01, s
4	159.9, C	
5	121.1, C	
6	126.1, CH	8.12, dd (7.9, 1.2)
7	127.4, CH	7.55, dd (7.9, 7.1)
8	134.8, CH	7.83, ddd (8.1, 7.1, 1.2)
9	127.2, CH	7.62, d (8.1)
10	147.4, C	
11	169.3, C	
12	60.4, CH	5.41, dd (11.1, 4.9)
13a	33.3, CH$_2$	3.41, dd (14.3, 4.9)
13b		3.32, dd (14.3, 11.1)
14	126.1, C	
15	129.8, CH	6.87, d (8.4)
16	115.3, CH	6.54, d (8.4)
17	156.2, C	
18	115.3, CH	6.54, d (8.4)
19	129.8, CH	6.87, d (8.4)
20	52.6, CH$_3$	3.69, s

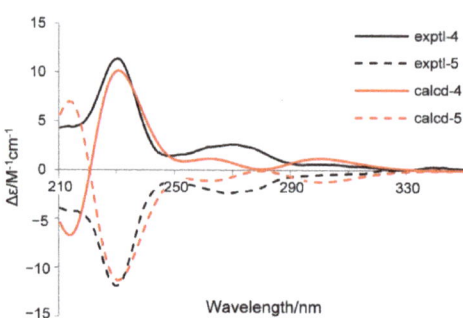

Figure 4. Experimental and calculated ECD spectra of **4** and **5** in MeOH.

Mariculture is often threatened by harmful algal blooms and pathogenic bacteria. Compounds **1–5** and dankasterone A were assayed for inhibition of the three microalgae *Chattonella marina*, *Heterosigma akashiwo*, and *Prorocentrum donghaiense* [35], and the results are shown in Table 4. Isolates **1**, **4**, **5**, and dankasterone A could inhibit the three microalga species with the IC_{50} values ranging from 0.57 to 9.1 µg/mL. The noticeable activities of **1** and dankasterone A suggested that the steroid moiety seemed to be the key pharmacophore. In combination with the weak activities of **2/3**, the slightly higher activities of **1** than those of dankasterone A indicated that the 2-hydrazinylbenzoic acid unit appeared weak to increase the activities. In addition, their inhibition against four marine-derived bacterial pathogens including *Vibrio anguillarum*, *Vibrio harveyi*, *Vibrio parahaemolyticus*, and *Vibrio splendidus* was detected using the disk diffusion method [36]. We found that **1**, **4**, **5**, and dankasterone A showed moderate inhibition against *V. harveyi* and *V. parahaemolyticus*, and their inhibition zone diameters exceeded 10 mm at 20 µg/disk. The MIC values of active molecules were also measured, but only those of **4** and **5** (8 µg/mL) appeared lower than 10 µg/mL. A structure–activity relationship analysis revealed that both enantiomerization of **4** and **5** and addition of 2-hydrazinylbenzoic acid to dankasterone A had almost no influence on the antibacterial activities. In view of the above inhibitory effects of **1**, **4**, **5**, and dankasterone A on the microalgal and bacterial species, their toxicities to the marine zooplankton *Artemia salina* were also tested. All the isolates possess low toxicities, with LC_{50} values being higher that 40 µg/mL.

Table 4. Inhibition of marine microalgae and marine-derived bacteria.

Compounds	IC_{50} (µg/mL)			Inhibitory Zone Diameter (mm) at 20 µg/disk				LC_{50} (µg/mL)
	C. marina	*H. akashiwo*	*P. donghaiense*	*V. anguillarum*	*V. harveyi*	*V. parahaemolyticus*	*V. splendidus*	*A. salina*
1	1.2	3.7	0.68	0	11	12	0	58
2/3	17	>100	5.4	0	0	7.0	9.7	>100
4	2.8	8.1	0.57	7.0	13	11	7.3	>100
5	9.1	9.0	1.2	0	13	11	7.0	>100
dankasterone A	1.9	4.6	1.0	7.0	12	12	0	43
$K_2Cr_2O_7$	0.60	2.4	1.2					18
chloramphenicol				18	29	28	23	

3. Materials and Methods

3.1. General Experimental Procedures

Melting points were measured with an SGW X-4 micro melting point apparatus (Shanghai Precision & Scientific Instrument Co., Ltd, Shanghai, China). Optical rotations were determined on an SGW-3 polarimeter (Shanghai Shenguang Instrument Co., Ltd., Shanghai, China). UV and ECD spectra were measured on a Chirascan CD spectrometer

(Applied Photophysics Ltd., Surrey, UK). IR spectra were recorded on a Nicolet iS50 FT-IR spectrometer (Thermo Fisher Scientific, Waltham, MA, USA). 1D and 2D NMR spectra were acquired on a Bruker Avance III 500 NMR spectrometer (Bruker Corp., Billerica, MA, USA). Low and high resolution ESI mass spectra were obtained on an Agilent G6230 (Agilent Technologies Inc., Santa Clara, CA, USA) or a Waters ACQUITY TOF mass spectrometer (Waters Corp., Milford, MA, USA). Agilent 1260 HPLC system (Agilent Technologies Inc., Santa Clara, CA, USA) with an Eclipse SB-C18 (5 μm, 9.4 × 250 mm) column or a (R, R) Whelk-O1 chiral column (10 μm, 4.6 × 250 mm) was used for HPLC separation. Silica gel (200–300 mesh, Qingdao Haiyang Chemical Co. Qingdao, China), RP-18 (AAG12S50, YMC Co. Ltd., Kyoto, Japan), and Sephadex LH-20 (GE Healthcare, Uppsala, Sweden) were employed for column chromatography (CC). Precoated silica gel plates (GF-254, Qingdao Haiyang Chemical Co., Qingdao, China) were used for thin-layer chromatography (TLC). Gaussian 09 software (IA32W-G09RevC.01, Gaussian, Inc., Wallingford, CT, USA) was applied to quantum chemical calculations.

3.2. Fungal Material and Fermentation

Penicillium oxalicum 13–37 was isolated from deep sea cold seep sediments. The species was identified by morphology and by analysis of the ITS regions of its rDNA, whose sequence data have been deposited at GenBank with the accession number MT898464. Its fermentation was carried out statically at room temperature for 30 days in 200 × 1 L Erlenmeyer flasks, each containing 50 g rice, 2 g glucose, 0.6 g peptone, 0.5 g yeast extract, 0.3 g monosodium glutamate, 0.1 g NaBr, 50 mL pure water, and 50 mL natural seawater from the coast of Yantai, China.

3.3. Extraction and Isolation

At the end of the above fermentation, the mycelia were dried in the shade and then exhaustively extracted with CH_2Cl_2 and MeOH (1:1, *v/v*). After removing organic solvents by evaporation under vacuum, the residue was partitioned between EtOAc and H_2O to give an EtOAc-soluble extract (536 g). The extract was subjected to silica gel CC for separation with step-gradient solvent systems consisting of petroleum ether (PE)/EtOAc (50:1 to 0:1) and then CH_2Cl_2/MeOH (10:1 to 0:1). Based on TLC analysis, eight fractions (Frs. 1-8) were obtained. Fr. 5 eluted with PE/EtOAc (1:1) and was further purified by CC on RP-18 (MeOH/H_2O, 93:7 to 49:1) to give two subfractions, Fr. 5-1 and 5-2. Fr. 5-1 eluted with MeOH/H_2O (93:7) and was further purified by Sephadex LH-20 (CH_2Cl_2/MeOH, 1:1) CC and semipreparative HPLC (acetonitrile/H_2O, 19:1 to 49:1) to obtain dankasterone A (13.4 mg). Fr. 5-2 eluted with MeOH/H_2O (49:1) and was further purified by Sephadex LH-20 (MeOH) CC to afford **1** (9.4 mg). Fr. 6 eluted with EtOAc and was further purified by CC on RP-18 MeOH/H_2O (7:3) and was further purified by Sephadex LH-20 (MeOH) CC as well as semipreparative HPLC (acetonitrile/H_2O, 23:27) to obtain a mixture of **2** and **3** (totally 24.7 mg). Fr. 7 eluted with CH_2Cl_2/MeOH (20:1) and was further purified by CC on RP-18 (MeOH/H_2O, 3:2) and Sephadex LH-20 (MeOH) and semipreparative HPLC (acetonitrile/H_2O, 3:7) as well as chiral HPLC (hexane/EtOH, 7:3) to give **4** (1.2 mg) and its enantiomer **5** (1.4 mg).

Penoxahydrazone A (**1**): yellow crystals; mp 207–209 °C; $[\alpha]^{27}_D$ +142 (*c* 0.024, MeOH); UV (MeOH) λ_{max} ($\Delta\varepsilon$) 401 (4.5), 222 (4.3) nm; IR (KBr) v_{max} 3446, 2959, 1681, 1603, 1261, 1223, 1148, 1024, 978, 754 cm^{-1}; ^{1}H and ^{13}C NMR data (Table 1); HRESIMS *m/z* 581.3357 [M + Na]$^+$ (calculated for $C_{35}H_{46}N_2O_4Na$, 581.3355).

Penoxahydrazone B/C (**2/3**): brown powder; IR (KBr) v_{max} 3415, 2921, 2852, 1669, 1647, 1243, 1020, 755 cm^{-1}; ^{1}H and ^{13}C NMR data (Table 2); HRESIMS m/z 283.0695 [M + Na]$^+$ (calculated for $C_{13}H_{12}N_2O_4Na$, 283.0689) and 283.0691 [M + Na]$^+$ (calculated for $C_{13}H_{12}N_2O_4Na$, 283.0689).

Penoxazolone A/B (**4/5**): colorless oil; $[\alpha]^{28}_D$ +169 (*c* 0.040, MeOH) for **4** and −176 (*c* 0.050, MeOH) for **5**; UV (MeOH) λ_{max} ($\Delta\varepsilon$) 226 (4.1), 272 (3.4) nm for **4** and 226 (4.3), 272 (3.6) nm for **5**; IR (KBr) v_{max} 3441, 2921, 2853, 1670, 1572, 1416, 1013 cm^{-1}; ^{1}H and ^{13}C

NMR data (Table 3); HRESIMS m/z 347.1013 [M + Na]$^+$ (calculated for C$_{18}$H$_{16}$N$_2$O$_4$Na, 347.1008).

3.4. X-ray Crystallographic Analysis

Yellow crystals of **1** were obtained from a solution of EtOH with a drop of water. Crystallographic data were collected at 100 K using Cu Kα radiation (λ = 1.54178Å) on a Bruker APEX DUO diffractometer equipped with an APEX II CCD. The structure of **1** was solved by direct methods with the SHELXS-97 software package. All non-hydrogen atoms were refined anisotropically with SHELXL-97 and SHELXL-2014 using full-matrix least-squares, and refinements of the H atoms in calculated positions were performed using a riding model. Molecular graphics were calculated with PLATON [37]. Crystallographic data have been deposited in the Cambridge Crystallographic Data Centre as CCDC 2,024,007 for **1**. These data can be obtained free of charge via http://www.ccdc.cam.ac.uk/data_request/cif (or from the CCDC, 12 Union Road, Cambridge CB21EZ, U.K.; fax: + 44-1223-336-033; e-mail: deposit@ccdc.cam.ac.uk).

3.5. Crystal Data for Penoxahydrazone A (1)

Crystal data is as follows: 2(C$_{35}$H$_{46}$N$_2$O$_4$)•H$_2$O, M = 1135.49, a = 14.7945(4) Å, b = 9.4752(2) Å, c = 23.3965(6) Å, α = 90°, β = 98.7230(10)°, γ = 90°, V = 3241.80(14) Å^3, T = 100.(2) K, space group $P1211$, Z = 2, μ(Cu Kα) = 0.604 mm^{-1}, 60,835 reflections measured, 12,787 independent reflections (R_{int} = 0.0347). The final R_1 values were 0.0427 ($I > 2\sigma(I)$). The final $wR(F^2)$ values were 0.1171 ($I > 2\sigma(I)$). The final R_1 values were 0.0433 (all data). The final $wR(F^2)$ values were 0.1179 (all data). The goodness of fit on F^2 was 1.032. Flack parameter = 0.01(4).

3.6. Computational Details

Conformational searches for compounds **2–5** were operated via the Dreiding force field in MarvinSketch software (optimization limit = normal, diversity limit = 0.1; MarvinSketch with Calculator Plugins for Structure Property Prediction and Calculation, Marvin, Version 6.2.2, 2014, ChemAxon, Budapest, Hungary). Regardless of the rotation of methyl and hydroxy groups, the energy-minimized conformers (Figures S1–S4) within a 3 kcal/mol energy threshold from the global minimum were generated after conformational optimization at the B3LYP/6-31+G(d,p) level in DMSO for **2** and **3** and at the B3LYP/6-31G(d) level in MeOH for **4** and **5** using Gaussian 09 software [31]. The ^{1}H and ^{13}C NMR data of each conformer of **2** and **3** were computed at the B3LYP/6-31+G(d,p) level in DMSO through the gauge-independent atomic orbital (GIAO) method, while the ECD spectrum of each conformer of **4** and **5** was calculated at the B3LYP/6-31G(d) level in MeOH via the time-dependent density function theory (TD-DFT) method and then drawn by SpecDis software with sigma = 0.25 and UV-shift = −8 nm. The overall calculated ^{1}H and ^{13}C NMR data and ECD curves of each compound were produced by Boltzmann weighting. All of the above calculations were performed with the integral equation formalism variant (IEF) of the polarizable continuum model (PCM) as implemented in Gaussian 09.

4. Conclusions

Five new dinitrogen-bearing metabolites have been isolated and identified from a cold-seep-derived strain of *P. oxalicum*, and they display high novelty due to the unprecedented linkages. As phenylhydrazone derivatives, **1** features a special steroid framework, while tautomers **2** and **3** contain a furan ring bonding to the azo group. It seems that this fungal strain has the ability to form phenylhydrazones through adding 2-hydrazinylbenzoic acid to ketones or aldehydes. The discovery of penoxahydrazones A–C (**1–3**) adds greatly to the diversity of phenylhydrazone derivatives. As quinazoline derivatives, enantiomers **4** and **5** possess a unique linkage between quinazoline alkaloid and cinnamic acid units. These metabolites with more or less antimicroalgal and antibacterial activities are structurally different from those isolated from the *P. oxalicum* strains of other origin, which demonstrates that deep-sea-derived fungi actually feature the potential to produce novel metabolites and further underpins the significance of chemically exploring the extreme-environment-derived fungi, such as those from the deep sea cold seep.

Supplementary Materials: The following are available online at https://www.mdpi.com/1660-3397/19/1/9/s1, Tables S1–S4: Sarotti's DP4+ sheets. Figures S1–S4: energy-minimized conformers, Figures S5–S26: 1D/2D NMR and HRMS spectra.

Author Contributions: B.-G.W. and N.-Y.J. conceived the ideas. Y.-P.L. performed the experiments aided by S.-T.F., Z.-Z.S., and N.-Y.J. X.-N.L. analyzed the X-ray crystallographic diffraction data. Y.-P.L., Z.-Z.S., N.-Y.J., and B.-G.W. wrote the manuscript. All authors have read and agreed to the published version of the manuscript.

Funding: This work was financially supported by the National Key R&D Program of China (2018YFC0310800), the Taishan Scholar Project (tsqn201909164 and ts201511060), the Shuangbai Plan of Yantai (2018-3), and the Youth Innovation Promotion Association of CAS (Y201734). The authors acknowledge the support of the Research Vessel KEXUE of the National Major Science and Technology Infrastructure from the Chinese Academy of Sciences (KEXUE2018G28, for sampling).

Institutional Review Board Statement: Not applicable.

Informed Consent Statement: Not applicable.

Data Availability Statement: The data presented in this study are available in the supplementary material.

Conflicts of Interest: The authors declare no conflict of interest.

References

1. Caneschi, W.L.; Sanchez, A.B.; Felestrino, É.B.; de Carvalho Lemes, C.G.; Cordeiro, I.F.; Fonseca, N.P.; Villa, M.M.; Vieira, I.T.; Moraes, L.Â.G.; de Almeida Barbosa Assis, R.; et al. Serratia liquefaciens FG3 isolated from a metallophyte plant sheds light on the evolution and mechanisms of adaptive traits in extreme environments. *Sci. Rep.* **2019**, *9*, 18006. [CrossRef] [PubMed]
2. Bérdy, J. Bioactive microbial metabolites. *J. Antibiot.* **2005**, *58*, 1–26. [CrossRef] [PubMed]
3. Ding, T.; Zhou, Y.; Qin, J.J.; Yang, L.L.; Zhang, W.D.; Shen, Y.H. Chemical constituents from wetland soil fungus *Penicillium oxalicum* GY1. *Fitoterapia* **2020**, *142*, 104530. [CrossRef] [PubMed]
4. Bian, X.Q.; Bai, J.; Hu, X.L.; Wu, X.; Xue, C.M.; Han, A.H.; Su, G.Y.; Hua, H.M.; Pei, Y.H. Penioxalicin, a novel 3-nor-2,3-seco-labdane type diterpene from the fungus *Penicillium oxalicum* TW01-1. *Tetrahedron Lett.* **2015**, *56*, 5013–5016. [CrossRef]
5. Liu, B.; Wang, H.F.; Zhang, L.H.; Liu, F.; He, F.J.; Bai, F.J.; Hua, H.M.; Chen, G.; Pei, Y.H. Isolation of a new compound from *Penicillium oxalicum*. *Chem. Nat. Compd.* **2016**, *52*, 821–823. [CrossRef]
6. Hu, X.L.; Bian, X.Q.; Wu, X.; Li, J.Y.; Hua, H.M.; Pei, Y.H.; Han, A.H.; Bai, J. Penioxalamine A, a novel prenylated spiro-oxindole alkaloid from *Penicillium oxalicum*. *Tetrahedron Lett.* **2014**, *55*, 3864–3867. [CrossRef]
7. Ren, Y.; Chao, L.H.; Sun, J.; Chen, X.N.; Yao, H.N.; Zhu, Z.X.; Dong, D.; Liu, T.; Tu, P.F.; Li, J. Two new polyketides from the fungus *Penicillium oxalicum* MHZ153. *Nat. Prod. Res.* **2018**, *33*, 347–353. [CrossRef]
8. Seetharaman, P.; Gnanasekar, S.; Chandrasekaran, R.; Chandrakasan, G.; Syed, A.; Hodhod, M.S.; Ameen, F.; Sivaperumal, S. Isolation of limonoid compound (Hamisonine) from endophytic fungi *Penicillium oxalicum* LA-1 (KX622790). *Environ. Sci. Pollut. Res.* **2017**, *24*, 21272–21282. [CrossRef]
9. Yuan, L.; Huang, W.Z.; Zhou, K.; Wang, Y.D.; Dong, W.; Du, G.; Gao, X.M.; Ma, Y.H.; Hu, Q.F. Butyrolactones derivatives from the fermentation products of a plant entophytic fungus *Penicillium oxalicum*. *Nat. Prod. Res.* **2015**, *29*, 1914–1919. [CrossRef]
10. Li, Q.Q.; Dang, L.Z.; Zhang, Y.P.; Jiang, J.X.; Zhang, C.M.; Xiang, N.J.; Yang, H.Y.; Du, G.; Duan, Y.Q. Isocoumarins from the fermentation products of a plant entophytic fungus *Penicillium oxalicum*. *J. Asian Nat. Prod. Res.* **2015**, *17*, 876–881. [CrossRef]
11. Yang, Z.; Huang, N.Y.; Xu, B.; Huang, W.F.; Xie, T.P.; Cheng, F.; Zou, K. Cytotoxic 1,3-thiazole and 1,2,4-thiadiazole alkaloids from *Penicillium oxalicum*: Structural elucidation and total synthesis. *Molecules* **2016**, *21*, 232. [CrossRef] [PubMed]
12. Shi, S.; Guo, K.B.; Wang, X.Y.; Chen, H.; Min, J.B.; Qi, S.H.; Zhao, W.; Li, W.R. Toxicity study of oxalicumone A, derived from a marine-derived fungus *Penicillium oxalicum*, in cultured renal epithelial cells. *Mol. Med. Rep.* **2017**, *15*, 2611–2619. [CrossRef] [PubMed]
13. Bao, J.; Zhang, X.Y.; Dong, J.J.; Xu, X.Y.; Nong, X.H.; Qi, S.H. Cyclopentane-condensed chromones from marine-derived fungus *Penicillium oxalicum*. *Chem. Lett.* **2014**, *43*, 837–839. [CrossRef]
14. Bao, J.; Luo, J.F.; Qin, X.C.; Xu, X.Y.; Zhang, X.Y.; Tu, Z.C.; Qi, S.H. Dihydrothiophene-condensed chromones from a marine-derived fungus *Penicillium oxalicum* and their structure–bioactivity relationship. *Bioorg. Med. Chem. Lett.* **2014**, *24*, 2433–2436. [CrossRef]
15. Sun, Y.L.; Bao, J.; Liu, K.S.; Zhang, X.Y.; He, F.; Wang, Y.F.; Nong, X.H.; Qi, S.H. Cytotoxic dihydrothiophene-condensed chromones from the marine-derived fungus *Penicillium oxalicum*. *Planta Med.* **2013**, *79*, 1474–1479. [CrossRef]

16. Li, X.; Li, X.M.; Zhang, P.; Wang, B.G. A new phenolic enamide and a new meroterpenoid from marine alga-derived endophytic fungus *Penicillium oxalicum* EN-290. *J. Asian Nat. Prod. Res.* **2015**, *17*, 1204–1212. [CrossRef]
17. Zhang, P.; Li, X.M.; Liu, H.; Li, X.; Wang, B.G. Two new alkaloids from *Penicillium oxalicum* EN-201, an endophytic fungus derived from the marine mangrove plant Rhizophora stylosa. *Phytochem. Lett.* **2015**, *2015*. *13*, 160–164. [CrossRef]
18. Wang, P.L.; Lib, D.Y.; Xie, L.R.; Wu, X.; Li, Z.L. Novel decaturin alkaloids from the marine-derived fungus *Penicillium oxalicum*. *Nat. Prod. Commun.* **2013**, *8*, 1397–1398. [CrossRef]
19. Chen, L.; Bi, Y.X.; Li, Y.P.; Li, X.X.; Liu, Q.Y.; Ying, M.G.; Zheng, Q.H.; Du, L.; Zhang, Q.Q. Secalonic acids H and I, two new secondary metabolites from the marine-derived fungus *Penicillium oxalicum*. *Heterocycles* **2017**, *94*, 1766–1774.
20. Chen, L.; Lu, Z.H.; Liu, Q.Y.; Zheng, Q.H.; Du, L.; Zhang, Q.Q. Secalonic acids J–M, four new secondary metabolites from the marine-derived fungus *Penicillium oxalicum*. *Heterocycles* **2019**, *98*, 155–965.
21. Liu, B.; Wang, H.F.; Zhang, L.H.; Liu, F.; He, F.J.; Bai, J.; Hua, H.M.; Chen, G.; Pei, Y.H. New compound with DNA Topo I inhibitory activity purified from *Penicillium oxalicum* HSY05. *Nat. Prod. Res.* **2015**, *29*, 2197–2202. [CrossRef] [PubMed]
22. Wang, P.L.; Li, D.Y.; Xie, L.R.; Wu, X.; Hua, H.M.; Li, Z.L. Two new compounds from a marine-derived fungus *Penicillium oxalicum*. *Nat. Prod. Res.* **2013**, *28*, 290–293. [CrossRef] [PubMed]
23. Pimenta, E.F.; Vita-Marques, A.M.; Tininis, A.; Seleghim, M.H.R.; Sette, L.D.; Veloso, K.; Ferreira, A.G.; Williams, D.E.; Patrick, B.O.; Dalisay, D.S.; et al. Use of experimental design for the optimization of the production of new secondary metabolites by two *Penicillium* species. *J. Nat. Prod.* **2010**, *73*, 1821–1832. [CrossRef] [PubMed]
24. Orsi, W.D.; Edgcomb, V.P.; Christman, G.D.; Biddle, J.F. Gene expression in the deep biosphere. *Nature* **2013**, *499*, 205–208. [CrossRef] [PubMed]
25. Orsi, W.D.; Richards, T.A.; Santoro, A.E. Cellular maintenance processes that potentially underpin the survival of subseafloor fungi over geological timescales. *Estuar. Coast. Shelf Sci.* **2015**, *164*, A1–A9. [CrossRef]
26. Amagata, T.; Tanaka, M.; Yamada, T.; Doi, M.; Minoura, K.; Ohishi, H.; Yamori, T.; Numata, A. Variation in cytostatic constituents of a sponge-derived *Gymnascella dankaliensis* by manipulating the carbon source. *J. Nat. Prod.* **2007**, *70*, 1731–1740. [CrossRef]
27. Cheng, P.; Xu, K.; Chen, Y.C.; Wang, T.T.; Chen, Y.; Yang, C.L.; Ma, S.Y.; Liang, Y.; Ge, H.M.; Jiao, R.H. Cytotoxic aromatic polyketides from an insect derived *Streptomyces* sp. NA4286. *Tetrahedron Lett.* **2019**, *60*, 1706–1709. [CrossRef]
28. Song, Y.P.; Shi, Z.Z.; Miao, F.P.; Fang, S.T.; Yin, X.L.; Ji, N.Y. Tricholumin A, a highly transformed ergosterol derivative from the alga-endophytic fungus *Trichoderma asperellum*. *Org. Lett.* **2018**, *20*, 6306–6309. [CrossRef]
29. Blair, L.M.; Sperry, J. Natural products containing a nitrogen−nitrogen bond. *J. Nat. Prod.* **2013**, *76*, 794–812. [CrossRef]
30. Han, M.; Liu, X.; Zhang, X.; Pang, Y.; Xu, P.; Guo, J.; Liu, Y.; Zhang, S.; Ji, S. 5-Hydroxymethyl-2-vinylfuran: A biomass-based solvent-free adhesive. *Green Chem.* **2017**, *19*, 722–728. [CrossRef]
31. Frisch, M.J.; Trucks, G.W.; Schlegel, H.B.; Scuseria, G.E.; Robb, M.A.; Cheeseman, J.R.; Scalmani, G.; Barone, V.; Mennucci, B.; Petersson, G.A.; et al. *Gaussian 09, Revision C.01*; Gaussian, Inc.: Wallingford, CT, USA, 2010.
32. Grimblat, N.; Zanardi, M.M.; Sarotti, A.M. Beyond DP4: An improved probability for the stereochemical assignment of isomeric compounds using quantum chemical calculations of NMR shifts. *J. Org. Chem.* **2015**, *80*, 12526–12534. [CrossRef] [PubMed]
33. Rao, K.R.; Raghunadh, A.; Mekala, R.; Meruva, S.B.; Pratap, T.V.; Krishna, T.; Kalita, D.; Laxminarayana, E.; Prasad, B.; Pal, M. Glyoxylic acid in the reaction of isatoic anhydride with amines: A rapid synthesis of 3-(un)substituted quinazolin-4(3h)-ones leading to rutaecarpine and evodiamine. *Tetrahedron Lett.* **2014**, *55*, 6004–6006. [CrossRef]
34. Allegretta, G.; Weidel, E.; Empting, M.; Hartmann, R.W. Catechol-based substrates of chalcone synthase as a scaffold for novel inhibitors of PqsD. *Eur. J. Med. Chem.* **2015**, *90*, 351–359. [CrossRef] [PubMed]
35. Song, Y.P.; Miao, F.P.; Fang, S.T.; Yin, X.L.; Ji, N.Y. Halogenated and nonhalogenated metabolites from the marine-alga-endophytic fungus *Trichoderma asperellum* cf44-2. *Mar. Drugs* **2018**, *16*, 266. [CrossRef]
36. Miao, F.P.; Liang, X.R.; Yin, X.L.; Wang, G.; Ji, N.Y. Absolute configurations of unique harziane diterpenes from *Trichoderma* species. *Org. Lett.* **2012**, *14*, 3815–3817. [CrossRef]
37. Pu, D.B.; Zhang, X.J.; Bi, D.W.; Gao, J.B.; Yang, Y.; Li, X.L.; Lin, J.; Li, X.N.; Zhang, R.H.; Xiao, W.L. Callicarpins, two classes of rearranged *ent*-clerodane diterpenoids from *Callicarpa* plants blocking NLRP3 inflammasome-induced pyroptosis. *J. Nat. Prod.* **2020**, *83*, 2191–2199. [CrossRef]

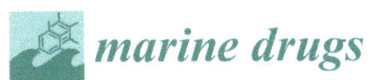

Article

Antimicrobial and Antioxidant Polyketides from a Deep-Sea-Derived Fungus *Aspergillus versicolor* SH0105

Lu-Jia Yang [1,2], Xiao-Yue Peng [1,2], Ya-Hui Zhang [1,2], Zhi-Qing Liu [1,2], Xin Li [1,2], Yu-Cheng Gu [3], Chang-Lun Shao [1,2], Zhuang Han [4,*] and Chang-Yun Wang [1,2,*]

1. Key Laboratory of Marine Drugs, The Ministry of Education of China, School of Medicine and Pharmacy, Institute of Evolution & Marine Biodiversity, Ocean University of China, Qingdao 266003, China; yanglujia@stu.ouc.edu.cn (L.-J.Y.); pengxiaoyue@stu.ouc.edu.cn (X.-Y.P.); zhangyahui@stu.ouc.edu.cn (Y.-H.Z.); liuzhiqing@ouc.edu.cn (Z.-Q.L.); lixin8962@ouc.edu.cn (X.L.); shaochanglun@ouc.edu.cn (C.-L.S.)
2. Laboratory for Marine Drugs and Bioproducts, Qingdao National Laboratory for Marine Science and Technology, Qingdao 266237, China
3. Jealott's Hill International Research Centre, Syngenta, Bracknell, Berkshire RG42 6EY, UK; yucheng.gu@syngenta.com
4. Institute of Deep-sea Science and Engineering, Chinese Academy of Science, Sanya 572000, China
* Correspondence: zhuanghan@idsse.ac.cn (Z.H.); changyun@ouc.edu.cn (C.-Y.W.); Tel.: +86-0898-88215868 (Z.H.); +86-0532-8203-1536 (C.-Y.W.)

Received: 9 November 2020; Accepted: 9 December 2020; Published: 11 December 2020

Abstract: Fifteen polyketides, including four new compounds, isoversiol F (**1**), decumbenone D (**2**), palitantin B (**7**), and 1,3-di-*O*-methyl-norsolorinic acid (**8**), along with 11 known compounds (**3–6** and **9–15**), were isolated from the deep-sea-derived fungus *Aspergillus versicolor* SH0105. Their structures and absolute configurations were determined by comprehensive spectroscopic data, including 1D and 2D NMR, HRESIMS, and ECD calculations, and it is the first time to determine the absolute configuration of known decumbenone A (**6**). All of these compounds were evaluated for their antimicrobial activities against four human pathogenic microbes and five fouling bacterial strains. The results indicated that 3,7-dihydroxy-1,9-dimethyldibenzofuran (**14**) displayed obvious inhibitory activity against *Staphylococcus aureus* (ATCC 27154) with the MIC value of 13.7 µM. In addition, the antioxidant assays of the isolated compounds revealed that aspermutarubrol/violaceol-I (**15**) exhibited significant 1,1-diphenyl-2-picrylhydrazyl (DPPH) radical scavenging activity with the IC_{50} value of 34.1 µM, and displayed strong reduction of Fe^{3+} with the ferric reducing antioxidant power (FRAP) value of 9.0 mM under the concentration of 3.1 µg/mL, which were more potent than ascorbic acid.

Keywords: *Aspergillus versicolor*; deep-sea-derived fungus; polyketide; antimicrobial activity; antioxidant activity

1. Introduction

Marine-sourced microbes have been deemed as one of the important resources for the discovery of drug lead compounds, with increasing number of diverse new bioactive natural products reported in recent years [1]. A series of remarkable progress have been made in the exploitation of marine microbial resources using various technical strategies, for instance, epigenetic modification [2,3], coculture [4,5], and genome mining [6,7]. The genus *Aspergillus* was widely distributed in marine environment and marine-derived *Aspergillus* species was home to a crucial reservoir for producing new bioactive chemical molecules to promote the development of marine drugs [8,9]. So far, plenty of novel and active secondary metabolites have been reported from *Aspergillus*, such as anticancer plinabulin (NPI-2358) [10], α-glucosidase inhibitor aspergillusol A [11], and antiviral ochraceopone A and isoasteltoxin [12]. Inspiringly, plinabulin (NPI-2358) was an inhibitor of tubulin polymerization in third phase of clinical study to treat metastatic advanced nonsmall cell lung cancer (NSCLC) [13]. It was noteworthy that the studies of microbial secondary metabolites from extreme marine environments like deep sea have been gradually brought to the forefront in recent decades [14–16]. More and more new bioactive natural products have been discovered from the deep-sea derived *Aspergillus*, e.g., antifungal versicoloids A and B [17], cytotoxic penicillenols A1 and B1 [18], and anti-inflammatory cyclopenin [19].

As a part of our continuous research for marine bioactive natural products, a variety of bioactive compounds have been obtained from marine-derived *Aspergillus* genus [20], such as antibacterial (−)-sydonic acid [21], anti-RSV 22-*O*-(*N*-Me-L-valyl)-21-*epi*-aflaquinolone B [22], and antituberculous asperversiamides A–C [23]. Recently, a deep-sea-derived fungus *Aspergillus versicolor* SH0105 isolated from a Mariana Trench sediment sample (−5455 m) attracted our attention owing to its EtOAc extract of the fungal culture exhibiting antibacterial activity. The further chemical investigation on the EtOAc extract led to the isolation of four new polyketides (**1–2** and **7–8**), along with 11 known compounds (**3–6** and **9–15**) (Figure 1). Herein, we report the isolation, structure elucidation, and biological activities of these compounds.

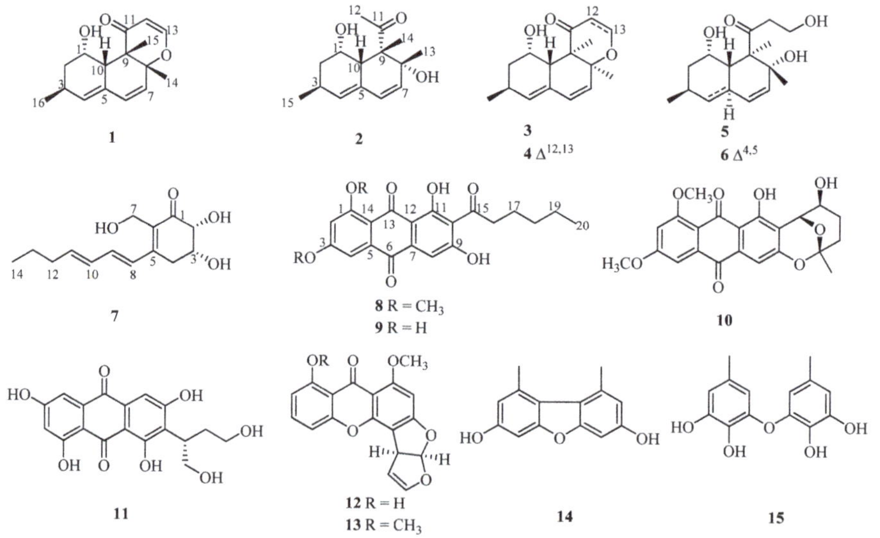

Figure 1. The structures of isolated compounds **1–15**.

2. Results and Discussion

Isoversiol F (**1**) was obtained as a yellowish oil with a molecular formula of $C_{16}H_{20}O_3$ on the basis of the HRESIMS at *m/z* 261.1492 [M + H]$^+$ (calcd for 261.1485) (Figure S9), displaying the same molecular formula with the coisolated 12,13-dedihydroversiol (**4**), which was first isolated from the marine-derived *Aspergillus* sp. SCS-KFD66 [24]. The ^{1}H NMR, ^{13}C NMR, and HSQC spectra of **1** (Table 1 and Figures S2–S4) revealed the presence of one carbonyl (δ_C 200.2), one olefinic quaternary carbon (δ_C 130.3), five olefinic methine, two sp^3 quaternary carbons (with one oxygenated (δ_C 86.2)), one methylene (δ_C 38.8, δ_H 1.30 and 2.00), three methines (including one oxymethine δ_C 67.5, δ_H 5.20), and three methyls. These structural features were also very similar to those of **4**. The ^{1}H-^{1}H COSY interactions and the key HMBC correlations from H-4 to C-2, C-6, C-10, and C-16, from H-13 to C-8 and C-11, from H$_3$-14 to C-7 and C-9, and from H$_3$-15 to C-8, C-9, C-10, and C-11 in **1** demonstrated the same planar structure with **4** (Figure 2 and Figures S5 and S6). The obvious distinctions were the chemical shifts of the oxymethine (δ_C 67.5 and δ_H 5.20) and methyl (δ_C 17.2 and δ_H 1.28) in **1** replaced the oxymethine (δ_C 66.8 and δ_H 3.95) and methyl (δ_C 13.5 and δ_H 1.17) in **4**, respectively, which manifested that compound **1** should be a diastereoisomer of **4**.

Table 1. The ^{1}H and ^{13}C NMR data of **1–2** and **7**.

No.	**1** [a]		**2** [b]		**7** [b]	
	δ_C, Type	δ_H (J in Hz)	δ_C, type	δ_H (J in Hz)	δ_C, Type	δ_H (J in Hz)
1	67.5, CH	5.20, m	67.3, CH	4.22, m	199.6, C	
2	38.8, CH$_2$	2.00, m; 1.30, m	40.8, CH$_2$	1.85, m; 1.22, m	76.8, CH	4.31, d (3.0)
3	25.9, CH	2.56, m	26.9, CH	2.53, m	70.9, CH	4.41, m
4	136.6, CH	5.71, brs	134.9, CH	5.58, brs	33.8, CH$_2$	3.01, dd (18.2, 3.5) 2.90, dd (18.2, 3.5)
5	130.3, C		132.7, C		151.0, C	
6	130.5, CH	6.00, d (9.8)	129.6, CH	5.94, d (9.8)	132.5, C	
7	127.6, CH	5.64, d (9.8)	134.1, CH	5.35, d (9.8)	54.5, CH$_2$	4.40, d (11.6) 4.58, d (11.6)
8	86.2, C		75.2, C		128.4, CH	6.88, m
9	49.4, C		58.9, C		139.3, CH	6.87, m
10	41.9, CH	2.65, q (3.3)	43.3, CH	2.88, q (3.3)	132.3, CH	6.33, ddq (15.1, 8.4, 1.4)
11	200.2, C		216.3, C		142.3, CH	6.11, dt (15.1, 7.2)
12	106.5, CH	5.31, d (5.9)	30.8, CH$_3$	2.28, s	36.1, CH$_2$	2.19, dq (7.2, 1.4)
13	158.4, CH	7.05, d (5.9)	26.5, CH$_3$	1.12, s	23.3, CH$_2$	1.50, qt (7.4, 1.4)
14	21.0, CH$_3$	1.47, s	15.2, CH$_3$	1.44, s	14.0, CH$_3$	0.96, t (7.4)
15	17.2, CH$_3$	1.28, s	21.6, CH$_3$	1.02, d (7.1)		
16	21.2, CH$_3$	1.04, q (7.1)				

[a], [b] Recorded at 600 MHz for ^{1}H NMR and 150 MHz for ^{13}C NMR in CDCl$_3$ and MeOH-d_4, respectively.

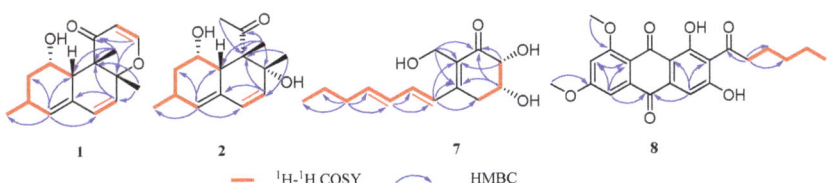

Figure 2. The key ^{1}H-^{1}H COSY and HMBC correlations of **1–2** and **7–8**.

The relative configuration of **1** was determined by coupling constants, 1D NOE and 2D NOESY spectra. The small coupling constant of $J_{H-1, H-10}$ = 3.3 Hz reflected the *syn*-relationship of H-1 and H-10. In the NOE spectrum, the irradiation of H$_3$-15 (δ_H 1.28) led to the signal increase of H-1 (δ_H 5.20) and H$_3$-16 (δ_H 1.04), suggesting that H$_3$-15, H$_3$-16, and H-1 should be positioned at the same planar (Figure 3 and Figure S8). Besides, in the NOESY spectrum, the correlation was also observed between H-10 and H$_3$-14 indicating the same face of these protons (Figure 3 and Figure S7). Thus, the relative configuration of **1** was assumed as 1*S**,3*S**,8*R**,9*S**,10*S**. The Mosher method was applied to determine the absolute configuration of **1**, however, it failed. Fortunately, the absolute configuration of **1** was resolved by ECD calculations. Its experimental ECD spectrum agreed with that of calculated 1*S*,3*S*,8*R*,9*S*,10*S*-**1**, which exhibited negative Cotton effect at around 230 nm and positive Cotton effect at around 260 nm (Figure 4 and Figure S32). Therefore, the absolute configuration of **1** was assigned as 1*S*,3*S*,8*R*,9*S*,10*S*. Compound **1** was a derivative of versiol [25], therefore, we named it as isoversiol F, which followed the reported isoversiols A–E [26].

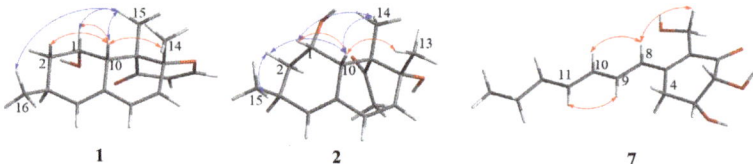

Figure 3. The NOE (blue) and NOESY (red) correlations of **1**–**2** and **7**.

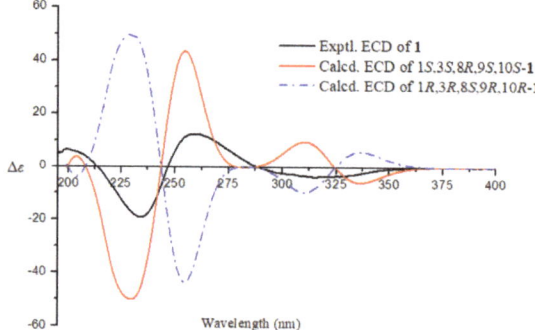

Figure 4. The experimental and calculated ECD spectra of **1**.

Decumbenone D (**2**) was also obtained as a yellowish oil and assigned the molecular formula $C_{15}H_{22}O_3$ by HRESIMS at *m/z* 233.1543 [M − H_2O + H]$^+$ (calcd for 233.1536) (Figure S18), with five degrees of unsaturation. The NMR data of **2** (Table 1 and Figures S10–S12) indicated the presence of one ketone carbonyl (δ_C 216.3), four olefinic signals (one quaternary), two sp^3 quaternary carbons (with one oxygenated), three methines (including one oxymethine δ_C 67.3, δ_H 4.22), one methylene (δ_C 40.8, δ_H 1.85 and 1.22), and four methyl groups. These spectroscopic features suggested the presence of a similar skeleton with those of coisolated decumbenone A (**6**), which was first discovered from the fungus *Penicillium decumbens* [27]. The distinct differences were the existence of an additional methyl group (δ_C 30.8 and δ_H 2.28) in **2**, and the absence of two methylenes (including one oxygenated) of the side chain in **6**, indicating an acetyl group [CH_3CO-] of the side chain at C-9 in **2** replaced the 3-hydroxypropionyl group [$HOCH_2CH_2CO-$] in **6**, which was verified by the HMBC correlations from H-12 to C-1 and C-9 (Figure 2 and Figure S14).

The relative configuration of **2** was also determined by coupling constants, 1D NOE, and 2D NOESY spectra. The small coupling constant of $J_{H-1, H-10}$ = 3.3 Hz demonstrated the same side of H-1 and H-10. In the 1D NOE experiment measured in CDCl$_3$ (Figure 3 and Figure S17), the irradiation of H$_3$-14 (δ_H 1.46) enhanced the signal of H-10 (δ_H 2.98), and the irradiation of H-10 and H$_3$-15 (δ_H 1.05) simultaneously resulted the enhancement of H-2b (δ_H 1.32), implying that H$_3$-14, H$_3$-15, and H-10 should be placed at the same face (Figure 3). In addition, the NOESY cross-peaks between H-10 and H$_3$-13 indicated that these protons also should be coplanar (Figure 3 and Figure S15). Herein, the relative configuration of **2** was deduced as 1S^*,3S^*,8R^*,9S^*,10S^*. The calculated ECD spectrum of 1S,3S,8R,9S,10S-**2** matched the experimental carve of **2** (Figure 5 and Figure S33). Therefore, the absolute configuration of **2** was assumed as 1S,3S,8R,9S,10S. It was worth mentioning that only the relative stereochemistry of the known compound **6** was assumed by Fujii et al. [27]. Herein, we firstly determined the absolute configuration of **6** as 1S,3S,8R,9R,10S by comparing the experimental and calculated ECD spectra (Figure 5 and Figure S35).

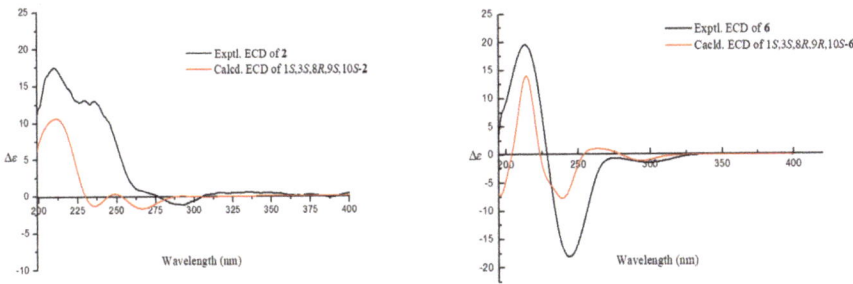

Figure 5. The experimental and calculated ECD spectra of **2** and **6**.

Palitantin B (**7**) was isolated as a yellow solid. Its molecular formula was suggested to be $C_{14}H_{20}O_4$ according to its HRESIMS at *m/z* 253.1442 [M + H]$^+$ (calcd for 253.1434) (Figure S25), with five degrees of unsaturation. The ^{1}H NMR, ^{13}C NMR data of **7** (Table 1 and Figures S19 and S20) displayed the presence of one carbonyl group, six olefinic carbons, two oxymethines, four methylenes, and one methyl group. In the ^{1}H-^{1}H COSY spectrum, the cross-peaks of H-2/H-3/H-4 and correlations between H-8 to H-14 demonstrated a residue of [–OCHCH(O)CH$_2$–] and an aliphatic spin system C-8 to C-14, respectively, which was also verified by the corresponding HMBC correlations (Figure 2 and Figures S22 and S23). The observed HMBC correlations from H-8 to C-4, C-5, and C-6 and from H-7 to C-1, C-5, and C-6 suggested the aliphatic chain should be located at C-5 and the hydroxymethyl linked at C-6 (Figure 2). Because of the demand of five degrees of unsaturation, an additional ring should be proposed, which was confirmed by the HMBC correlations from H-3 to C-1 and C-5, and H-2 to C-1 and C-6 (Figure 2). Hence, the planar structure of **7** was determined, which was similar with the known palitantin isolated from a plant endophytic *A. fumigatiaffinis* [28], except that the saturated bond at C-5/C-6 in palitantin was replaced by a double bond in **7**.

The relative configuration of **7** was determined by coupling constants and NOESY correlations. The coupling constant of $J_{H-2, H-3}$ = 3.0 Hz suggested the *syn*-relationship of H-2 and H-3. The *E*-configuration of the two double bonds was elucidated by the large coupling constant $J_{H-10, H-11}$ = 15.1 Hz and the NOESY correlations of H-9/H-11 and H-8/H-10 (Figure 3 and Figure S24). The absolute configuration of **7** was investigated by quantum chemical TDDFT calculations of its ECD spectrum. The experimental ECD spectrum was consistent with the calculated one of 2*R*,3*R*-**7** (Figure 6 and Figure S34), suggesting the absolute configuration of **7** as 2*R*,3*R*.

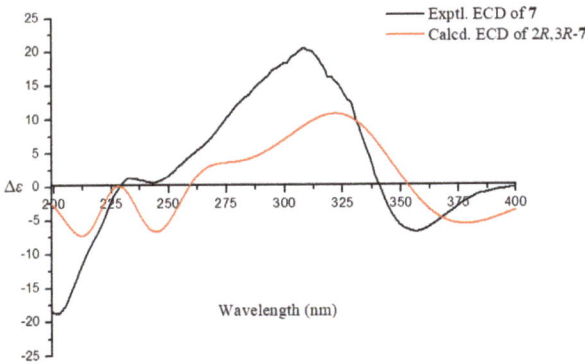

Figure 6. The experimental and calculated ECD spectra of **7**.

1,3-Di-*O*-methyl-norsolorinic acid (**8**) was isolated as a red powder and assigned the molecular formula as $C_{22}H_{22}O_7$ based on its HRESIMS data (Figure S31), including 12 degrees of unsaturation.

The ^{1}H NMR spectrum (Table 2 and Figure S26) displayed one active hydrogen signal (δ_C 13.9), three aromatic protons (δ_C 6.99 (d, J = 2.5 Hz), 7.08 (s), 7.24 (d, J = 2.5 Hz)), two oxymethyl groups, four methylenes, and one methyl. The ^{13}C NMR spectrum (Table 2 and Figure S27) showed the presence of 3 carbonyl groups and 12 aromatic carbons. These spectroscopic features were analogous to those of coisolated norsolorinic acid (**9**), which was obtained from the fungus *Emericella navahoensis* [29], except for two additional oxymethyl groups in **8**. The HMBC correlations from these two oxymethyl groups to C-1 and C-3 revealed that they were attached to C-1 and C-3, respectively (Figure 2 and Figure S30). Therefore, the structure of **8** was determined.

Table 2. The ^{1}H and ^{13}C NMR data of **8** in DMSO-d_6.

No.	δ_C, Type	δ_H (J in Hz)	No.	δ_C, Type	δ_H (J in Hz)
1	163.1, C		13	183.5, C	
2	104.6, CH	6.99, d (2.5)	14	113.8, C	
3	164.9, C		15	203.2, C	
4	104.9, CH	7.24, d (2.5)	16	43.7, CH$_2$	2.74, t (7.3)
5	133.7, C		17	22.6, CH$_2$	1.54, dd (8.5, 5.6)
6	181.8, C		18	30.7, CH$_2$	1.25, m
7	136.4, C		19	21.9, CH$_2$	1.25, m
8	106.6, CH	7.08, s	20	13.8, CH$_3$	0.83, t (7.0)
9	163.0, C		1-OCH$_3$	56.6, CH$_3$	3.91, s
10	121.6, C		3-OCH$_3$	56.2, CH$_3$	3.99, s
11	161.3, C		11-OH		13.9, s
12	109.1, C				

The structures of all known compounds, versiol (**3**) [25], 12,13-dedihydroversiol (**4**) [24], decumbenones B (**5**) and A (**6**) [27], norsolorinic acid (**9**) [29], 6,8-di-*O*-methylaverufin (**10**) [30], versiconol (**11**) [31], sterigmatocystin (**12**) [32], *O*-methylsterigmatocystin (**13**) [33], 3,7-dihydroxy-1,9-dimethyldibenzofuran (**14**) [34], aspermutarubrol/violaceol-I (**15**) [35,36], were elucidated by NMR, MS data and comparing with those of reported literature.

Antimicrobial resistance phenomenon is still a global issue, which is threatening the human's life [37,38], indicating that it is very urgent to discover new antimicrobial molecules or mechanisms. In this study, all the isolated compounds **1–15** were evaluated for their antimicrobial activities against four human pathogenic microbes and five fouling bacterial strains. The results suggested that compound **14** displayed strong inhibitory activity against *Staphylococcus aureus* (ATCC 27154) with the MIC value of 13.7 µM, which was comparable to the positive control ciprofloxacin (MIC = 9.4 µM), and presented moderate inhibitory activity against *Aeromonas salmonicida* (ATCC 7965D) with the same MIC value of 13.7 µM (sea nine 211, MIC = 1.4 µM; Table S1). In addition, the antioxidant assays of the isolated compounds were carried out by DPPH radicals scavenging and FRAP models. The results revealed that **15** exhibited significant DPPH radical scavenging activity with the IC$_{50}$ value of 34.1 µM and displayed strong reduction of Fe^{3+} with the FRAP value of 9.0 mM under the concentration of 3.1 µg/mL; thus, **15** was more potent than the positive control ascorbic acid (DPPH, IC$_{50}$ = 115.1 µM; FRAP = 5.6 mM under 3.1 µg/mL; Table S2). However, the radical scavenging effects of **1–14** were less than 50% under the concentration of 50 µg/mL.

3. Materials and Methods

3.1. General Experimental Procedures

The Optical rotations were measured on a JASCO P-1020 digital polarimeter (Jasco Corp., Tokyo, Japan). UV spectra were recorded by a Milton Roy UV–VIS spectrophotometer (Hitachi, Tokyo, Japan). IR spectra were performed on a Nicolet-Nexus-470 spectrometer using KBr pellets (Thermo Electron, Waltham, MA, USA). NMR spectra were tested by a JEOL JEMECP NMR spectrometer (600 MHz for ^{1}H NMR, 150 MHz for ^{13}C NMR and 500 MHz for NOE spectra, JEOL, Tokyo, Japan) using tetramethylsilane (TMS) as an internal standard. ESIMS spectra were measured on a Micromass Q-TOF spectrometer (Waters Corp., Manchester, UK). ECD spectra were obtained on a JASCO J-815 circular dichroism spectrometer (JASCO Electric Co., Ltd., Tokyo, Japan). In the biological assay, the optical densities (OD) were acquired by a multimode reader Spark 10M (Tecan, Männedorf, Switzerland). Semipreparative HPLC was performed on a Hitachi L-2000 HPLC system coupled with a Hitachi L-2455 photodiode array detector and a Kromasil C_{18} semipreparative HPLC column (250 mm × 10 mm, 5 μm). Silica gel (Qingdao Haiyang Chemical Group Co., Qingdao, China) and Sephadex LH-20 (Amersham Biosciences Inc., Piscataway, NJ, USA) were used for column chromatography (CC). Precoated silica gel GF254 plates (Yantai Zifu Chemical Group Co., Yantai, China) were used for thin layer chromatography (TLC).

3.2. Fungal Material

The fungal strain *A. versicolor* SH0105 was isolated from a deep-sea sediment sample collected at a depth of 5455 m from the Mariana Trench. The strain was deposited in the Key Laboratory of Marine Drugs, the Ministry of Education of China, School of Medicine and Pharmacy, Ocean University of China, Qingdao, China. The fungal strain was identified as *A. versicolor* according to its morphological features, amplification and sequencing of the DNA sequences of the ITS region, and construction of phylogenetic tree by MEGA 7.0 (Temple University, Philadelphia, PA, USA; Figure S1). The sequence data was submitted to NCBI with the GeneBank accession number MT620963.

3.3. Fermentation, Extraction, and Isolation

The fungal strain was cultured on rice solid medium (100 × 1000 mL Erlenmeyer flasks, each containing 80 g of rice and 80 mL of sea water) for 60 days at 25 °C. The fermented rice substrate was extracted three times with ethyl acetate (EtOAc) and concentrated under the vacuum evaporation to yield an organic extract (85 g). Then, the extract was performed on the silica gel vacuum liquid chromatography (VLC) eluting by a gradient of petroleum ether (PE)—EtOAc (100%, 90%, 70%, 50%, and 0% PE) and 10% EtOAc-MeOH to give six fractions (Fr.1–Fr.6). Fr.3 was subjected to the octadecyl silane (ODS) column with MeOH-H_2O (15–100%) to afford four subfractions (Fr.3A–Fr.3D). Fr.3A was separated by Sephadex LH-20 column chromatography (CC) eluting with MeOH and then purified by semipreparative HPLC (75% MeOH-H_2O) to obtain **1** (2 mg), **2** (4 mg), **3** (18 mg), and **4** (4 mg). Fr.3B was repeatedly isolated by silica gel CC eluting with PE-EtOAc to produce **12** (10 mg) and **13** (8 mg). Fr.3C was subjected to Sephadex LH-20 CC and then performed on HPLC (60% MeOH-H_2O) to yield **14** (5 mg) and **15** (38 mg). Fr.3D was chromatographed on silica gel CC and recrystallized to give **8** (6 mg) and **9** (12 mg). Fr.4 was also fractionated on ODS column with MeOH-H_2O (15–100%) to obtain three subfractions (Fr.4A–Fr.4C). Fr.4A was subjected to Sephadex LH-20 CC (50% CH_2Cl_2-MeOH) to obtain two subfractions (Fr.4A1–Fr.4A2). Fr.4A1 was purified on HPLC (45% MeOH-H_2O) to yield **7** (14 mg). Fr.4A2 was reseparated by silica gel CC and HPLC (60% MeOH-H_2O) to provide **5** (65 mg) and **6** (26 mg). Fr.4B was isolated on silica gel CC and further eluted with Sephadex LH-20 CC (50% CH_2Cl_2-MeOH) to afford **9** (6 mg) and **11** (9 mg).

Isoversiol F (**1**): yellowish oil; $[\alpha]_D^{20}$ − 11 (*c* 0.1, MeOH); UV (MeOH) λ_{max} (log ε) 236 (1.48) nm; IR (KBr) v_{max} 3734, 2360, 1699, 1539, 1033 cm^{-1}; ^{1}H and ^{13}C NMR see Table 1; HRESIMS *m/z* 261.1492 [M + H]$^+$ (calcd for $C_{16}H_{21}O_3$, 261.1485).

Decumbenone D (**2**): yellowish oil; $[\alpha]_D^{20}$ +70.8 (*c* 0.1, MeOH); UV (MeOH) λ_{max} (log ε) 283 (1.93) nm; IR (KBr) v_{max} 3444, 2958, 2360, 1687, 1380, 1113 cm^{-1}; ^{1}H and ^{13}C NMR see Table 1; HRESIMS *m/z* 233.1543 [M + H_2O + H]$^+$ (calcd for $C_{15}H_{21}O_2$, 233.1536).

Palitantin B (**7**): yellow solid; $[\alpha]_D^{20}$ +53.2 (*c* 0.1, MeOH); UV (MeOH) λ_{max} (log ε) 321(2.66) nm; IR (KBr) v_{max} 3748, 2361, 1658, 1598, 987 cm^{-1}; ^{1}H and ^{13}C NMR see Table 1; HRESIMS *m/z* 253.1442 [M + H]$^+$ (calcd for $C_{14}H_{21}O_4$, 253.1434); 275.1262 [M + Na]$^+$ (calcd for $C_{14}H_{20}O_4Na$, 275.1254).

1,3-Di-O-methyl-norsolorinic acid (**8**): red powder; UV (CHCl$_3$) λ_{max} (log ε) 245 (1.24), 260 (1.05), 340 (0.65) nm; IR (KBr) v_{max} 3362, 2362, 1683, 1423, 1059 cm^{-1}; ^{1}H and ^{13}C NMR see Table 2; HRESIMS m/z 397.1282 [M + H]$^+$ (calcd for C$_{22}$H$_{21}$O$_7$, 397.1293).

3.4. ECD Calculations

The Merck molecular force field (MMFF94S) was used to conformational searches of compounds **1–2** and **6–7** during theoretical ECD calculations. All conformers were optimized twice by the basis set at the B3LYP/6-31G (d) and B3LYP/6-311+G (d) levels using the Gaussian 09 (Gaussian Inc., Wallingford, CT, USA) [39]. The ECD spectrum was calculated by the time-dependent density functional theory (TD-DFT) method at B3LYP/6-311++G (2d, p) level and simulated by Boltzmann distributions in SpecDis 1.62 (University of Würzburg, Würzburg, Germany) [40].

3.5. Biological Assays

3.5.1. Antimicrobial Assay

The antimicrobial assays were evaluated using a broth microdilution method in 96-well polystyrene microtiter plates Costar 3599 (Corning Inc., New York, NY, USA) according to the standard of Clinical and Laboratory Standards Institute (CLSI) [41]. Three pathogenic bacterial strains, *Staphylococcus aureus* (ATCC 27154), *Escherichia coli* (ATCC 25922), and *Pseudomonas aeruginosa* (ATCC 10145); five fouling bacterial strains, *P. fulva* (ATCC 31418), *Aeromonas salmonicida* (ATCC 7965D), *Photobacterium angustum* (ATCC 33975), *Enterobacter cloacae* (ATCC 39978), and *E. hormaechei* (ATCC 700323); and one pathogenic fungal strain *Candida albicans* (ATCC 76485) were used as the test strains. First, the tested pathogenic bacteria, fouling bacteria, and pathogenic fungus were inoculated in 10 mL of LB (yeast extract 5 g/L, peptone 10 g/L, NaCl 10 g/L), 2216E (Hopebio, Qingdao, China), and YM (Hopebio, Qingdao, China) liquid medium, respectively, and cultivated at 37 °C for 12 h to yield the initial microbial liquids. The microbial density was adjusted to 0.5 MacFarland and then diluted 1000 times using the corresponding broth to obtain the tested microbial suspension with an inoculum density of 1 ×10^5 cfu/mL. The tested compounds were dissolved in 100% DMSO to obtain the mother solution with the initial concentration of 1 mg/mL. Following the principle of twofold serial dilution, each well contained 5 µL of tested compounds and 195 µL of the microbial suspension to obtain the final measured concentration of 25–0.098 µg/mL. Finally, the plates were incubated at 37 °C for 24 h and the optical density of each well was recorded by microplate reader (Tecan, Männedorf, Switzerland) at 600 nm. MIC represents the minimal inhibitory concentration of compound without visible microbial growth. The antimicrobial assays were performed in triplicate. Broad-spectrum antimicrobial ciprofloxacin and commercial antifouling sea-nine 211 were used as positive controls for pathogenic and fouling microbial strains, respectively. DMSO was used as a negative control.

3.5.2. Antioxidant Activity

The DPPH radical scavenging assay and ferric reducing antioxidant power assay (FRAP) were used to evaluate the antioxidant activities of the isolated compounds [42]. The samples and positive control ascorbic acid were dissolved in DMSO with final concentrations of 100, 50, 25, 12.5, and 6.25 µg/mL. DPPH was dissolved in anhydrous ethanol (EtOH) with the concentrations of 0.05 mg/mL. Fe^{3+}-TPTZ solution consisted of 2 mmol/L FeCl$_3$ and 2,4,6-Tris(2-pyridyl)-s-triazine (TPTZ), respectively. Tested samples (100 µL) were added to 100 µL of fresh DPPH or Fe^{3+}-TPTZ solution, then reacted in the dark for 30 min. The optical density (OD) was measured by a multimode reader Spark 10 M (Tecan, Männedorf, Switzerland) at 517 and 593 nm, respectively. The EtOH and DMSO were employed as a blank and negative control, respectively. The IC$_{50}$ values were calculated on the software of GraphPad Prism 5 (GraphPad Software Inc., San Diego, CA, USA).

4. Conclusions

Deep-sea derived fungi are potential resources to seek for structural novel and diverse biological natural products. In the present study, chemical investigation of the deep-sea-derived fungus *A. versicolor* SH0105 led to the isolation of four new polyketides (**1–2** and **7–8**), along with 11 known compounds (**3–6** and **9–15**), which enriched the diversity of secondary metabolites from the deep-sea-derived *Aspergillus*. The structures and absolute configurations of new compounds were elucidated by comprehensive spectroscopic data and ECD calculations, and it is the first time to determine the absolute configuration of known decumbenone A (**6**). In the bioactive assays, compound **14** displayed obvious inhibitory activity against *S. aureus* (ATCC 27154) and **15** exhibited significant DPPH radical scavenging activity and displayed strong reduction of Fe^{3+}, which were more potent than ascorbic acid, indicating the prospect to discovery of chemical entities with antimicrobial and antioxidant activities from the deep-sea medicinal microbial resources.

Supplementary Materials: The following are available online at http://www.mdpi.com/1660-3397/18/12/636/s1. Figure S1: The neighbor-joining phylogenetic tree of the fungus *A. versicolor* SH0105: Figure S2 to Figure S31: The HRESIMS and 1D and 2D NMR spectra of new compounds **1–2** and **7–8**; Figure S32 to Figure S35: The lowest-energy conformers of compounds **1–2** and **6–7** in ECD calculations; Table S1 and Table S2: The data of antimicrobial and antioxidant activities.

Author Contributions: L.-J.Y. contributed to extraction, isolation, structural elucidation, and manuscript preparation; X.-Y.P. contributed to the fermentation of the fungus; Y.-H.Z. contributed to the ECD calculations; Z.-Q.L. and X.L. contributed to the evaluation of bioactivities of the isolated compounds; Y.-C.G. and C.-L.S. contributed to the critical reading of the manuscript; Z.H. and C.-Y.W. designed the project and manuscript writing. All authors have read and agreed to the published version of the manuscript.

Funding: This work was supported by the Shandong Provincial Natural Science Foundation (Major Basic Research Projects), China (ZR2019ZD18), the Program of Open Studio for Druggability Research of Marine Natural Products, Pilot National Laboratory for Marine Science and Technology (Qingdao, China) Directed by Kai-Xian Chen and Yue-Wei Guo, and the Taishan Scholars Program, China.

Acknowledgments: This paper is dedicated to Youyou Tu, the 2015 Nobel Prize Laureate of Physiology or Medicine on the occasion of her 90th birthday. Lu-Jia Yang is thankful for the Syngenta-OUC-PhD Studentship.

Conflicts of Interest: The authors declare no conflict of interest.

References

1. Carroll, A.R.; Copp, B.R.; Davis, R.A.; Keyzers, R.A.; Prinsep, M.R. Marine natural products. *Nat. Prod. Rep.* **2020**, *37*, 175–223. [CrossRef]
2. Zhang, Z.Z.; He, X.Q.; Wu, G.W.; Liu, C.C.; Lu, C.J.; Gu, Q.Q.; Che, Q.; Zhu, T.J.; Zhang, G.J.; Li, D.H. Aniline-tetramic acids from the deep-sea-derived fungus *Cladosporium sphaerospermum* L3P3 cultured with the HDAC inhibitor SAHA. *J. Nat. Prod.* **2018**, *81*, 1651–1657. [CrossRef]
3. Wu, J.S.; Yao, G.S.; Shi, X.H.; Rehman, S.U.; Xu, Y.; Fu, X.M.; Zhang, X.L.; Liu, Y.; Wang, C.Y. Epigenetic agents trigger the production of bioactive nucleoside derivatives and bisabolane sesquiterpenes from the marine-derived fungus *Aspergillus versicolor*. *Front. Microbiol.* **2020**, *11*, 85. [CrossRef]
4. Yu, M.L.; Li, Y.X.; Banakar, S.P.; Liu, L.; Shao, C.L.; Li, Z.Y.; Wang, C.Y. New metabolites from the co-culture of marine-derived actinomycete *Streptomyces rochei* MB037 and fungus *Rhinocladiella similis* 35. *Front. Microbiol.* **2019**, *10*, 915. [CrossRef] [PubMed]
5. Peng, X.Y.; Wu, J.T.; Shao, C.L.; Li, Z.Y.; Chen, M.; Wang, C.Y. Co-culture: Stimulate the metabolic potential and explore the molecular diversity of natural products from microorganisms. *Mar. Life. Sci. Technol.* **2020**. [CrossRef]
6. Li, Z.Y.; Zhu, D.Y.; Shen, Y.M. Discovery of novel bioactive natural products driven by genome mining. *Drug. Discov. Ther.* **2018**, *12*, 318–328. [CrossRef] [PubMed]
7. Liu, Q.; Liu, Z.Y.; Sun, C.L.; Shao, M.W.; Ma, J.Y.; Wei, X.Y.; Zhang, T.Y.; Li, W.J.; Ju, J.H. Discovery and biosynthesis of atrovimycin, an antitubercular and antifungal cyclodepsipeptide featuring vicinal-dihydroxylated cinnamic acyl chain. *Org. Lett.* **2019**, *21*, 2634–2638. [CrossRef] [PubMed]
8. Zhao, C.Y.; Liu, H.S.; Zhu, W.M. New natural products from the marine-derived *Aspergillus* fungi—A review. *Acta Microbiol. Sin.* **2016**, *56*, 331–362. [CrossRef]

9. Wang, K.W.; Ding, P. New bioactive metabolites from the marine-derived fungi *Aspergillus*. *Mini-Rev. Med. Chem.* **2018**, *18*, 1072–1094. [CrossRef] [PubMed]
10. Nicholson, B.; Lloyd, K.; Miller, B.R.; Palladino, M.A.; Kiso, Y.; Hayashi, Y.; Neuteboom, S.T.C. NPI-2358 is a tubulin-depolymerizing agent: In-vitro evidence for activity as a tumor vascular-disrupting agent. *Anti-Cancer Drug.* **2006**, *17*, 25–31. [CrossRef] [PubMed]
11. Ingavat, N.; Dobereiner, J.; Wiyakrutta, S.; Mahidol, C.; Ruchirawat, S.; Kittakoop, P. Aspergillusol A, an α-glucosidase inhibitor from the marine-derived fungus *Aspergillus aculeatus*. *J. Nat. Prod.* **2009**, *72*, 2049–2052. [CrossRef] [PubMed]
12. Wang, J.F.; Wei, X.Y.; Qin, X.C.; Tian, X.P.; Li, K.M.; Zhou, X.F.; Yang, X.W.; Wang, F.Z.; Zhang, T.Y.; Tu, Z.C.; et al. Antiviral merosesquiterpenoids produced by the Antarctic fungus *Aspergillus ochraceopetaliformis* SCSIO 05702. *J. Nat. Prod.* **2016**, *79*, 59–65. [CrossRef] [PubMed]
13. Cimino, P.J.; Huang, L.; Du, L.H.; Wu, Y.P.; Bishop, J.; Dalsing-Hernandez, J.; Kotlarczyk, K.; Gonzales, P.; Carew, J.; Nawrocki, S.; et al. Plinabulin, an inhibitor of tubulin polymerization, targets KRAS signaling through disruption of endosomal recycling. *Biomed. Rep.* **2019**, *10*, 218–224. [CrossRef] [PubMed]
14. Zhang, X.Y.; Zhang, Y.; Xu, X.Y.; Qi, S.H. Diverse deep-sea fungi from the south China sea and their antimicrobial activity. *Curr. Microbiol.* **2013**, *67*, 525–530. [CrossRef] [PubMed]
15. Wang, Y.T.; Xue, Y.R.; Liu, C.H. A brief review of bioactive metabolites derived from deep-sea fungi. *Mar. Drugs.* **2015**, *13*, 4594–4616. [CrossRef] [PubMed]
16. Wilson, Z.E.; Brimble, M.A. Molecules derived from the extremes of life: A decade later. *Nat. Prod. Rep.* **2020**. [CrossRef] [PubMed]
17. Wang, J.F.; He, W.J.; Huang, X.L.; Tian, X.P.; Liao, S.R.; Yang, B.; Wang, F.Z.; Zhou, X.J.; Liu, Y.H. Antifungal new oxepine-containing alkaloids and xanthones from the deep-sea-derived fungus *Aspergillus versicolor* SCSIO 05879. *J. Agr. Food. Chem.* **2016**, *64*, 2910–2916. [CrossRef]
18. Wang, J.; Yao, Q.F.; Amin, M.; Nong, X.H.; Zhang, X.Y.; Qi, S.H. Penicillenols from a deep-sea fungus *Aspergillus restrictus* inhibit *Candida albicans* biofilm formation and hyphal growth. *J. Antibiot.* **2017**, *70*, 763–770. [CrossRef]
19. Wang, L.Y.; Li, M.J.; Lin, Y.Z.; Du, S.W.; Liu, Z.Y.; Ju, J.H.; Suzuki, H.; Sawada, M.; Umezawa, K. Inhibition of cellular inflammatory mediator production and amelioration of learning deficit in flies by deep sea *Aspergillus* derived cyclopenin. *J. Antibiot.* **2020**, *73*, 622–629. [CrossRef]
20. Liu, L.; Zheng, Y.Y.; Shao, C.L.; Wang, C.Y. Metabolites from marine invertebrates and their symbiotic microorganisms: Molecular diversity discovery, mining, and application. *Mar. Life. Sci. Technol.* **2019**, *1*, 60–94. [CrossRef]
21. Li, D.; Xu, Y.; Shao, C.L.; Yang, R.Y.; Zheng, C.J.; Chen, Y.Y.; Fu, X.M.; Qian, P.Y.; She, Z.G.; Voogd, N.J.D.; et al. Antibacterial bisabolane-type sesquiterpenoids from the sponge-derived fungus *Aspergillus* sp. *Mar. Drugs.* **2012**, *10*, 234–241. [CrossRef] [PubMed]
22. Chen, M.; Shao, C.L.; Meng, H.; She, Z.G.; Wang, C.Y. Anti-respiratory syncytial virus prenylated dihydroquinolone derivatives from the gorgonian-derived fungus *Aspergillus* sp. XS-20090B15. *J. Nat. Prod.* **2014**, *77*, 2720–2724. [CrossRef] [PubMed]
23. Hou, X.M.; Liang, T.M.; Guo, Z.Y.; Wang, C.Y.; Shao, C.L. Discovery, absolute assignments, and total synthesis of asperversiamides A–C and their potent activity against *Mycobacterium marinum*. *Chem. Commun.* **2019**, *55*, 1104–1107. [CrossRef] [PubMed]
24. An, C.L.; Kong, F.D.; Ma, Q.Y.; Xie, Q.Y.; Yuan, J.Z.; Zhou, L.M.; Dai, H.F.; Yu, Z.F.; Zhao, Y.X. Chemical constituents of the marine-derived fungus *Aspergillus* sp. SCS-KFD66. *Mar. Drugs.* **2018**, *16*, 468. [CrossRef] [PubMed]
25. Fukuyama, K.; Tsukihara, T.; Katsube, Y. Structure of versiol, a new metabolite from *Aspergillus versicolor*. *Tetrahedron Lett.* **1976**, *3*, 189–190. [CrossRef]
26. Cho, N.; Ransom, T.T.; Sigmund, J.; Cichewicz, R.H.; Goetz, M.; Beutler, J.A. Growth inhibition of colon cancer and melanoma cells by versiol derivatives from a *Paraconiothyrium* species. *J. Nat. Prod.* **2017**, *80*, 2037–2044. [CrossRef]
27. Fujii, Y.; Asahara, M.; Ichinoe, M.; Nakajima, H. Fungal melanin inhibitor and related compounds from *Penicillium decumbens*. *Phytochemistry* **2002**, *60*, 703–708. [CrossRef]
28. Ola, A.R.B.; Tawo, B.D.; Belli, H.L.L.; Proksch, P.; Tommy, D.; Hakim, E.H. A new antibacterial polyketide from the endophytic fungi *Aspergillus fumigatiaffinis*. *Nat. Prod. Commun.* **2018**, *13*, 1573–1574. [CrossRef]

29. Yamazaki, M.; Satoh, Y.; Maebayashi, Y.; Horie, Y. Monoamine oxidase inhibitors from a fungus, *Emericella navahoensis*. *Chem. Pharm. Bull.* **1988**, *36*, 670–675. [CrossRef]
30. Shao, C.L.; Wang, C.Y.; Wei, M.Y.; Li, S.D.; She, Z.G.; Gu, Y.C.; Lin, Y.C. Structural and spectral assignments of six anthraquinone derivatives from the mangrove fungus (ZSUH-36). *Magn. Reson. Chem.* **2008**, *46*, 886–889. [CrossRef]
31. Steyn, P.S.; Vleggaar, R.; Wessels, P.L. Structure and carbon-13 nuclear magnetic resonance assignments of versiconal acetate, versiconol acetate, and versiconol, metabolites from cultures of *Aspergillus parasiticus* treated with dichlorvos. *J. Chem. Soc. Perkin Trans.* **1979**, *1*, 451–459. [CrossRef]
32. Lee, Y.M.; Li, H.Y.; Hong, J.; Cho, H.Y.; Bae, K.S.; Kim, M.A.; Kim, D.K.; Jung, J.H. Bioactive metabolites from the sponge-derived fungus *Aspergillus versicolor*. *Arch. Pharm. Res.* **2010**, *33*, 231–235. [CrossRef] [PubMed]
33. Cox, R.H.; Cole, R.J. Carbon-13 nuclear magnetic resonance studies of fungal metabolites, aflatoxins, and sterigmatocystins. *J. Org. Chem.* **1977**, *42*, 112–114. [CrossRef] [PubMed]
34. Tanahashia, T.; Takenaka, Y.; Nagakura, N.; Hamada, N. Dibenzofurans from the cultured lichen mycobionts of *Ecanora cinereocarnea*. *Phytochemistry* **2001**, *8*, 1129–1134. [CrossRef]
35. Taniguchi, M.; Kaneda, N.; Shibata, K.; Kamikawa, T. Isolation and biological activity of aspermutarubrol, a self-growth inhibitor from *Aspergillus sydowi*. *Agr. Biol. Chem.* **1978**, *42*, 1629–1630. [CrossRef]
36. Nakamaru, T.; Shiojiri, H.; Kawai, K.; Nozawa, Y.; Maebayashi, Y.; Yamazaki, M. The effects of toxic metabolites violaceol I and II from *Emericella violacea* on mitochondrial respiration. *Mycotoxins*. **1984**, *19*, 30–33. [CrossRef]
37. Chakraborty, M.; Chakraborty, A.; Mukherjee, P. Antibiotic resistance: The global crisis. *J. Pharm. Res* **2020**, *9*, 12–16. [CrossRef]
38. Dugassa, J.; Shukuri, N. Review on antibiotic resistance and its mechanism of development. *J. Health Med. Nurs.* **2017**, *1*, 1–17.
39. Frisch, M.J.; Trucks, G.W.; Schlegel, H.B.; Scuseria, G.E.; Robb, M.A.; Cheeseman, J.R.; Scalmani, G.; Barone, V.; Mennucci, B.; Petersson, G.A.; et al. *Gaussian 09, Revision D.01*; Gaussian Inc.: Wallingford, CT, USA, 2013.
40. Bruhn, T.; Schaumloffel, A.; Hemberger, Y.; Bringmann, G. SpecDis: Quantifying the comparison of calculated and experimental electronic circular dichroism spectra. *Chirality* **2013**, *25*, 243–249. [CrossRef]
41. Clinical and Laboratory Standards Institute (CLSI). *Performance Standards for Antimicrobial Susceptibility Testing*; Twenty-Second Informational Supplement M100-S22; Clinical and Laboratory Standards Institute: Wayne, PA, USA, 2012.
42. Aktumsek, A.; Zengin, G.; Guler, G.O.; Cakmak, Y.S.; Duran, A. Antioxidant potentials and anticholinesterase activities of methanolic andaqueous extracts of three endemic *Centaurea* L. species. *Food. Chem. Toxicol.* **2013**, *55*, 290–296. [CrossRef]

Publisher's Note: MDPI stays neutral with regard to jurisdictional claims in published maps and institutional affiliations.

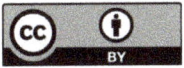

© 2020 by the authors. Licensee MDPI, Basel, Switzerland. This article is an open access article distributed under the terms and conditions of the Creative Commons Attribution (CC BY) license (http://creativecommons.org/licenses/by/4.0/).

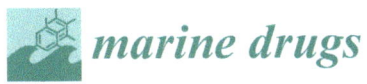

Review

Progress in Research on Bioactive Secondary Metabolites from Deep-Sea Derived Microorganisms

Ya-Nan Wang [1,2,3], Ling-Hong Meng [1,2,*] and Bin-Gui Wang [1,2,4,*]

1. Key Laboratory of Experimental Marine Biology, Institute of Oceanology, Chinese Academy of Sciences, Nanhai Road 7, Qingdao 266071, China; wangyn@qdio.ac.cn
2. Laboratory of Marine Biology and Biotechnology, Qingdao National Laboratory for Marine Science and Technology, Wenhai Road 1, Qingdao 266237, China
3. College of Earth Science, University of Chinese Academy of Sciences, Yuquan Road 19A, Beijing 100049, China
4. Center for Ocean Mega-Science, Chinese Academy of Sciences, Nanhai Road 7, Qingdao 266071, China
* Correspondence: menglh@ms.qdio.ac.cn (L.-H.M.); wangbg@ms.qdio.ac.cn (B.-G.W.); Tel.: +86-532-8289-8890 (L.-H.M.); +86-532-8289-8553 (B.-G.W.)

Received: 29 October 2020; Accepted: 30 November 2020; Published: 2 December 2020

Abstract: Deep sea has an extreme environment which leads to biodiversity of microorganisms and their unique physical and biochemical mechanisms. Deep-sea derived microorganisms are more likely to produce novel bioactive substances with special mechanism of action for drug discovery. This article reviews secondary metabolites with biological activities such as anti-tumor, anti-bacterial, anti-viral, and anti-inflammatory isolated from deep-sea fungi and bacteria during 2018–2020. Effective methods for screening and obtaining natural active compounds from deep-sea microorganisms are also summarized, including optimizing the culture conditions, using genome mining technology, biosynthesis and so on. The comprehensive application of these methods makes broader prospects for the development and application of deep sea microbial bioactive substances.

Keywords: deep-sea fungi; deep-sea actinomycetes; secondary metabolites; bioactivity

1. Introduction

Deep sea is one of the latest extreme environments developed on earth. The deep sea is an environment with extreme features including: (1) For every 10 m of increase in depth, the pressure increases by one atmosphere, so the water pressure is higher than 1000 atmospheres in the deep sea trench; (2) The temperature decreases with depth, which is usually around 2 °C on the deep sea bottom; (3) The seawater oxygen concentration mainly depends on the absorption of oxygen at the sea-air interface, the photosynthesis rate of autotrophs in the true light layer, and rate of consumption of marine life respiration; (4) The light intensity is close to zero below the depth of 250 m [1]. In conclusion, deep sea has the characteristics of extreme ecological environment, including high pressure, low temperature, lack of oxygen and darkness. The cold seeps, hydrothermal and seamounts of the world deep-sea locations may worth favoring for bioprospection. Deep-sea microbes have unique biological metabolic pathways to deal with extreme ecological environments, especially stress. Many deep-sea microbes are hypertrophic or pressure-sensitive. Existing research methods limit the cultivation of these steps [2].

Over the past fifty years, more than 30,000 marine natural products have been discovered, of which about 2% are derived from deep-sea microorganisms [3]. Based on our review of the literature, the number of marine natural products from deep-sea have increased since then, but they are still a small percentage of the total amount found. Also, we found that most recent researches on bioactive secondary metabolites are derived from bacteria and fungi in deep-sea environment. So, this review mainly covers natural products from deep-sea derived fungi and bacteria who were almost isolated from sediment or sea water. Among the natural products, people pay the most attention to compounds with antibacterial activity, especially for their application in the field of biotechnology and pharmaceuticals. The discovery of antibiotics with new structures is very important for dealing with the spread of resistant bacteria [4]. To a large extent, it is related to the isolation and cultivation of unknown deep-sea microorganisms and the discovery of related secondary metabolites. Although it is supposed that microorganisms are huge in number and rich in diversity in these environments [5], few have been characterized so far [6]. In fact, the discovery of deep-sea microbial diversity can lead to the discovery of compounds with new biological activities, further promoting the drug development process [7]. The first antibacterial natural product isolated from deep-sea sediments was a glial toxin produced by the metabolism of a fungus species, *Penicillium* sp., isolated from the Seto Inland Sea, Japan, which inhibits the growth of Gram-positive bacteria *Staphylococcus aureus* and *Bacillus subtilis* [8].

In the past three years, the development of deep-sea exploration and molecular biology provided technical support for the exploitation of deep-sea microbial natural products. To enable researchers to better understand the research work in these fields, this article summarized the characteristics of secondary metabolites isolated from deep-sea microorganisms and their biological activities in 2018–2020, as well as research methods for diversity of secondary metabolites from deep-sea microorganisms.

2. Secondary Metabolites from Deep-Sea Derived Fungi

Recent studies have shown that fungi from the extreme environments are potential producers for clinically important natural products [9] and may be the next frontier of drug discovery [10].

According to the references, 829 (194 novel) natural products were discovered from deep-sea derived fungi in the past three years, 79 among which showed biological activities (Table 1). Most of these compounds were isolated from species of two genera of fungi, *Penicillium* sp. (23, accounting for 30.26% of the total compounds) and *Aspergillus* sp. (16, accounting for 21.05% of the total compounds) (Figure 1).

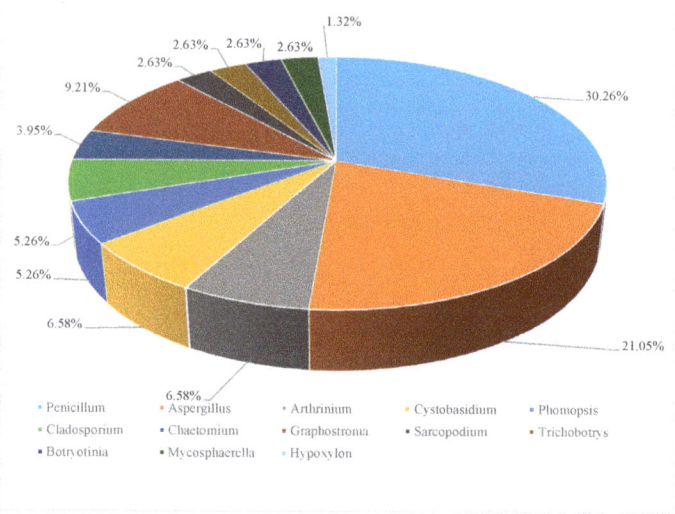

Figure 1. Distribution of deep-sea derived fungi in secondary metabolites discovery. (*Data based on the statistics of references [11–38]).

Table 1. Bioactive Natural products from deep-sea derived fungi in 2018–2020.

Bioactivity	Fungal Species	Structural Class	Number	Depth (m)	Region	Source	Reference
antiallergic	*Botryotinia fuckeliana*	diterpenoid	79	5572	Western Pacific Ocean	sea water	[38]
antibacterial	*Aspergillus penicillioides*	steroid	32, 33	2038	South China Sea	sediment	[23]
antibacterial	*Mycosphaerella* sp. SCSIO z059	iron (III) chelator	34	1330	Okinawa Trough	sediment	[24]
antibacterial	*Mycosphaerella* sp. SCSIO z059	dimerum acid	35	1330	Okinawa Trough	sediment	[24]
antibacterial	*Penicillium* sp. YPGA11	polyketide	36–38	4500	West Pacific	sea water	[25]
antibacterial	*Penicillium canescens* SCSIO z053.	polyketide	39, 40	1387	Okinawa Trough	sediment	[26]
antibacterial	*Aspergillus versicolor*	sesquiterpene	41–44	1487	South China Sea	sediment	[27]
antibacterial	*Aspergillus fumigatus*	alkaloid	45, 46	3614	India Ocean	sediment	[28]
antibacterial	*Penicillium bioburgeianum*	alkaloid	47	2226	South China Sea	sediment	[29]
antibacterial	*Arthrinium* sp. UJNMF0008	alkaloid	25, 48–51	3858	South China Sea	sediment	[19]
antibacterial	*Aspergillus* sp. SCSIO06786	phenol	52–56	4762	India Ocean	sediment	[30]
antibacterial	*Penicillium crustosum* *	phenol	55–58	526	Prydz Bay	sediment	[31]
antifood allergic	*Graphostroma* sp. MCCC 3A00421	polyketide	76–78	2721	Atlantic	hydrothermal sulfide	[37]
antifungal	*Aspergillus fumigatus*	alkaloid	63	3614	India Ocean	sediment	[28]
anti-inflammatory	*Trichobotrys effuse*	polyketide	64, 65	1428	South China Sea	sediment	[34]
anti-inflammatory	*Graphostroma* sp. MCCC 3A00421	sesquiterpenoid	66–69	2721	Atlantic	hydrothermal sulfide	[35]
anti-inflammatory	*Cystobasidium laryngis*	alkaloid	70–75	4317	India Ocean	sediment	[36]
antituberculosis	*Aspergillus fischeri*	polyketide	60–63	3000	India Ocean	sediment	[33]
cytotoxic	*Penicillium citreonigrum*	polyketide	1, 2	2910	Southeast India Ocean	sediment	[11]
cytotoxic	*Phomopsis lithocarpus*	polyketide	3, 4	3606	India Ocean	sediment	[12]
cytotoxic	*Chaetomium globosum*	polyketide	5, 6	2476	South China Sea	sediment	[13]
cytotoxic	*Penicillium chrysogenum*	polyketide	7–15	2076	South Atlantic Ocean	sediment	[14]
cytotoxic	*Hypoxylon rubiginosum*	polyketide	16–19	4188	South China Sea	sediment	[15]
cytotoxic	*Penicillium griseofulvum*	sesquiterpene	20	1420	India Ocean	sediment	[16]
cytotoxic	*Botryotinia fuckeliana*	diterpene	21	5572	West Pacific	sea water	[17]
cytotoxic	*Phomopsis tersa*	meroterpenoid	22, 23	3000	India Ocean	sediment	[18]
cytotoxic	*Chaetomium globosum*	alkaloid	24	2476	South China Sea	sediment	[13]
cytotoxic	*Arthrinium* sp. UJNMF0008	alkaloid	25	3858	South China Sea	sediment	[19]
cytotoxic	*Cladosporium sphaerospermum*	alkaloid	26	4571	East India Ocean	sediment	[20]
cytotoxic	*Cladosporium sphaerospermum*	alkaloid	27–29	6562	Mariana Trench	sediment	[21]
cytotoxic	*Sarcopodium* sp. FKJ-0025	phenol	30, 31	200	Kagoshima coast	sediment	[22]

* refers to a mixed culture of the Antarctic deep-sea-derived fungus *Penicillium crustosum* PRB-2 and the mangrove-derived fungus *Xylaria* sp. HDN13-249.

2.1. Antitumoral Secondary Metabolites

Compounds **1–32** were isolated from deep-sea fungi from different sea areas and showed varying degrees of antitumor activity.

Compounds **1–4** (Figure 2) are all polyketides. New compounds 2-hydroxyl-3pyrenocine-thio propanoic acid (**1**) and 5, 5-dichloro-1-(3, 5dimethoxyphenyl)-1, 4-dihydroxypentan-2-one (**2**), containing sulfur or chlorine atoms, were isolated from the ethyl acetate extract of *Penicillium citreonigrum*. Compound **1** existed in the form of C-2′ epimers with a ratio of 1:2 (2′R:2′S). It showed potent cytotoxicity against human hepatocellular carcinoma cell (HCC) line Bel7402 and human fibrosarcoma cell line HT1080. The IC_{50} (50% inhibiting concentration) values were 7.63 ± 1.46 and 10.22 ± 1.32 µM, respectively. Compound **2** exhibited an IC_{50} value of 16.53 ± 1.67 µM against human fibrosarcoma tumor cell HT1080 [11]. Benzophenone derivatives tenellone H (**3**) and compound AA03390 (**4**) were isolated from the extract of a fungus *Phomopsis lithocarpus* derived from Indian Ocean sediments, compound **3** exhibited moderate cytotoxic activity against human HCC line and human non-small cell lung cancer cell (NSCLC) line A549, with IC_{50} values of 16.0 ± 0.1 and 17.6 ± 0.3 µM, respectively. Compound **4** showed weak cytotoxic activity against human HCC cell line HepG-2, human breast cancer cell line MCF-7, human neuronal cancer cell line SF-268 and human NSCLC line A549 [12].

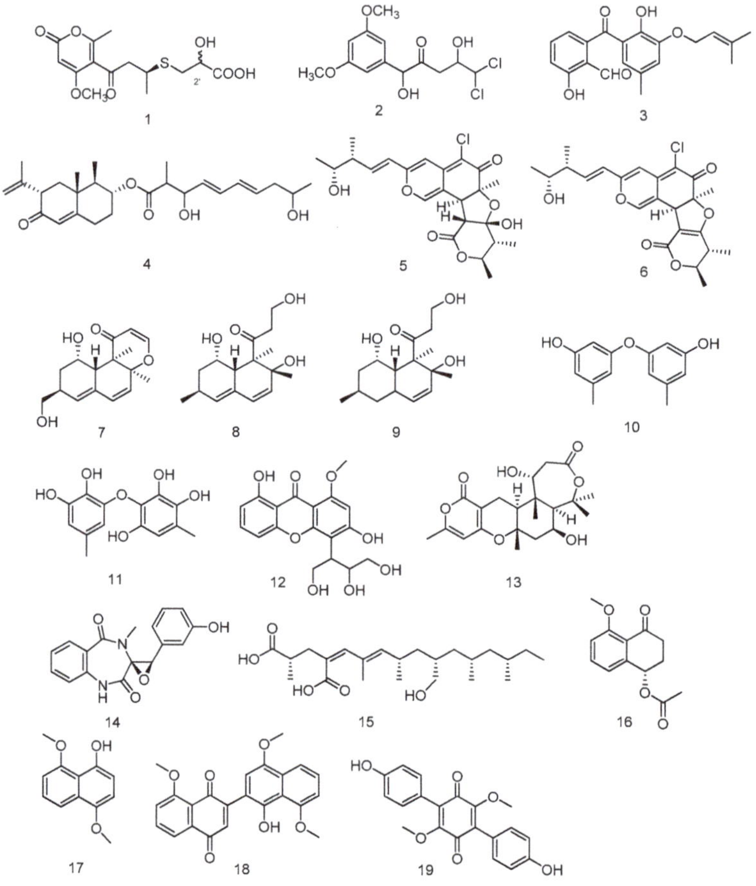

Figure 2. Structures of polyketides with antitumor activity.

Chaetomium globosum HDN151398 was isolated from deep-sea sediments in the South China Sea, and its metabolites chaetomugilin A (**5**) and chaetomugilin C (**6**) (Figure 2) showed broad-spectrum cytotoxic activities. Compound **5** exhibited significant cytotoxic activity against human promyelocytic leukemia cell line HL-60 and human colorectal cancer cells HCT-116, with IC_{50} values of 6.4 and 6.1 µM, respectively. While compound **6** exhibited IC_{50} values of 6.6 and 5.7 µM against HL-60 and HCT-116, respectively [13].

Peniciversiols A (**7**), decumbenone A (**8**), decumbenone B (**9**), 3, 3′-dihydroxy-5, 5′-dimethyldiphenyl ether (**10**), violaceol-II (**11**), 3, 8-dihydroxy-4-(2, 3-dihydroxy-1-hydroxymethylpropyl)-1-methoxyxanthone (**12**), asperdemin (**13**), cyclopenol (**14**) and radiclonic acid (**15**) were isolated from the ethyl acetate extract of *Penicillium chrysogenum* MCCC 3A00292. Their structures were shown in Figure 2. Compound **7** was a versiol-type analogue featuring a 2, 3-dihydropyran-4-one ring and showed significant cytotoxic activity against human Bladder cancer cell line BIU-87 with the IC_{50} value of 10.21 µM. Meanwhile compounds **10**, **14** and **15** also had selective inhibition against BIU-87 with IC_{50} values of 16.41, 8.34 and 12.47 µM, respectively. Compounds **8**, **9**, **11** and **16** exhibited selective inhibitory effect against human esophageal cell line ECA109 with IC_{50} values of 12.41, 15.60, 8.95 and 7.70 µM, respectively. Compounds **12**–**15** had selective inhibition against human Hepatocellular carcinoma cell line BEL-7402. The IC_{50} values were 15.94, 12.75, 7.81 and 13.75, respectively [14].

Hypoxylon rubiginosum FS521, a higher fungi species, was isolated from deep-sea sediments in the South China Sea. From its ethyl acetate extract, hypoxone A (**16**), 4, 8-dimethoxy-1-naphthol (**17**), 1′-hydroxy-4′, 8, 8′-trimethoxy[2, 2′]binaphthalenyl-1, 4-dione (**18**) and 3, 6-dimethylatromentin (**19**) were isolated. Compounds **17** and **18** were new natural products. Compound **18** exhibited significant selective inhibitory effects against human glioblastoma carcinoma cell line SF-268, human breast cancer cell line MCF-7, human liver cancer cell line HepG-2 and human lung cancer cell line A549 with IC_{50} values of 1.9, 3.2, 2.5, and 5.0 µM, respectively. Compounds **16**, **17** and **19** showed weak inhibition against the four tumor cell lines with IC_{50} values ranging from 18.89 to 69.62 µM [15].

Penigrisacid D (**20**) is a sesquiterpene isolated from the extract of *Penicillium griseofulvum*, which showed a weak inhibitory activity against esophageal cancer cell line ECA-109, with an IC_{50} value of 28.7 µM [16]. Aphidicolin A8 (**21**) is a diterpene isolated from the extract of *Botryotinia fuckeliana* derived from Western Pacific seawater samples, which induced human bladder cancer cell T24 and human promyelocytic leukemia cell HL-60 apoptosis by DNA damage, with the IC_{50} values of 2.5 µM and 6.1 µM, respectively [17]. Photoroids A (**22**) and B (**23**) were isolated from the extract of the fungus *Phomopsis tersa*. They are both heteroterpenes containing a 6/6/6/6 tetracyclic system which forms Ortho-Quinone methides (o-QMs) intermediates through a rare Diels-Alder reaction. Compounds **22** and **23** (Figure 3) showed moderate cytotoxicity against four human cancer cell lines: SF-268, MCF-7, HepG-2 and A549 [18].

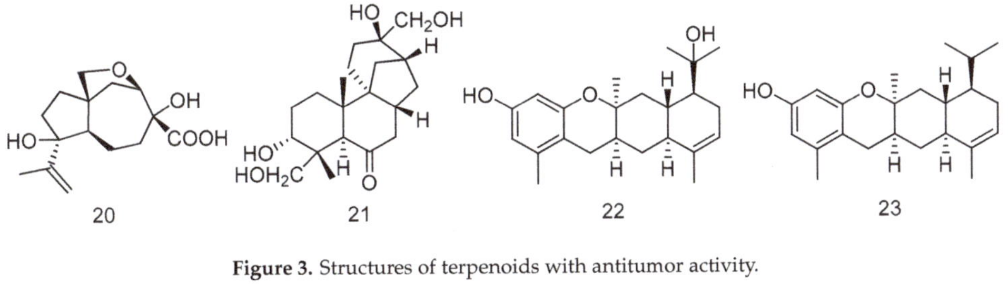

Figure 3. Structures of terpenoids with antitumor activity.

N-glutarylchaetoviridins (**24**) is an azaphilone alkaloid containing glutamine residues isolated from *Chaetomium globosum* HDN151398. Compound **24** exhibited significant cytotoxic activity against human gastric cancer cell line MGC-803 and human ovarian cancer cell line HO-8910, with IC_{50} values of 6.6 and 9.7 µM, respectively [13]. Apiosporamide (**25**) is also an alkaloid, isolated from the extract of

Arthrinium sp. UJNMF0008 derived from sediments of the South China Sea. It exihibited cytotoxicity against two human osteosarcoma cell lines (U2OS and MG63) with IC_{50} values of 19.3 and 11.7 μM [19].

Cladodionen (**26**) was isolated from the extract of *Cladosporium sphaerospermum* derived from the Indian Ocean deep sea sediments, and cladosins I–K (**27–30**) (Figure 4) were isolated from the extract of *Cladosporium sphaerospermum* derived from Mariana Trench. Compound **26** showed cytotoxic activity against human promyelocytic leukemia cell line HL-60, with the IC_{50} value of 28.6 μM [20]. Compounds **27–29** showed different levels of cytotoxic activity against human chronic myelogenous leukemia cell line K562 and human promyelocytic leukemia cell line HL-60, with IC_{50} values ranging from 2.8 to 7.8 μM [21].

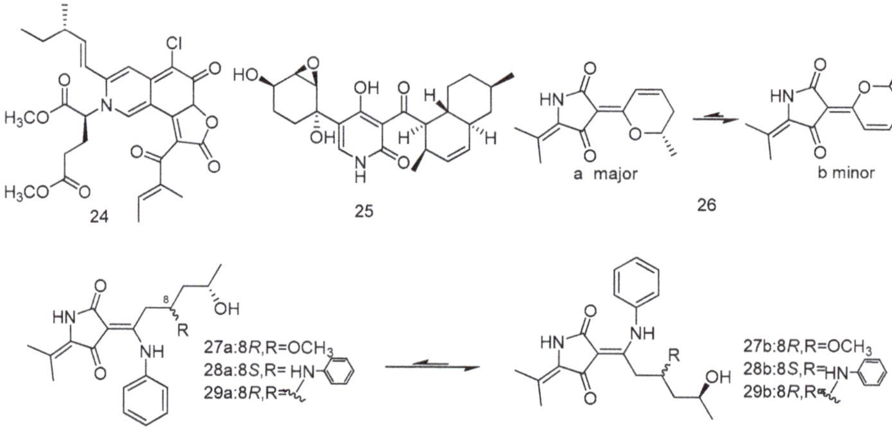

Figure 4. Structures of alkaloids with antitumor activity.

Sarcopodinols A (**30**) and B (**31**) (Figure 5) were isolated from the fungus *Sarcopodium* sp. FKJ-0025 isolated from coastal sediments of Kagoshima. Compound **30** had weak cytotoxicity towards human T-lymphocytic leukemia Jurkat cell line, with the IC_{50} value of 47 μg/mL. Compound **31** exhibited an IC_{50} value of 37 μg/mL against HL-60 cell line, 47 μg/mL against Jurkat cell line, and 66 μg/mL against human pancreatic cancer Panc1 cell [22].

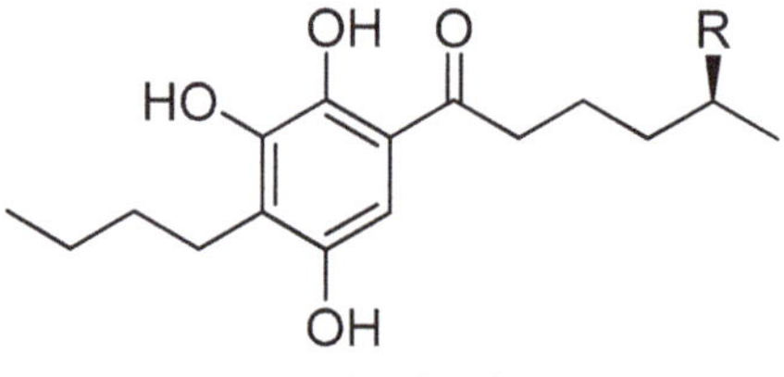

Figure 5. Structures of other compounds with antitumor activity.

2.2. Antmicrobial Secondary Metabolites

2.2.1. Antibacterial Secondary Metabolites

Compounds **32–62** are secondary metabolites with antibacterial activity isolated from fungi extracts from different deep-sea environments.

7β, 8β-epoxy-(22E, 24R)-24-methylcholesta-4, 22-diene-3, 6-dione (**32**) and ergosta-4, 6, 8(14), 22-tetraene-3-one (**33**) (Figure 6) were steroids isolated from the extract of *Aspergillus penicillioides* SD-311 from deep sea-sediment collected of the South China Sea. Compound **32** could inhibit *Vibrio anguillarum* with the MIC (minimum inhibitory concentration) value of 32.0 mg/mL. And compound **33** showed antibacterial activity against *Edwardsiella tarda* and *Micrococcus luteus* with MIC values both of 16 mg/mL [23].

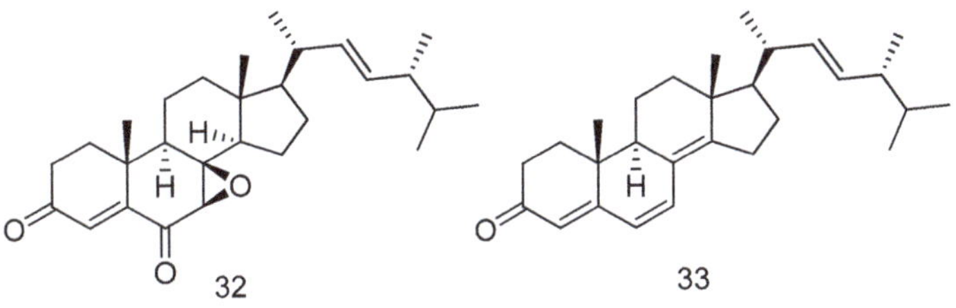

Figure 6. Structures of steroids with antibacterial activity.

Mycosphazine A (**34**) was isolated from the extract of *Mycosphaerella* sp. SCSIO z059. It is a new a new iron(III) chelator of coprogen-type siderophore which could greatly promote the biofilm formation of *Bacillus amyloliquefaciens* with the rate of about 249% at concentration of 100 μg·mL^{-1}. Its alkaline hydrolysate was a new epimer of dimerum acid, mycosphazine B (**35**) (Figure 7) which showed the same activity with the rate of about 524% at concentration of 100 μg·mL^{-1} [24].

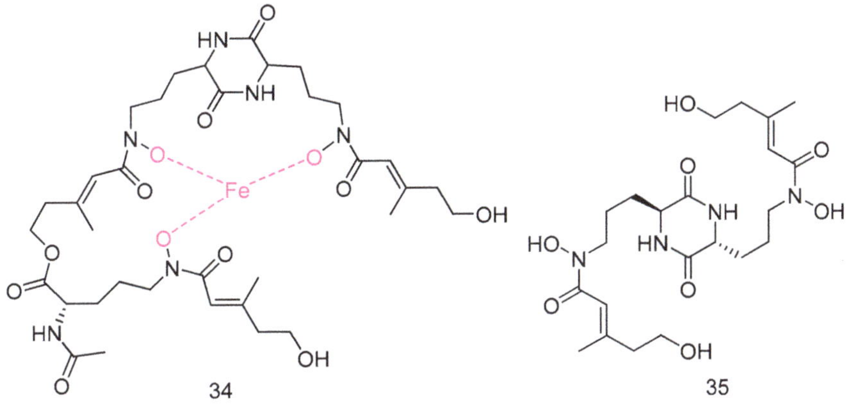

Figure 7. Structures of Mycosphazine A and B.

Peniginsengins C–E (**36–38**) (Figure 8) were new farnesylcyclohexenones isolated from the extract of *Penicillium* sp. YPGA11 from the sea water in the Yapu Trench. They showed activity against methicillin-resistant *Staphylococcus aureus* (Methicillin-resistant *Staphylococcus aureus* (MRSA), and anti-methicillin-sensitive *Staphylococcus aureus* (Methicillin-Sensitive *Staphylococcus aureus*, MSSA), with the MICvalues ranging from 8 μg/mL to 64 μg/mL [25].

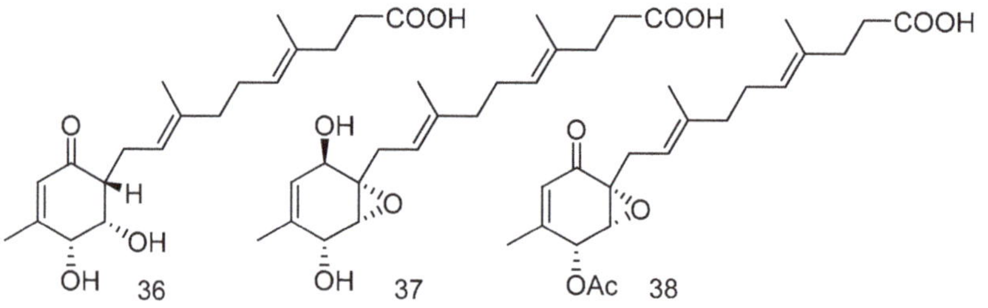

Figure 8. Structures of farnesylcyclohexenones with antibacterial activity.

Canescenin A–B (**39–40**) (Figure 9) were isolated from the extract of *Penicillium canescens* SCSIO z053 derived from the deep-sea sediment of Okinawa Trough. Both of the compounds showed weak antibacterial activities toward *B. amyloliquefaciens* and *P. aeruginosa* at 100 µM [24].

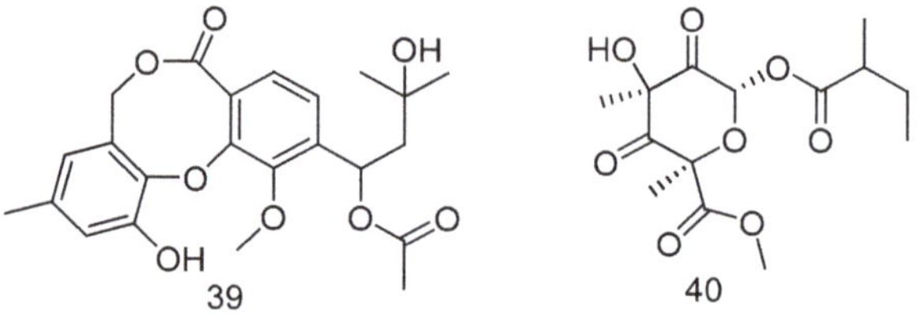

Figure 9. Structures of Canescenin A–B.

Four bisabolane-type sesquiterpenoid derivatives *ent*-aspergoterpenin C (**41**), 7-*O*-methylhydroxysydonic acid (**42**), hydroxysydonic acid (**43**) and sydonic acid (**44**) (Figure 10) were isolated from *Aspergillus versicolor* derived from the deep-sea sediment of South China Sea. Compounds **41–42** had strong antibacterial activity, whose MIC values against *Escherichia coli*, *Edwardsiella tarda*, *Vibrio harveyi* and *Vibrio parahaemolyticus* were all below or equal to 8.0 µg/mL. Moreover, compound **43** exihibited antibacterial activities against *Aeromonas hydrophila*, *Escherichia coli*, *Vibrio anguillarum* and *Vibrio harveyi*, with the MIC value of 4.0 µg/mL, equal to the positive control Chloramphenicol [25].

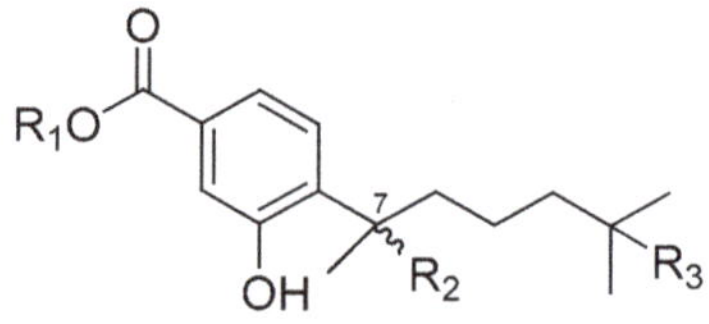

41 $R_1=CH_3, R_2=OH, R_3=OH(7R)$
42 $R_1=H, R_2=OCH_3, R_3=OH(7R)$
43 $R_1=H, R_2=OH, R_3=OH$
44 $R_1=H, R_2=OH, R_3=H(7S)$

Figure 10. Structures of bisabolane-type sesquiterpenoid with antibacterial activity.

Fumigatosides E (**45**) and F (**46**) (Figure 11) were quinazoline-containing indole alkaloids, isolated from the extract of *Aspergillus fumigatus* from the deep-sea sediments of the Indian Ocean. Both of them showed potent antibacterial activities. The MIC values of compound **45** against *Acinetobacter baumannii* ATCC 19606, *Acinetobacter baumannii* ATCC 15122, *Staphylococcus aureus*

ATCC 16339 and *Klebsiella pneumoniae* ATCC 14578 were: 12.5 ± 0.042, 6.25 ± 0.035, 6.25 ± 0.13, 12.5 ± 0.098 µg/mL, and the MIC value of compound **46** against *Acinetobacter baumannii* was 6.25 ± 0.033 µg/mL [26].

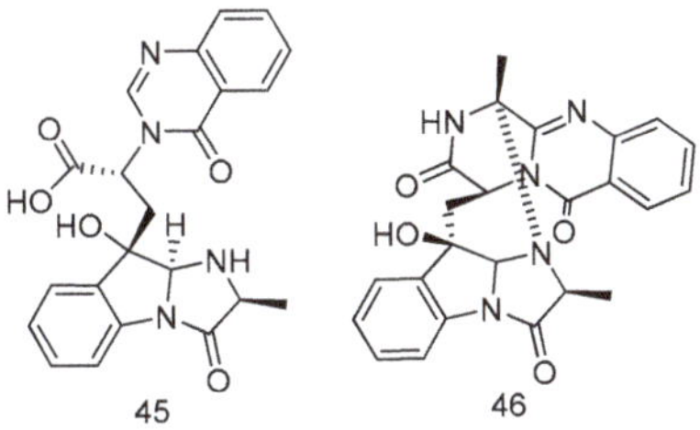

Figure 11. Structures of quinazoline-containing indole alkaloids with antibacterial activity.

Penicillenol A2 (**47**) (Figure 12) was isolated from the extract of *Penicillium biourgeianum* isolated from the sediments of the South China Sea with an inhibitory effect on MSSA. The diameter of inhibitory zone (ZD) is 6.75 ± 0.25 mm. Besides, the synergy of compound **47** with penicillin G sodium (Pen), cefotaxime sodium (Ctx) and oxacillin sodium (Oxa) was studied by plate count and Kirby-Bordisk diffusion method. It was found that, in comparison with the control group, the reduction of bacteria in the experimental group using Pen (10 U mL^{-1}), Ctx (15 U mL^{-1}) and Oxa (1 U mL^{-1}) was less than 1 log $^{CFU/mL}$. Compared with using compound **30** alone, the reduction of viable bacteria in the experimental group using both the above drugs and compound **47** was greater than or equal to 2 log CFU/mL. Therefore, the combination of compound **30** and β-lactam antibiotics had a synergistic effect, which can increase the sensitivity of MRSA to β-lactam antibiotics [27].

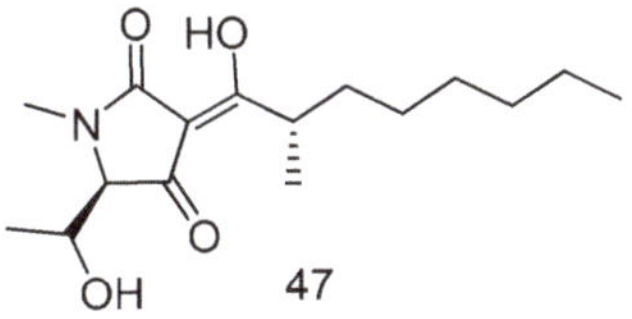

Figure 12. Structure of Penicillenol A2.

Pyridone alkaloids, apiosporamide (**25**) and arthpyrones F–K (**48–51**) (Figure 13), were isolated from the extract of *Arthrinium* sp. UJNMF0008 from the sediments of South China Sea, which showed moderate to strong antibacterial activity against *Mycobacterium smegmatis* and *Staphylococcus aureus*, with the IC$_{50}$ values ranging from 1.66–42.8 µM [19].

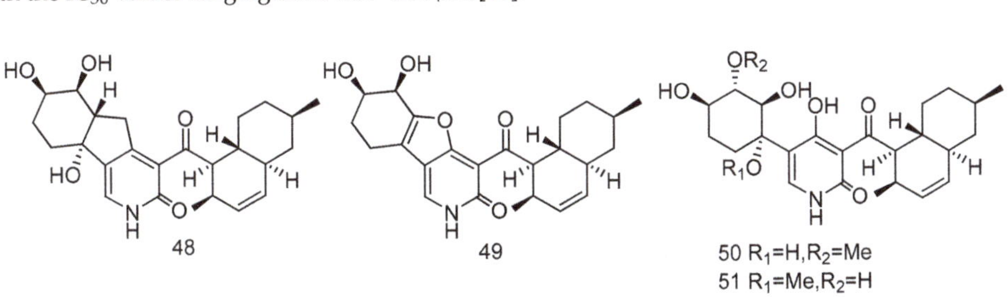

Figure 13. Structures of pyridone alkaloids with antibacterial activity.

3, 5-dimethoxytoluene (**52**), 3, 3′-dihydroxy-5, 5′-dimethyldiphenyl ether (**53**), 3, 4-dihydroxyphenylacetic acid methyl ester (**54**) (Figure 14) were isolated from the extract of *Aspergillus* sp. SCSIO06786 from deep-sea sediments in the Indian Ocean. Compounds **52** and **53** with 50 µg/disc showed inhibition zones against *S. aureus*, MRSA and *E. faecalis*. Compound **54** with 50 µg/disc inhibited the growth of MRSA. In addition, their MIC was tested and the results showed that it was between 3.13–12.5 µg/mL [30]. Penixylarins B–C (**55**–**56**), 1, 3-dihydroxy-5-(12-hydroxyheptadecyl)benzene (**57**), and 1, 3dihydroxy-5-(12-sulfoxyheptadecyl)benzene (**58**) (Figure 14) were isolated from a mixed culture of the Antarctic deep-sea-derived fungus *Penicillium crustosum* PRB-2 with a fungus *Xylaria* sp. HDN13-249. Compounds **55**–**58** showed activities against *Bacillus tuberculosis*, *B. subtilis* or *Vibrio parahaemolyticus*, MIC values ranging from 6.25 to 100 µM. Among them, the MIC value of compound **56** against *B. tuberculosis* was 6.25 µM, showing the anti-tuberculosis potential [31].

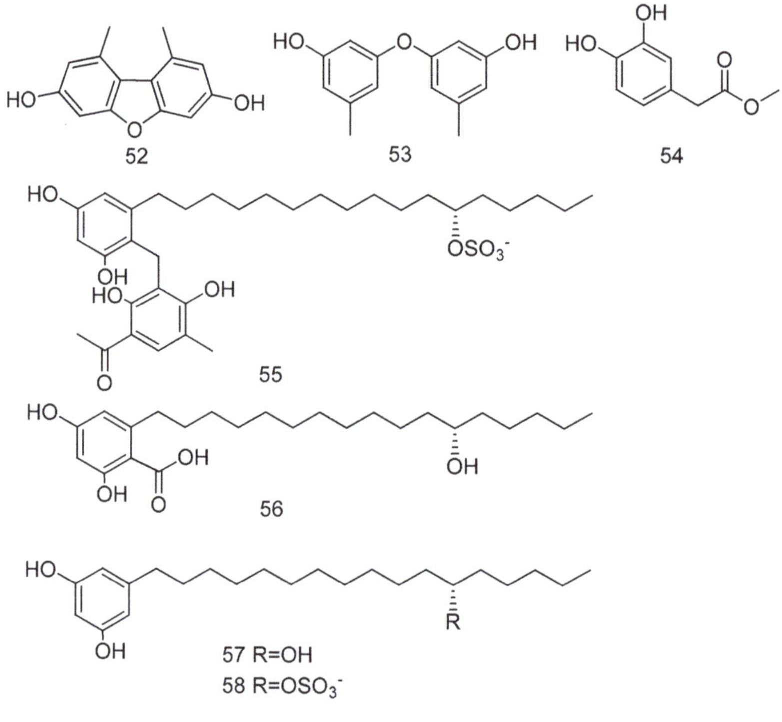

Figure 14. Structures of phenols with antibacterial activity.

The tyrosine phosphatase (Mptp) secreted by *Mycobacterium tuberculosis* is an important virulence factor of *Mycobacterium tuberculosis* and recognized to be an important target to treat tuberculosis. Tyrosine phosphatase is secreted by *Mycobacterium tuberculosis*, which has two functional phosphatases, PTP A and B (MptpA and MptpB) and enters the cytoplasm of macrophages, preventing the activation of the host's immune system and regulating the survival of the bacilli in the host [32]. Compounds **59**–**62** (Figure 15) were polyacrylate derivatives with long hydrophobic chains, isolated from the extract of *Aspergillus fischeri* derived from deep sea sediments in Indian Ocean. Compounds **59**–**62** inhibited *M. tuberculosis* protein tyrosine phosphatase B (MptpB) through non-competitive inhibition, with IC_{50} values of 5.1, 12, 4.0 and 11 µM, respectively [33].

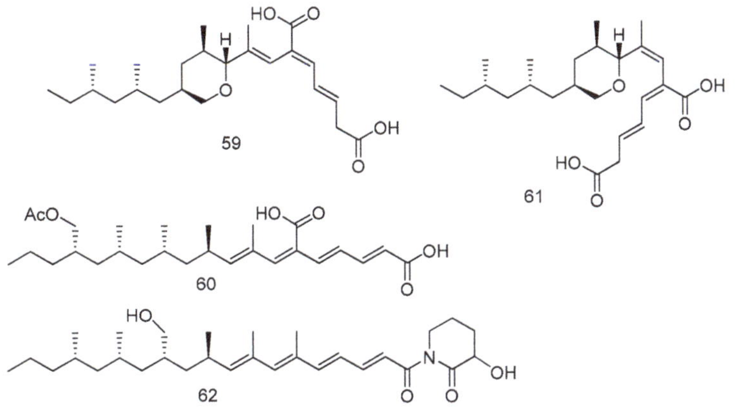

Figure 15. Structures of polypropionate derivatives with antituberculosis activity.

2.2.2. Antifungal Secondary Metabolites

Quinazoline-containing indole alkaloid, fumigatoside F (**63**) (Figure 16), was isolated from the extract of *Aspergillus fumigatus* derived from deep-sea sediments of the Indian Ocean. The MIC values against *Fusarium oxysporum* f. sp. *cucumerinu* and *Fusarium oxysporum* f. sp. *momordicae* were 25 ± 0.04 and 1.565 ± 0.098 µg/mL, respectively [28].

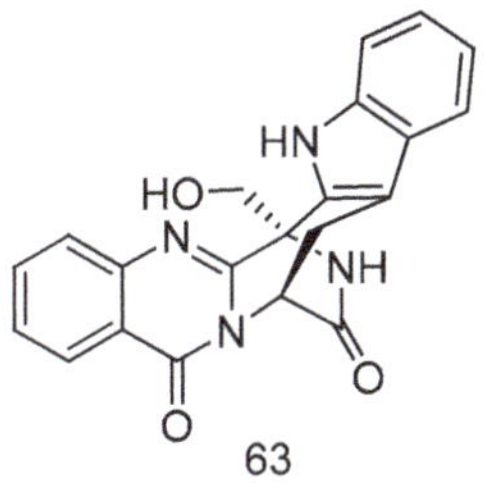

Figure 16. Structure of fumigatoside F.

2.3. Secondary Metabolites with Other Bioactivities

In addition to antitumoral and antimicrobial activity, secondary metabolites of deep-sea fungi reported in recent years also have anti-inflammatory and anti-food allergic activities. Compounds **64–69** were secondary metabolites from deep-sea fungi with anti-inflammatory activity.

Trieffusols C (**64**) and D (**65**) (Figure 17) were isolated from the extract of *Trichobotrys effuse* from deep-sea sediments of the South China Sea with inhibition of nitric oxide (NO) production in murine macrophages. Their IC_{50} values were 51.9 and 55.9 µM, which is equivalent to the positive control aminoguanidine (IC_{50}: 24.8 µM) [34].

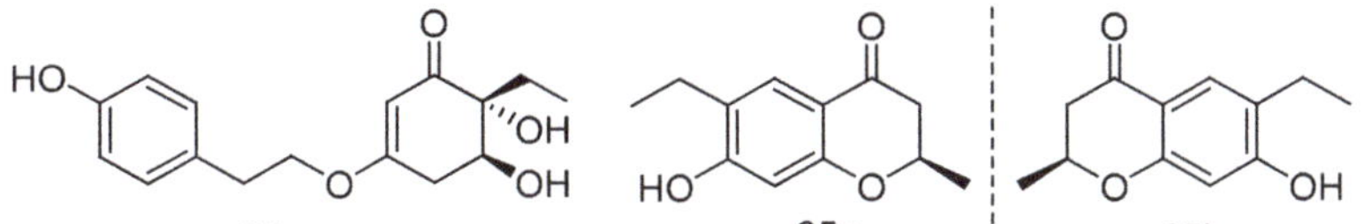

Figure 17. Molecular structures of Trieffusols C and D.

Graphostromane D (**66**), graphostromane F (**67**), graphostromane I (**68**) and (1R, 4S, 5S, 7S, 9R, 10S, 11R)-guaiane-9, 10, 11, 12-tetraol (**69**) (Figure 18) were sesquiterpenoids isolated from the extract of *Graphostroma* sp. MCCC 3A00421 derived from hydrothermal sulfide deposit. Compound **50** showed anti-infammatory activity against LPS-induced NO production in RAW264.7 macrophages, with an IC$_{50}$ value of 14.2 µM, even stronger than that of positive contrast. Meanwhile compound **66, 68** and **69** exhibited weak anti-infammatory activities, with the IC$_{50}$ values of 72.9, 79.1, and 88.2 µM [35].

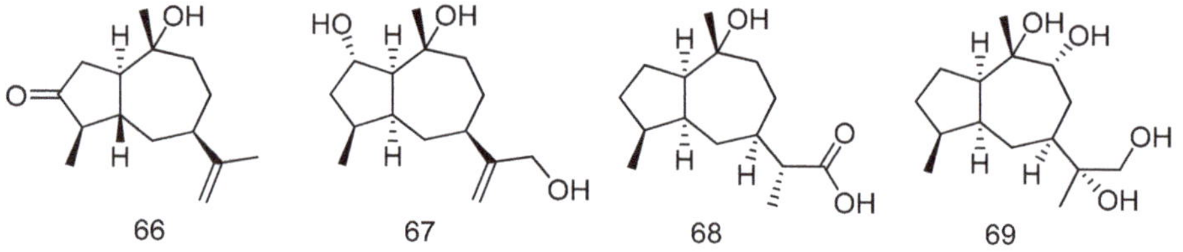

Figure 18. Molecular structures of sesquiterpenoids.

Phenazine derivatives, 6-[1-(2-aminobenzoyloxy)ethyl]-1-phenazinecarboxylic acid (**70**), saphenol (**71**), (R)-saphenic acid (**72**), phenazine-1-carboxylic acid (**73**), 6-(1-hydroxyehtyl)phenazine-1-carboxylic acid (**74**) and 6-acetyl-phenazine-1-carboxylic acid (**75**) (Figure 19), were isolated from the extract of *Cystobasidium laryngis*, which inhibits the NO in mouse macrophage RAW 264.7 cells induced by Lipopolysaccharide (LPS), and does not affect the viability of RAW 264.7 cells at a concentration of up to 30 µg/mL. Compounds **72, 74, 75** showed similar inhibitory effects, of which compound **74** had the most obvious inhibitory effect, with the concentration for 50% of maximal effect (EC$_{50}$) value of 19.6 µM. Methylated compound **74** and oxidized compound **75** showed no significant differences in activity mentioned above, but their strength was twice as strong as compound **70** (EC$_{50}$ = 46.8 µM) substituted with 2-aminobenzoic acid. In addition, when there is no functional group substitution at C-6 of phenazine (**73**, EC$_{50}$ = 76.1 µM), the activity is the lowest [36].

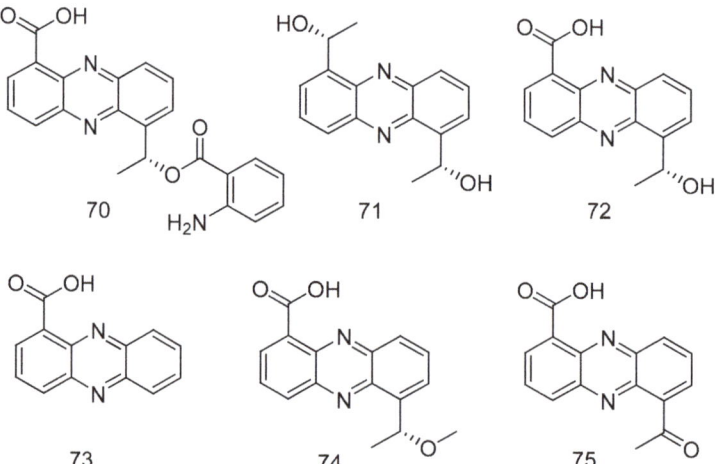

Figure 19. Structures of phenazine derivatives with anti-inflammatory activity.

The occurrence of food allergic diseases may be related to excessive immune response. Allergens are usually harmless foods such as milk, eggs, fish, peanuts and grains [39]. Acute hypersensitivity is triggered by factors released by mast cells when allergens interact with membrane-bound immune proteins (IgE) [40].

Polyketides **76–78** (Figure 20) were isolated from *Graphostroma* sp. MCCC 3A00421 derived from hydrothermal sulfide, which showed antifood allergic activity. Reticulol (**76**) showed effective inhibition of immunoglobulin E-mediated rat basophilic leukemia-2H3 cells (RBL-2H3) degranulation, with an IC_{50} value of 13.5 µM, which was about seven times stronger than the commercially available anti-food allergy drug loratadine (IC_{50} = 91.6 µM), while 7, 8-dihydroxy -3-methyl-3, 4-dihydroisocoumarin (**77**) and hydroxyemodin (**78**) showed weaker effects, with IC_{50} values of 154.1 and 139.3 µM [37].

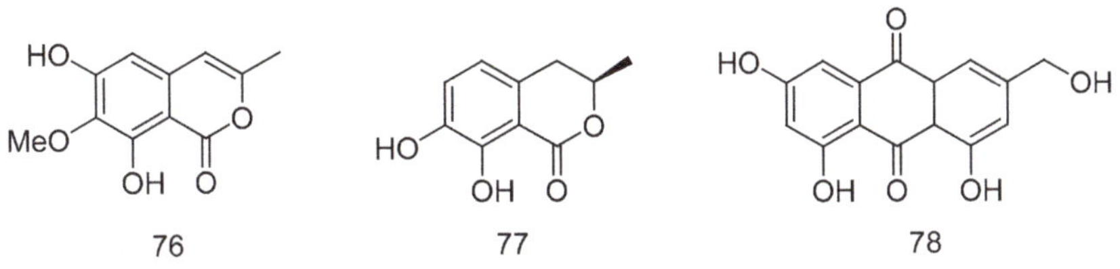

Figure 20. Structures of polyketides with antifood allergic activity.

Botryotin A (**79**) (Figure 21) was isolated from *Botryotinia fuckeliana* derived from deep-sea water of the Western Pacific Ocean, which showed moderate antiallergic effect with the IC_{50} value of 0.2 mM [38].

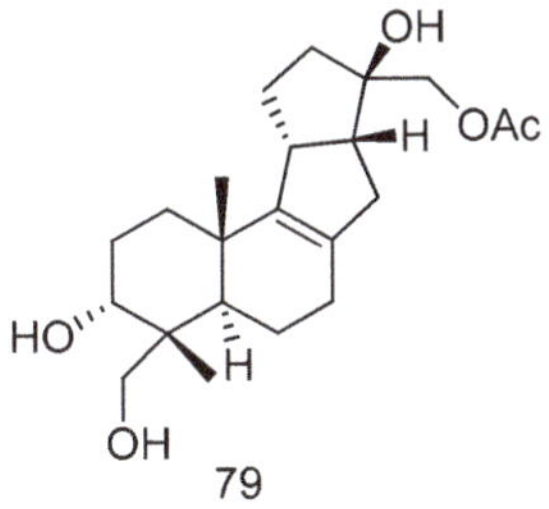

Figure 21. Structure of Botryotin A.

3. Secondary Metabolites from Deep-Sea Derived Bacteria

Bacteria from deep-sea sediments are a good source of marine natural products, and their secondary metabolites are usually novel in structure with significant biological activities [41–45]. In particular, actinomycetes are currently proven to be the most important sources of biologically active natural products with clinical or pharmaceutical applications [46]. According to the references, 40 (16 novel) natural products were discovered from deep-sea derived bacteria in the past three years, 19 among which showed biological activities (Table 2).

Table 2. Bioactive Natural products from deep-sea derived bacteria in 2018–2020.

Bioactivity	Bacterial Species	STRUCTRUAL CLASS	Number	Depth (m)	Region	Source	Reference
anti-allergic effect	Saccharopolyspora cebuensis	polyketide	98	2875	Atlantic	sediment	[47]
cytotoxic	Saccharopolyspora cebuensis	polyketide	80	2875	Atlantic	sediment	[47]
cytotoxic	Nonomuraea sp. AKA32	polyketide	81–83	800	Sagami Bay	sea water	[48]
cytotoxic	Ochrobactrum sp. OUCMDZ-2164	polyketide	84	2000	South China Sea	sea water	[49]
cytotoxic	Ochrobactrum sp. OUCMDZ-2164	polyketide	85	2000	South China Sea	sea water	[50]
cytotoxic	Streptomyces cyaneofuscatus	alkaloid	86, 87	2000	Biscay Bay	solitary coral	[51]
antibacterial	Streptomyces sp. SCSIO ZS0098	peptide	88	3000	South China Sea	sediment	[52]
antibacterial	Streptomyces atratus	peptide	89	3536	South China Sea	sediment	[53]
antibacterial	Streptomyces cyaneofuscatus	polyketide	90, 91	1500	Avilés submarine Canyon	gorgonian coral	[54]
antibacterial	Nocardiopsis sp. HB-J378	polyketide	92–94	—	—	Theonella sp.	[55]
antibacterial	Streptomycetes sp. strain SMS636.	alkaloid	95, 96	3000	South China Sea	sediment	[56]
anti-BCG	Streptomycetes sp. strain SMS636.	alkaloid	96	3000	South China Sea	sediment	[56]
inhibit the cell damage	Alcanivorax sp. SHA4	alkaloid	97	5180	West Atlantic	sediment	[57]

3.1. Antitumoral Secondary Metabolites

Compounds **80–87** all showed potent cytotoxic activity.

Cebulactam A2 (**80**) (Figure 22) was a polyketide isolated from the extract of *Saccharopolyspora cebuensis* derived from Atlantic deep-sea sediments, which had a weak antiproliferative effect on human cervical cancer cell Hela and human lung cancer cell H1299, the inhibition rates (20.00 μg/mL) were 35.0 and 31.0%, respectively [47].

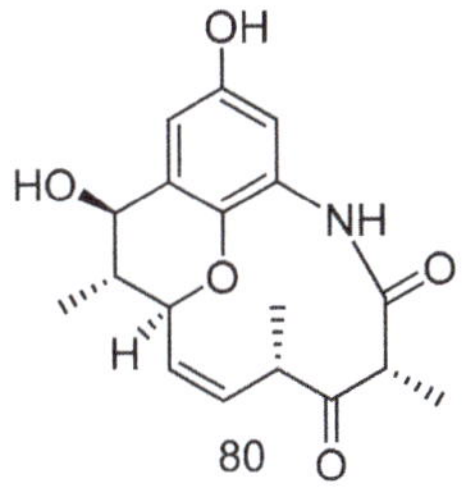

Figure 22. Structure of Cebulactam A2.

Akazamicin (**81**), actinofuranone C (**82**) and N-formylanthranilic acid (**83**) (Figure 23) were isolated from the extract of *Nonomuraea* sp. AKA32 derived from seawater of Sagami Bay in Japan. Compounds **81** and **82** showed the same level of cytotoxic activity against B16 melanoma cells, with IC_{50} values of 1.7 and 1.2 μM, respectively. Compound **83** showed about 10 times lower cytotoxic activity than that of compounds **81** and **82**. The cytotoxic activity of these three compounds against human liver cancer cells Hep G2 and human colorectal adenocarcinoma cells Caco-2 was not obvious, with IC_{50} values ranging from 10 to 200 μM [48].

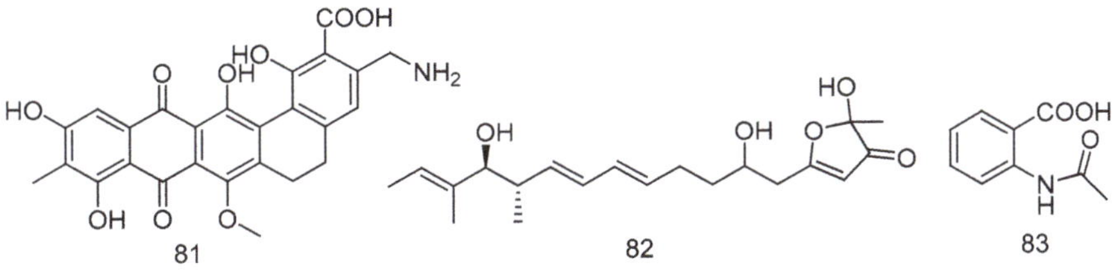

Figure 23. Structures of aromatic polyketides with antitumor activity.

Trienomycins J–H (**84–85**) (Figure 24) were isolated from the extract of *Ochrobactrum* sp. OUCMDZ-2164 derived from deep-sea water of the South China Sea. Compound **84** exhibited antitumor activity against human breast cancer cells (MCF-7) with 61.5% inhibition rate at 10 μmol/L [49]. Compound **85** showed cytotoxic activity against human lung carcinoma cell line (A549) and human leukemia cell line (K562) with IC_{50} values of 15 and 23 μM, respectively [50].

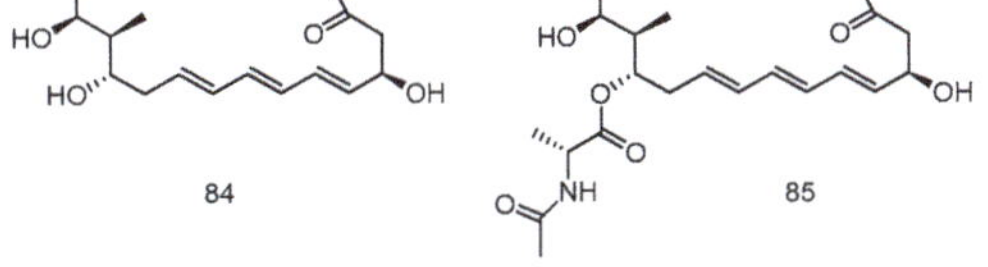

Figure 24. Structures of Ansamycins with antitumor activity.

(*S*)-3-hydroxy-N-(1-hydroxy-3-oxobutan-2-yl) quinoline-2-carboxamide (**86**) and 3-hydroxyquinoline-2-carboxamide (**87**) (Figure 25), were isolated from a solitary coral derived *Streptomyces cyaneofuscatus* from Biscay Bay of north Atlantic. The IC$_{50}$ values towards human liver cancer cell HepG2 were 15.6 and 51.5 µM, respectively [51].

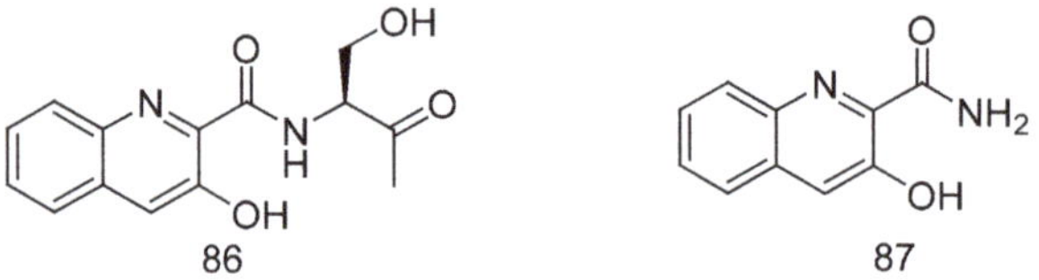

Figure 25. Structures of (*S*)-3-hydroxy-N-(1-hydroxy-3-oxobutan-2-yl) quinoline-2-carboxamide and 3-hydroxyquinoline-2-carboxamide.

3.2. Antimicrobial Secondary Metabolites

Compounds **88**–**96** all showed potent antibacterial activity.

Aborycin (**88**) was a lasso peptide isolated and identified from the deep-sea-derived microbe *Streptomyces* sp. SCSIO ZS0098 which was isolated from the deep-sea sediments of the South China Sea. Shao et al. [52] identified the aborycin biosynthetic gene cluster (abo) on the basis of genomic sequence analysis, and then heterologously expressed in *Streptomyces coelicolor* to obtain compound **86**. The compound had moderate bacteriostatic activity against 13 *Staphylococcus aureus* strains from various sources, with MIC values between 8.0–128 µg/mL. The MIC values of compound **88** against *Enterococcus faecalis* and *Bacillus thuringiensis* were 8.0 µg/mL and, 2.0 µg/mL, respectively. In addition, compound **88** had significant antibacterial activity against the poultry pathogen *Enterococcus enterococci* (MIC = 0.5 µg/mL) [44]. Atratumycin (**89**) was also a peptide isolated from the extract of *Streptomyces atratus* from deep-sea sediments of the South China Sea, which is a cyclic dipeptide that has activity against *Mycobacterium tuberculosis*, whose MIC values were 3.8 and 14.6 µM against *M. tuberculosis* H37Ra and H37Rv [53].

Compounds **90**–**94** are all polyketides. Anthracimycin B (**90**) and anthracimycin (**91**) (Figure 26) were isolated from the extract of *Streptomyces cyaneofuscatus* isolated from a gorgonian coral collected in the 1500 m Avilis submarine canyon. They were sensitive to Gram-positive pathogens MRSA, MSSA, vancomycin-sensitive *Enterococcus faecium* and vancomycin-sensitive *Enterococcus faecalis* and all showed strong antibacterial effects. The MIC value of compound **90** was less than 0.03 µg/mL, and the MIC value of compound **91** was between 0.125–8 µg/mL. Compound **90** also had anti-tuberculosis activity, with the MIC value of 1–2 µg/mL [54].

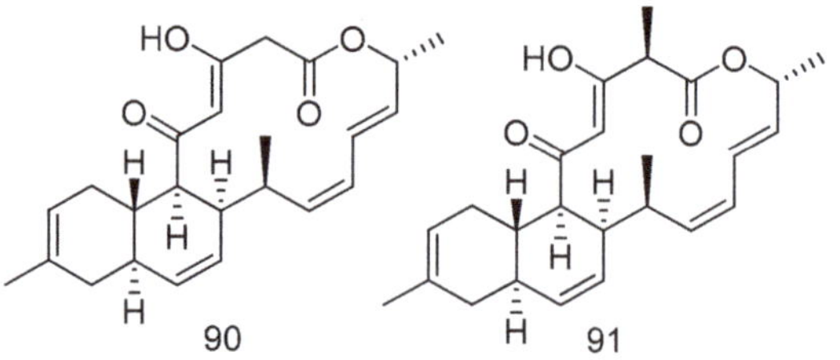

Figure 26. Structures of anthracimycin B and anthracimycin.

Nocardiopsistins A–C (**92**–**94**) (Figure 27) were isolated from the extract of *Nocardiopsis* sp. HB-J378 isolated from a deep-sea sponge *Theonella* sp. Compound **93** had the same MIC (3.12 µg/mL) as the positive control chloramphenicol, while compounds **92** and **94** had moderate anti-MRSA activity (MIC = 12.5 µg/mL) [55].

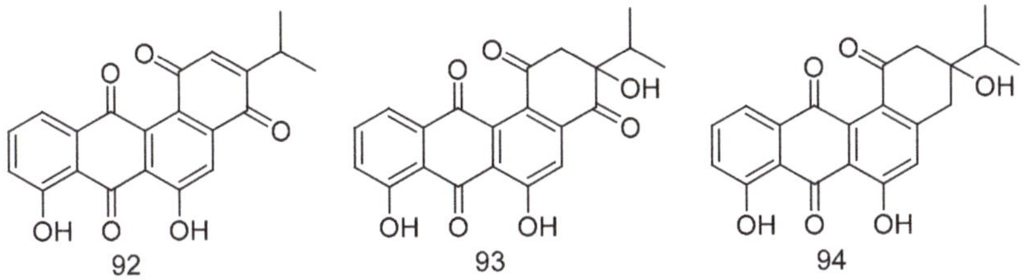

Figure 27. Structures of nocardiopsistins A–C.

1-N-methyl-(E, Z)-albonoursin (**95**) and streptonigrin (**96**) (Figure 28) were alkaloids isolated from the extract of *Streptomycetes* sp. strain SMS636 from deep-sea sediments in the South China Sea. Compound **95** showed moderate antibacterial activity towards *Staphylococcus aureus* and MRSA, with MIC values of 12.5 and 25 µg/mL, respectively. The MIC value of compound **96** was 0.78 µg/mL for *Staphylococcus aureus* and MRSA, and had anti-BCG (Bacillus Calmette-Guérin, BCG) activity with a MIC value of 1.25 µg/mL [56].

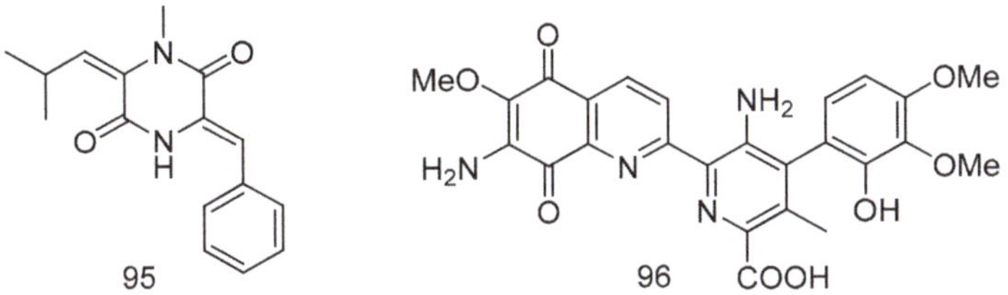

Figure 28. Structures of 1-N-methyl- (E, Z)-albonoursin and streptonigrin.

3.3. Other Bioactive Secondary Metabolites

Acantimycic acid (**97**) was an alkaloid with good neuroprotection. It was isolated from the extract of *Alcanivorax* sp. SHA4 from deep-sea sediments of the Western Pacific and could inhibit the cell damage caused by glutamic acid to PC12 cells. The protective effect was more obvious at low concentration [57]. Indol-3-carbaldehyde (**98**) was isolated from the extract of *Saccharopolyspora cebuensis* derived from Atlantic deep-sea sediments. It showed weak anti-allergic effect with the IC_{50} value of 55.75 µg/mL [47]. The structures of compounds **97** and **98** are shown in Figure 29.

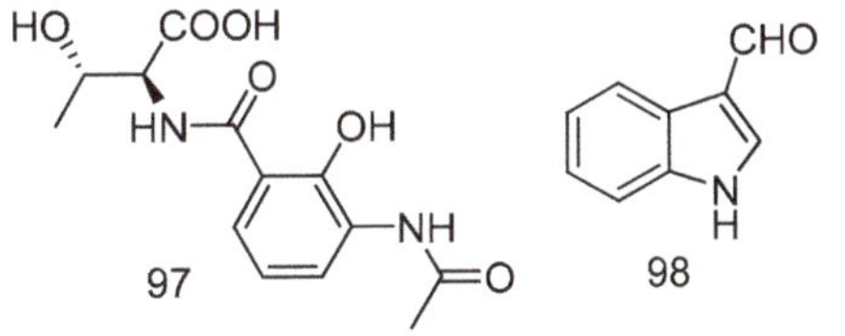

Figure 29. Structures of acantimycic acid and Indol-3-carbaldehyde.

4. Research Methods for Diversity of Secondary Metabolites from Deep-Sea Microorganisms

4.1. Isolation and Cultivation of Deep-Sea Microorganisms

Marine microorganisms have the following characteristics: (1) can grow and/or form spores in the marine environment; (2) form a symbiotic relationship with other marine organisms; or (3) adapt and evolve at the genetic level or have metabolic activity in the marine environment [58]. It is estimated that the diversity of marine fungi exceeds 10,000 species [59,60], but so far only about 1250 species have been described [61,62]. However, deep-sea microbial research starts late for its difficulties in collection and cultivation, so people face more challenges in the exploration of its secondary metabolites.

4.1.1. Sample Pretreatment

In natural samples without pretreatment, the isolation frequency of bacteria is higher than that of fungi [63]. Different pretreatment methods should be adopted for different target strains to improve the isolation efficiency.

Because the actinomycete spores have a certain heat resistance, dry and wet heat treatment can effectively reduce other bacterial contamination [64–68]. Dry heat treatment can inactivate bacteria, and at the same time induce the germination of actinomycetes spores to a certain extent; the principle of wet heat treatment is to denature and inactivate non-target strain proteins in the sample by heating in a water bath. In addition to heat treatment, the commonly used pretreatment methods include chemical reagent treatment [69], differential centrifugation [70] and so on.

Microwave treatment can not only significantly increase the number of isolated alkaliphilic and halophilic marine actinomycetes, but also significantly increase the isolation of rare marine actinomycetes. Ding et al. [71] used 120 W, 2450 MHz microwave and ice-water mixture to process one part of the suspension in the treatment of sea mud samples. After gradient dilution, they were applied to three separate media. In the seven samples after microwave treatment, the number of rare alkaliphilic marine actinomycetes in four samples and the halophilic marine actinomycetes in three samples increased significantly. Therefore, microwave processing also has certain application value.

4.1.2. Medium Selection and Improvement

When the strains are separated, the medium as a nutrient source plays an important role in the growth and metabolism of the strains. Different culture media provide different carbon and nitrogen sources for different microorganisms to grow, so it is necessary to select the appropriate culture media for microorganism screening.

For fungi, we usually use common media such as: Potato Dextrose Agar Medium (PDA), Czapek Dox Agar Medium (CDA), Sabouraud Dextrose Agar Medium (SDA), Corn Meal Agar Medium (CMA), Malt Extract Agar Medium (MEA), yeast malt agar medium (YM), etc. He et al. [72] used the above-mentioned six media (all added chloramphenicol and streptomycin sulfate to inhibit growth of bacteria) to separate samples from the deep-sea sediment samples of Yapu Trench. In their study, YM media was the best from the perspective of the isolation ability of six different media, which obtained nine kinds of fungi; followed by PDA which allowed the retrieval of eight different fungal species. The worst were CMA (three kinds) and CDA (two kinds).

For bacteria, according to the main components of the medium, it can be divided into marine agar medium (MA), synthetic medium for selective isolation of actinomycetes (Actinomycete Isolation Agar, AIA), starch medium, natural ingredient medium, high salt medium and other media (Table 3). Chen et al. [73] used the 23 media in the table to isolate bacteria in the 4000 m deep-sea sediments of the South China Sea, and most of natural products from the strains obtained from the deep sea sediment environment, are antibiotic, cytotoxins, with high efficiency enzyme activity, and tolerant for unfavorable environment, degradation of refractory pollutants and other characteristics suitable for the unique marine extreme environment.

Table 3. Different kinds of medium and their components.

Type of Medium	Name of Medium	Composition of Medium
marine agar medium (MA)	MA; BD Difco™ MAB MAE MAJ	① marine bacteria medium2216E ② 50%MA medium ③ 20%MA medium ④ 10%MA medium
Actinomycete Isolation Agar (AIA)	AIA; BD Difco™ AIAB AIAE	① selective medium for actinomycetes ② 50%AIA medium ③ 20%AIA medium
natural ingredient medium	acid microbial medium (AM) Maltose-Yeast-Peptone Medium (MYP) nutrient medium® R2AB; BD Difco™ R2AJ	① $MgSO_4$ 7 H_2O 0.50 g, $(NH_4)_2SO_4$ 0.40 g, K_2HPO_4 0.20 g, KCl 0.10 g, $FeSO_4·7H_2O$ 0.01 g, yeast extract 0.25 g ② maltose extract 5.0 g, yeast extract 5.0 g, peptone 5.0 g, NaCl 3.0 g ③ peptone 10.0 g, yeast extract 5.0 g, maltose extract 5.0 g, casein amino acid 5.0 g, beef extract 2.0 g, glycerin 2.0 g, Tween 80 50.0 mg, $MgSO_4·7H_2O$ 1.0 g ④ 50%R2A medium ⑤ 5%R2A medium
starch medium	MA starch medium (MAS) 50%MA starch medium (MABS) 20%MA starch medium (MAES) 10%MA starch medium (MAJS) 5%MA starch medium (MATS)	① MA, 1% (m/V) soluble starch ② MAB, 1% (m/V) soluble starch ③ MAE, 1% (m/V) soluble starch ④ MAJ, 1% (m/V) soluble starch ⑤ 5% MA, 1% (m/V) soluble starch
high-salinity medium	high-salinity AIA medium (AIAS) high-salinity beef extract medium (BFSM) high-salinity casein medium (CAAM) high-salinity iron-containing medium (YJSF)	① AIA 10.0 g, NaCl 100.0 g, crude salt extract5.0 g, $SrCl_2$ 2.0 g ② beef extract 2.0 g, $CaCO_3$ 1.0 g, crude salt extract 5.0 g, Na_2MoO_4 5.0 g, soluble starch 2.0 g, NaCl 100.0 g ③ casein hydrolysate 1.0 g, KCl 2.0 g, $MgSO_4·7H_2O$ 2.0 g, NaCl 100.0 g, crude salt extract 10.0 g, gluconate 1.0 g; trisodium citrate1.0 g, yeast extract 1.0 g, $KMnO_4$ 2.0 g (sterilize alone) ④ MA 15.0 g, $CaCO_3$ 5.0 g, NaCl 100.0 g, $FeCl_2$ 0.5 g (filter sterilization), $FeSO_4$ 0.5 g (filter sterilization)
other medium	SN ZANT	① $NaNO_3$ 0.75 g, K_2HPO_4 0.0159 g, EDTA-2Na 0.0056 g, Na_2CO_3 0.0104 g, 50% sea water, Vitamin B12 0.001 g(filter sterilization), cyano trace metal solution 1×10^{-6} sterilize alone (acetic acid 6.25 g, ammonium ferric citrate 6.0 g, $MnCl_2·4H_2O$ 1.4 g, $Na_2MoO_4·2H_2O$ 0.39 g, $Co(NO_3)_2·6H_2O$ 0.025 g, $ZnSO_3·7H_2O$ 0.222 g) ② $NaHCO_3$ 2.0 g, $NaH_2PO_4·2H_2O$ 0.05 g, $NaNO_3$ 0.5 g, $CaCl_2$ 0.02 g, $MgSO_4·7H_2O$ 0.05 g, KCl 0.1 g, A5 solution 1×10^{-6}(H_3BO_3 2.86 g, $MnCl·4H_2O$ 1.80 g, $ZnSO_4·7H_2O$ 0.22 g, $Na_2MoO_4·2H_2O$ 0.3 g, $CuSO_4·5H_2O$ 0.08 g)

4.2. Screening Methods of Deep-Sea Natural Products

One of the keys to develop and utilize biological resources is how to obtain bioactive natural products from cultivable deep-sea microorganisms. Traditional natural product activity screening method is also suitable for the activity screening of deep-sea microbial metabolites, which mainly tracks the active substances in the cultivation broth. In addition, commonly used methods include model screening for specific target modeling and evaluation, and gene screening based on microbial natural product synthesis gene clusters.

4.2.1. In Vivo Screening Methods

In vivo screening models mainly refer to animal models and Serum pharmacology models. Animal models can mimic clinical features such as physiology and pathology similar to those of patients. Serum pharmacology models can help prove the true positive compounds, whether they are original drugs or metabolites [74]. Therefore, in vivo experiments have an irreplaceable role in activity screening. However, due to its time-consuming, low throughput, and large sample consumption, it is less used in preliminary screening.

4.2.2. Cell and Receptor/Enzyme Model Screening Methods

Cell and receptor/enzyme model screening is used for target screening, and is usually established as a specific and effective model on pharmacology at the cellular or molecular level.

Compared with simple chemical methods, evaluation of biological activity of natural products based on cell models can not only simulate the human physiological environment, but it can also explore and evaluate the biological activity and mechanism of natural products at multiple targets; compared with animal experiments in vivo, it not only shorten the experimental time, but greatly reduces the experimental cost [75]. The most commonly used cell models are human cancer cell lines, such as: A54, MCF7, HepG2, Caov-3, PANC-1 and so on. In addition, there are other models at the cellular level to test other bioactivities. Xu et al. used hemolysis assay on sheep red blood cell to test the anti-complement activity of 42 strains of marine actinomycetes isolated from Dalian Xinghai Bay mud samples, and further isolated three small molecular compounds with weak anti-complement activity from extract of strain DUT11 [76].

Receptors or enzymes related to various physiological and pathological processes in the body are considered to be one of the main targets of drug action [74]. Liu et al. tested IC_{50} values of the polypropionate derivatives against MptpB to show their antituberculosis activities [33]. ACE2 has been shown to be the main receptor for SARS-CoV S protein to infect cells [77]. Deng et al. showed that baicalin had an inhibitory activity against ACE with the IC_{50} value of 2.24 mM [78].

4.2.3. Virtual and Gene Screening Methods

Virtual screening based on compound structural diversity, that is, using computer programs to screen bioactive compounds from existing virtual libraries. And compounds with higher chemical structure spatial diversity are more suitable for virtual library establishment [79].

Gene screening breaks through the traditional active screening model. Because the secondary metabolite synthetic gene clusters with similar structures have a certain degree of similarity, the strains that produce the target compound can be obtained from nature by screening specific gene clusters.

Polyketide compounds are catalyzed by a type of polyketide synthetase (PKS) which is widely present in nature. Polyketide synthetase can generally be divided into three types according to its protein structure and catalytic mechanism, namely type I, type II and type III [80]. Type I PKS includes type I modular PKS (bacteria) and type I repeat PKS (fungi). A typical type I module PKS is a multifunctional complex enzyme composed of modules. Each module contains a unique and non-repetitive structural domain, which mainly contains acyltransferase (acyltransferase, AT), β-keto synthase (ketosynthase, KS) responsible for catalyzing the formation of carbon-carbon bonds and extending the main chain, and acyltransferase cylcar-rier protein (acyltransferase cylcar-rier protein, ACP) responsible for receiving and transporting acyl units provided by the AT domain), these three domains constitute the smallest catalytic module and are also the three essential domains of PKS.

Non-ribosomal peptide synthetase (NRPS) is also widely present in bacteria, fungi and plants, and uses different amino acids as substrates to catalyze the production of condensed peptides. NRPS is mainly composed of different independent modules. Each module contains an adenylation structural functional domain (andeylation, A) that selects and activates special amino acids, and loads aminoacyl residues into the sulfhydryl structural functional domain (thiolation, T), and the condensation domain (C) of peptide compounds that polymerize activated amino acids to produce amides.

In fungi, the genes encoding PKS and NRPS can be aggregated to produce type I repeat PKS units (KS, AT, DH, CMeT, KR and ACP domains) and NRPS units (A, T and C domains) PKS-NRPS hybrid enzyme. PKS-NRPS has the function of catalyzing the combination of PKS products and NRPS products, thereby producing more abundant natural products-PKS-NRPS hybrid compounds [81]. Such PKS-NRPS hybrid compounds are often a class of natural products with complex and diverse structures and a wide range of biological activities. They not only play an important role in the survival and prosperity of the host in the natural environment, but also is an important source for the discovery of active lead compounds with potential applications.

Jiang et al. [82] applied the type I polyketide synthase (PKS-I) gene screening system and DNA sequence similarity comparison to select positive *Actinoplanes* sp. from 32 strains of marine actinomycetes. *Actinoplanes* sp. FIM060065 was one of them. And from its fermentation broth researchers obtained a macrolide compound homogenous to tiacumicin B by High Performance Liquid Chromatography (HPLC) preparation, which showed strong antibacterial activity towards Gram-positive bacteria, such as *Clostridium difficile, Streptococcus pneumoniae, Bifidobacterium*, etc. Vanessa Rédou et al. [83] isolated 124 filamentous fungi and 59 yeasts from sediments in the Canterbury basin of New Zealand. The PKS-NRPS analysis results showed that there was no PKS-NRPS hybrid gene in the yeast genome; compared with yeast, filamentous fungal isolates from deep seabed sediments have greater bioactive compound synthesis potential, but they have fewer bioactive compound genes than those isolated from shallower depths.

4.3. Secondary Metabolite Discovery Based on Synthetic Biology

Synthetic biology is a multidisciplinary disruptive study leading a new generation of biotechnology revolution, in which gene editing takes an important part. Gene editing has unique advantages in establishing an artificially regulated biosynthetic system, further mining new natural product resources of actinomycetes, solving the bottleneck of existing natural products and developing derivatives. Recently, CRISPR (clustered regularly interspaced short palindromic repeats)/Cas9 system, known as "magic scissor", was found to improve the efficiency of gene editing.

Elizabeth J. Culp et al. [84] applied CRISPR/Cas9 system to 11 actinomycete strains, knocked out the common streptomycin and streptomycin genes, produced a variety of hidden rare antibiotics, and constructed a platform that can be widely used to stimulate the potential of microbial secondary metabolism. Indra Roux et al. [85] established the first CRISPRa system for filamentous fungi and discovered the *mic* cluster product, dehydromicroperfuranone. Meanwhile, factors affecting the efficiency of the system was also studied.

5. Conclusions and Perspective

Although the research on secondary metabolites of deep-sea microbes started later than that in other environments [9], it has drawn much more attention, and natural products with novel structures and good biological activities have been discovered in the past three years. From our literature review, fungi seem to be the focus of most isolations from the deep-sea for bioprospection of metabolites with biological activities; also, producers of higher diversity and amount of compounds. Among bacteria, actinomycetes seem to be studied more deeply in natural product research, and they have shown the potential to become biological resources with novel structures and good biological activities. When it comes to structural classes, polyketides showed a broad spectrum of bioactivities, such as antitumor, antibacterial, anti-inflammatory and antifood allergic.

The rapid development of deep sea exploration and bioinformatics has provided solid technical support for the chemical diversity and bioactivity diversity of secondary metabolites of deep sea microorganisms, but there are still many challenges, such as activation of specific biosynthetic gene clusters and heterologous expression, directed transformation of synthetic gene clusters, design of virtual screening libraries for natural products, and how to solve the problem of yield of active compounds.

Deep-sea microbial natural product resources are still a virgin land that needs to be developed urgently. Reasonable and green applied research will contribute more power to drug discovery.

Author Contributions: Y.-N.W. prepared the manuscript; L.-H.M. and B.-G.W. supervised the research work and revised the manuscript. All authors have read and agreed to the published version of the manuscript.

Funding: This work was funded by the Strategic Priority Research Program of the Chinese Academy of Sciences (Grant No. XDA22050401), and the Natural Science Foundation of China (Grant No. 41976090). L.-H.M. thanks the Youth Innovation Promotion Association of the Chinese Academy of Sciences (2017250). B.-G.W. acknowledges the support of Taishan Scholar Project from Shandong Province.

Conflicts of Interest: The authors declare no conflict of interest.

References

1. Tortorella, E.; Tedesco, P.; Esposito, F.P.; January, G.G.; Fani, R.; Jaspars, M.; Pascale, D. Antibiotics from Deep-Sea Microorganisms: Current Discoveries and Perspectives. *Mar. Drugs* **2018**, *16*, 355. [CrossRef] [PubMed]
2. Jebbar, M.; Franzetti, B.; Girard, E.; Oger, P. Microbial diversity and adaptation to high hydrostatic pressure in deep-sea hydrothermal vents prokaryotes. *Extremophiles* **2015**, *19*, 721–740. [CrossRef] [PubMed]
3. Skropeta, D.; Wei, L. Recent advances in deep-sea natural products. *Nat. Prod. Rep.* **2014**, *31*, 999–1025. [CrossRef] [PubMed]
4. Ventola, C.L. The Antibiotic Resistance Crisis: Part 1: Causes and threats. *Pharm. Ther.* **2015**, *40*, 277–283.
5. Mahé, S.; Rédou, V.; Le Calvez, T.; Vandenkoornhuyse, P.; Burgaud, G. Fungi in Deep-Sea Environments and Metagenomics. In *The Ecological Genomics of Fungi*; John Wiley & Sons, Inc.: Hoboken, NJ, USA, 2013; pp. 325–354.
6. Sharma, S.; Fulke, A.B.; Chaubey, A. Bioprospection of marine actinomycetes: Recent advances, challenges and future perspectives. *Acta Oceanol. Sin.* **2019**, *38*, 1–17. [CrossRef]
7. Bhatnagar, I.; Kim, S.-K. Immense Essence of Excellence: Marine Microbial Bioactive Compounds. *Mar. Drugs* **2010**, *8*, 2673–2701. [CrossRef] [PubMed]
8. Okutani, K. Gliotoxin produced by a strain of Aspergillus isolated from marine mud. *Nippon. Suisan Gakkaishi* **1977**, *43*, 995–1000. [CrossRef]
9. Muhammad, Z.A.; Ma, Y.N.; Xue, Y.R.; Liu, C.H. Deep-Sea Fungi Could Be the New Arsenal for Bioactive Molecules. *Mar. Drugs* **2020**, *18*, 9. [CrossRef]
10. Ibrar, M.; Ullah, M.W.; Manan, S.; Farooq, U.; Rafiq, M.; Hasan, F. Fungi from the extremes of life: An untapped treasure for bioactive compounds. *Appl. Microbiol. Biotechnol.* **2020**, *104*, 2777–2801. [CrossRef]
11. Tang, X.; Liu, S.-Z.; Yan, X.; Tang, B.-W.; Fang, M.; Wang, X.; Wu, Z.; Qiu, Y.-K. Two New Cytotoxic Compounds from a Deep-Sea Penicillium citreonigrum XT20-134. *Mar. Drugs* **2019**, *17*, 509. [CrossRef]
12. Xu, J.-L.; Liu, H.; Chen, Y.; Tan, H.-B.; Guo, H.; Xu, L.-Q.; Li, S.-N.; Huang, Z.-L.; Li, H.; Gao, X.-X.; et al. Highly Substituted Benzophenone Aldehydes and Eremophilane Derivatives from the Deep-Sea Derived Fungus Phomopsis lithocarpus FS508. *Mar. Drugs* **2018**, *16*, 329. [CrossRef] [PubMed]
13. Sun, C.; Ge, X.; Shah, M.; Zhou, L.; Yu, G.; Che, Q.; Zhang, G.; Peng, J.; Gu, Q.-Q.; Zhu, T.-J.; et al. New Glutamine-Containing Azaphilone Alkaloids from Deep-Sea-Derived Fungus Chaetomium globosum HDN151398. *Mar. Drugs* **2019**, *17*, 253. [CrossRef] [PubMed]
14. Niu, S.; Xia, M.; Chen, M.; Liu, X.; Li, Z.; Xie, Y.; Shao, Z.; Zhang, G. Cytotoxic Polyketides Isolated from the Deep-Sea-Derived Fungus Penicillium chrysogenum MCCC 3A00292. *Mar. Drugs* **2019**, *17*, 686. [CrossRef] [PubMed]
15. Zhang, J.; Chen, Y.; Liu, Z.; Guo, B.; Gao, X.; Liu, H.; Zhang, W. Cytotoxic Secondary Metabolites from a Sea-Derived Fungal Strain of Hypoxylon rubiginosum FS521. *Chin. J. Org. Chem.* **2020**, *40*, 1367. [CrossRef]
16. Xing, C.; Xie, C.-L.; Xia, J.-M.; Liu, Q.; Lin, W.-X.; Ye, D.-Z.; Liu, G.; Yang, X. Penigrisacids A–D, Four New Sesquiterpenes from the Deep-Sea-Derived Penicillium griseofulvum. *Mar. Drugs* **2019**, *17*, 507. [CrossRef]
17. Niu, S.; Xia, J.-M.; Li, Z.; Yang, L.-H.; Yi, Z.-W.; Xie, C.-L.; Peng, G.; Luo, Z.-H.; Shao, Z.; Yang, X. Aphidicolin Chemistry of the Deep-Sea-Derived Fungus Botryotinia fuckeliana MCCC 3A00494. *J. Nat. Prod.* **2019**, *82*, 2307–2331. [CrossRef]

18. Chen, S.C.; Liu, Z.M.; Tan, H.B.; Chen, Y.C.; Zhu, S.; Liu, H.X.; Zhang, W.M. Photeroids A and B, unique phenol–sesquiterpene meroterpenoids from the deep-sea-derived fungus Phomopsis tersa. *Org. Biomol. Chem.* **2020**, *18*, 642–645. [CrossRef]
19. Bao, J.; Zhai, H.; Zhu, K.; Yu, J.-H.; Zhang, Y.; Wang, Y.-Y.; Jiang, C.-S.; Zhang, X.-Y.; Zhang, Y.; Zhang, H. Bioactive Pyridone Alkaloids from a Deep-Sea-Derived Fungus *Arthrinium* sp. UJNMF0008. *Mar. Drugs* **2018**, *16*, 174. [CrossRef]
20. Liang, X.; Huang, Z.-H.; Ma, X.; Qi, S. Unstable Tetramic Acid Derivatives from the Deep-Sea-Derived Fungus Cladosporium sphaerospermum EIODSF 008. *Mar. Drugs* **2018**, *16*, 448. [CrossRef]
21. Zhang, Z.; He, X.; Wu, G.; Liu, C.; Lu, C.; Gu, Q.; Che, Q.; Zhu, T.; Zhang, G.; Li, D. Aniline-Tetramic Acids from the Deep-Sea-Derived Fungus Cladosporium sphaerospermum L3P3 Cultured with the HDAC Inhibitor SAHA. *J. Nat. Prod.* **2018**, *81*, 1651–1657. [CrossRef]
22. Matsuo, H.; Nonaka, K.; Nagano, Y.; Yabuki, A.; Fujikura, K.; Takahashi, Y.; Ōmura, S.; Nakashima, T. New metabolites, sarcopodinols A and B, isolated from deep-sea derived fungal strain *Sarcopodium* sp. FKJ-0025. *Biosci. Biotechnol. Biochem.* **2018**, *82*, 1323–1326. [CrossRef] [PubMed]
23. Chi, L.; Yang, S.-Q.; Li, X.-M.; Li, X.-D.; Wang, B.-G.; Li, X. A new steroid with 7β,8β-epoxidation from the deep sea-derived fungus Aspergillus penicillioides SD-311. *J. Asian Nat. Prod. Res.* **2020**, 1–8. [CrossRef] [PubMed]
24. Huang, Z.-H.; Liang, X.; Qi, S. A new iron(III) chelator of coprogen-type siderophore from the deep-sea-derived fungus Mycosphaerella sp. SCSIO z059. *Chin. J. Nat. Med.* **2020**, *18*, 243–249. [CrossRef]
25. Cheng, Z.; Xu, W.; Liu, L.; Li, S.; Yuan, W.; Luo, Z.; Zhang, J.; Cheng, Y.; Li, Q. Peniginsengins, B–E, New Farnesylcyclohexenones from the Deep Sea-Derived Fungus *Penicillium* sp. YPGA11. *Mar. Drugs* **2018**, *16*, 358. [CrossRef] [PubMed]
26. Dasanayaka, S.A.H.K.; Nong, X.-H.; Liang, X.; Liang, J.-Q.; Amin, M.; Qi, S. New dibenzodioxocinone and pyran-3,5-dione derivatives from the deep-sea-derived fungus Penicillium canescens SCSIO z053. *J. Asian Nat. Prod. Res.* **2020**, *22*, 338–345. [CrossRef] [PubMed]
27. Li, X.-D.; Yin, X.; Li, X.; Wang, B.; Li, X. Antimicrobial Sesquiterpenoid Derivatives and Monoterpenoids from the Deep-Sea Sediment-Derived Fungus Aspergillus versicolor SD-330. *Mar. Drugs* **2019**, *17*, 563. [CrossRef] [PubMed]
28. Salendra, L.; Luo, X.; Lin, X.; Liao, S.; Wang, J.; Zhou, X.; Yang, B.; Liu, Y. Bioactive Novel Indole Alkaloids and Steroids from Deep Sea-Derived Fungus *Aspergillus fumigatus* SCSIO 41012. *Molecules* **2018**, *23*, 2379. [CrossRef]
29. Li, S.; Mou, Q.; Xu, X.; Qianqian, M.; Leung, P.H.M. Synergistic antibacterial activity between penicillenols and antibiotics against methicillin-resistant Staphylococcus aureus. *R. Soc. Open Sci.* **2018**, *5*, 172466. [CrossRef]
30. Pang, X.; Lin, X.; Zhou, X.; Yang, B.; Tian, X.; Wang, J.; Xu, S.; Liu, Y. New quinoline alkaloid and bisabolane-type sesquiterpenoid derivatives from the deep-sea-derived fungus *Aspergillus* sp. SCSIO06786. *Fitoterapia* **2020**, *140*, 104406. [CrossRef]
31. Yu, G.; Sun, Z.; Peng, J.; Zhu, M.; Che, Q.; Zhang, G.; Zhu, T.; Gu, Q.; Li, D. Secondary Metabolites Produced by Combined Culture of Penicillium crustosum and a *Xylaria* sp. *J. Nat. Prod.* **2019**, *82*, 2013–2017. [CrossRef]
32. Xiao, Z.E.; Lin, S.E.; Huang, X.S.; Xia, G.P.; Li, H.X.; Lu, Y.J.; She, Z.G. The mPtpB Enzyme Inhibitors Derived from the Mangrove Fungi of the South China Sea. Abstracts of Papers. In Proceedings of the Ninth National Conference on Marine Biotechnology and Innovative Drugs, ChiFeng, China, 6 August 2014.
33. Liu, Z.; Wang, Q.; Li, S.; Cui, H.; Sun, Z.; Chen, D.; Lu, Y.-J.; Liu, H.; Zhang, W. Polypropionate Derivatives with Mycobacterium tuberculosis Protein Tyrosine Phosphatase B Inhibitory Activities from the Deep-Sea-Derived Fungus Aspergillus fischeri FS452. *J. Nat. Prod.* **2019**, *82*, 3440–3449. [CrossRef] [PubMed]
34. Chen, S.-C.; Liu, Z.; Chen, Y.; Tan, H.-B.; Li, S.-N.; Liu, H.; Zhang, W.-M.; Zhu, S. Highly Substituted Phenol Derivatives with Nitric Oxide Inhibitory Activities from the Deep-Sea-Derived Fungus Trichobotrys effuse FS524. *Mar. Drugs* **2020**, *18*, 134. [CrossRef] [PubMed]
35. Lee, H.-S.; Kang, J.S.; Choi, B.-K.; Shin, H.J.; Lee, H.-S.; Lee, Y.-J.; Lee, J.; Shin, H.J. Phenazine Derivatives with Anti-Inflammatory Activity from the Deep-Sea Sediment-Derived Yeast-Like Fungus Cystobasidium laryngis IV17-028. *Mar. Drugs* **2019**, *17*, 482. [CrossRef] [PubMed]
36. Niu, S.; Xie, C.-L.; Xia, J.-M.; Luo, Z.-H.; Shao, Z.; Yang, X. New anti-inflammatory guaianes from the Atlantic hydrotherm-derived fungus *Graphostroma* sp. MCCC 3A00421. *Sci. Rep.* **2018**, *8*, 530. [CrossRef]

37. Niu, S.; Liu, Q.; Xia, J.-M.; Xie, C.-L.; Luo, Z.-H.; Shao, Z.; Liu, G.; Yang, X. Polyketides from the Deep-Sea-Derived Fungus *Graphostroma* sp. MCCC 3A00421 Showed Potent Antifood Allergic Activities. *J. Agric. Food Chem.* **2018**, *66*, 1369–1376. [CrossRef]
38. Niu, S.; Xie, C.-L.; Xia, J.-M.; Liu, Q.-M.; Peng, G.; Liu, G.; Yang, X. Botryotins A–H, tetracyclic diterpenoids representing three carbon skeletons from a Deep-Sea-Derived. *Org. Lett.* **2019**, *22*, 580–583. [CrossRef]
39. Bochner, B.S.; Rothenberg, M.E.; Boyce, J.A.; Finkelman, F. Advances in mechanisms of allergy and clinical immunology in 2012. *J. Allergy Clin. Immunol.* **2013**, *131*, 661–667. [CrossRef]
40. Kay, A.B. Overview of 'Allergy and allergic diseases: With a view to the future'. *Br. Med Bull.* **2000**, *56*, 843–864. [CrossRef]
41. Abdel-Mageed, W.M.; Milne, B.F.; Wagner, M.; Schumacher, M.; Sandor, P.; Pathom-Aree, W.; Goodfellow, M.; Bull, A.T.; Horikoshi, K.; Ebel, R.; et al. Dermacozines, a new phenazine family from deep-sea dermacocci isolated from a Mariana Trench sediment. *Org. Biomol. Chem.* **2010**, *8*, 2352–2362. [CrossRef] [PubMed]
42. Huang, H.; Yang, T.; Ren, X.; Liu, J.; Song, Y.; Sun, A.; Ma, J.; Wang, B.; Zhang, Y.; Huang, C.; et al. Cytotoxic Angucycline Class Glycosides from the Deep Sea Actinomycete Streptomyces lusitanus SCSIO LR32. *J. Nat. Prod.* **2012**, *75*, 202–208. [CrossRef] [PubMed]
43. Li, S.; Tian, X.; Niu, S.; Zhang, W.; Chen, Y.-C.; Zhang, H.; Yang, X.; Zhang, W.; Li, W.; Zhang, S.; et al. Pseudonocardians A–C, New Diazaanthraquinone Derivatives from a Deap-Sea Actinomycete *Pseudonocardia* sp. SCSIO 01299. *Mar. Drugs* **2011**, *9*, 1428–1439. [CrossRef] [PubMed]
44. Sato, S.; Iwata, F.; Yamada, S.; Kawahara, H.; Katayama, M. Usabamycins A-C: New anthramycin-typeanalogues from a marine-derived actinomycete. *Bioorganic Med. Chem. Lett.* **2011**, *21*, 7099–7101. [CrossRef] [PubMed]
45. Zhang, W.; Liu, Z.; Li, S.; Yang, T.; Zhang, Q.; Ma, L.; Tian, X.; Zhang, H.; Huang, C.; Zhang, S.; et al. Spiroindimicins A–D: New Bisindole Alkaloids from a Deep-Sea-Derived Actinomycete. *Org. Lett.* **2012**, *14*, 3364–3367. [CrossRef] [PubMed]
46. Bérdy, J. Bioactive Microbial Metabolites. *J. Antibiot.* **2005**, *58*, 1–26. [CrossRef] [PubMed]
47. Xie, C.-L.; Niu, S.; Xia, J.-M.; Peng, K.; Zhang, G.-Y.; Yang, X.-W. Saccharopolytide A, a new cyclic tetrapeptide with rare 4-hydroxy-proline moieties from the deep-sea derived actinomycete Saccharopolyspora cebuensis MCCC 1A09850. *Nat. Prod. Res.* **2017**, *32*, 1627–1631. [CrossRef]
48. Yang, T.; Yamada, K.; Zhou, T.; Harunari, E.; Igarashi, Y.; Terahara, T.; Kobayashi, T.; Imada, C. Akazamicin, a cytotoxic aromatic polyketide from marine-derived *Nonomuraea* sp. *J. Antibiot.* **2019**, *72*, 202–209. [CrossRef]
49. Wang, C.; Cui, T.X.; Wang, D.Y.; Zhu, W.M. Trienomycin J, a new ansamycin from deep-sea derived bacterium *Ochrobactrum* sp. *Chin. Tradit. Herb. Drugs* **2019**, *23*, 5661–5665.
50. Fan, Y.; Wang, C.; Wang, L.; Chairoungdua, A.; Piyachaturawat, P.; Fu, P.; Zhu, W. New Ansamycins from the Deep-Sea-Derived Bacterium *Ochrobactrum* sp. OUCMDZ-2164. *Mar. Drugs* **2018**, *16*, 282. [CrossRef]
51. Ortiz-López, F.J.; Alcalde, E.; Sarmiento-Vizcaíno, A.; Díaz, C.; Cautain, B.; García, L.A.; Blanco, G.; Reyes, F. New 3-Hydroxyquinaldic Acid Derivatives from Cultures of the Marine Derived Actinomycete Streptomyces cyaneofuscatus M-157. *Mar. Drugs* **2018**, *16*, 371. [CrossRef]
52. Shao, M.; Ma, J.; Li, Q.; Ju, J. Identification of the Anti-Infective Aborycin Biosynthetic Gene Cluster from Deep-Sea-Derived *Streptomyces* sp. SCSIO ZS0098 Enables Production in a Heterologous Host. *Mar. Drugs* **2019**, *17*, 127. [CrossRef]
53. Yang, Z.-J.; Wei, X.; He, J.; Sun, C.; Ju, J.; Ma, J. Characterization of the Noncanonical Regulatory and Transporter Genes in Atratumycin Biosynthesis and Production in a Heterologous Host. *Mar. Drugs* **2019**, *17*, 560. [CrossRef] [PubMed]
54. Martín, J.; Martín, J.; Sarmiento-Vizcaíno, A.; De La Cruz, M.; García, L.A.; Blanco, G.; Reyes, F. Anthracimycin B, a Potent Antibiotic against Gram-Positive Bacteria Isolated from Cultures of the Deep-Sea Actinomycete Streptomyces cyaneofuscatus M-169. *Mar. Drugs* **2018**, *16*, 406. [CrossRef]
55. Xu, D.; Nepal, K.K.; Chen, J.; Harmody, D.; Zhu, H.; McCarthy, P.J.; Wright, A.E.; Wang, G. Nocardiopsistins A-C: New angucyclines with anti-MRSA activity isolated from a marine sponge-derived Nocardiopsis sp. HB-J378. *Synth. Syst. Biotechnol.* **2018**, *3*, 246–251. [CrossRef] [PubMed]
56. Xu, X.; Han, J.; Lin, R.; Polyak, S.W.; Song, F. Two New Piperazine-Triones from a Marine-Derived Streptomycetes sp. Strain SMS636. *Mar. Drugs* **2019**, *17*, 186. [CrossRef]
57. Zhang, D.S. Research on the Active Secondary Metabolites of Three Marine Microorganisms Based on Different Fermentation Methods. Master's Thesis, Zhejiang University, Hangzhou, China, 2019.

58. Pang, K.L.; Overy, P.D.; Jones, E.B.G.; da Luz Calado, M.; Burgaud, G.; Walker, K.A.; Johnson, A.J.; Kerr, G.R.; Cha, H.J.; Gerald, F.B. 'Marine fungi' and 'marine-derived fungi' in natural product chemistry research: Toward a new consensual definition. *Fungal Biol. Rev.* **2016**, *30*, 163–175. [CrossRef]
59. Jones, E.G. Are there more marine fungi to be described? *Bot. Mar.* **2011**, *54*, 343–354. [CrossRef]
60. Jones, E.B.G.; Pang, K.L. *Marine Fungi and Fungal-Like Organisms*; De Gruyter: Berlin, Germany, 2012; pp. 1–13.
61. Jones, E.G.; Suetrong, S.; Sakayaroj, J.; Bahkali, A.H.; Abdel-Wahab, M.A.; Boekhout, T.; Pang, K.-L. Classification of marine Ascomycota, Basidiomycota, Blastocladiomycota and Chytridiomycota. *Fungal Divers.* **2015**, *73*, 1–72. [CrossRef]
62. Raja, H.A.; Miller, A.N.; Pearce, C.J.; Oberlies, N.H. Fungal identification using molecular tools: A primer for the natural products research community. *J. Nat. Prod.* **2017**, *80*, 756–770. [CrossRef]
63. Seong, C.N.; Choi, J.H.; Baik, K.S. An improved selective isolation of rare Actinomycetes from forest soil. *J. Microbiol.* **2001**, *39*, 17–23.
64. Wang, H.Y.; Liu, J.; Zhao, S.J. Study on the isolation of marine actinomycetes in the sediments of Nanji Island. *Mar. Sci.* **2010**, *34*, 48–51.
65. Wang, F.; Xu, X.X.; Qu, Z.; Wang, C.; Lin, H.P.; Xie, Q.Y.; Ruan, J.S.; Sun, M.; Hong, K. Nonomuraea wenchangensis sp.nov. isolated from mangrove rthizosphere soil. *Int. J. Syst. Evol. Microbiol.* **2011**, *61*, 1304–1308. [CrossRef] [PubMed]
66. Xi, L.J.; Zhang, L.M.; Ruan, J.S.; Huang, Y. Micromonospora rhizosphaerae sp. nov. isolated from mangrove rhizosphere soil. *Int. J. Syst. Evol. Microbiol.* **2011**, *61*, 320–324.
67. Lin, L.; Tan, Y.; Chen, F.F.; Zhou, H.X.; Wang, Y.G.; He, W.Q.; Wang, Y. Diversity of cultivable actinomycetes in sediments of Laohutan, Bohai Sea, Dalian. *Acta Microbiol. Sin.* **2011**, *51*, 262–269.
68. Xi, L.J.; Zhang, L.M.; Ruan, J.S.; Huang, Y. *Nonomuraea maritima* sp. nov., isolated from coastal sediment. *Int. J. Syst. Evol. Microbiol.* **2011**, *61*, 2740–2744. [CrossRef] [PubMed]
69. Li, J.; Yang, J.; Zhu, W.Y.; He, J.; Tian, X.P.; Xie, Q.; Zhang, S.; Li, W.J. Nocardiopsis coralliicola sp. nov., isolated from the gorgonian coral, Menella praelonga. *Int. J. Syst. Evol. Microbiol.* **2012**, *62*, 1653–1658. [CrossRef] [PubMed]
70. Maldonado, L.A.; Stach, J.E.M.; Pathom-Aree, W.; Ward, A.C.; Bull, A.T.; Goodfellow, M. Diversity of cultivable actinobacteria in geographically widespread marine sediments. *Antonie van Leeuwenhoek* **2005**, *87*, 11–18. [CrossRef]
71. Ding, Y.B.; Cai, C.J.; Mu, Y.L.; Shan, Y.Q.; Lu, X.H.; Jiang, Q. The effect of microwave treatment on the separation of alkali and halophilic marine actinomycetes. *Bull. Microbiol.* **2012**, *39*, 407–414.
72. He, G.Y.; Xu, W.; Guo, S.S.; Liu, W.H.; Luo, Z.H. Study on the cultivable fungal diversity and denitrification ability of deep-sea sediments in Yapu Trench. *J. Appl. Oceanogr.* **2018**, *37*, 230–238.
73. Chen, R.W.; Wang, K.X.; He, Y.Q.; Tian, X.P.; Long, L.J. Diversity of culturable bacteria in a deep-sea sediment sample from the South China Sea. *Biol. Resour.* **2018**, *40*, 321–333.
74. Wang, B.; Deng, J.; Gao, Y.; Zhu, L.; He, R.; Xu, Y. The screening toolbox of bioactive substances from natural products: A review. *Fitoterapia* **2011**, *82*, 1141–1151. [CrossRef]
75. Bu, L.N. Screening and Evaluation of Active Ingredients of Natural Products Based On in vitro Cell Model Screening. Master's Thesis, Lanzhou University, Lanzhou, China, 2013.
76. Xu, X.N.; Cui, H.T.; Chen, L.Y.; Su, C.; Bai, F.W.; Zhao, X.Q. Screening of marine actinomycetes with anti-complement activity and isolation of their active substances. *J. Appl. Environ. Biol.* **2018**, *24*, 1295–1300.
77. Ou, H.L.; Li, L.J. Research progress of renin angiotensin system in newly emerging respiratory infectious diseases. *Mod. Pract. Med.* **2019**, *1*, 1–3.
78. Deng, Y.F.; Aluko, R.E.; Jin, Q.; Zhang, Y.; Yuan, L.J. Inhibitory activities of baicalin against renin and angiotensin-converting enzyme. *Pharm. Biol.* **2011**, *50*, 401–406. [CrossRef] [PubMed]
79. Yibo, L. Designing natural product-like virtual libraries using deep molecule generative models. *J. Chin. Pharm. Sci.* **2018**, *27*, 451–459. [CrossRef]
80. Shen, B. Polyketide biosynthesis beyond the type I, II and III polyketide synthase paradigms. *Curr. Opin. Chem. Biol.* **2003**, *7*, 285–295. [CrossRef]
81. Evans, B.S.; Robinson, S.J.; Kelleher, N.L. Surveys of non-ribosomal peptide and polyketide assembly lines in fungi and prospects for their analysisin vitro and in vivo. *Fungal Genet. Biol.* **2011**, *48*, 49–61. [CrossRef]
82. Jiang, H.L.; Fang, Z.K.; Chen, M.H.; Peng, F.; Jiang, H.; Lian, Y.Y. Gene screening of macrolide-producing bacteria and research on their metabolites. *Nat. Prod. Res. Dev.* **2017**, *29*, 1895–1899.

83. Rédou, V.; Navarri, M.; Meslet-Cladière, L.; Barbier, G.; Burgaud, G. Species Richness and Adaptation of Marine Fungi from Deep-Subseafloor Sediments. *Appl. Environ. Microbiol.* **2015**, *81*, 3571–3583. [CrossRef]
84. Culp, E.J.; Yim, G.; Waglechner, N.; Wang, W.; Pawlowski, A.C.; Wright, G.D. Hidden antibiotics in actinomycetes can be identified by inactivation of gene clusters for common antibiotics. *Nat. Biotechnol.* **2019**, *37*, 1149–1154. [CrossRef]
85. Roux, I.; Woodcraft, C.; Hu, J.; Wolters, R.; Gilchrist, C.L.M.; Chooi, Y.-H. CRISPR-Mediated Activation of Biosynthetic Gene Clusters for Bioactive Molecule Discovery in Filamentous Fungi. *ACS Synth. Biol.* **2020**, *9*, 1843–1854. [CrossRef]

Publisher's Note: MDPI stays neutral with regard to jurisdictional claims in published maps and institutional affiliations.

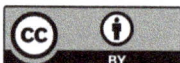

© 2020 by the authors. Licensee MDPI, Basel, Switzerland. This article is an open access article distributed under the terms and conditions of the Creative Commons Attribution (CC BY) license (http://creativecommons.org/licenses/by/4.0/).

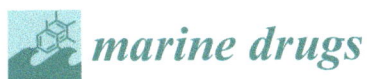

Article

Antibacterial Alkaloids and Polyketide Derivatives from the Deep Sea-Derived Fungus *Penicillium cyclopium* SD-413

Yan-He Li [1,2,3], Xiao-Ming Li [1,2,4], Xin Li [1,2,4], Sui-Qun Yang [1,2,4], Xiao-Shan Shi [1,2,4], Hong-Lei Li [1,2,4,*] and Bin-Gui Wang [1,2,3,4,*]

1. Key Laboratory of Experimental Marine Biology, Institute of Oceanology, Chinese Academy of Sciences, Nanhai Road 7, Qingdao 266071, China; liyanhe@qdio.ac.cn (Y.-H.L.); lixmqd@qdio.ac.cn (X.-M.L.); lixin@qdio.ac.cn (X.L.); yangsuiqun@qdio.ac.cn (S.-Q.Y.); Shixs@qdio.ac.cn (X.-S.S.)
2. Laboratory of Marine Biology and Biotechnology, Qingdao National Laboratory for Marine Science and Technology, Wenhai Road 1, Qingdao 266237, China
3. College of Marine Sciences, University of Chinese Academy of Sciences, Yuquan Road 19A, Beijing 100049, China
4. Center for Ocean Mega-Science, Chinese Academy of Sciences, Nanhai Road 7, Qingdao 266071, China
* Correspondence: lihonglei@qdio.ac.cn (H.-L.L.); wangbg@ms.qdio.ac.cn (B.-G.W.); Tel.: +86-532-8289-8553 (B.-G.W.)

Received: 19 October 2020; Accepted: 2 November 2020; Published: 6 November 2020

Abstract: Nine secondary metabolites (**1**–**9**), including two new polyketide derivatives 9-dehydroxysargassopenilline A (**4**) and 1,2-didehydropeaurantiogriseol E (**5**), along with seven known related secondary metabolites (**1**–**3** and **6**–**9**), were isolated and identified from the deep sea-derived fungus *Penicillium cyclopium* SD-413. Their structures were elucidated on the basis of 1D/2D NMR spectroscopic and mass spectrometric analysis and the absolute configurations were determined by the combination of NOESY correlations and time-dependent density functional (TDDFT) ECD calculations. Compounds **1**–**9** inhibited some pathogenic bacteria including *Escherichia coli*, *E. ictaluri*, *Edwardsiella tarda*, *Micrococcus luteus*, *Vibrio anguillarum*, and *V. harveyi*, with MIC (minimum inhibitory concentration) values ranging from 4 to 32 µg/mL.

Keywords: *Penicillium cyclopium*; marine sediment-derived fungus; quinazoline alkaloid; polyketide derivatives; antibacterial activity

1. Introduction

Marine sediment-derived fungi have received considerable attention as a valuable resource of bioactive metabolites with diversified chemical structures including alkaloids, peptides, polyketides, and terpenoids [1–6]. These natural products are characterized by intriguing biological properties such as anticancer, antifouling, antimicrobial, antioxidant, and antiviral activities [4–9].

In our continuing excavation to identify new bioactive metabolites from deep sea-derived fungi [7–12], the fungus *Penicillium cyclopium* SD-413, which was obtained from a sediment sample collected from the East China Sea, was screened out for chemical investigations. As a result, two new polyketide derivatives, 9-dehydroxysargassopenilline A (**4**) and 1,2-didehydropeaurantiogriseol E (**5**), along with seven known related metabolites (**1**–**3** and **6**–**9**) (Figure 1), were isolated and identified from the culture extract of the fungus. Chemical structures of the isolated compounds were established by detailed interpretation of 1D/2D NMR spectroscopic and mass spectrometric data and the absolute configurations of compounds **4** and **5** were determined by ECD calculations. All of these compounds were evaluated for antibacterial activities against some human and fish pathogenic bacteria. Herein, the details of isolation, structure elucidation, and biological activities of compounds **1**–**9** are described.

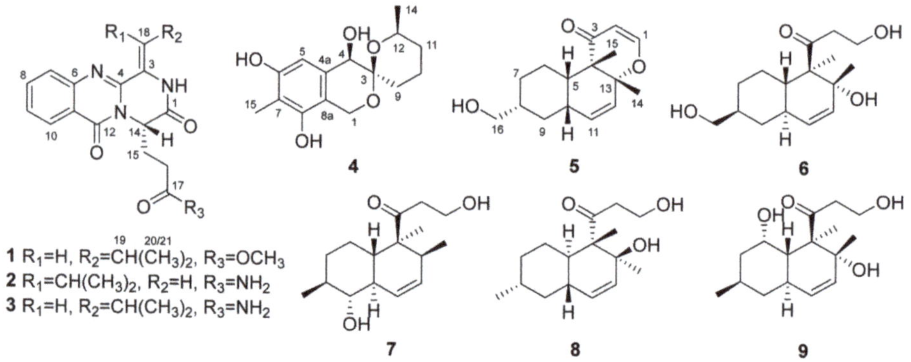

Figure 1. Structures of compounds 1–9.

2. Results and Discussion

2.1. Structure Elucidation of the Isolated Compounds

Compounds **1** and **2** were originally treated as new quinazoline alkaloids during the preparation of this manuscript, and their structures were elucidated by detailed analysis of NMR spectroscopic and high-resolution mass spectrometric data. However, when the manuscript was ready for submission, Cao and co-workers reported three new quinazoline-containing diketopiperazines, namely polonimides A–C, from the marine-derived fungus *Penicillium polonicum* HBU-114 [13]. Among them, polonimides A and B had virtually identical NMR data to those of compounds **1** and **2**, respectively. The NMR data of polonimides A and B were recorded on a Bruker AV-600 spectrometer, whereas for compounds **1** and **2**, the data were acquired on a Bruker Avance 500 spectrometer. For future reference, our NMR data of compounds **1** and **2** are listed in the Supporting Information (Figures S1–S11, Table S1).

The molecular formula of 9-dehydroxysargassopenilline A (**4**) was determined to be $C_{15}H_{20}O_5$ on the basis of HRESIMS data (six degrees of unsaturation, Figure S12). The NMR spectroscopic data (Table 1, Figures S13 and S14) revealed the presence of 15 carbon atoms, which were clarified into two methyls, four methylenes, three methines, and six non-protonated carbons. Extensive analysis of its ^1H and ^{13}C NMR data revealed that compound **4** is a derivative of 6,6-spiroketal, very similar to sargassopenilline A, which was previously isolated from the axenic culture of the marine alga-derived fungus *Penicillium thomii* KMM4645 [14]. However, signals at δ_H 4.15 and δ_C 66.1 for an oxygenated methine (CH-9) in the NMR spectra of sargassopenilline A disappeared in those of compound **4**, while resonances for an additional methylene at δ_H 1.40/1.94 and δ_C 29.4 were observed in the NMR spectra of compound **4** (Table 1). The above observation disclosed that the oxymethine (CH-9) of sargassopenilline A was replaced by a methylene group in compound **4**. This deduction was further verified by the proton-proton spin-coupling system from C-9 to C-12 and C-14 established by the COSY and HSQC analysis of compound **4** (Figures S15 and S16), as well as by the key HMBC correlations from H-1 and H$_2$-9 to C-3 (Figure 2 and Figure S17). Thus, the planar structure of compound **4** was determined as shown in Figure 1.

Table 1. ^{1}H and ^{13}C NMR data of compounds 4 and 5 (measured in DMSO-d_6).

No.	4		No.	5	
	δ_H (J in Hz) [a]	δ_C, Type [b]		δ_H (J in Hz) [a]	δ_C, Type [b]
1α	4.34, d (14.7)	58.2, CH$_2$	1	7.26, d (5.9)	157.9, CH
1β	4.49, d (14.7)		2	5.19, d (5.9)	105.6, CH
3		95.7, C	3		199.0, C
4	4.09, d (8.5)	69.6, CH	4		47.4, C
4a		133.8, C	5	1.59, m	42.2, CH
5	6.55, s	104.4, CH	6α	1.13, m	26.4, CH$_2$
6		154.3, C	6β	2.75, m	
7		108.9, C	7α	1.00, m	29.4, CH$_2$
8		149.7, C	7β	1.77, m	
8a		112.6, C	8	1.48, m	40.7, CH
9α	1.40, m	29.4, CH$_2$	9α	0.81, m	35.0, CH$_2$
9β	1.94, m		9β	1.85, m	
10α	1.61, m	18.5, CH$_2$	10	1.89, m	40.1, CH
10β	1.80, m		11	5.48, dd (10.1, 2.1)	131.4, CH
11α	1.11, m	31.9, CH$_2$	12	5.67, dd (10.1, 2.1)	128.3, CH
11β	1.55, m		13		85.3, C
12	3.75, m	66.9, CH	14	1.37, s	21.6, CH$_3$
14	1.01, d (6.3)	21.6, CH$_3$	15	1.15, s	13.9, CH$_3$
15	1.95, s	8.6, CH$_3$	16	3.22, m	66.3, CH$_2$
4-OH	4.57, d (8.5)		16-OH	4.42, br	
6-OH	8.93, s				
8-OH	8.08, s				

[a] Measured at 500 MHz; [b] measured at 125 MHz.

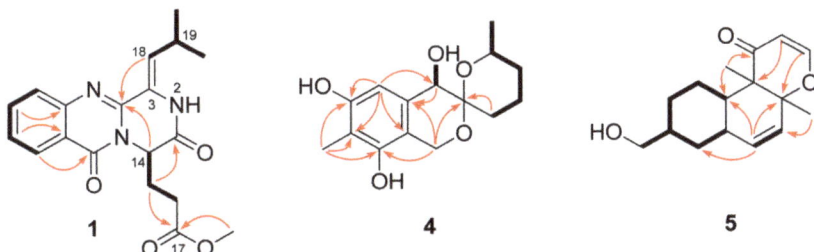

Figure 2. Key COSY (bold lines) and HMBC (arrows) correlations of compounds 1, 4, and 5.

The relative configuration of compound 4 was assigned by analysis of NOESY data (Figure 3 and Figure S18). The key NOE correlations from H-4 to H-9α and H-12 oriented these protons to the same face of the molecule. The absolute configuration of compound 4 was established by the TDDFT-ECD calculation in Gaussian 09 [15]. After geometry optimization, the minimum energy conformers were obtained, and then the TDDFT method at the B3LYP/6-31G level was employed to generate the calculated ECD spectrum of compound 4 (Figure 4). The experimental ECD spectrum of compound 4 exhibited excellent accordance with that calculated for the absolute configuration (3R, 4R, 12S) in compound 4 (Figure 4), which established the absolute configuration of compound 4.

1,2-Didehydropeaurantiogriseol E (5) was isolated as a colorless oil and its HRESIMS data (Figure S19) gave the molecular formula as $C_{16}H_{22}O_3$. The ^{1}H and ^{13}C NMR data (Table 1, Figures S20 and S21) of compound 5 showed a close relationship to that of peaurantiogriseol E, a derivative of polyketide isolated from *Penicillium aurantiogriseum* [16]. However, signals for two methylenes (C-1 and C-2) in the NMR spectra of peaurantiogriseol E were not present in those of compound 5. Instead, two olefinic methines at $\delta_{C/H}$ 157.9/7.26 (CH-1) and $\delta_{C/H}$ 105.6/5.19 (CH-2) were observed in the NMR spectra of compound 5 (Figures S20–S24). Furthermore, the HMBC correlations (Figure 2 and Figure S24) from H-1 to C-13 and from H-2 to C-4 revealed the presence of dihydropyranone ring in compound **5**.

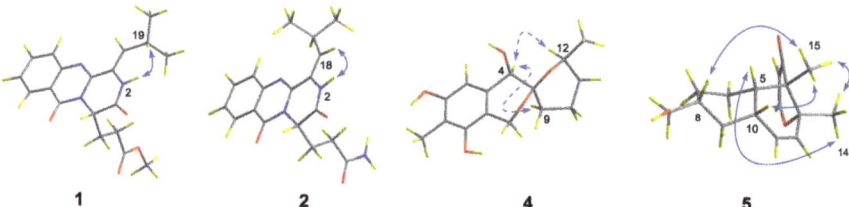

Figure 3. Key NOESY correlations for **1, 2, 4**, and **5** (solid lines: β-orientation; dashed lines: α-orientation).

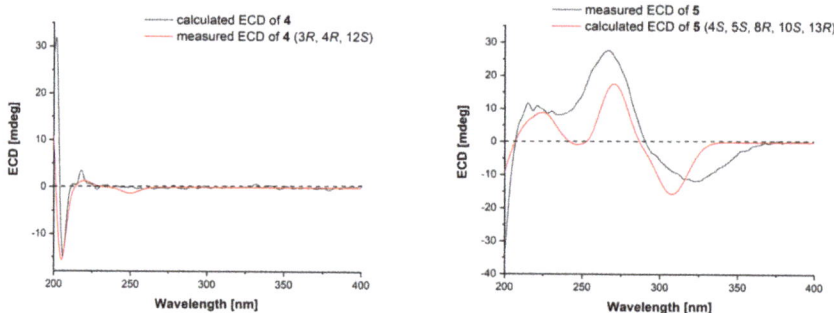

Figure 4. Experimental and calculated ECD spectra of compounds **4** and **5**.

The relative configuration of compound **5** was established by analysis of NOESY data (Figure 3 and Figure S25). The key NOE correlations from H-14 to H-5 and H-15 and from H-15 to H-8 and H-10 located these groups on the same side of the molecule. Similarly, the absolute configuration of compound **5** was determined by the TDDFT-ECD calculation in Gaussian 09 [15]. The TDDFT-ECD spectrum calculated at the B3LYP/6-31G level for the isomer (4S, 5S, 8R, 10S, 13R) of compound **5** matched well with the experimental ECD spectrum (Figure 4).

In addition to the two new secondary metabolites (**4** and **5**) and three known quinazoline alkaloids (**1–3**), four known derivatives of polyketide (**6–9**) were also isolated from the culture extract of the fungus *P. cyclopium* SD-413. By detailed spectroscopic analysis as well as comparisons with reported data, the structures of compounds **3** and **6–9** were identified as aurantiomide C (**3**) [17], craterellone D (**6**) [18], peaurantiogriseol A (**7**) [16], aspermytin A (**8**) [19], and 1-(2,8-dihydroxy-1,2,6-trimethyl-1,2,6,7,8,8a-hexahydronaphthalen-1-yl)-3-hydroxy-1-propanone (**9**) [20], respectively.

2.2. Antibacterial Activities of the Isolated Compounds

The obtained compounds **1–9** were evaluated for antibacterial activities against 2 human pathogenic bacteria (*Escherichia coli* and *Staphylococcus aureus*) and 10 fish pathogenic bacteria (*Aeromonas hydrophila*, *Edwardsiella ictaluri*, *E. tarda*, *Micrococcus luteus*, *Pseudomonas aeruginosa*, *Vibrio alginolyticus*, *V. anguillarum*, *V. harveyi*, *V. parahemolyticus*, and *V. vulnificus*). Compounds **1–3** exhibited inhibitory activities against *E. coli*, *E. ictaluri*, *E. tarda*, and *V. harveyi*, with MIC values ranging from 4.0 to 32 μg/mL (Table 2), while compound **4** showed potent inhibitory activity against *M. luteus*, with an MIC value of 4.0 μg/mL, and compound **5** showed potent activities against *V. anguillarum* and *V. harveyi*, each with an MIC value of 4.0 μg/mL. These results indicated that the formation of dihydropyranone ring (**5** vs. **6–9**) in structures strengthened their effects against *V. anguillarum* and *V. harveyi*. However, the tested compounds were inactive against the remaining microorganisms.

Table 2. Antibacterial activities of compounds 1–9 (MIC, μg/mL).

Strains	1	2	3	4	5	6	7	8	9	Chl [a]
Escherichia coli	8.0	4.0	8.0	n.a.	16	8.0	n.a.	32	16	2.0
Edwardsiella tarda	8.0	8.0	8.0	16	n.a.	32	16	32	8.0	2.0
Edwardsiella ictaluri	8.0	8.0	8.0	n.a.	n.a.	n.a.	32	16	n.a.	0.5
Micrococcus luteus	32	n.a.	n.a.	4.0	32	n.a.	32	n.a.	n.a.	2.0
Vibrio harveyi	8.0	8.0	32	n.a.	4.0	8.0	n.a.	32	32	0.5
Vibrio anguillarum	n.a.	n.a.	n.a.	32	4.0	32	16	32	n.a.	1.0

[a] Chl: chloramphenicol (positive control); n.a.: no activity (MIC > 64 μg/mL).

3. Experimental Section

3.1. General Experimental Procedures

Optical rotations: an Optical Activity AA-55 polarimeter (Optical Activity Ltd., Cambridgeshire, UK); UV spectra: a PuXi TU-1810 UV-visible spectrophotometer (Shanghai Lengguang Technology Co. Ltd., Shanghai, China); ECD spectra: a JASCO J-715 spectropolarimeter (JASCO, Tokyo, Japan); NMR spectra: a Bruker Avance 500 spectrometer (Bruker Biospin Group, Karlsruhe, Germany); mass spectra: an API QSTAR Pulsar 1 mass spectrometer (Applied Biosystems, Foster City, CA, USA); analytical HPLC: a Dionex HPLC system, equipped with P680 pump (Dionex, Sunnyvale, CA, USA); and TLC: silica gel GF254 precoated plates (Qingdao Haiyang Chemical Group Corporation, Qingdao, China). Column chromatography (CC): 100–200 mesh and 200–300 mesh silica gel (SiO_2; Qingdao Haiyang Chemical Group Corporation), 40–63 μm RP-18 reverse-phase Si gel (Merck, Darmstadt, Germany), and Sephadex LH-20 (Merck, Darmstadt, Germany). All solvents were distilled prior to use.

3.2. Fungal Material

The fungus *Penicillium cyclopium* SD-413 was isolated from a marine sediment sample collected from the East China Sea in May 2017. It was identified using a molecular biological protocol described in our previous report [21] by DNA amplification and the sequencing of the ITS (internal transcribed spacer) region. The sequenced data derived from the fungal strain were deposited in GenBank (accession no. MN818582). A BLAST search result showed that the sequence was most similar (99%) to the sequence of *Penicillium cyclopium* (accession no. MT990551.1). The strain is preserved at the Key Laboratory of Experimental Marine Biology, Institute of Oceanology, Chinese Academy of Sciences (IOCAS).

3.3. Fermentation

For the purpose of chemical composition analysis, the fresh mycelia of *P. cyclopium* SD-413 were grown on PDA (potato dextrose agar) medium at 28 °C for five days and then cultivated in a 1 L conical flask (100 flasks) with solid rice medium (each flask contained 70 g rice; 0.1 g corn flour; 0.3 g peptone; 0.1 g sodium glutamate; and 100 mL naturally sourced and filtered seawater, which was obtained from the Huiquan Gulf of the Yellow Sea near the campus of Institute of Oceanology, Chinese Academy of Sciences (IOCAS), pH 6.5–7.0) for 30 days at room temperature.

3.4. Extraction and Isolation

The whole fermented cultures were extracted four times with EtOAc. The solvents were evaporated under reduced pressure to yield an organic extract (71.2 g), which was fractionated by vacuum liquid chromatography (VLC) on silica gel eluting with different solvents of increasing polarity from petroleum ether (PE) to MeOH to yield nine fractions (Frs. 1–9) based on TLC and HPLC analysis. Fr. 5 (6.65 g), eluted with PE-EtOAc (2:1), was further purified by CC over Lobar LiChroprep RP-18 with a MeOH-H_2O gradient (from 10:90 to 100:0) to yield ten subfractions (Fr. 5.1–5.10). Fr. 5.6 (126.1 mg) was further purified by CC on Sephadex LH-20 (MeOH) and then by semi-preparative

HPLC (55% MeOH-H$_2$O, 5 mL/min) to yield compounds **3** (5.9 mg, t_R 22.5 min) and **4** (20.7 mg, t_R 27.3 min). Fr. 7 (23.52 g), eluted with CH$_2$Cl$_2$-MeOH (20:1), was further purified by CC on silica gel, eluting with a PE-EtOAc gradient (from 5:1 to 2:1), to yield two subfractions (Fr. 7.1 and Fr. 7.2). Fr. 7.1 (12.91 g) was further purified by CC over Lobar LiChroprep RP-18 with a MeOH-H$_2$O gradient (from 10:90 to 100:0) to yield ten subfractions (Fr. 7.1.1–7.1.10). Fr. 7.1.6 (100.9 mg) was purified by CC on silica gel eluting with a CH$_2$Cl$_2$-MeOH gradient (from 200:1 to 20:1), and then by CC on Sephadex LH-20 (MeOH), obtained compounds **6** (16.1 mg) and **7** (10.7 mg). Fr. 7.1.7 was further purified by CC over RP-18 eluting with a MeOH-H$_2$O gradient (10:90 to 100:0) and by semi-preparative HPLC (MeOH-H$_2$O, 60% to 85%, 5 mL/min) to obtain **1** (8.3 mg, t_R 18.1 min), **2** (8.2 mg, t_R 22.3 min), and **5** (29.3 mg, t_R 26.7 min). Fr. 7.2 (10.42 g) was further purified by CC over Lobar LiChroprep RP-18 with a MeOH-H$_2$O gradient (from 10:90 to 100:0) to yield ten subfractions (Fr. 7.2.1–7.2.10). Fr. 7.2.3 (201.3 mg) was purified by CC on silica gel eluting with a CH$_2$Cl$_2$-MeOH gradient (from 200:1 to 20:1) and then by CC on Sephadex LH-20 (MeOH) to obtain compounds **8** (64.6 mg) and **9** (12.9 mg).

Polonimide A (**1**): Amorphous powder; $[\alpha]_D^{20}$ = +67.3 (*c* 0.10, CHCl$_3$); UV (MeOH) λ_{max} (log ε) 212 (7.32), 312 (4.48) nm; ECD (0.33 mg/mL, MeOH) λ_{max} ($\Delta\varepsilon$) 227 (+25.18), 250 (−16.35), 274 (−3.28), 295 (−6.27), 329 (+4.20) nm; ^{1}H and ^{13}C NMR data, Table S1; HRESIMS *m/z* 356.1609 [M + H]$^+$ (calcd for C$_{19}$H$_{22}$N$_3$O$_4$, 356.1607), 378.1438 [M + Na]$^+$ (calcd for C$_{19}$H$_{21}$N$_3$O$_4$Na, 378.1436).

Polonimide B (**2**): Amorphous powder; $[\alpha]_D^{20}$ = +14.2 (*c* 0.15, CHCl$_3$); UV (MeOH) λ_{max} (log ε) 212 (7.32), 312 (4.48) nm; ECD (0.26 mg/mL, MeOH) λ_{max} ($\Delta\varepsilon$) 223 (+21.59), 246 (−18.10), 271 (−1.34), 295 (−5.81), 326 (+6.74) nm; ^{1}H and ^{13}C NMR data, Table S1; HRESIMS *m/z* 341.1609 [M + H]$^+$ (calcd for C$_{18}$H$_{21}$N$_4$O$_3$, 341.1608).

9-Dehydroxysargassopenilline A (**4**): Amorphous powder; $[\alpha]_D^{20}$ = −83.5 (*c* 0.10, MeOH); UV (MeOH) λ_{max} (log ε) 235 (3.25), 282 (3.10) nm; ECD (7.21 mM, MeOH) λ_{max} ($\Delta\varepsilon$) 202 (+31.83), 206 (−17.93), 218 (+3.45), 229 (−0.51) nm; ^{1}H and ^{13}C NMR data, Table [1]; HRESIMS *m/z* 279.1236 [M + H]$^+$ (calcd for C$_{15}$H$_{19}$O$_5$, 279.1238).

1,2-Didehydropeaurantiogriseol E (**5**): Amorphous powder; $[\alpha]_D^{20}$ = −40.3 (*c* 0.12, MeOH); UV (MeOH) λ_{max} (log ε) 201 (2.49), 254 (1.95) nm; ECD (7.11 mM, MeOH) λ_{max} ($\Delta\varepsilon$) 215 (+11.73), 235 (+8.04), 267 (+27.67), 324 (−11.74) nm; ^{1}H and ^{13}C NMR data, Table [1]; HRESIMS *m/z* 263.1644 [M + H]$^+$ (calcd for C$_{16}$H$_{23}$O$_3$, 263.1642).

3.5. Antibacterial Assays

Antibacterial evaluation against human pathogenic bacteria (*Escherichia coli* and *Staphylococcus aureus*) and fish pathogenic bacteria (*Aeromonas hydrophila*, *Edwardsiella ictaluri*, *E. tarda*, *Micrococcus luteus*, *Pseudomonas aeruginosa*, *Vibrio alginolyticus*, *V. anguillarum*, *V. harveyi*, *V. parahemolyticus*, and *V. vulnificus*) was carried out by the microplate assay with a microplate assay with three repetitions [22]. The bacteria including *A. hydrophila*, *E. ictaluri*, *E. coli*, *E. tarda*, *M. luteus*, *S. aureus*, *V. harveyi*, and *V. parahemolyticus* were incubated in LB medium (1% peptone, 1% NaCl, 0.5% yeast extract powder in distilled water), while the rest of the bacteria in assay were incubated in TSB medium (1.5% tryptone, 0.5% soytone, 0.5% NaCl in distilled water). The pathogenic bacteria and fish pathogenic strains were provided by the Institute of Oceanology, Chinese Academy of Sciences. Chloramphenicol was used as positive control against bacteria.

3.6. Computational Section

Conformational searches were performed via molecular mechanics using the MM+ method in HyperChem software (Version 8.0, Hypercube, Inc., Gainesville, FL, USA), and the geometries were further optimized at B3LYP/6-31G(d) level via Gaussian 09 software (Version D.01; Gaussian, Inc.: Wallingford, CT, USA) [15] to give the energy-minimized conformers. After that, the optimized conformers were subjected to the calculations of ECD spectra using TDDFT at B3LYP/6-31G level. Solvent effects of the MeCN solution were evaluated at the same DFT (density functional theory) level using the SCRF/PCM (polarizable continuum model) method.

4. Conclusions

In summary, chemical investigations of the deep sea-derived fungus *P. cyclopium* SD-413 provided two new polyketide derivatives, 9-dehydroxysargassopenilline A (**4**) and 1,2-didehydropeaurantiogriseol E (**5**), along with seven known related secondary metabolites (**1–3** and **6–9**). The structures of these compounds were elucidated on the basis of NMR spectroscopic and mass spectrometric analysis and the absolute configurations of compounds **4** and **5** were established by the TDDFT-ECD calculation. Compounds **1–5** exhibited inhibitory activities against some tested human and fish pathogenic bacteria, with MIC values ranging from 4.0 to 32 µg/mL. These compounds might be used as leading compounds for the development of agents against the pathogenic bacteria.

Supplementary Materials: The following are available online at http://www.mdpi.com/1660-3397/18/11/553/s1. Figure S1: HRESIMS spectrum of compound **1**. Figure S2: ^{1}H NMR (500 MHz, DMSO-d_6) spectrum of compound **1**. Figure S3: ^{13}C NMR (125 MHz, DMSO-d_6) and DEPT spectra of compound **1**. Figure S4: COSY spectrum of compound **1**. Figure S5: HSQC spectrum of compound **1**. Figure S6: HMBC spectrum of compound **1**. Figure S7: NOESY spectrum of compound **1**. Figure S8: HRESIMS spectrum of compound **2**. Figure S9: ^{1}H NMR (500 MHz, DMSO-d_6) spectrum of compound **2**. Figure S10: ^{13}C NMR (125 MHz, DMSO-d_6) and DEPT spectra of compound **2**. Figure S11: NOESY spectrum of compound **2**. Table S1: ^{1}H and ^{13}C NMR data of compounds **1** and **2**. Figure S12: HRESIMS spectrum of compound **4**. Figure S13: ^{1}H NMR (500 MHz, DMSO-d_6) spectrum of compound **4**. Figure S14: ^{13}C NMR (125 MHz, DMSO-d_6) and DEPT spectra of compound **4**. Figure S15: COSY spectrum of compound **4**. Figure S16: HSQC spectrum of compound **4**. Figure S17: HMBC spectrum of compound **4**. Figure S18: NOESY spectrum of compound **4**. Figure S19: HRESIMS spectrum of compound **5**. Figure S20: ^{1}H NMR (500 MHz, DMSO-d_6) spectrum of compound **5**. Figure S21: ^{13}C NMR (125 MHz, DMSO-d_6) and DEPT spectra of compound **5**. Figure S22: COSY spectrum of compound **5**. Figure S23: HSQC spectrum of compound **5**. Figure S24: HMBC spectrum of compound **5**. Figure S25: NOESY spectrum of compound **5**.

Author Contributions: Y.-H.L. performed the experiments for the isolation, structure elucidation, antibacterial evaluation, and prepared the manuscript; X.-M.L. performed the 1D and 2D NMR experiments; X.L. performed the ECD calculations, S.-Q.Y. and X.-S.S. participated in the structure elucidation; H.-L.L. jointly contributed to supervise the research and revised the manuscript; B.-G.W. supervised the research work and revised the manuscript. All authors have read and agreed to the published version of the manuscript.

Funding: This research work was financially supported by the Strategic Priority Research Program of the Chinese Academy of Sciences (Grant No. XDA22050401), the National Natural Science Foundation of China (31700043), and the Aoshan Scientific and Technological Innovation Project of Qingdao National Laboratory for Marine Science and Technology (No. 2016ASKJ14). B.-G.W. acknowledges the support of the Research Vessel KEXUE from the National Major Science and Technology Infrastructure from the Chinese Academy of Sciences (KEXUE2018G28) and the Taishan Scholar Project from Shandong Province. H.-L.L. appreciates the support of the Qingdao National Laboratory for Marine Science and Technology (OF2019NO03).

Acknowledgments: The authors appreciate the High Performance Computing Environment Qingdao Branch of Chinese Academy of Science (CAS)—High Performance Computing Center of Institute of Oceanology of CAS for CPU time. H.-L.L. acknowledges the Young Scientists Partner Program of Shenyang Branch of Chinese Academy of Sciences-Shandong Academy of Sciences for project supporting.

Conflicts of Interest: The authors declare no conflict of interest.

References

1. Carroll, A.R.; Copp, B.R.; Davis, R.A.; Keyzers, R.A.; Prinsep, M.R. Marine natural products. *Nat. Prod. Rep.* **2020**, *37*, 175–223. [CrossRef] [PubMed]
2. Daletos, G.; Ebrahim, W.; Ancheeva, E.; El-Neketi, M.; Song, W.G.; Lin, W.H.; Proksch, P. Natural products from deep-sea-derived fungi-A new source of novel bioactive compounds? *Curr. Med. Chem.* **2018**, *25*, 186–207. [CrossRef] [PubMed]
3. Chen, S.C.; Liu, Z.M.; Tan, H.B.; Chen, Y.C.; Li, S.N.; Li, H.H.; Guo, H.; Zhu, S.; Liu, H.X.; Zhang, W.M. Tersone A–G, new pyridone alkaloids from the deep-sea fungus *Phomopsis tersa*. *Mar. Drugs* **2019**, *17*, 394. [CrossRef] [PubMed]
4. Jiang, W.; Ye, P.; Chen, C.T.; Wang, K.; Liu, P.; He, S.; Wu, X.; Gan, L.; Ye, Y.; Wu, B. Two novel hepatocellular carcinoma cycle inhibitory cyclodepsipeptides from a hydrothermal vent crab-associated fungus *Aspergillus clavatus* C2WU. *Mar. Drugs* **2013**, *11*, 4761–4772. [CrossRef] [PubMed]

5. Yao, Q.; Wang, J.; Zhang, X.; Nong, X.; Xu, X.; Qi, S. Cytotoxic polyketides from the deep-sea-derived fungus *Engyodontium album* DFFSCS021. *Mar. Drugs* **2014**, *12*, 5902–5915. [CrossRef] [PubMed]
6. Niu, S.W.; Liu, D.; Shao, Z.Z.; Proksch, P.; Lin, W.H. Eremophilane-type sesquiterpenoids in a deep-sea fungus *Eutypella* sp. activated by chemical epigenetic manipulation. *Tetrahedron* **2018**, *74*, 7310–7325. [CrossRef]
7. Li, X.D.; Li, X.M.; Yin, X.L.; Li, X.; Wang, B.G. Antimicrobial sesquiterpenoid derivatives and monoterpenoids from the deep-sea sediment-derived fungus *Aspergillus versicolor* SD-330. *Mar. Drugs* **2019**, *17*, 563. [CrossRef]
8. Huang, Z.; Nong, X.; Ren, Z.; Wang, J.; Zhang, X.; Qi, S. Anti-HSV-1, antioxidant and antifouling phenolic compounds from the deep-sea-derived fungus *Aspergillus versicolor* SCSIO 41502. *Bioorg. Med. Chem. Lett.* **2017**, *27*, 787–791. [CrossRef]
9. Niu, S.; Si, L.; Liu, D.; Zhou, A.; Zhang, Z.; Shao, Z.; Wang, S.; Zhang, L.; Zhou, D.; Lin, W. Spiromastilactones: A new class of influenza virus inhibitors from deep-sea fungus. *Eur. J. Med. Chem.* **2016**, *108*, 229–244. [CrossRef]
10. Li, X.D.; Li, X.; Li, X.M.; Xu, G.M.; Liu, Y.; Wang, B.G. 20-Nor-isopimarane epimers produced by *Aspergillus wentii* SD-310, a fungal strain obtained from deep sea sediment. *Mar. Drugs* **2018**, *16*, 440. [CrossRef] [PubMed]
11. Chi, L.P.; Li, X.M.; Li, L.; Li, X.; Wang, B.G. New antibacterial thiodiketopiperazines from the deep sea-derived fungus *Epicoccum nigrum* SD-388. *Chem. Biodiver.* **2020**, *17*, e2000320. [CrossRef] [PubMed]
12. Li, X.L.; Chi, L.P.; Navarro-Vázquez, A.; Hwang, S.; Schmieder, P.; Li, X.M.; Li, X.; Yang, S.Q.; Lei, X.X.; Wang, B.G.; et al. Stereochemical elucidation of natural products from residual chemical shift anisotropies in a liquid crystalline phase. *J. Am. Chem. Soc.* **2020**, *142*, 2301–2309. [CrossRef]
13. Guo, X.C.; Zhang, Y.H.; Gao, W.B.; Pan, L.; Zhu, H.J.; Cao, F. Absolute configurations and chitinase inhibitions of quinazoline-containing diketopiperazines from the marine-derived fungus *Penicillium polonicum*. *Mar. Drugs* **2020**, *18*, 479. [CrossRef]
14. Zhuravleva, O.I.; Sobolevskaya, M.P.; Afiyatullov, S.S.; Kirichuk, N.N.; Denisenko, V.A.; Dmitrenok, P.S.; Yurchenko, E.A.; Dyshlovoy, S.A. Sargassopenillines A–G, 6,6-spiroketals from the alga-derived fungi *Penicillium thomii* and *Penicillium lividum*. *Mar. Drugs* **2014**, *12*, 5930–5943. [CrossRef] [PubMed]
15. Frisch, M.J.; Trucks, G.W.; Schlegel, H.B.; Scuseria, G.E.; Robb, M.A.; Cheeseman, J.R.; Scalmani, G.; Barone, V.; Mennucci, B.; Petersson, G.A.; et al. *Gaussian 09, Revision D.01*; Gaussian, Inc.: Wallingford, CT, USA, 2013.
16. Ma, Y.H.; Li, J.; Huang, M.X.; Liu, L.; Wang, J.; Lin, Y.C. Six new polyketide decalin compounds from mangrove endophytic fungus *Penicillium aurantiogriseum* 328#. *Mar. Drugs* **2015**, *13*, 6306–6318. [PubMed]
17. Xin, Z.H.; Fang, Y.C.; Du, L.; Zhu, T.J.; Duan, L.; Chen, J.; Gu, Q.Q.; Zhu, W.M. Aurantiomides A–C, quinazoline alkaloids from the sponge-derived fungus *Penicillium aurantiogriseum* SP0-19. *J. Nat. Prod.* **2007**, *70*, 853–855. [CrossRef]
18. Guo, H.; Feng, T.; Li, Z.H.; Liu, J.K. Five new polyketides from the basidiomycete *Craterellus odoratus*. *Nat. Prod. Bioprospect.* **2012**, *2*, 170–173. [CrossRef]
19. Tsukamoto, S.; Miura, S.; Yamashita, Y.; Ohta, T. Aspermytin A: A new neurotrophic polyketide isolated from a marine-derived fungus of the genus *Aspergillus*. *Bioorg. Med. Chem. Lett.* **2004**, *14*, 417–420. [CrossRef]
20. Fujii, Y.; Asahara, M.; Ichinoe, M.; Nakajima, H. Fungal melanin inhibitor and related compounds from *Penicillium decumbens*. *Phytochemistry* **2002**, *60*, 703–708. [CrossRef]
21. Wang, S.; Li, X.M.; Teuscher, F.; Li, D.L.; Diesel, A.; Ebel, R.; Proksch, P.; Wang, B.G. Chaetopyranin, a benzaldehyde derivative, and other related metabolites from *Chaetomium globosum*, an endophytic fungus derived from the marine red alga *Polysiphonia urceolata*. *J. Nat. Prod.* **2006**, *69*, 1622–1625. [CrossRef]
22. Song, F.; Liu, X.; Guo, H.; Ren, B.; Chen, C.; Piggott, A.M.; Yu, K.; Gao, H.; Wang, Q.; Liu, M.; et al. Brevianamides with antitubercular potential from a marine-derived isolate of *Aspergillus versicolor*. *Org. Lett.* **2012**, *14*, 4770–4773. [CrossRef] [PubMed]

Publisher's Note: MDPI stays neutral with regard to jurisdictional claims in published maps and institutional affiliations.

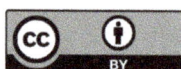

© 2020 by the authors. Licensee MDPI, Basel, Switzerland. This article is an open access article distributed under the terms and conditions of the Creative Commons Attribution (CC BY) license (http://creativecommons.org/licenses/by/4.0/).

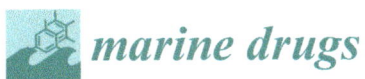

Article

Lipopeptide Epimers and a Phthalide Glycerol Ether with AChE Inhibitory Activities from the Marine-Derived Fungus *Cochliobolus Lunatus* SCSIO41401

Yu Dai [1,†], Kunlong Li [1,2,†], Jianglian She [1], Yanbo Zeng [3], Hao Wang [3], Shengrong Liao [1,2], Xiuping Lin [1,2], Bin Yang [1,2], Junfeng Wang [1,2], Huaming Tao [4], Haofu Dai [3], Xuefeng Zhou [1,2,*] and Yonghong Liu [1,2,5,*]

1. CAS Key Laboratory of Tropical Marine Bio-resources and Ecology, Guangdong Key Laboratory of Marine Materia Medica, South China Sea Institute of Oceanology, Chinese Academy of Sciences, Guangzhou 510301, China; daiyu15@mails.ucas.ac.cn (Y.D.); likunlong16@mails.ucas.edu.cn (K.L.); shejianglian20@mails.ucas.ac.cn (J.S.); ljrss@126.com (S.L.); xiupinglin@hotmail.com (X.L.); yangbin@scsio.ac.cn (B.Y.); wangjunfeng@scsio.ac.cn (J.W.)
2. Southern Marine Science and Engineering Guangdong Laboratory (Guangzhou), Guangzhou 511458, China
3. Research and Development of Natural Product from Li Folk Medicine, Institute of Tropical Bioscience and Biotechnology, Chinese Academy of Tropical Agriculture Sciences, Haikou 571101, China; zengyanbo@itbb.org.cn (Y.Z.); wanghao@itbb.org.cn (H.W.); daihaofu@itbb.org.cn (H.D.)
4. School of Traditional Chinese Medicine, Southern Medical University, Guangzhou 510515, China; taohm@smu.edu.cn
5. Wuya College of Innovation, Shenyang Pharmaceutical University, Shenyang 110016, China
* Correspondence: xfzhou@scsio.ac.cn (X.Z.); yonghongliu@scsio.ac.cn (Y.L.)
† These authors contributed equally to this work.

Received: 16 September 2020; Accepted: 28 October 2020; Published: 30 October 2020

Abstract: A pair of novel lipopeptide epimers, sinulariapeptides A (**1**) and B (**2**), and a new phthalide glycerol ether (**3**) were isolated from the marine algal-associated fungus *Cochliobolus lunatus* SCSIO41401, together with three known chromanone derivates (**4–6**). The structures of the new compounds, including the absolute configurations, were determined by comprehensive spectroscopic methods, experimental and calculated electronic circular dichroism (ECD), and $Mo_2(OAc)_4$-induced ECD methods. The new compounds **1–3** showed moderate inhibitory activity against acetylcholinesterase (AChE), with IC_{50} values of 1.3–2.5 µM, and an in silico molecular docking study was also performed.

Keywords: lipopeptides; phthalide; *Cochliobolus lunatus*; absolute configurations; AChE inhibitory

1. Introduction

In order to survive in a highly competitive environment, many marine organisms can produce an array of biologically-active secondary metabolites, many of which exert cytotoxic or chemical defense activity [1]. The production of metabolites targeting cholinesterase enzymes among sessile organisms—such as sponge, coral, and algae—represent an additional advantage in a survival strategy against different predators and/or fouling invertebrates [2].

Cholinesterase enzymes, such as acetylcholinesterase (AChE), are widely expressed throughout the animal kingdom, from land to sea. AChE is the key enzyme for the termination of neurotransmission in cholinergic pathways, and AChE inhibition is an effective approach for the symptomatic treatment for Alzheimer's disease (AD) [3,4].

In our recent efforts to search for bioactive natural products from marine-derived fungi, one endophytic fungus—*Cochliobolus lunatus* SCSIO41401—was isolated from the alga *Coelarthrum* sp., collected in Yongxing Island, in the South China Sea. In our previous work, several cytotoxic and antibacterial eremophilane sesquiterpenes [5] and anti-influenza spirostaphylotrichins [6] were discovered from this fungus SCSIO41401, when it was fermented with liquid medium. In order to discover more diverse and bioactive compounds from this strain, a fermentation with a solid rice medium was recently undertaken, and six natural products were obtained from this strain for the first time (Figure 1). Three of them were identified as new compounds with AChE-inhibitory activity. Described herein are the isolation, structure determination, and biological evaluation of these compounds.

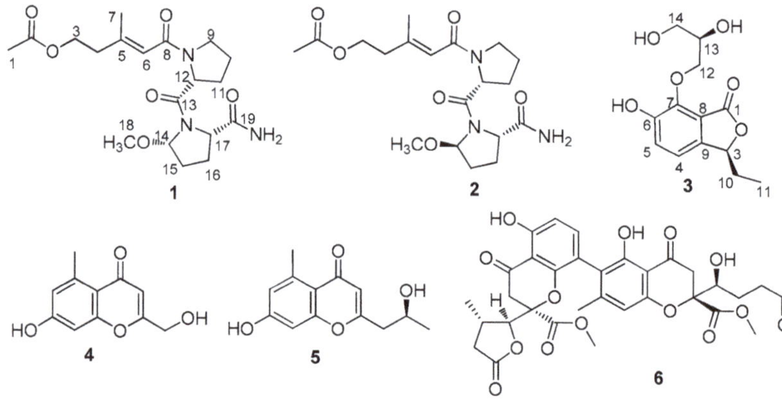

Figure 1. Compounds 1–6, isolated from fungal strain SCSIO41401.

2. Results

2.1. Structure Elucidation

Compound **1** was obtained as a brown oil. The HRESIMS (*m/z* 418.1951 [M + Na]$^+$) data suggested a molecular formula of $C_{19}H_{29}N_3O_6$, revealing seven degrees of unsaturation. The analysis of the NMR data showed the presence of three methyls (including one oxygenated), seven methylenes (including one oxygenated), four methines (including one olefinic), one olefinic carbon, and four carbonyl carbons (Table 1). Combined with the 1D-NMR data, the ^1H-^1H COSY correlations of H-9/H-10/H-11/H-12 and the HMBC correlations from H-9 to C-12/C-8, H-11 to C-13, and H-12 to C-8/C-13 indicated the presence of one Pro residue. On the other hand, the ^1H-^1H COSY correlations of H-14/H-15/H-16/H-17, and the HMBC correlations of H-14 with C-13/C-17, H-16 with C-19, H-17 with C-13/C-19, and H-18 to C-14 suggested the presence of another amino acid residue, 5-methoxy-prolinamide (Me-O-Pro-NH$_2$). Moreover, the HMBC correlations of H-11/H-12/H-14/H-17 with C-13 confirmed the connection of two amino acid residues. The ^1H-^1H COSY correlations from H-3 to H-4, and the HMBC correlations from H-1/H-3 to C-2, H-4/H-6 to C-5, H-7 to C-4/C-5/C-6 displayed the presence of the branched chain. The HMBC correlations from H-6/ H-9/H-12 to C8 showed the connection of the branched chain with the C-8 amino acid group. Thus, the planar structure of **1** was determined, as shown in Figure 2.

Table 1. ^{13}C and ^{1}H NMR data for **1–3** in CD$_3$OD (δ_C and δ_H are given in ppm).

Pos.	1		2		3	
	δ_C [a]	δ_H, (J in Hz) [b]	δ_C [c]	δ_H, (J in Hz) [d]	δ_C [c]	δ_H, (J in Hz) [d]
1	20.8 CH$_3$	2.02 s	20.8 CH$_3$	2.02 s	172.0 C	
2	173.0 C		172.9 C			
3	63.3 CH$_2$	4.22 t (6.5)	63.2 CH$_2$	4.22 t (6.5)	83.3 CH	5.39 dd (7.0, 4.2)
4	40.4 CH$_2$	2.43 t (6.5)	40.3 CH$_2$	2.43 t (6.5)	118.5 CH	7.05 d (8.4)
5	150.7 C		150.7 C		127.1 CH	7.19 d (8.4)
6	121.2 CH	5.72 brd (1.0)	121.2 CH	5.73 brd (1.0)	156.1 C	
7	18.4 CH$_3$	2.13 d (1.5)	18.4 CH$_3$	2.13 d (1.5)	146.9 C	
8	169.5 C		169.5 C		140.8 C	
9	39.8 CH$_2$	3.23 t (7.0)	39.8 CH$_2$	3.24 t (6.3)	119.3 C	
10	26.0 CH$_2$	1.63 m	25.4 CH$_2$	1.66 m	28.9 CH$_2$	2.11 m, 1.79 m
11	27.7 CH$_2$	1.93 m/1.81 m	27.2 CH$_2$	1.98 m/1.84 m	8.9 CH$_3$	0.97 t (7.0)
12	55.8 CH	4.24 t (5.0)	56.4 CH	4.14 t (4.2)	77.0 CH$_2$	4.31 dd (10.5, 3.5) 4.19 dd (10.5, 6.3)
13	169.3 C		170.4 C		72.0 CH	3.95 m
14	89.3 CH	5.44 t (8.0)	88.5 CH	5.26 d (4.9)	63.9 CH$_2$	3.75 m, 3.69 m
15	31.0 CH$_2$	1.87 m	31.7 CH$_2$	1.90 m		
16	26.1 CH$_2$	2.34 m	25.9 CH$_2$	2.16 m 2.11 m		
17	58.7 CH	4.37 t (7.0)	60.5 CH	4.24 t (7)		
18	56.8 CH$_3$	3.38 s	57.4 CH$_3$	3.37 s		
19	172.4 C		173.5 C			

[a] in 125 MHz, [b] in 500 MHz, [c] in 175 MHz, [d] in 700 MHz.

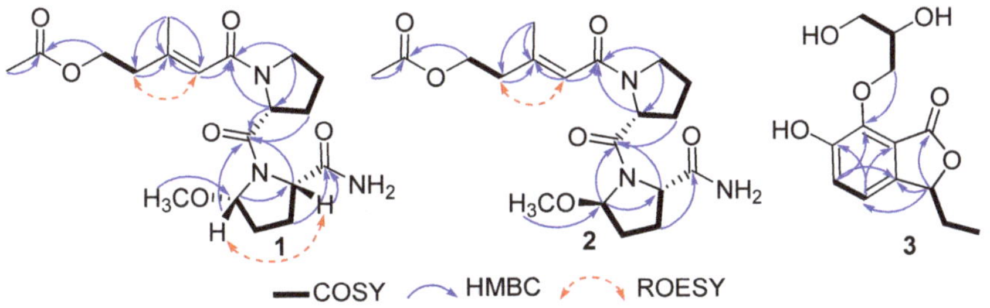

Figure 2. The key HMBC, COSY, and ROESY correlations of **1–3**.

Compound **2** was isolated as a brown oil. Its molecular formula was reported to be same as **1** by HRESIMS (m/z 418.1958 [M + Na]$^+$), which required seven degrees of unsaturation. The ^{1}H-^{1}H COSY correlations of H-9/H-10/H-11/H-12, and the HMBC correlations of H-9 with C-12/C-8, H-11 with C-13, and H-12 with C-8/C-13 indicated the presence of one Pro residue. In addition, the ^{1}H-^{1}H COSY correlations of H-14/H-15/H-16/H-17, and the HMBC correlations of H-14 with C-13/C-17, H-16 with C-19, H-17 with C-13/C-19, and H-18 to C-14 suggested the presence of another amino acid residue, 5-methoxy-prolinamide (Me-O-Pro-NH$_2$). All of those indicated that compounds **1** and **2** were a pair of epimers.

The configurations of the Δ^5 double bond of **1** and **2** were deduced as *E*, based on the ROESY correlation of H$_2$-4/H-6 (Figure 2). The ROESY correlation of H-14 with H-17 indicated that H-14/H-17 were co-facial in **1**. In order to further determine the absolute configuration of C-12/C-14/C-17 of **1**, ECD calculations with four truncated models—12R*,14S*,17S*-**1** and 12S*,14S*,17S*-**1**—were used. Based on the time-dependent density functional theory (TD-DFT), the Boltzmann-weighted ECD curves of 12R,14S,17S-**1** gave the best agreement (Figure 3A), which led to the determination of the 12R,14S,17S absolute configurations of **1**. Comparing the NMR spectra of **1** and **2**, the ROESY correlation of H-14 with H-17 was not observed in **2**. Additionally, the difference in the coupling constant and the splitting of the peaks of H-14 indicated that **2** should be an epimer of **1** at C-14.

From a biosynthetic point of view, the absolute configurations of **2** were suggested to be 12R*,14R*,17S*. The Boltzmann-weighted ECD curves of 12R,14R,17S-**2** gave the best agreement with the experimental CD (Figure 3B). Thus, the structures of the two lipopeptide epimers were identified as shown in Figure 1, and were named sinulariapeptides A (**1**) and B (**2**).

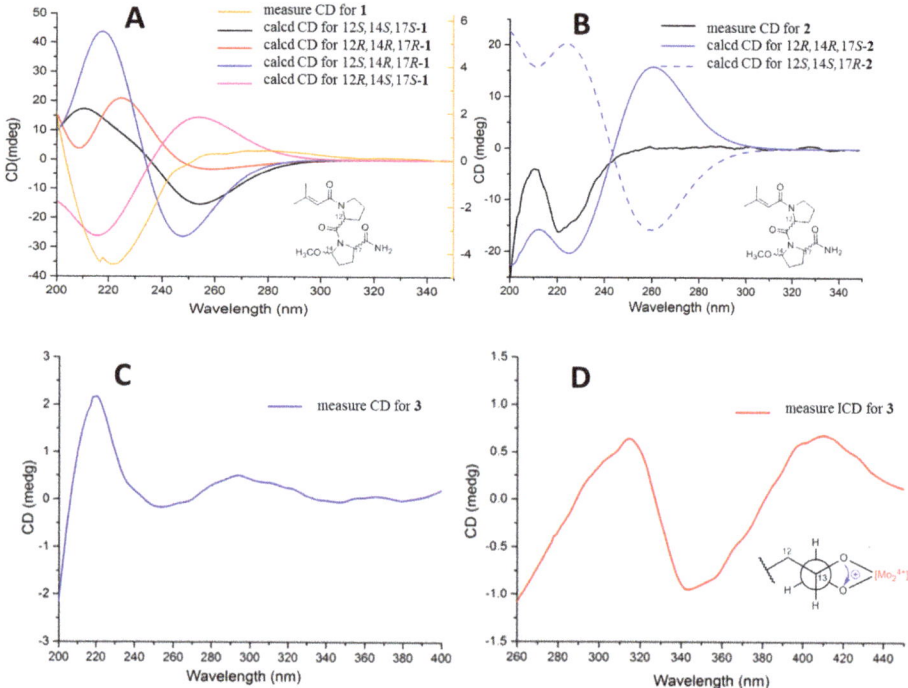

Figure 3. (**A**) Experimental CD spectra of **1**, and the calculated ECD spectra of its truncated models. (**B**) Experimental CD spectra of **2**, and the calculated ECD spectra of its truncated models. (**C**) Experimental CD spectra of **3** in MeOH. (**D**) Induced CD (ICD) spectra from the Mo$_2$-complexes of **3** in DMSO.

Compound **3** was obtained as a brown oil. The molecular formula was determined as $C_{13}H_{16}O_6$ by HRESIMS (m/z 291.0838 [M + Na]$^+$). The NMR spectra indicated the presence of one methy, three methenes, four methines (including two olefinic and two oxygenated), four aromatic quaternary carbons, and a ketone carbonyl carbon (Table 1). A comparison of its ^{1}H and ^{13}C NMR data with those of (S)-3-ethyl-6,7-dihydroxyphthalide, another phthalide compound we obtained in this strain previously [5], indicated that they shared the same substructure [7,8]. The difference was the replacement of a glycerol ether substituent at C-7, which was further confirmed by the COSY correlations from H-4/H-5; H-12/H-13/H-14 (Figure 2), and the HMBC correlations (Figure 2) from H-12 to C-7. Thus, the planar structure of **3** was established.

The absolute configurations of **3** were determined by the CD method. The CD of the α,β-unsaturated γ-lactone rings with a chiral γ-carbon shows Cotton effects associated with the π→π* transition in the region 200–235 nm, and the n→π* transition in the region 235–270 nm [9–12]. Compound **3** showed a positive π→π* Cotton effect at 217 nm, and a negative n→π* Cotton effect at 259 nm, indicating the S absolute configuration at C-3 (Figure 3C) [9,10]. The stereogenic center of C-13 was characterized by the dimolybdenum induced CD (ICD) analysis. In the ICDs conducted by Snatzke's method [13,14] using dimolybdenum tetraacetate (Mo$_2$(OAc)$_4$) in DMSO, the Mo$_2$-complex of **3** gave positive CD bands II (408 nm) and IV (around 313 nm) (Figure 3D), and confirmed that C-13 was (*R*)-configured. Finally, the absolute configurations of **3** were assigned as 3*S*, 13*R*.

In addition, the structures of three known compounds (**4–6**) were elucidated by the analysis of the spectral data (Figures S27–S32), as well as through comparison with those reported in the literature. They were identified as 2-(2′-Hydroxypropyl)-5-methyl-7-hydroxychromone (**4**) [15], orthosporin (**5**) [16], and bipolarinone (**6**) [17], respectively (Figure 1). All of these compounds are benzopyrone derivates, while compound **6** contains two benzopyrone moieties.

2.2. Bioassays

The new compounds **1–3** were evaluated for their cytotoxicities against several human cancer cell lines: K562, BEL-7402, SGC-7901, A549, and Hela. However, none of the compounds showed obvious inhibitory activity against those cells at a concentration of 50 μM in the preliminary screening (an inhibition rate less than 30%).

In the screening assay of the AChE inhibitory activities, compounds **1–3** showed moderate inhibitory activity, with IC_{50} values of 1.8 ± 0.12, 1.3 ± 0.11, and 2.5 ± 0.21 μM, respectively, in which huperzine A was used as a positive control (IC_{50} 0.30 ± 0.06 μM). The preliminary kinetic study of **1** towards AChE suggested the noncompetitive inhibition mode (Figure S33).

2.3. Molecular Docking

In order to gain an insight into the molecular interactions between compounds **1–3** and AChE, the crystal structure of the recombinant human Acetylcholinesterase enzyme (rhAChE, PDB ID: 4EY7) [18] was selected and subjected to an in silico molecular docking analysis with **1–3**, using the induced-fit module in the Schrödinger software suite [19]. As the docking results showed in Figure 4A, **1–3** were obviously able to bind to the active pocket of AChE, with TYR124 as the center of the binding site of AChE. The carbonyl group at C-8 connected to the Pro residue in the structures of **1** and **2** formed a hydrogen bond interaction with the active site residue TYR124 of AChE. Although the $CONH_2$-19 group of **1** and **2** formed a hydrogen bond interaction with the different residues, SER125 and GLU202, respectively, there is no significant difference in the docking effects of AChE with **1** and **2**. In the docking model of AChE and **3**, a hydrogen bond interaction was formed with the active site residues TYR124 and PHE295. Moreover, the phthalide ring of **3** played a key role to form a π–π stacking interaction with TRP286.

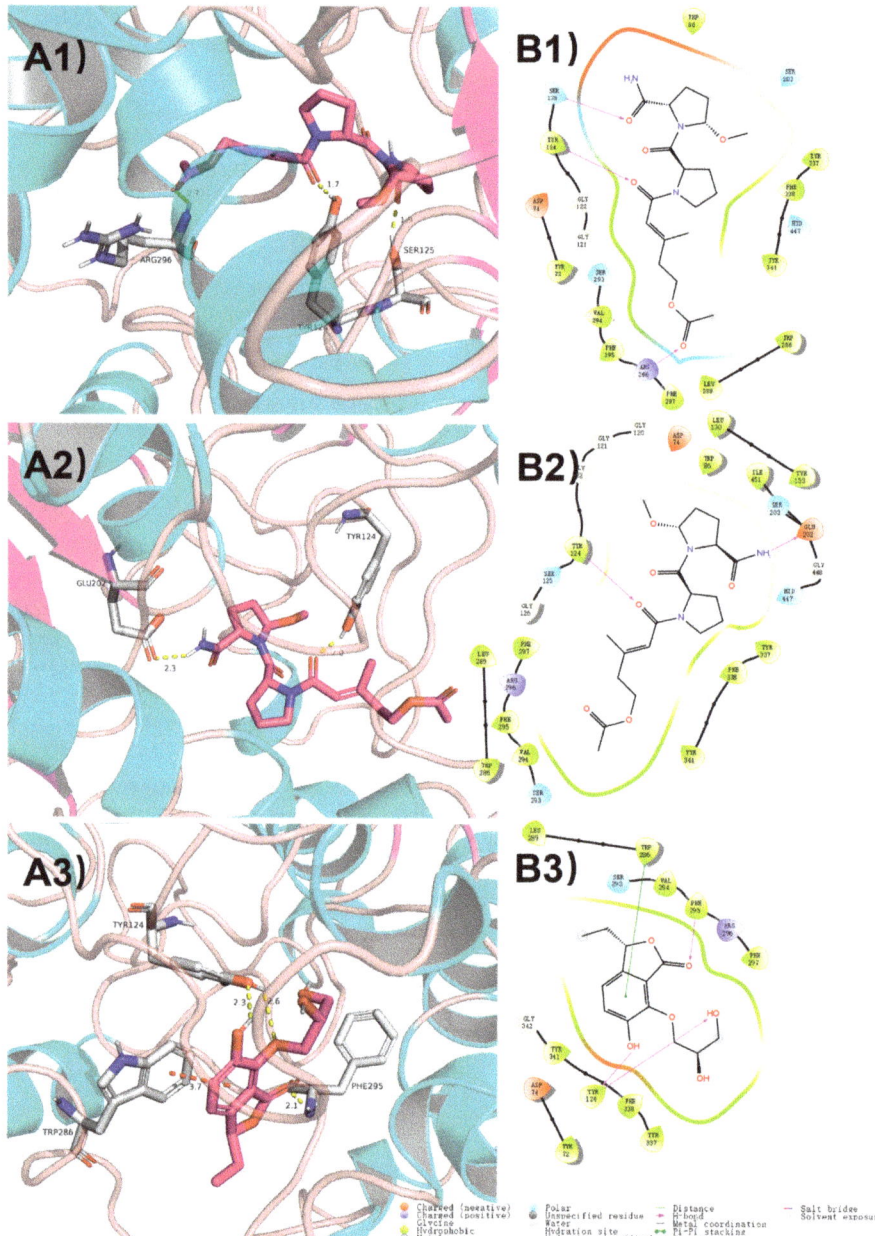

Figure 4. Molecular docking of **1**–**3** with AChE (PDB code: 4EY7). The binding sites of the molecules **1** (**A1**), **2** (**A2**) and **3** (**A3**) with the AChE protein. The 2D interaction details of the predicted binding mode of **1** (**B1**), **2** (**B2**) and **3** (**B3**) with the AChE.

3. Materials and Methods

3.1. General Experimental Procedures

The UV spectra were recorded on a UV-2600 UV-Vis spectrophotometer (Shimadzu, Japan). The optical rotations were measured using a PerkinElmer MCP-500 Polarimeter (Anton, Austria). The HRESIMS data were recorded on a Bruker maXis Q-TOF in positive/negative ion mode (Bruker, Fällanden, Switzerland). The NMR spectra were obtained on a Bruker Avance spectrometer (Bruker) operating at 500 and 700 MHz for ^{1}H NMR, and 125 and 175 MHz for ^{13}C NMR, using tetramethylsilane (TMS) as an internal standard. The chemical shifts were given as δ values, with J values reported in Hz. TLC plates with silica gel GF254 (0.4–0.5 mm, Qingdao Marine Chemical Factory, Qingdao, China) were used for the analytical and preparative TLC. The column chromatography was carried out on silica gel (200–300 mesh, Jiangyou Silica Gel Development Co., Yantai, China), YMC Gel ODS-A (12 nm, S-50 μm YMC, MA, USA) and Sephadex LH-20 (40–70 μm, Amersham Pharmacia Biotech AB, Uppsala, Sweden). The semi-preparative HPLC was carried on HTACHI L2130 with YMC ODS SERIES (YMC-Pack ODS-A, 250 × 10 mm I.D., S-5 μm, 12 nm) and the analysis HPLC was carried on a shimadzu LC-10ATvp with YMC ODS SERIES (YMC-Pack ODS-A, 250 × 4.6 mm I.D., S-5 μm, 12 nm). Spots were detected on the TLC under UV light, or by heating after spraying with the mixed solvent of saturated vanillin and 5% H_2SO_4 in H_2O. The artificial sea salt was a commercial product (Guangzhou Haili Aquarium Technology Company, Guangzhou, China).

3.2. Fungal Material

The fungal strain SCSIO41401 was isolated from a marine alga *Coelarthrum* sp. collected in Yongxing Island, South China Sea [5]. The strain was identified as *Cochliobolus lunatus* SCSIO41401, according to the ITS region sequence. The producing strain was stored on Medium B (malt extract: 15 g, sea salt: 24.4 g, agar: 15 g, water: 1 L and pH: 7.4–7.8) agar slants at 4 °C, and then deposited at the Key Laboratory of Tropical Marine Bio-resources and Ecology, Chinese Academy of Science.

3.3. Fermentation and Extraction

The seed culture was prepared by inoculating spores of the strain *Cochliobolus lunatus* SCSIO41401 into a 1000 mL flask containing 10 mL seed medium (malt extract: 15 g, sea salt: 10 g, distilled water: 1 L and pH: 7.4–7.8), and incubated at 25 °C on a rotary shaker (178 rpm) for 3 days. In total, 10 mL seed culture was then transferred into 1 L × 48 conical flasks with solid rice medium (each flask contained 200 g rice, 2.5 g sea salt and 210 mL naturally-sourced water), and the large scale fermentation of the strain was carried out at 25 °C for 30 days. The total rice culture was crushed and extracted with EtOAc three times. The EtOAc extract was evaporated under reduced pressure to afford a crude extract. The extract was suspended in MeOH and then partitioned with equivoluminal petroleum ether to separate the oil. Finally, the MeOH solution was concentrated, yielding a black extractive (256.4 g).

3.4. Extraction and Purification

The crude extract was subjected to silica gel column chromatography eluting with CH_2Cl_2/MeOH (v/v 100:0–0:100) to give twelve fractions (Fr.1–Fr.12). Fr.6 was subjected to reversed phase medium-pressure liquid chromatography (MPLC) with MeOH/H_2O (v/v 2:8 to 10:0) to offer thirteen sub-fractions. Fr.6-4 was further purified by semi-preparative reverse phase (SP-RP) HPLC with MeOH/H_2O (v/v 45:55, 2.0 mL/min) to yield compound **5** (t_R = 27.0 min, 105.8 mg, with purity of 98.5%). Fr.6-11 was purified by SP-RP HPLC with MeOH/H_2O (v/v 57:43, 3.0 mL/min) to yield compound **6** (t_R = 30.0 min, 6.2 mg, with a purity of 95.5%). Fr.7 was subjected to reversed phase MPLC with MeOH/H_2O (v/v 1:9 to 10:0) to offer fifteen sub-fractions. Fr.7-8 was further purified by semi-preparative reverse phase (SP-RP) HPLC with CH_3CN/H_2O (v/v 25:75, 2.0 mL/min) to yield compounds **4** (t_R = 12.8 min, 10.4 mg, with a purity of 98.0%), **2** (t_R = 15.7 min, 7.0 mg, with a purity of 97.8%), **1** (t_R = 18.6 min, 13.1 mg, with purity of 98.4%), and **3** (t_R = 26.5 min, 6.3 mg, with purity of 98.0%).

Compound **1**: brown oil; $[\alpha]_D^{25}$ +5.1 (c 0.198, MeOH); UV (MeOH) λmax (log ε) 210 (3.18) nm. For ^{1}H and ^{13}C NMR spectroscopic data, see Table 1; (+)-HRESEMS m/z 418.1951 [M + Na]$^+$ (Calcd for $C_{19}H_{29}NaO_6$, 418.1949) (Figures S1–S9).

Compound **2**: brown oil; $[\alpha]_D^{25}$ −0.48 (c 0.101, MeOH); UV (MeOH) λmax (log ε) 200 (3.24) nm. For ^{1}H and ^{13}C NMR spectroscopic data, see Table 1; (+)-HRESEMS m/z 418.1958 [M + Na]$^+$ (Calcd for $C_{19}H_{29}NaO_6$, 418.1949) (Figures S10–S18).

Compound **3**: brown oil; $[\alpha]_D^{25}$ +2.4 (c 0.062, MeOH); UV (MeOH) λmax (log ε) 204 (3.10), 310 (2.26) nm; CD (0.33 mg/mL, MeOH) λmax (Δε) 217 (0.79), 259 (−0.07), 291 (0.15) nm. For ^{1}H and ^{13}C NMR spectroscopic data, see Table 1; (+)-HRESEMS m/z 291.0838 [M + Na]$^+$ (Calcd for $C_{13}H_{16}NaO_6$, 291.0839) (Figures S19–S26).

3.5. ECD Calculations for the Truncated Models of 1 and 2

The relative configurations of **1** and **2** were established initially on the basis of their ROESY spectra. The Molecular Merck force field (MMFF) and density functional theory (DFT)/time-dependent density functional theory (TDDFT) calculations of **1** and **2** were performed with the Spartan'14 software and Gaussian 09 software, respectively, using default grids and convergence criteria. A MMFF conformational search generated low energy conformers with a Boltzmann population of over 5% (the relative energy within 6 kcal/mol) [20], which were subjected to geometry optimization using the DFT method at the B3LYP/6-31G(d,p) level in MeOH using the conductor-like polarizable continuum model (CPCM). The overall theoretical calculation of the ECD was conducted in MeOH using time-dependent density functional theory at the B3LYP/6-31 + G(d,p) level for the stable conformers of **1** and **2**. The rotatory strengths for a total of 30 excited states were calculated. The ECD spectra of the different conformers were generated using the programmes SpecDis 1.6 (University of Würzburg, Würzburg, Germany) and Prism 5.0 (GraphPad Software Inc., La Jolla, CA, US) with a half-bandwidth of 0.3–0.4 eV, according to the Boltzmann-calculated contribution of each conformer after the UV correction.

3.6. Bioactivity Assay

Five human cancer cell lines—K562, BEL-7402, SGC-7901, A549, and Hela—were purchased from Shanghai Cell Bank, Chinese Academy of Sciences. Compounds **1–3** were evaluated for their cytotoxicities against those cell lines according to the reported methyl thiazolyl tetrazolium (MTT) method [5]. Briefly, the cancer cells were cultured in RPMI1640 media supplemented with 10% phosphate-buffered saline (FBS). The cells were seeded at a density of 400 to 800 cells/well in 384-well plates, and then incubated with the tested compounds in one concentration of 50 μM for the preliminary screening, with 5-flurouracil as the positive control. After 72 h treatment, MTT reagent was added, and the OD value of each well was measured at 570 nm with an Envision 2104 multilabel reader (PerkinElmer). If the tested compound showed an obvious inhibitory activity with an inhibition rate of more than 30% in the preliminary screening test, the further screening with more concentrations was then performed. However, none of the compounds showed significant activity in the preliminary screening.

The inhibitory effects of compounds **1–3** on acetylcholinesterase (AChE, human-recombinant, purchased by Sigma-Aldrich, St. Louis, MO, USA, Catalog Number C1682) were measured in vitro in 96-well plates according to the modified Ellman methods [21]. Briefly, 0.2 Units of AChE were dissolved in 0.1M potassium phosphate buffer (pH 7.4), and compounds **1–3** dissolved in DMSO (with final concentrations of 8, 4, 2, 1, 0.5, 0.25 μM) were added to each well of a 96-well plate. Acetylthiocholine iodide and 5,5'-dithiobis (2-nitrobenzoic acid) were then added for a final concentration of 50 μM. The reaction was carried out for 30 min at 30 °C. The absorbance was measured at 410 nm by an Envision 2104 multilabel reader (PerkinElmer), and the IC_{50} value was calculated using Prism 5.0

(GraphPad Software Inc.). Huperzine A was used as the positive control, with an IC_{50} value of 0.30 ± 0.06 μM.

3.7. Molecular Docking Analysis

The Schrödinger 2017-1 suite (Schrödinger Inc., New York, NY, USA) was employed to perform the docking analysis [19]. The structure of AChE (PDB code: 4EY7) [18] was used as a starting model—with all of the waters and the N-linked glycosylated saccharides removed—and was constructed following the Protein Prepare Wizard workflow in Maestro 11-1. The prepared ligands were then flexibly docked into the receptor using the induced-fit module with the default parameters. The figures were generated using PyMol molecular graphics software (Schrödinger 2017-1, Schrödinger Inc., New York, NY, USA).

4. Conclusions

Three new compounds—a pair of lipopeptide epimers (**1** and **2**) and a phthalide glycerol ether (**3**)—were isolated from the marine algal-associated fungus *Cochliobolus lunatus* SCSIO41401. Their structures, including their absolute configurations, were determined by comprehensive spectroscopic methods, together with experimental, calculated, and $Mo_2(OAc)_4$-induced ECD methods. The in vitro bioassay and in silico docking study revealed compounds **1–3** to be moderate AChE inhibitors.

Supplementary Materials: The following are available online at http://www.mdpi.com/1660-3397/18/11/547/s1, Figures S1–S26: ^{1}H NMR, ^{13}C NMR, DEPT, HSQC, HMBC, COSY, ROESY, UV and HRESIMS spectra of compounds **1–3**. Figures S27–S32: ^{1}H NMR and ^{13}C NMR, spectra of compounds **4–6**. Figure S33: Preliminary Lineweaver–Burk plots for the AChE inhibition with **1**.

Author Contributions: Conceptualization, X.Z. and Y.L.; Formal analysis, J.S., Y.Z., H.W. and S.L.; Investigation, Y.D. and K.L.; Methodology, J.W. and H.T.; Project administration, H.D. and Y.L.; Resources, X.L. and B.Y.; Writing—original draft, Y.D. and K.L.; Writing—review and editing, X.Z. All authors have read and agreed to the published version of the manuscript.

Funding: This research was funded by grants from the National Natural Science Foundation of China (81973235, 21977102), Guangdong Basic and Applied Basic Research Foundation (2019B151502042), Key-Area Research and Development Program of Guangdong Province (2020B1111030005), the Special Funds for Promoting Economic Development (Marine Economic Development) of Guangdong Province (No. [2019]A28, [2020]033, [2020]037, [2020]039), Guangdong Local Innovation Team Program (2019BT02Y262), Key Special Project for Introduced Talents Team of Southern Marine Science and Engineering Guangdong Laboratory (Guangzhou) (GML2019ZD0406), and Liao Ning Revitalization Talents Program (XLYC1802037).

Acknowledgments: This paper is in honour of Peter Proksch, for the dedication of his research career, and his contribution to marine natural product chemistry. We are grateful to the analytical facilities (Z. Xiao, A. Sun, Y. Zhang, et al.) at SCSIO.

Conflicts of Interest: The authors declare no conflict of interest. The funders had no role in the design of the study; in the collection, analyses, or interpretation of data; in the writing of the manuscript, or in the decision to publish the results.

References

1. Puglisi, M.P.; Sneed, J.M.; Ritson-Williams, R.; Young, R. Marine chemical ecology in benthic environments. *Nat. Prod. Rep.* **2019**, *36*, 410–429. [CrossRef] [PubMed]
2. Moodie, L.W.K.; Sepčić, K.; Turk, T.; Frangež, R.; Svenson, J. Natural cholinesterase inhibitors from marine organisms. *Nat. Prod. Rep.* **2019**, *36*, 1053–1092. [CrossRef] [PubMed]
3. Zagorska, A.; Jaromin, A. Perspectives for New and More Efficient Multifunctional Ligands for Alzheimer's Disease Therapy. *Molecules* **2020**, *25*, 3337. [CrossRef] [PubMed]
4. Prasasty, V.; Radifar, M.; Istyastono, E. Natural Peptides in Drug Discovery Targeting Acetylcholinesterase. *Molecules* **2018**, *23*, 2344. [CrossRef] [PubMed]
5. Fang, W.; Wang, J.; Wang, J.; Shi, L.; Li, K.; Lin, X.; Min, Y.; Yang, B.; Tang, L.; Liu, Y.; et al. Cytotoxic and Antibacterial Eremophilane Sesquiterpenes from the Marine-Derived Fungus *Cochliobolus lunatus* SCSIO41401. *J. Nat. Prod.* **2018**, *81*, 1405–1410. [CrossRef] [PubMed]

6. Wang, J.; Chen, F.; Liu, Y.; Liu, Y.; Li, K.; Yang, X.; Liu, S.; Zhou, X.; Yang, J. Spirostaphylotrichin X from a Marine-Derived Fungus as an Anti-influenza Agent Targeting RNA Polymerase PB2. *J. Nat. Prod.* **2018**, *81*, 2722–2730. [CrossRef] [PubMed]
7. Chou, T.H.; Chen, I.S.; Hwang, T.L.; Wang, T.C.; Lee, T.H.; Cheng, L.Y.; Chang, Y.C.; Cho, J.Y.; Chen, J.J. Phthalides from Pittosporum illicioides var. illicioides with inhibitory activity on superoxide generation and elastase release by neutrophils. *J. Nat. Prod.* **2008**, *71*, 1692–1695. [CrossRef] [PubMed]
8. Pang, X.; Lin, X.; Yang, J.; Zhou, X.; Yang, B.; Wang, J.; Liu, Y. Spiro-Phthalides and Isocoumarins Isolated from the Marine-Sponge-Derived Fungus *Setosphaeria* sp. SCSIO41009. *J. Nat. Prod.* **2018**, *81*, 1860–1868. [CrossRef] [PubMed]
9. Lee, C.L.; Chang, F.R.; Hsieh, P.W.; Chiang, M.Y.; Wu, C.C.; Huang, Z.Y.; Lan, Y.H.; Chen, M.; Lee, K.H.; Yen, H.F. Cytotoxic ent-abietane diterpenes from Gelonium aequoreum. *Phytochemistry* **2008**, *69*, 276–287. [CrossRef] [PubMed]
10. Gawronski, J.K.; van Oeveren, A.; vanderDeen, H.; Leung, C.W.; Feringa, B.L. Simple circular dichroic method for the determination of absolute configuration of 5-substituted 2(5H)-furanones. *J. Org. Chem.* **1996**, *61*, 1513–1515. [CrossRef]
11. Beecham, A.F. The CD of α,β-unsaturated lactones. *Tetrahedron* **1972**, *28*, 5543–5554. [CrossRef]
12. Uchida, I.; Kuriyama, K. The π-π circular dichroism of δβ-unsaturated γ-lactones. *Tetrahedron Lett.* **1974**, *15*, 3761–3764. [CrossRef]
13. Wang, J.; Liang, Z.; Li, K.; Yang, B.; Liu, Y.; Fang, W.; Tang, L.; Zhou, X. Ene-yne Hydroquinones from a Marine-derived Strain of the Fungus Pestalotiopsis neglecta with Effects on Liver X Receptor Alpha. *J. Nat. Prod.* **2020**, *83*, 1258–1264. [CrossRef] [PubMed]
14. Chen, X.W.; Li, C.W.; Cui, C.B.; Hua, W.; Zhu, T.J.; Gu, Q.Q. Nine new and five known polyketides derived from a deep sea-sourced *Aspergillus* sp. 16-02-1. *Mar. Drugs* **2014**, *12*, 3116–3137. [CrossRef] [PubMed]
15. Kimura, Y.; Shiojima, K.; Nakajima, H.; Hamasaki, T. Structure and Biological Activity of Plant Growth Regulators Produced by *Penicillium* sp.No.31f. *J. Agric. Chem. Soc. Jpn.* **1992**, *56*, 1138–1139.
16. Gao, L.; Xu, X.; Yang, J. Chemical constituents of the roots of *Rheum officinale*. *Chem. Nat. Compd.* **2013**, *49*, 603–605. [CrossRef]
17. Maha, A.; Rukachaisirikul, V.; Phongpaichit, S.; Poonsuwan, W.; Sakayaroj, J. Dimeric chromanone, cyclohexenone and benzamide derivatives from the endophytic fungus *Xylaria* sp. PSU-H182. *Tetrahedron* **2016**, *72*, 2874–2879. [CrossRef]
18. Cheung, J.; Rudolph, M.J.; Burshteyn, F.; Cassidy, M.S.; Gary, E.N.; Love, J.; Franklin, M.C.; Height, J.J. Structures of Human Acetylcholinesterase in Complex with Pharmacologically Important Ligands. *J. Med. Chem.* **2012**, *55*, 10282–10286. [CrossRef] [PubMed]
19. Zhou, X.; Liang, Z.; Li, K.; Fang, W.; Tian, Y.; Luo, X.; Chen, Y.; Zhan, Z.; Zhang, T.; Liao, S.; et al. Exploring the Natural Piericidins as Anti-Renal Cell Carcinoma Agents Targeting Peroxiredoxin 1. *J. Med. Chem.* **2019**, *62*, 7058–7069. [CrossRef] [PubMed]
20. Frisch, M.J.; Trucks, G.W.; Schlegel, H.B.; Scuseria, G.E.; Robb, M.A.; Cheeseman, J.R.; Scalmani, G.; Barone, V.; Mennucci, B.; Petersson, G.A.; et al. *Gaussian 09, Revision D.01*; Gaussian, Inc.: Wallingford, CT, USA, 2013.
21. Ellman, G.L.; Courtney, K.D.; Andres, V.; Featherstone, R.M. A New and Rapid Colorimetric Determination of Acetylcholinesterase Activity. *Biochem. Pharmacol.* **1961**, *7*, 88–90. [CrossRef]

Publisher's Note: MDPI stays neutral with regard to jurisdictional claims in published maps and institutional affiliations.

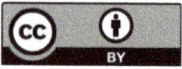

© 2020 by the authors. Licensee MDPI, Basel, Switzerland. This article is an open access article distributed under the terms and conditions of the Creative Commons Attribution (CC BY) license (http://creativecommons.org/licenses/by/4.0/).

MDPI
St. Alban-Anlage 66
4052 Basel
Switzerland
Tel. +41 61 683 77 34
Fax +41 61 302 89 18
www.mdpi.com

Marine Drugs Editorial Office
E-mail: marinedrugs@mdpi.com
www.mdpi.com/journal/marinedrugs

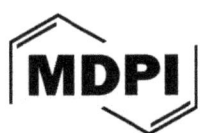

www.ingramcontent.com/pod-product-compliance
Lightning Source LLC
LaVergne TN
LVHW070158100526
838202LV00015B/1963